Anterior Knee Pain and Patellar Instability

Vicente Sanchis-Alfonso (Ed)

Anterior Knee Pain and Patellar Instability

With 240 Figures
including 108 Color Plates

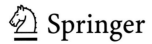 Springer

Vicente Sanchis-Alfonso, MD, PhD (Member of the
  International Patellofemoral Study Group/Member
  of the ACL Study Group)
Department of Orthopaedic Surgery
Hospital Arnau de Vilanova
Valencia
Spain

British Library Cataloguing in Publication Data
Anterior knee pain and patellar instability
  1. Patellofemoral joint - Dislocation 2. Patella -
  Dislocation 3. Knee - Diseases 4. Knee - Wounds and injuries
  5. Knee - Surgery 6. Pain - Physiological aspects
  I. Sanchis-Alfonso, Vicente
  617.5′82
ISBN-10: 1846280036

Library of Congress Control Number: 2005925983

ISBN-10: 1-84628-003-6   e-ISBN 1-84628-143-1
ISBN-13: 978-1-84628-003-0

Printed on acid-free paper

Printed in Singapore   (SPI/KYO)

9 8 7 6 5 4 3 2 1

Springer Science+Business Media
springeronline.com

To my father. In memoriam (†)

Foreword

Anterior knee pain is one of the really big problems in my specialty, sports orthopaedic surgery, but also in all other types of orthopaedic surgery. Many years ago Sakkari Orava in Finland showed that among some 1311 Finnish runners, anterior knee pain was the second most common complaint. In young school girls around 15 years of age, anterior knee pain is a common complaint. In ballet classes of the same age, as much as 60-70% of the students complain of anterior knee pain. It is therefore an excellent idea of Dr. Sanchis-Alfonso to publish a book about anterior knee pain and patello-femoral instability in the active young.

He has been able to gather a group of extremely talented experts to help him write this book. I am particularly happy that he has devoted so much space to the non-operative treatment of anterior knee pain. During my active years as a knee surgeon, one of my worst problems was young girls referred to me for surgery of anterior knee pain. Girls that had already had 8-12 surgeries for their knee problem — surgeries that had rendered them more and more incapacitated after each operation. They now came to me for another operation. In all these cases, I referred them to our pain clinic for careful analysis, and pain treatment followed by physical therapy. All recovered but had been the victims of lots of unnecessary knee surgery before they came to me.

I am also happy that Suzanne Werner in her chapter refers to our study on the personality of these anterior knee patients. She found that the patients differ from a normal control group of the same age. I think this is very important to keep in mind when you treat young patients with anterior knee pain.

In my mind physical therapy should always be the first choice of treatment. Not until this treatment has completely failed and a pain clinic recommends surgery, do I think surgery should be considered.

In patello-femoral instability the situation is different. When young patients suffer from frank dislocations of the patella, surgery should be considered. From my many years of treating these types of patients, I recommend that the patients undergo an arthroscopy before any attempts to treat the instability begin. The reason is that I have seen so many cases with normal X-rays that have 10-15 loose bodies in their knees. If these pieces consist of just cartilage, they cannot be seen on X-ray. When a dislocated patella jumps back, it often hits the lateral femoral condyle with considerable force. Small cartilage pieces are blasted away as well from femur as from the patella. If they are overlooked they will eventually lead to blockings of the knee in the future.

The role of the medial patello-femoral ligament can also not be overstressed. When I was taught to operate on these cases, this ligament was not even known.

I also feel that when patellar instability is going to be operated on, it is extremely important that the surgeon carefully controls in what direction the instability takes place. All instability is not in lateral direction. Some patellae have medial instability. If someone performs a routine lateral release in a case of medial instability, he will end up having to repair the lateral retinaculum in order to treat the medial dislocation that eventually occurs. Hughston and also Teitge have warned against this in the past.

It is a pleasure for me to recommend this excellent textbook by Dr. Vicente Sanchis-Alfonso.

Ejnar Eriksson, MD, PhD
Professor Emeritus of Sports Medicine
Karolinska Institute, Stockholm, Sweden

Preface

This book reflects my deep interest in the pathology of the knee, particularly that of the extensor mechanism, and to bring to the fore the great importance I give to the concept of subspecialization, this being the only way to confront the deterioration and mediocrity of our speciality, Orthopaedic Surgery; and to provide our patients with better care. In line with the concept of subspecialization, this book necessarily required the participation of various authors. In spite of this, I do not think there is a lack of cohesion between the chapters. Now, there are certain variations in form, but not in basic content, regarding some topics dealt with by different authors. It is thus evident that a few aspects remain unclear, and the controversy continues.

With this work, we draw upon the most common pathology of the knee, even though the most neglected, the least known and the most problematic (Black Hole of Orthopaedics). To begin with, the terminology is confusing (The Tower of Babel). Our knowledge of its etiopathogeny is also limited, with the consequence that its treatment is of the most complex among the different pathologies of the knee. On the other hand, we also face the problem of frequent and serious diagnostic errors that can lead to unnecessary interventions. The following data reflect this problem: 11% of patients in my series underwent unnecessary arthroscopy, and 10% were referred to a psychiatrist by physicians who had previously been consulted.

Unlike other publications, this work gives great weight to etiopathogeny; the latest theories are presented regarding the pathogeny of anterior knee pain and patellar instability, although in an eminently clinical and practical manner. In agreement with John Hunter, I think that to know the effects of an illness is to know very little; to know the cause of the effects is what is important. Nonetheless, we forget neither the diagnostic methods nor therapeutic alternatives, both surgical and non-surgical, emphasizing minimal intervention and non-surgical methods. Similarly, much importance is given to anterior knee pain following ACL reconstruction. Further, the participation of diverse specialists (orthopaedic surgeons, physiotherapists, radiologists, biologists, pathologists, bioengineers, and plastic surgeons), that is, their multidisciplinary approach, assures us of a wider vision of this pathology. The second part of this monograph is given over to discussion of complex clinical cases that are presented. I reckon we learn far more from our own errors, and those of other specialists, than from our successes. We deal with oft-operated patients with sequelae due to interventions, adequate or otherwise, but which have become complicated. The diagnoses arrived at are explained, and how the cases were resolved (*"Good results come from experience, experience from bad results"*, Professor Erwin Morscher).

Nowadays we are plunged into the *"Bone and Joint Decade"* (2000-2010). The WHO's declared aim is to make people aware of the great incidence of musculoskeletal pathology and to reduce both economic and social costs. These same goals I have laid out in this book. Firstly, we are mindful of the soaring incidence of this pathology, and the impact on young people, athletes, workers, and the economy. Secondly, to improve prevention and diagnosis in order to reduce the economic and social costs of this pathology. The final objective is to improve health care in these patients. This, rather than being an objective, should point the way forward.

Anterior Knee Pain and Patellar Instability is addressed to orthopaedic surgeons (both general and those specialized in knee surgery), specialists in sports medicine and physiotherapists.

We feel thus that with this approach, this monograph will fill an important gap in the literature of pathology of the extensor mechanism of the knee. However, we do not intend to substitute any work on patellofemoral pathology, but rather to complement existing literature (*"All in all, you're just another brick in the wall"*, Pink Floyd, The Wall). Although the information contained herein will evidently require future revision, it serves as an authoritative reference on one of the most problematic entities current in pathology of the knee. We trust that the reader will find the work useful, and consequently, be indirectly valuable for patients.

Vicente Sanchis-Alfonso, MD, PhD
Valencia, Spain
February 2005

Acknowledgments

I wish to express my sincere gratitude to my friend and colleague, Dr Donald Fithian, who I met in 1992 during my stay in San Diego CA, for all I learned, together with his help, for which I will be forever grateful; to Professor Ejnar Eriksson for writing the foreword; to Dr Scott Dye for writing the epilogue, to Nicolás Fernández for his valuable photographic work, and also to Stan Perkins for his inestimable collaboration, without whom I would not have managed to realize a considerable part of my projects. My gratitude also goes out to all members of the International Patellofemoral Study Group for their constant encouragement and inspiration.

Further, I have had the privilege and honor to count on the participation of outstanding specialists who have lent prestige to this monograph. I thank all of them for their time, effort, dedication, amiability, as well as for the excellent quality of their contributing chapters. All have demonstrated generosity in sharing their great clinical experience in clear and concise form. I am in debt to you all. Personally, and on behalf of those patients who will undoubtedly benefit from this work, thank you.

Last but not least, I am extremely grateful to both Springer in London for the confidence shown in this project, and to Barbara Chernow and her team for completing this project with excellence from the time the cover is opened until the final chapter is presented.

Vicente Sanchis-Alfonso, MD, PhD

Contents

Section I
Etiopathogenic Bases and Therapeutic Implications

Section II
Clinical Cases Commented

Contributors

Håkan Alfredson, MD, PhD
Associate Professor
Umeå University
Sports Medicine Unit
Department of Surgical and
Perioperative Science
Umeå, Sweden

Francisco Aparisi-Rodriguez, MD, PhD
Department of Radiology
Hospital Universitario La Fe
Valencia, Spain

Carlos M. Atienza-Vicente, Mch Eng,
PhD
Orthopaedic Biomechanics Group
Instituto de Biomecánica de Valencia
(IBV)
Universidad Politécnica de Valencia
Valencia, Spain

Kim Bennell, BAppSc(physio), PhD
Centre for Health, Exercise and Sports
Medicine
School of Physiotherapy
Faculty of Medicine, Dentistry and
Health Sciences
University of Melbourne
Australia

Roland M. Biedert, MD
Member of the "International
Patellofemoral Study Group"
Associate Professor, University of Basle
Swiss Federal Institute of Sports
Orthopaedics & Sport Traumatology
Magglingen, Switzerland

Matthew Close, BA
Steadman Hawkins Sports Medicine
Foundation
Vail, Colorado, USA

Jill L. Cook
Musculoskeletal Research Centre
La Trobe University School of
Physiotherapy
Melbourne, Australia

Mario Comín-Clavijo, Mch Eng, PhD
Orthopaedic Biomechanics Group
Instituto de Biomecánica de Valencia
(IBV)
Universidad Politécnica de Valencia
Valencia, Spain

Scott F. Dye, MD
Member of the "International
Patellofemoral Study Group"
Associate Clinical Professor of
Orthopaedic Surgery
University of San Francisco
San Francisco, California, USA

Ejnar Eriksson, MD, PhD
Professor Emeritus of Sports Medicine
Karolinska Institute
Stockholm, Sweden

Donald C. Fithian, MD
Member of the "International
Patellofemoral Study Group"
Kaiser Permanente Medical Group
El Cajon, California, USA

László Hangody, MD, PhD, DSc
Uzsoki Hospital
Orthopaedic & Trauma Department
Budapest, Hungary

Christopher D. Harner, MD
Medical Director
Center for Sports Medicine
Department of Orthopaedic Surgery
University of Pittsburgh Medical Center
Pittsburgh, PA, USA

Kimberly Hydeman, BA
Steadman Hawkins Sports Medicine
Foundation
Vail, Colorado, USA

Jon Karlsson, MD, PhD
Department of Orthopaedics
Sahlgrenska University Hospital
Göteborg, Sweden

Karim M. Khan
Department of Family Practice & School
of Human Kinetics
University of British Columbia
Vancouver, Canada

Jüri Kartus, MD, PhD
Department of Orthopaedics
NÄL-Hospital
Trollhättan, Sweden

Sung-Jae Kim, MD, PhD, FACS
Arthroscopy and Joint Research Institute
Department of Orthopaedic Surgery
Yonsei University College of Medicine
Seoul, Korea

Sumant G. Krishnan, MD
W.B. Carrell Memorial Clinic
Dallas, Texas, USA

Scott Lawrance, PT, ATC
The Shelbourne Clinic at Methodist
Hospital
Indianapolis, Indiana, USA

Ronny Lorentzon, MD, PhD
Professor
Umeå University
Sports Medicine Unit
Department of Surgical and
Perioperative Science
Umeå, Sweden

Vicente Martinez-Sanjuan, MD, PhD
Profesor of Radiology
Universidad Cardenal Herrera
ERESA-Hospital General Universitario
MR and CT Unit
Valencia, Spain

**Jenny McConnell, Grad Dip Manip Ther,
MBiomedEng**
Centre for Health, Exercise and Sports
Medicine
School of Physiotherapy
Faculty of Medicine, Dentistry and
Health Sciences
University of Melbourne
Australia
McConnell and Clements Physiotherapy
Sydney, Australia

Peter J. Millett, MD, MSc
Harvard Medical School
Brigham & Women's Hospital
Boston, MA, USA

Eric Montesinos-Berry, MD
Department of Orthopaedics
Hospital Arnau de Vilanova
Valencia, Spain

Carmen Monserrat
Department of Radiology
Hospital Arnau de Vilanova
Valencia, Spain

Tomas Movin, MD, PhD
Department of Orthopaedics
Karolinska University Hospital
Karolinska Institutet
Stockholm, Sweden

Maurice Y. Nahabedian, MD, FACS
Associate Professor of Plastic Surgery
Georgetown University Hospital
Washington, USA

Eiki Nomura, MD
Department Director
Orthopaedic Surgery
Kawasaki Municipal Hospital
Kawasaki, Japan

Ron Noy, MD
The Shelbourne Clinic at Methodist
Hospital
Indianapolis, Indiana, USA

Fermín Ordoño, MD, PhD
Department of Neurophysiology
Hospital Arnau de Vilanova
Valencia, Spain

Jaime M. Prat-Pastor, MD, PhD
Orthopaedic Biomechanics Group
Instituto de Biomecánica de Valencia
(IBV)
Universidad Politécnica de Valencia
Valencia, Spain

Carlos Puig-Abbs, MD
Orthopaedic Surgeon
Department of Orthopaedics
Hospital Universitario Dr Peset
Valencia, Spain

Fernando Revert-Ros
Patología Molecular
Fundación Valenciana de
Investigaciones Biomédicas
Valencia, Spain

Esther Roselló-Sastre, MD, PhD
Pathologist
Department of Pathology
Hospital Universitario Dr. Peset
Valencia, Spain

Vicente Sanchis-Alfonso, MD, PhD
Member of the International
Patellofemoral Study Group and Member
of the ACL Study Group
Staff Orthopaedic Surgeon
Department of Orthopaedics
Hospital Arnau de Vilanova
Valencia, Spain

Juan Saus-Mas
Patología Molecular
Fundación Valenciana de
Investigaciones Biomédicas
Valencia, Spain

K. Donald Shelbourne, MD
The Shelbourne Clinic at Methodist
Hospital
Indianapolis, Indiana, USA

J. Richard Steadman, MD
Steadman Hawkins Sports Medicine
Foundation
Vail, Colorado, USA

Alfredo Subías-López, MD
Department of Orthopaedics
Hospital Lluís Alcanyís
Játiva, Valencia, Spain

Robert A. Teitge, MD
Member of the "International
Patellofemoral Study Group"
Department of Orthopaedics
Wayne State University School of
Medicine
Detroit, Michigan, USA

Roger Torga-Spak, MD
Instituto Universitario CEMIC
Buenos Aires, Argentina

Iván Udvarhelyi, MD
Uzsoki Hospital
Orthopaedic & Trauma Department
Budapest, Hungary

Damien Van Tiggelen, PT
Department of Rehabilitation Sciences
and Physical Therapy
Faculty of Medicine
University of Gent
Gent, Belgium
Department of Traumatology and
Rehabilitation
Military Hospital of Base Queen Astrid
Brussels, Belgium

Tracy M. Vogrin
Center for Sports Medicine
Department of Orthopaedic Surgery
University of Pittsburgh Medical
Center
Pittsburgh, PA, USA

Suzanne Werner, PT, PhD
Associated Professor
Dpt Physical Therapy
Karolinska Institutet & Section Sports
Medicine
Karolinska Hospital
Stockholm, Sweden

Kenneth J. Westerheide, MD
Center for Sports Medicine
Department of Orthopaedic Surgery
University of Pittsburgh Medical
Center
Pittsburgh, PA, USA

Tine Willems
Department of Rehabilitation Sciences
and Physical Therapy
Faculty of Medicine
University of Gent
Gent, Belgium

Erik Witvrouw, PT, PhD
Department of Rehabilitation Sciences
and Physical Therapy
Faculty of Medicine
University of Gent
Gent, Belgium

Mark A. Young
Musculoskeletal Research Centre
La Trobe University School of
Physiotherapy
Melbourne, Australia

I

Etiopathogenic Bases and Therapeutic Implications

1

Background: Patellofemoral Malalignment versus Tissue Homeostasis

Myths and Truths about Patellofemoral Disease

Vicente Sanchis-Alfonso

Introduction

Anterior knee pain[a] is the most common knee complaint seen in adolescents and young adults, in both the athletic and nonathletic population, although in the former, its incidence is higher. The rate is around 9% in young active adults.[69] Its incidence is 5.4% of the total injuries and as high as a quarter of all knee problems treated at a sports injury clinic.[16] Nonetheless, I am convinced that not all cases are diagnosed and hence the figure is bound to be even higher. Furthermore, it is to be expected that the number of patients with this complaint will increase because of the increasing popularity of sport practice. On the other hand, a better understanding of this pathology by orthopedic surgeons and general practitioners should lead to this condition being diagnosed more and more frequently. Females are particularly predisposed to it.[14] Anatomic factors such as increased pelvic width and resulting excessive lateral thrust on the patella, and postural and sociological factors such as wearing high heels and sitting with legs adducted can influence the incidence and severity of this condition in women.[29] Moreover, it is a nemesis to both the patient and the treating physician, creating chronic disability, limitation from participation in sports, sick leave, and generally diminished quality of life.

Special mention should be made of the term "patellar tendonitis," closely related to anterior knee pain. In 1998, *Arthroscopy* published an article by Nicola Maffulli and colleagues[52] that bore the title "Overuse tendon conditions: Time to change a confusing terminology." Very aptly, these authors concluded that the clinical syndrome characterized by pain (diffuse or localized), tumefaction, and a lower sports performance should be called "tendinopathy."[52] The terms tendinitis, paratendinitis, and tendinosis should be used solely when in possession of the results of an excision biopsy. Therefore the pervasive clinical diagnosis of patellar tendinitis, which has become the paradigm of overuse tendon injuries, would be incorrect. Furthermore, biopsies in these types of pathologies do not prove the existence of chronic or acute inflammatory infiltrates, which clearly indicate the presence of tendinitis. Patellar tendinopathy is a frequent cause for anterior knee pain, which can turn out to be frustrating for physicians as well as for athletes, for whom this lesion can well mean the end of their sports career. This means that in this monograph we cannot leave out a discussion of this clinical entity, which is dealt with in depth in Chapters 15 and 16.

Finally, anterior knee pain is also a well-documented complication and the most common complaint after anterior cruciate ligament (ACL) reconstruction. Because of the upsurge of all kinds of sports, ACL injuries have become increasingly common and therefore their surgical

---

[a] Term that describes pain in which the source is either within the patellofemoral joint or in the support structures around it.

treatment is currently commonplace.[b] The incidence of anterior knee pain after ACL reconstruction with bone-patellar tendon-bone (B-PT-B) autografts is from 4% to 40% .[24] In this sense, we must remember that the tissue most commonly used for ACL reconstruction, according to the last survey of the ACL Study Group (May 29–June 4, 2004, Forte Village Resort, Sardinia, Italy), is the B-PT-B.[9] Moreover, anterior knee pain is also a common complaint, from 6% to 12.5% after 2 years, with the use of hamstring grafts.[4,11,48,65] For the reasons mentioned above, we believe it is interesting to carry out a detailed analysis in this book of the appearance of anterior knee pain secondary to ACL reconstructive surgery, underscoring the importance of treatment, and especially, prevention. In order not to fall into the trap of dogmatism, the problem is analyzed by different authors from different perspectives (see Chapters 17 to 19).

The Problem

In spite of its high incidence, anterior knee pain syndrome is the most neglected, the least known, and the most problematic pathological knee condition. This is why the expression "Black Hole of Orthopedics" that Stanley James used to refer to this condition is extremely apt to describe the current situation. On the other hand, our knowledge of the causative mechanisms of anterior knee pain is limited, with the consequence that its treatment is one of the most complex among the different pathologies of the knee. As occurs with any pathological condition, and this is not an exception, for the correct application of conservative as well as operative therapy, it is essential to have a thorough understanding of the pathogenesis of the same (see Chapters 2, 3, 4, 8, and 11). This is the only way to prevent the all-too-frequent stories of multiple failed surgeries and demoralized patients, a fact that is relatively common for the clinical entity under scrutiny in this book as compared with other pathological processes affecting the knee (see Chapters 20 and 21).

Finally, diagnostic errors, which can lead to unnecessary interventions, are relatively frequent in this pathologic condition. As early as 1922, in the German literature, Georg Axhausen[5] stated that *chondromalacia* can simulate a meniscal lesion resulting in the removal of normal menisci. In this connection, Tapper and Hoover,[66] in 1969, suspected that over 20% of women who did badly after an open meniscectomy had a patellofemoral pathology. Likewise, John Insall,[41] in 1984, stated that patellofemoral pathology was the most common cause of meniscectomy failure in young patients, especially women. Obviously, this failure was a result of an erred diagnosis and, consequently, of a mistakenly indicated surgery. At present, the problem of diagnostic confusion is still the order of the day. The following data reflect this problem. In my surgical series 11% of patients underwent unnecessary arthroscopic meniscal surgery, which, far from eradicating the symptoms, had worsened them. An improvement was obtained, however, after realignment surgery of the extensor mechanism. Finally, 10% of patients in my surgical series were referred to a psychiatrist by physicians who had previously been consulted.

The question we ask ourselves is: Why is there less knowledge about this kind of pathology than about other knee conditions? According to the International Patellofemoral Study Group (IPSG),[42] there are several explanations: (1) The biomechanics of the patellofemoral joint is more complex than that of other structures in the knee; (2) the pathology of the patella arouses less clinical interest than that of the menisci or the cruciate ligaments; (3) there are various causes for anterior knee pain; (4) there is often no correlation between symptoms, physical findings, and radiological findings; (5) there are discrepancies regarding what is regarded as "normal;" and (6) there is widespread terminological confusion ("the Tower of Babel"). As regards what is considered "normal" or "abnormal" it is interesting to mention the work by Johnson and colleagues,[45] who makes a gender-dependent analysis of the clinical assessment of asymptomatic knees. We discuss some of the conclusions of this interesting study below.

In 1995, the prevailing confusion led to the foundation by John Fulkerson of the United States and Jean-Yves Dupont of France of the IPSG in order to advance in the knowledge of the patellofemoral joint disorders by intercultural exchange of information and ideas. The

---

[b] In the general population, an estimated one in 3000 individuals sustains an ACL injury per year in the United States,[37] corresponding to an overall injury rate of approximately 80,000[32] to 100,000[37] injuries annually. The highest incidence is in individuals 15 to 25 years old who participate in pivoting sports.[32]

condition is of such high complexity that even within this group there are antagonistic approaches and theories often holding dogmatic positions. Moreover, to stimulate research efforts and education regarding patellofemoral problems John Fulkerson created in 2003 the Patellofemoral Foundation. The Patellofemoral Foundation sponsors the "Patellofemoral Research Excellence Award" to encourage outstanding research leading to improved understanding, prevention, and treatment of patellofemoral pain or instability. I want to emphasize the importance to improve prevention and diagnosis in order to reduce the economic and social costs of this pathology (see Chapters 6, 8, and 17). Moreover this foundation sponsors the "Patellofemoral Traveling Fellowship" to promote better understanding and communication regarding patellofemoral pain, permitting visits to several centers, worldwide, that offer opportunities to learn about the complexities of patellofemoral pain.

This chapter provides an overview of the most important aspects of etiopathogenesis of anterior knee pain and analyzes some myths and truths about patellofemoral disease.

Historical Background: Internal Derangement of the Knee and Chondromalacia Patellae; Actual Meaning of Patellar Chondral Injury

Anterior knee pain in young patients has historically been associated with the terms "internal derangement of the knee" and "chondromalacia patellae." In 1986, Schutzer and colleagues[63] published a paper in the Orthopedic Clinics of North America about the CT-assisted classification of patellofemoral pain. The authors of that paper highlight the lack of knowledge that besets this clinical entity when they associate the initials of internal derangement of the knee (IDK) with those of the phrase "*I Don't Know*," and those of chondromalacia patellae (CMP) with those of "*Could be – May be – Possibly be*." Although we think that nowadays this is certainly an exaggeration, it is true that the analogy helps us underscore the controversies around this clinical entity, or at least draw people's attention to it.

The expression "internal derangement of the knee" was coined in 1784 by British surgeon William Hey.[50] This term was later discredited by the German school surgeon Konrad Büdinger, Dr. Billroth's assistant in Vienna, who in 1906

described fissuring and degeneration of the patellar articular cartilage of spontaneous origin,[7] and in 1908 in another paper described similar lesions of traumatic origin.[8] Although Büdinger was the first to describe chondromalacia, this term was not used by Büdinger himself. Apparently it was Koenig who in 1924 used the term "chondromalacia patellae" for the first time, although according to Karlson this term had already been used in Aleman's clinic since 1917.[1,28] What does seem clear is that it was Koenig who popularized the term. Büdinger considered that the expression "internal derangement of the knee" was a "wastebasket" term. And he was right since the expression lacks any etiological, therapeutic, or prognostic implication.

Until the end of the 1960s anterior knee pain was attributed to chondromalacia patellae. Stemming from the Greek *chondros* and *malakia*, this term translates literally as "softened patellar articular cartilage." However, in spite of the fact that the term "chondromalacia patellae" has historically been associated with anterior knee pain, many authors have failed to find a connection between both.[12,49,59] In 1978, Leslie and Bentley reported that only 51% of patients with a clinical diagnosis of chondromalacia had changes on the patellar surface when were examined by arthroscopy.[49] In 1991, Royle and colleagues[59] published in *Arthroscopy* a study in which they analyzed 500 arthroscopies performed in a 2-year period, with special reference made to the patellofemoral joint. In those patients with pain thought to be arising from this joint, 63% had "chondromalacia patellae" compared with a 45% incidence in those with meniscal pathological findings at arthroscopy. They concluded that patients with anterior knee pain do not always have patellar articular changes, and patellar pathology is often asymptomatic (Figure 1.1). In agreement with this, Dye[18] did not feel any pain during arthroscopic palpation of his extensive lesion of the patellar cartilage without intraarticular anesthesia. In this regard it would be remembered that the articular cartilage is devoid of nerve fibers and, therefore, cannot hurt.

Surgeons often refer to patellar cartilage changes as chondromalacia, using poor defined grades. According to the IPSG[42] we should use the term chondral or cartilage lesion, and rather than resorting to grades in a classification, providing a clear description of the injury (e.g., appearance, depth, size, location, acute vs. chronic clinical status). Although hyaline cartilage cannot be the

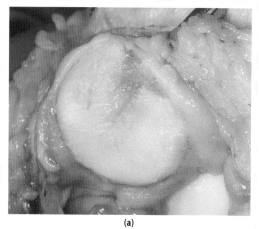

(a)

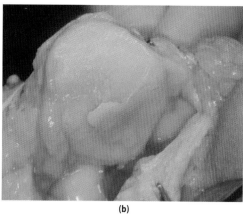

(b)

Figure 1.1. The intensity of preoperative pain is not related to the seriousness or the extension of the chondromalacia patellae found during surgery. The most serious cases of chondromalacia arise in patients with a recurrent patellar dislocation who feel little or no pain between their dislocation episodes **(a)**. Chondral lesion of the patella with fragmentation and fissuring of the cartilage in a patient with PFM that consulted for anterior knee pain **(b)**.

source of pain in itself, damage of articular cartilage can lead to excessive loading of the subchondral bone, which, due to its rich innervation, could be a potential source of pain. Therefore, a possible indication for very selected cases could be a resurfacing procedure such as mosaicplasty (see Chapter 12) or periostic autologous transplants (see Chapter 13).

According to the IPSG,[42] the term chondromalacia should not be used to describe a clinical condition; it is merely a descriptive term for morphologic softening of the patellar articular cartilage. In conclusion, this is a diagnosis that can be made only with visual inspection and palpation by open or arthroscopic means and it is

irrelevant. In short, chrondromalacia patellae is not synonymous with patellofemoral pain. Thus, the term chondromalacia, is also, using Büdinger's own words, a wastebasket term as it is lacking in practical utility. In this way, the following ominous 1908 comment from Büdinger about "internal derangement of the knee" could be applied to chondromalacia:[22] "[It] will simply not disappear from the surgical literature. It is the symbol of our helplessness in regards to a diagnosis and our ignorance of the pathology."

Although I am aware of the fact that traditions die hard, the term "chondromalacia patellae" should be excluded from the clinical terminology of current orthopedics for the reasons I have expressed. Almost one century has elapsed and this term is still used today, at least in Spain, by clinicians, by the staff in charge of codifying the different pathologies for our hospitals' databases, as well as by private health insurers' lists of covered services.

Patellofemoral Malalignment

In the 1970s anterior knee pain was related to the presence of patellofemoral malalignment (PFM).[c] In 1968, Jack C. Hughston (Figure 1.2) published an article on subluxation of the patella, which represented a major turning point in the recognition and treatment of patellofemoral disorders.[35] In 1974, Al Merchant, in an attempt to better understand patellofemoral biomechanics, intro-

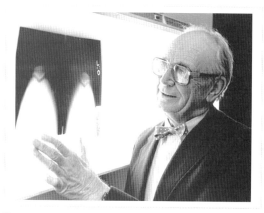

Figure 1.2. Jack C. Hughston, MD (1917–2004). One of the founding fathers of Sports Medicine. (Reproduced with permission from the *Journal of Athletic Training*, 2004; 39: 309.)

---

[c] We define PFM as an abnormality of patellar tracking that involves lateral displacement or lateral tilt of the patella, or both, in extension, that reduces in flexion.

duced the axial radiograph of the patellofemoral joint.[54] The same author suggested, also in 1974, the lateral retinacular release as a way of treating recurrent patellar subluxation.[55] In 1975, Paul Ficat, from France, popularized the concept of patellar tilt, always associated with increased tightness of the lateral retinaculum, which caused excessive pressure on the lateral facet of the patella, leading to the "lateral patellar compression syndrome" ("*Syndrome d'Hyperpression Externe de la Rotule*").[21] According to Ficat lateral patellar compression syndrome would cause hyperpressure in the lateral patellofemoral compartment and hypopressure in the medial patellofemoral compartment. Hypopressure and the disuse of the medial patellar facet would cause malnutrition and early degenerative changes in the articular cartilage because of the lack of normal pressure and function. This may explain why early chondromalacia patellae is generally found in the medial patellar facet. Hyperpression also would favor cartilage degeneration, which might explain the injury of the lateral facet. Two years later, in 1977, Ficat and Hungerford[22] published *Disorders of the Patellofemoral Joint,* a classic of knee extensor mechanism surgery and the first book in English devoted exclusively to the extensor mechanism of the knee. In the preface of the book these authors refer to the patellofemoral joint as "the forgotten compartment of the knee." This shows what the state of affairs was in those days. In fact, before the 1970s only two diagnoses were used relating to anterior knee pain or patellar instability: chondromalacia patellae and recurrent dislocation of the patella. What is more, the initial designs for knee arthroplasties ignored the patellofemoral joint. In 1979, John Insall published a paper on "patellar malalignment syndrome"[38] and his technique for proximal patellar realignment, used to treat this syndrome.[39] According to Insall lateral loading of the patella is increased in malalignment syndrome. In some cases, this causes chondromalacia patellae, but it does not necessarily mean that chondromalacia is the cause of pain.[41] In this way, in 1983 Insall and colleagues reported that anterior knee pain correlates better to malalignment rather than with the severity of chondromalacia found during surgery.[40] Fulkerson and colleagues have also emphasized the importance of PFM and excessively tight lateral retinaculum as a source of anterior knee pain.[25,26,63] Finally, in 2000, Ronald Grelsamer,[31] from the IPSG, stated that malalignment appears to be a necessary but not sufficient condition for the onset of anterior knee pain.[d] According to Grelsamer,[31] pain seems to be set off by a trigger (i.e., traumatism). In this sense, Grelsamer[30] tells his patients that "people with malaligned knees are akin to someone riding a bicycle on the edge of a cliff. All is well until a strong wind blows them off the cliff, which may or may not ever happen." Although it is more common to use the term malalignment as a malposition of the patella on the femur some authors, as Robert A Teitge, from the IPSG, use the term malalignment as a malposition of the knee joint between the body and the foot with the subsequent effect on the patellofemoral mechanics (see Chapter 11).

In a previous paper[61] we postulated that PFM, in some patients with patellofemoral pain, produces a favorable environment for the onset of symptoms, and neural damage would be the main "provoking factor" or "triggering factor." Overload or overuse may be another triggering factor. In this sense, in our surgical experience, we have found that in patients with symptoms in both knees, when the more symptomatic knee is operated on, the symptoms in the contralateral less symptomatic malaligned knee disappear or decrease in many cases, perhaps because we have reduced the load in this knee; that is, it allows us to restore joint homeostasis. In this connection, Thomee and colleagues suggested that chronic overloading and temporary overuse of the patellofemoral joint, rather than malalignment, contribute to patellofemoral pain.[68]

For many years, PFM has been widely accepted as an explanation for the genesis of anterior knee pain and patellar instability in the young patient. Moreover, this theory had a great influence on orthopedic surgeons, who developed several surgical procedures to "correct the malalignment." Unfortunately, when PFM was diagnosed it was treated too often by means of surgery. A large amount of surgical treatments has been described, yielding extremely variable results. Currently, however, the PFM concept is questioned by many, and is not universally accepted to account for the presence of anterior knee pain and/or patellar instability.

---

[d] However, many patients with patellofemoral pain have no evidence of malalignment, whatsoever.[68] Therefore if PFM is a necessary condition for the presence of patellofemoral pain, how could patellofemoral pain be occurring in patients without malalignment?

At present, most of the authors agree that only a small percentage of patients with patellofemoral pain have truly malalignment and are candidates for surgical correction of malalignment for resolution of symptoms. In fact, the number of realignment surgeries has dropped dramatically in recent years, due to a reassessment of the paradigm of PFM. Moreover, we know that such procedures are, in many cases, unpredictable and even dangerous; they may lead to reflex sympathetic dystrophy, medial patellar dislocations, and iatrogenous osteoarthrosis (see Chapters 20 and 21). We should recall here a phrase by doctor Jack Hughston, who said: "There is no problem that cannot be made worse by surgery" (see Chapters 20 to 23). Among problems with the knee, this statement has never been more relevant than when approaching the extensor mechanism. Therefore, we must emphasize the importance of a correct diagnosis (see Chapters 6 and 7) and nonoperative treatment (see Chapters 9 and 10).

Criticism

The great problem of the PFM concept is that not all malalignments, even of significant proportions, are symptomatic. Even more, one knee may be symptomatic and the other not, even though the underlying malalignment is entirely symmetrical (Figure 1.3). On the other hand,

patients with normal patellofemoral alignment on computed tomography (CT) can also suffer from anterior knee pain (Figure 1.4). Therefore, PFM cannot explain all the cases of anterior knee pain, so other pathophysiological processes must exist. Moreover, PFM theory cannot adequately explain the variability of symptoms experienced by patients with anterior knee pain syndrome.

Finally, we must also remember that it has been demonstrated that there are significant differences between subchondral bone morphology and geometry of the articular cartilage surface of the patellofemoral joint, both in the axial and sagittal planes[6] (Figure 1.5). Therefore, a radiographical PFM may not be real and it could induce us to indicate a realignment surgery than could provoke involuntarily an iatrogenic PFM leading to a worsening of preoperative symptoms. This would be another point against the universal acceptance of the PFM theory. Moreover, this could explain also the lack of predictability of operative results of realignment surgery.

Critical Analysis of Long-term Follow-up of Insall's Proximal Realignment for PFM: What Have We Learned?

In agreement with W.S. Halsted, I think that the operating room is "a laboratory of the highest order." As occurs with many surgical techniques, and realignment surgery is not an exception,

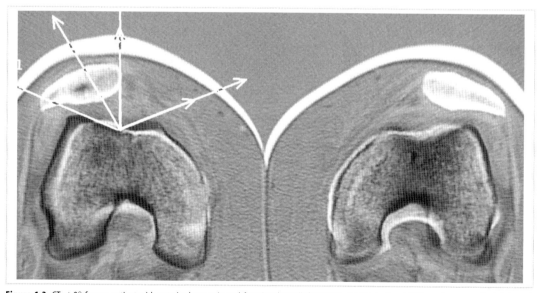

Figure 1.3. CT at 0° from a patient with anterior knee pain and functional patellofemoral instability in the right knee; however, the left knee is completely asymptomatic. In both knees the PFM is symmetric.

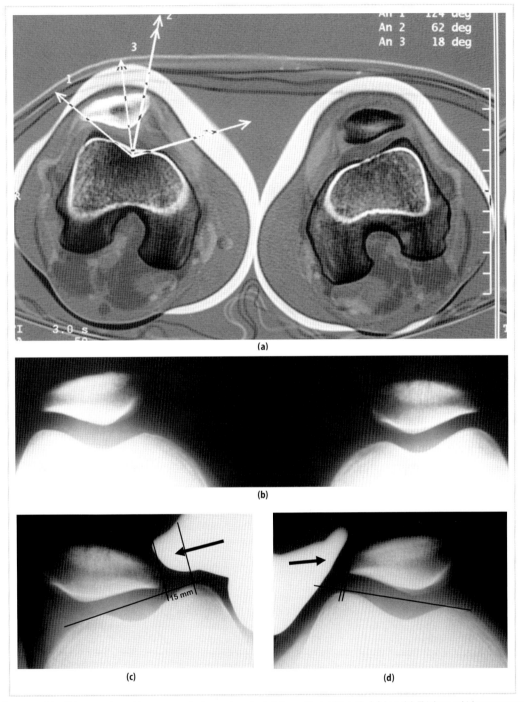

Figure 1.4. CT at 0° from a patient with severe anterior knee pain and patellofemoral instability in the left knee **(a)**. This knee, which was operated on two years ago, performing an Insall's proximal realignment, was very symptomatic in spite of the correct patellofemoral congruence. Fulkerson test for medial subluxation was positive. Nevertheless, the right knee was asymptomatic despite the PFM. Conventional radiographs were normal and the patella was seen well centered in the axial view of Merchant **(b)**. Axial stress radiograph of the left knee **(c)** allowed us to detect an iatrogenic medial subluxation of the patella (medial displacement of 15 mm). Note axial stress radiograph of the right knee **(d)**. The symptomatology disappeared after surgical correction of medial subluxation of the patella using iliotibial tract and patellar tendon for repairing the lateral stabilizers of the patella.

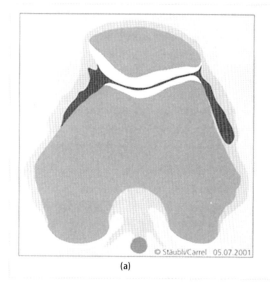
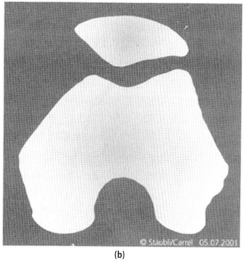

(a)   (b)

Figure 1.5. Scheme of gadolinium-enhanced MR arthrotomogram of the left knee in the axial plane. Note perfect patellofemoral congruence **(a)**. Note patellofemoral incongruence of the osseous contours **(b)**. (Reprinted from *Clin Sports Med*, 21, HU Staeubli, C Bosshard, P Porcellini, et al., Magnetic resonance imaging for articular cartilage: Cartilage-bone mismatch, pp. 417–433, 2002, with permission from Elsevier.)

after wide usage, surgeons may question the basic tenets and may devise clinical research to test the underlying hypothesis, in our case the PFM concept.

In this way we have evaluated retrospectively 40 Insall's proximal realignments (IPR) performed on 29 patients with isolated symptomatic PFM.[e] The average follow-up after surgery was 8 years (range 5–13 years). The whole study is presented in detail in Chapter 2.

One of the objectives of this study was to analyze whether there is a relationship between the presence of PFM and the presence of anterior knee pain or patellar instability.

In my experience IPR provides a satisfactory centralization of the patella into the femoral trochlea in the short-term follow-up.[60] However, this satisfactory centralization of the patella is lost in the CT scans performed in the long-term follow-up in almost 57% of the cases. That is, IPR does not provide a permanent correction in all the cases. Nonetheless, this loss of centralization does not correlate with a worsening of clinical

results. Furthermore, I have not found, in the long-term follow-up, a relation between the result, satisfactory versus nonsatisfactory, and the presence or absence of postoperative PFM. I postulate that PFM could influence the homeostasis negatively, and that realignment surgery could allow the restoring of joint homeostasis when nonoperative treatment of symptomatic PFM fails. Realignment surgery temporarily would unload inflamed peripatellar tissues, rather than permanently modify PFM. Moreover, according to Dye, rest and physical therapy are most important in symptoms resolution than realignment itself. Once we have achieved joint homeostasis, these PFM knees can exist happily within the envelope of function without symptoms. Moreover, in my series, 12 patients presented with unilateral symptoms. In 9 of them the contralateral asymptomatic knee presented a PFM and only in 3 cases was there a satisfactory centralization of the patella into the femoral trochlea.

We can conclude that not all patellofemoral malaligned knees show symptoms, which is not surprising, as there are numerous examples of asymptomatic anatomic variations. Therefore, PFM is not a sufficient condition for the onset of symptoms, at least in postoperative patients. Thus, no imaging study should give us an indication for surgery. History and physical exam must

---

[e] We define the term "isolated symptomatic PFM" as anterior knee pain or patellar instability, or both, with abnormalities of patellar tracking during physical examination verified with CT scans at 0° of knee flexion, but with no associated intra-articular abnormality demonstrated arthroscopically.

point toward surgery and imaging only to allow us to confirm clinical impression (see Chapter 6).

Relevance of our Findings

To think of anterior knee pain or patellar instability as somehow being necessarily tied to PFM is an oversimplification that has positively stultified progress toward better diagnosis and treatment. The great danger in using PFM as a diagnosis is that the unsophisticated or unwary orthopedic surgeon may think that he or she has a license or "green light" to correct it with misguided surgical procedures that very often make the patients' pain worse (see Chapters 20 and 21).

Tissue Homeostasis Theory

In the 1990s, Scott F. Dye, of the University of California, San Francisco, and his research group, came up with the tissue homeostasis theory.[17,19] The initial observation that led to the development of the tissue homeostasis theory of patellofemoral pain was made by Dye, when a patient with complaints of anterior knee pain without evidence of chondromalacia or malalignment underwent a technetium 99m methylene diphosphonate bone scan evaluation of the knees in an attempt to assess the possible presence of covert osseous pathology. The bone scan of that individual manifested an intense diffuse patellar uptake in the presence of normal radiographic images. This finding revealed the presence of a covert osseous metabolic process of the patella in a symptomatic patient with anterior knee pain and normal radiographic findings.

The tissue homeostasis theory is in agreement with the ideas exposed by John Hilton (1807–1876) in his famous book *Rest and Pain*:[50] "The surgeon will be compelled to admit that he has no power to repair directly any injury . . . it is the prerogative of Nature alone to repair . . . his chief duty consists of ascertaining and removing those impediments with thwart the effort of Nature." Moreover, this is in agreement with the ideas exposed by Thomas Sydenhan (1624–1689), "the father of English Medicine," and a cardinal figure in orthopedics in Britain and the world, who looked back to Hippocrates, who taught that Nature was the physician of our diseases. According to Sydenhan the doctor's task was to supplement, not to supplant Nature.[50]

The tissue homeostasis theory states that joints are more than mechanical structures –

they are living, metabolically active systems. This theory attributes pain to a physiopathological mosaic of causes such as increase of osseous remodeling, increase of intraosseous pressure, or peripatellar synovitis that lead to a decrease of what he called "Envelope of Function" (or "Envelope of Load Acceptance").

According to Dye,[17] the Envelope of Function describes a range of loading/energy absorption that is compatible with tissue homeostasis of an entire joint system, that is, with the mechanisms of healing and maintenance of normal tissues. Obviously, the Envelope of Function for a young athlete will be greater than that of sedentary elderly individual. Within the Envelope of Function is the region termed Zone of Homeostasis (Figure 1.6A). Loads that exceed the Envelope of Function but are insufficient to cause a macrostructural failure are termed the Zone of Supraphysiological Overload (Figure 1.6A). If sufficiently high forces are placed across the patellofemoral system, macrostructural failure can occur (Figure 1.6A).

For Dye[17] the following four factors determine the Envelope of Function or Zone of Homeostasis: (1) anatomic factors (morphology, structural integrity and biomechanical characteristics of tissue); (2) kinematic factors (dynamic control of the joint involving proprioceptive sensory output, cerebral and cerebellar sequencing of motor units, spinal reflex mechanisms, and muscle strength and motor control); (3) physiological factors (the genetically determined mechanisms of molecular and cellular homeostasis that determine the quality and rate of repair of damaged tissues); and (4) treatment factors (type of rehabilitation or surgery received).

According to Dye, the loss of both osseous and soft tissue homeostasis is more important in the genesis of anterior knee pain than structural characteristics. To him, it matters little what specific structural factors may be present (i.e., chondromalacia patellae, PFM, etc.) as long as the joint is being loaded within its Envelope of Function, and is therefore asymptomatic. He suggests that patients with patellofemoral pain syndrome are often symptomatic due to supraphysiological loading of anatomically normal knees components.[17] In fact, patients with anterior knee pain often lack an easily identifiable structural abnormality to account for the symptoms. The Envelope of Function frequently diminishes after an episode of injury to the level

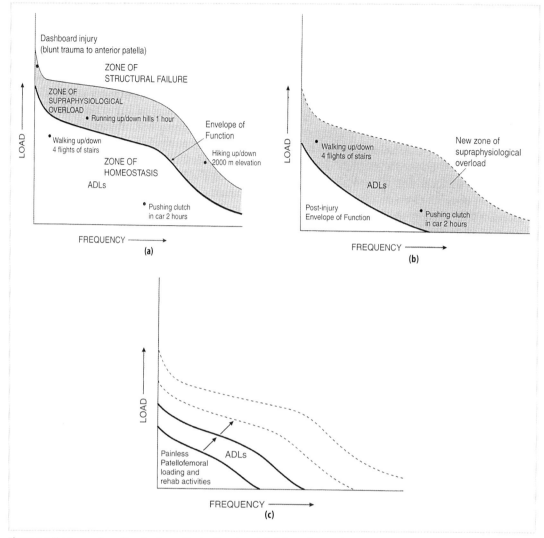

Figure 1.6. The Dye envelope of function theory. (Reprinted from *Operative Techniques in Sports Medicine*, 7, SF Dye, HU Staubli, RM Biedert, et al., Mosaic of pathophysiology causing patellofemoral pain: Therapeutic implications, pp. 46–54, 1999, with permission from Elsevier.)

where many activities of daily living previously well tolerated (e.g., stair climbing, sitting down in and arising out of chairs, pushing the clutch of a car) become sufficiently high (supraphysiological loads for that patient) to lead to subversion of tissue healing and continued symptoms (Figure 1.6B). Decreasing loading to within the newly diminished Envelope of Function allows normal tissue healing processes (Figure 1.6C).

Finally, according to Dye many instances of giving way, in patients with patellofemoral pain, could represent reflex inhibition of the quadriceps, which results from transient impingement of swollen, innervated peripatellar soft tissues, such as inflamed synovium in patients with normal alignment.

Clinical Relevance

Patients with an initial presentation of anterior knee pain frequently will respond positively to load restriction within their Envelope of Function and pain-free rehabilitation program. Moreover, Dye believes that enforced rest after realignment surgery could also be important in symptom resolution. Even if patients, parents, and trainers are apt to stubbornly reject any suggestion to introduce changes into the patient's activities and training routine demanding an urgent surgical procedure, orthopedic surgeons should under no circumstances alter their opinions and recommendations, however strong the pressure exerted upon them may be. Trainers, physical therapists, and physicians all have a high degree of responsibility and need to behave in an ethical way.

Patellofemoral Malalignment Theory versus Tissue Homeostasis Theory

In essence, the proponents of tissue homeostasis theory look at PFM as representing internal load shifting within the patellofemoral joint that may lower the threshold (i.e., decrease of the Envelope of Function) for the initiation and persistence of loss of tissue homeostasis leading to the perception of patellofemoral pain. Pain always denotes loss of tissue homeostasis. From this perspective, there is no inherent conflict between both theories. However, these are not two co-equal theories. Tissue homeostasis theory easily incorporates and properly assesses the clinical importance of possible factors of PFM, whereas the opposite is not true.

In conclusion, I truly believe that both theories are not exclusive, but complementary. In my experience, a knee with PFM can exist happily within its envelope of function, but once it is out, for example by overuse, training error, patterns of faulty sports movements, or traumatism, it can be harder to get back within it, and realignment surgery could be necessary in very selected cases.

Myths and Truths about Patellofemoral Disease

Myth: Anterior knee pain and patellar instability are always self-limited and therefore active treatment is unnecessary. The natural history of this pathological entity is always benign.

Traditionally, anterior knee pain syndrome is considered to be a self-limited condition without long-term sequelae. This is true of many cases but cannot be regarded as a golden rule. A large percentage of patients experience spontaneous recoveries; indeed, many patients remain asymptomatic even without specific treatment. In the case of some of our patients, 10 years elapsed from the onset of symptoms until the time of surgery; their symptoms not only

failed to improve but they worsened in spite of the passage of time and of the patient's restricting or even abandoning sports practice. These same patients obtained excellent or good results after correction of their symptomatic PFM, which persisted in the long-term follow-up (see Chapter 2). Milgrom and colleagues[57] performed a prospective study to determine the natural history of anterior knee pain caused by overactivity. At six years' follow-up, half of the knees originally with anterior knee pain were still symptomatic, but in only 8% of the originally symptomatic knees was the pain severe, hindering physical activity. Clinical experience shows that a prolonged and controlled active conservative treatment generally solves the problem. On the other hand, trying to negligently ignore the problem causes disability in some patients. Unfortunately, the patients' own ambition, as well as that of their parents and coaches, prevails over their doctor's judgment, which is necessarily based on avoiding for at least 3 to 6 months any sports movement that could cause pain. That is, the fact that this process is on occasion self-limited should not make us forget the need to indicate active treatment in all cases. This means that the process we are studying is reversible at least until a certain point has been reached. The question we ask ourselves is: Where is the point of no return?

Primary patellar dislocation is not a trivial condition either. It is true that with the passage of time the frequency of recurrent dislocations tends to diminish, but each episode is a potential source for a chondral injury.[31] A long-term assessment of patients (mean follow-up of 13 years) reveals that conservative treatment of patellar dislocation results in 44% of redislocations and 19% of late patellofemoral pain.[51]

Also, there are studies that establish a connection between PFM and patellofemoral and tibiofemoral osteoarthrosis.[28,43] Now, osteoarthrosis is a long-term hazard, both with or without a surgical procedure.[31] Davies and Newman[13] carried out a comparative study to evaluate the incidence of previous adolescent anterior knee pain syndrome in patients who underwent patellofemoral replacement for isolated patellofemoral osteoarthrosis in comparison with a matched group of patients who underwent unicompartmental replacement for isolated medial compartment osteoarthrosis. They found that the incidence of adolescent anterior knee pain syndrome and patellar instability was higher (p < 0.001) in the patients who underwent patellofemoral replacement for isolated patellofemoral osteoarthrosis (22% and 14% respectively) than in those who underwent unicompartmental replacement for isolated medial compartment osteoarthrosis (6% and 1% respectively). They conclude that anterior knee pain syndrome is not always a self-limiting condition given that it may lead to patellofemoral osteoarthrosis. On the other hand, Arnbjörnsson and colleagues[3] found a high incidence of patellofemoral degenerative changes (29%) after nonoperative treatment of recurrent dislocation of the patella (average follow-up time 14 years with a minimum follow-up time of 11 years and a maximum follow-up time of 19 years (range 11–19 years)). Bearing in mind that the mean age of the patients at follow-up was 39 years they conclude that recurrent dislocation of the patella seems to cause patellofemoral osteoarthrosis. In conclusion, PFM's natural history is not always benign.

Quite often, symptomatic PFM is associated with a patellar tendinopathy.[2] The latter has also been called a self-limited pathology. It has been shown that it is not a benign condition that subsides with time; that is, it is not a self-limited process in athletes.[53] Normally, the injury progresses and when it gets to Blazina's stage III it generally becomes irreversible and leads to the failure of conservative treatment.[53]

Myth: Anterior knee pain is related to growth and, therefore, once the patient has fully grown symptoms will disappear.

Anterior knee pain has also been related to growing pains. It is true that in young athletes during their maximum growth phase ("growth spurt") there can be an increase in the tension of the extensor mechanism as a consequence of some "shortcoming" or "delay" in its development vis-à-vis bone growth. There may exist also a delay in the development of the VMO with regard to other muscles in the knee and therefore a transient muscle imbalance may ensue. But it is also true that quite often parents tell us that the doctor their child saw told them that when the child stopped growing the symptoms would go away and that, nevertheless, these persist once the child has fully grown.

Myth: Anterior knee pain in adolescents is an expression of psychological problems.

Many physicians believe that anterior knee pain is a sign of psychological problems.

Consequently this condition has been associated with a moderate elevation of hysteria and, to a lesser degree, hypochondria with the problem in the knee being considered an unconscious strategy to confront an emotional conflict.[44] Likewise, it has been shown that, on some occasions, in adolescent women anterior knee pain with no evident somatic cause can represent a way to control solicitous or complacent parents.[44] What cannot be questioned is that anybody at whatever age can somatize or try to attract other people's attention through some disease. In spite of this, one should be very cautious when it comes to suggesting to parents that their child's problem is wholly psychological. Nonetheless, it has to be recognized that these types of patients present with a very particular psychological profile (see Chapter 6). Furthermore, there are patients with objective somatic problems who disproportionately exaggerate their pain because of some associate psychological component or secondary emotional or financial gains.

Unfortunately, in my personal current surgical series (84 patients, 102 knees) there are 8 patients (7 females and 1 male) who had been referred to a mental health unit. Strangely enough, these patients' problem was satisfactorily addressed by surgery, which shows that the problem was not psychological. In addition, both the histological and the immunohistochemical and immunochemical techniques-based studies of the lateral patellar retinacula of these patients showed objective alterations that made it possible for us to detect that the pain had a neuroanatomic base. In short, the orthopedic surgeon has the duty to rule out mechanical problems as well as other pathologies that may cause anterior knee pain before blaming the pain on emotional problems or feigning.

Myth: Patellofemoral crepitation is in itself an indication of disfunction.

A very common symptom that worries patients very much is patellofemoral crepitation. Crepitation is indicative of an articular cartilage lesion in the patella or in the femoral trochlea. Nonetheless, some patients who present with crepitation have a macroscopically intact cartilage at the moment of performing the arthroscopy.[30] The crepitation could be caused by alterations in the synovial or in other soft tissues.

The International Knee Documentation Committee (IKDC)[33] stated: "The knee is normal when crepitation is absent." However, this statement cannot be upheld after Johnson and colleagues[45] published their 1998 paper in *Arthroscopy* on the assessment of asymptomatic knees. Indeed, patellofemoral crepitation has a great incidence in asymptomatic women (94% in females versus 45% in males).[45] Patellofemoral crepitation has been associated with the lateral subluxation of the patella, but Johnson and colleagues[45] have observed that lateral subluxation of the patella in asymptomatic persons is more common in males than in females (35% vs. 19%). Crepitation is not always present in patients with significant pain. Furthermore, when it is present is does not necessarily cause anterior knee pain. In short, since crepitation is frequent in asymptomatic knees, its presence is more significant when it is absent from the contralateral knee or when there is some kind of asymmetry.

Myth: VMO is responsible for patellar stability.

It has been stated that the vastus medialis obliquus (VMO) is responsible for patellar stability, but we have not found convincing evidence in the literature for this belief; and, as ligaments are the joint stabilizers, this premise would appear to be faulty. In theory, the VMO resists lateral patellar motion, either by active contraction or by passive muscle resistance. In this way, in Farahmand's study,[20] lateral patellar force-displacement behavior was not affected by simulated muscle forces at any flexion angle from 15 to 75°. On the other hand, the orientation of the VMO varies greatly during knee flexion. The VMO's line of pull most efficiently resists lateral patellar motion when the knee is in deep flexion, at which time trochlear containment of the patella is independent of soft tissues influences (see Chapter 5).

It seems likely that operations that advance the VMO include tightening of the underlying medial patellofemoral ligament (MPFL), and it would be responsible for the success of the surgical technique (see Chapter 2). In this sense, we must note that the VMO tendon becomes confluent with the MPFL in the region of patellar attachment. Therefore, it would be more logical to protect the VMO and address the ligament deficiency surgically as needed (see Chapter 5).

Controversy: Should the Q angle be measured? If so, how should it be measured? Is this of any use?[31,58]

Another aspect that normally receives great importance in the physical examination of these patients is their Q angle, to the extent that some authors regard it as one of the criteria to be used for indicating a realignment surgery. Nonetheless, values considered to be normal vary greatly across the different studies carried out. In addition, there are no scientific criteria that correlate the incidence of patellofemoral pathology with the Q angle measure. Nowadays, some believe that the Q angle, as it is calculated, is not a very accurate way of measuring the patella's alignment since the measurement is made in extension and a laterally subluxating patella would lead to a falsely low measurement. In sum, even if Q angle measurement has traditionally been used in the clinical assessment of patients with a patellofemoral pathology, currently the usefulness of this measurement is uncertain in spite of the multiple studies performed to date. A realignment surgery must never be justified on the basis of a high Q angle (see Chapter 20, clinical case 1). The real controversy at present is how to measure the Q angle.

Myth: Lateral release is a minor risk-free surgical procedure.

Over the years, lateral retinacular release has been recommended for a number of specific patellofemoral conditions:[23] recurrent lateral patellar dislocations or subluxations, chronic lateral subluxation – fixed lateral position, excessive lateral pressure syndrome, lateral retinacular tightness, and retinacular neuromata. A possible explanation for this wide range of surgical indications could be that some orthopedic surgeons consider the lateral release as a minor risk-free surgical procedure. However, I believe in agreement with Ronald Grelsamer that "There is no such thing as minor surgery – only minor surgeons." Surprisingly, in a survey of the IPSG[23] on isolated lateral retinacular release, published in 2004 in *Arthroscopy*, most respondents (89%) indicated that this surgical procedure is a legitimate treatment, but only on rare occasions (1% to 2% of surgeries performed, less than 5 lateral releases a year). Furthermore, strong consensus (78%) existed that objective evidence should show lateral retinacular tension if a lateral release is to be performed.

Although lateral retinacular release is a simple procedure, it can lead to significant complications (see Chapters 20 and 21). In biomechanical studies, lateral release has been shown: (1) to reduce lateral tilt of the patella in cases in which tight lateral retinaculum is seen on CT scans,[27] (2) to increase passive medial displacement of the patella,[64,67] and (3) to increase passive lateral displacement of the patella.[15] Finally, in cadaver knees without preexisting lateral retinacular tightness, lateral release had no effect on articular pressures when the quadriceps were loaded.[34]

In conclusion, indiscriminate use of lateral release is of little benefit and can often cause increased symptoms. That is the reason why lengthening of the lateral retinaculum is the therapy chosen by authors such as Roland Biedert (see Chapter 20).

Reality: Patellofemoral pathology leads to diagnostic error and, therefore, to inappropriate treatments and to patients being subjected to multiple procedures and to a great deal of frustration.

All myths and controversies analyzed throughout the present chapter could lead the reader to attribute importance to things that in actual fact are unimportant (i.e., crepitation) or, on the contrary, to underrate or cast aside complaints like anterior knee pain or functional patellar instability, considering them to be either a psychological problem or a condition bound to subside with time. Sometimes we do not go far enough, which may lead us to overlook other pathologies (diagnostic errors leading to therapeutic errors). In other cases we overdo it and treat cases of malalignment that are not symptomatic. So we have seen patients with symptoms of instability who were treated for malalignment when what they really had was instability caused by a tear in their ACL.

We have also seen patients treated for a meniscal injury who really had isolated symptomatic PFM. In this connection it is important to point out that McMurray's test, traditionally associated with meniscal pathology, can lead to a medial-lateral displacement of the patella and also cause pain in patients with PFM. Finally, it is worrying to see how many patients are referred to outpatient orthopedic surgery practices in our hospitals with an MRI-based diagnosis of a tear in the posterior horn of the medial meniscus who during clinical examination present with anterior knee pain and no meniscal symptoms. It is a proven fact that given the overcrowding of outpatient units' orthopedic services and because of social pressure, as time passes doctors tend to conduct more superficial physical examinations and to order more MRIs. In this way we must remember the statement by Dr. Casscells:[10] "Technology: a good servant, but a bad master." According to Augusto Sarmiento, former Chairman of the American Academy of Orthopedic Surgeons (AAOS), MRIs are unfortunately replacing the physical examination when it comes to assessing a painful joint.[62] MRI is not a panacea and, what's more, it gives rise to false positives. Patients' great faith in technology and their skepticism regarding their doctors and an increasingly dehumanized medical practice has resulted in the failure of partial arthroscopic meniscectomies owing to a bad indication, in frustrated patients, and in the squandering of resources. In 1940, Karlson[46] wrote the following about chondromalacia patellae: "The diagnosis is difficult to make and the differential diagnosis of injury to the meniscus . . . causes special difficulties, as in both these ailments [meniscal and patellar pathology] there is a pressure tenderness over the medial joint space." Hughston endorsed these words when he stated, first in 1960 and then in 1984:[36] "The orthopedic surgeon who has not mistaken a recurrent subluxation of the patella for a torn meniscus has undoubtedly had a very limited and fortunate experience with knees and meniscectomies." Just think of the sheer amount of arthroscopies performed unnecessarily on the basis of a complaint of anterior knee pain!

Nowadays this problem has been magnified because of the relative ease with which meniscectomies are indicated and performed thanks to the benefits of arthroscopy. In a lecture delivered at the Conference of the Nordic Orthopaedic Federation held in Finland in 2000, Augusto Sarmiento stated that the number of unnecessary surgeries (including arthroscopies) carried out in our field in the United States is extremely high.[62] It is therefore essential to underscore the importance of physically examining the patient (see Chapter 6).

Finally, another source of frustration for the patient is the lack of communication with his or her doctor (dehumanized medicine), which may lead to unrealistic expectations. It is essential for the patient to understand the difficulties inherent in treating patellofemoral problems. This is the only way in which patients can be satisfied after surgery even if their symptoms do not disappear completely.

Reality: "Treatment should be customized."

It is very important to identify the pathological alteration responsible for the clinical aspect of this clinical entity to select the most effective treatment options based on clinical findings (made-to-measure treatment). This will yield the most satisfactory results. At present, minimal intervention (e.g., specific soft tissue excision of painful tissue[47]) and nonsurgical methods are emphasized (see Chapters 9 and 10). Obviously, if the etiology of patellofemoral pain and patellar instability is multifactorial, then the evaluation must be multifactorial, and the treatment should be multifactorial also.[56] This should lead to a simplified treatment plan. We must find out what is wrong and fix it; that is, we must address specific identifiable pathology (e.g., peripatellar synovitis, serious rotational alterations, etc.). In the few patients who require surgery, a minimalist surgical approach is the best in most cases.[19,47] We agree with the statement of Philip Wiles in 1952: "However important surgery may be now, it should be the aim of all doctors, including surgeons, to limit and ultimately abolish it." [50]

Conclusions

The pathology we discuss in the present monograph presents itself with a multifactorial etiology and a great pathogenic, diagnostic, and therapeutic complexity.

The consideration of anterior knee pain to be a self-limited condition in patients with an underlying neurotic personality should be banished from the orthopedic literature.

Our knowledge about anterior knee pain has evolved throughout the twentieth century. While until the end of the 1960s this pain was attributed to chrondromalacia patellae, a concept born at the beginning of the century, after that period it came to be connected with abnormal patellofemoral alignment. More recently, the pain was put down to a wide range of physiopathological processes such as peripatellar synovitis, the increment in intraosseous pressure, and increased bone remodeling. We are now at a turning point. New information is produced at breakneck speed. Nowadays, medicine in its entirety is being reassessed at the subcellular level, and this is precisely the line of thought we are following in the approach to anterior knee pain syndrome. Still to be seen are the implications that this change of mentality will have in the treatment of anterior knee pain syndrome in the future, but I am sure that these new currents of thought will open for us the doors to new and exciting perspectives that could potentially revolutionize the management of this troublesome pathological condition in the new millennium we have just entered. Clearly, we are only at the beginning of the road that will lead to understanding where anterior knee pain comes from.

References

1. Aleman, O. Chondromalacia post-traumatica patellae. *Acta Chir Scand* 1928; 63: 194.
2. Allen, GM, PG Tauro, and SJ Ostlere. Proximal patellar tendinosis and abnormalities of patellar tracking. *Skeletal Radiol* 1999; 28: 220–223.
3. Arnbjörnsson, A, N Egund, and O Rydling. The natural history of recurrent dislocation of the patella: Long-term results of conservative and operative treatment. *J Bone Joint Surg* 1992; 74-B: 140–142.
4. Aune, AK, I Holm, MA Risberg, et al. Four-strand hamstring tendon autograft compared with patellar tendon-bone autograft for anterior cruciate ligament reconstruction: A randomized study with two-year follow-up. *Am J Sports Med* 2001; 29: 722–728.
5. Axhausen, G. Zur Pathogenese der Arthritis deformans. *Arch Orthop Unfallchir* 1922; 20: 1.
6. Bosshard, C, HU Staubli, and W Rauschning. Konturinkongruenz von gelenkknorpeloberflachen und subchondralem knochen des femoropatellargelenkas in der sagittalen ebene. *Arthroskopie* 1997; 10: 72–76.
7. Budinger, K. Üeber ablösung von gelenkteilen und verwandte prozesse. *Dtsch Z Chir* 1906; 84: 311–365.
8. Budinger, K. Üeber traumatische knorpelrisse im kniegelenk. *Dtsch Z Chir* 1908; 92: 510.
9. Campbell, JD. Treatment trends with ACL, PCL, MCL, and cartilage problems 2004. *ACL Study Group Meeting*, Sardinia, Italy, 2004.
10. Casscells, SW. Technology: a good servant, but a bad master. *Arthroscopy* 1990; 6: 1–2.
11. Corry, IS, JM Webb, AJ Clingeleffer et al. Arthroscopic reconstruction of the anterior cruciate ligament: A comparison of patellar tendon autograft and four-strand hamstring tendon autograft. *Am J Sports Med* 1999; 27: 444–454.
12. Dandy, DJ, and H Poirier. Chondromalacia and the unstable patella. *Acta Orthop Scand* 1975; 46: 695–699.
13. Davies, G, and JH Newman. Does adolescent anterior knee pain lead to patellofemoral arthritis? *Tenth Congress European Society of Sports Traumatology, Knee Surgery and Arthroscopy*, Rome 23–27 April 2002, *Book of Abstracts*, p. 353.
14. DeHaven, KE, and DM Lintner. Athletic injuries: comparison by age, sport, and gender. *Am J Sports Med.* 1986; 14: 218–224.
15. Desio, SM, RT Burks, and KN Bachus. Soft tissue restraints to lateral patellar translation in the human knee. *Am J Sports Med* 1998; 26: 59–65.
16. Devereaux, MD, and SM Lachmann. Patello-femoral arthralgia in athletes attending a sports injury clinic. *Brit J Sports Medicine* 1984; 18: 18–21.
17. Dye, SF. The knee as a biologic transmission with an envelope of function: a theory. *Clin Orthop* 1996; 325: 10–18.
18. Dye, SF, GL Vaupel, and CC Dye. Conscious neurosensory mapping of the internal structures of the human

knee without intra-articular anesthesia. *Am J Sports Med* 1998; 26: 773–777.

19. Dye, SF, HU Staubli, RM Biedert et al. The mosaic of pathophysiology causing patellofemoral pain: Therapeutic implications. *Operative Techniques in Sports Medicine* 1999; 7: 46–54.

20. Farahmand, F, MN Tahmasbi, and AA Amis. Lateral force-displacement behaviour of the human patella and its variation with knee flexion: A biomechanical study in vitro. *J Biomech* 1998; 31: 1147–1152.

21. Ficat, P, C Ficat, and A Bailleux. Syndrome d`hyperpression externe de la rotule (S.H.P.E). *Rev Chir Orthop* 1975; 61: 39–59.

22. Ficat, P, and DS Hungerford. *Disorders of the Patello-Femoral Joint*. Baltimore: Williams & Wilkins, 1977.

23. Fithian, DC, EW Paxton, WR Post et al. Lateral retinacular release: A survey of the International Patellofemoral Study Group. *Arthroscopy* 2004; 20: 463–468.

24. Fu, FH, CH Bennett, CB Ma et al. Current trends in anterior cruciate ligament reconstruction. Part 2: Operative procedures and clinical correlations. *Am J Sports Med* 2000; 28: 124–130.

25. Fulkerson, JP. The etiology of patellofemoral pain in young, active patients: A prospective study. *Clin Orthop* 1983; 179: 129–133.

26. Fulkerson, JP, R Tennant, and JS Jaivin. Histologic evidence of retinacular nerve injury associated with patellofemoral malalignment. *Clin Orthop* 1985; 197: 196–205.

27. Fulkerson, JP, SF Schutzer, GR Ramsby et al. Computerized tomography of the patellofemoral joint before and after release and malalignment. *Arthroscopy* 1987; 3: 19–24.

28. Fulkerson, JP, and DS Hungerford. *Disorders of the Patellofemoral Joint*. Baltimore: Williams & Wilkins; 1990.

29. Fulkerson, JP, and EA Arendt. Anterior knee pain in females. *Clin Orthop* 2000; 372: 69–73.

30. Grelsamer, RP, and J McConnell. *The Patella. A Team Approach*. Gaithersburg, MD: Aspen, 1998.

31. Grelsamer, RP. Patellar malalignment. *J Bone Joint Surg* 2000; 82-A: 1639–1650.

32. Griffin, LY, J Agel, MJ Albohm et al. Noncontact anterior cruciate ligament injuries: Risk factors and prevention strategies. *J Am Acad Orthop Surg* 2000; 8: 141–150.

33. Hefti, F, W Muller, RP Jakob et al. Evaluation of knee ligament injuries with the IKDC form. *Knee Surg Sports Traumatol Arthrosc* 1993; 1: 226–234.

34. Huberti, HH, and WC Hayes. Contact pressures in chondromalacia patellae and the effects of capsular reconstructive procedures. *J Orthop Res* 1988; 6: 499–508.

35. Hughston, JC. Subluxation of the patella. *J Bone Joint Surg* 1968; 50-A: 1003–1026.

36. Hughston, JC, WM Walsh, and G Puddu. Patellar subluxation and dislocation. In *Saunders Monographs in Clinical Orthopaedics,* vol. 5. Philadelphia: WB Saunders, 1984.

37. Huston, LJ, ML Greenfield, and EM Wojtys. Anterior cruciate ligament injuries in the female athlete: Potential risk factors. *Clin Orthop* 2000; 372: 50–63.

38. Insall, J. "Chondromalacia Patellae": Patellar malalignment syndrome. *Orthop Clin North Am* 1979; 10: 117–127.

39. Insall, J, PG Bullough, and AH Burnstein. Proximal "tube" realignment of the patella for chondromalacia patellae. *Clin Orthop* 1979; 144: 63–69.

40. Insall, JN, P Aglietti, and AJ Tria Jr. Patellar pain and incongruence. II: Clinical application. *Clin Orthop* 1983; 176: 225–232.

41. Insall, *J. Surgery of the Knee*. New York: Churchill Livingstone, 1984 & 1993.

42. International Patellofemoral Study Group. Patellofemoral semantics: The Tower of Babel. *Am J Knee Surg* 1997; 10: 92–95.

43. Iwano, T, H Kurosawa, H Tokuyama et al. Roentgenographic and clinical findings of patellofemoral osteoarthritis. *Clin Orthop* 1990; 252: 190–197.

44. Johnson, LL. Arthroscopic Surgery: Principles and Practice. St. Louis: C.V. Mosby, 1986.

45. Johnson, LL, E van Dyk, JR Green et al. Clinical assessment of asymptomatic knees: Comparison of men and women. *Arthroscopy* 1998; 14: 347–359.

46. Karlson, S. Chondromalacia patellae. *Acta Chir Sacand* 1940; 83: 347–381.

47. Kasim, N, and JP Fulkerson. Resection of clinically localized segments of painful retinaculum in the treatment of selected patients with anterior knee pain. *Am J Sports Med* 2000; 28: 811–814.

48. Larson, RV. Complications and pitfalls in anterior cruciate ligament reconstruction with hamstring tendons. In Malek, MM, ed., *Knee Surgery: Complications, Pitfalls and Salvage*. New York: Springer-Verlag, 2001; 77–88.

49. Leslie, IJ, and G Bentley. Arthroscopy in the diagnosis of chondromalacia patellae. *Ann Rheum Dis* 1978; 37: 540–547.

50. Levay, D. *The History of Orthopaedics*. New Jersey: Parthenon Publishing Group, 1990.

51. Mäenpää, H, and MUK Lehto. Patellar dislocation: The long-term results of nonoperative management in 100 patients. *Am J Sports Med* 1997; 25: 213–217.

52. Maffulli, N, KM Khan, and G Puddu. Overuse tendon conditions: time to change a confusing terminology. *Arthroscopy* 1998; 14: 840–843.

53. Martens, M, P Wouters, A Burssens et al. Patellar tendinitis: Pathology and results of treatment. *Acta Orthop Scand* 1982; 53: 445–450.

54. Merchant, AC, RL Mercer, RH Jacobsen et al. Roentgenographic analysis of patellofemoral congruence. *J Bone Joint Surg* 1974; 56-A: 1391–1396.

55. Merchant, AC, and RL Mercer. Lateral release of the patella: A preliminary report. *Clin Orthop* 1974; 103: 40.

56. Merchant, AC. Thirty-three years in the PF joint: What have I learned? *VIII International Patellofemoral Study Group Meeting,* Florida, 2003.

57. Milgrom, C, A Finestone, N Shlamkovitch et al. Anterior knee pain caused by overactivity: A long-term prospective followup. *Clin Orthop* 1996; 331: 256–260.

58. Post, WR. Clinical evaluation of patients with patellofemoral disorders. *Arthroscopy* 1999; 15: 841–851.

59. Royle, SG, J Noble, DR Davies et al. The significance of chondromalacic changes on the patella. *Arthroscopy* 1991; 7: 158–160.

60. Sanchis-Alfonso, V, E Gastaldi-Orquín, and V Martinez-SanJuan. Usefulness of computed tomography in evaluating the patellofemoral joint before and after Insall's realignment: Correlation with short-term clinical results. *Am J Knee Surg* 1994; 7: 65–72.

61. Sanchis-Alfonso, V, and E Roselló-Sastre. Anterior knee pain in the young patient: What causes the pain? "Neural model." *Acta Orthop Scand*. 2003; 74: 697–703.

62. Sarmiento, A. The future of our specialty. *Acta Orthop Scand* 2000; 71: 574–579.

63. Schutzer, SF, GR Ramsby, and JP Fulkerson. Computed tomographic classification of patellofemoral pain patients. *Orthop Clin North Am* 1986; 17: 235–248.

64. Skalley, TC, GC Terry, and RA Teitge. The quantitative measurement of normal passive medial and lateral patellar motion limits. *Am J Sports Med* 1993; 21: 728–732.

65. Spicer, DD, SE Blagg, AJ Unwin et al. Anterior knee symptoms after four-strand hamstring tendon anterior cruciate ligament reconstruction. *Knee Surg Sports Traumatol Arthrosc* 2000; 8: 286–289.

66. Tapper, EM, and NW Hoover. Late results after meniscectomy. *J Bone Joint Surg* 1969; 51-A: 517–526.

67. Teitge, RA, WW Faerber, P Des Madryl et al. Stress radiographs of the patellofemoral joint. *J Bone Joint Surg* 1996; 78-A: 193–203.

68. Thomee, R, P Restrom, J Karlsson et al. Patellofemoral pain syndrome in young women. I: A clinical analysis of alignment, pain parameters, common symptoms and functional activity level. *Scand J Med Sci Sports* 1995; 5: 237–244.

69. Witvrouw, E, R Lysens, J Bellemans et al. Intrinsic risk factors for the development of anterior knee pain in an athletic population: A two-year prospective study. *Am J Sports Med* 2000; 28: 480–489.

2

Pathogenesis of Anterior Knee Pain and Patellar Instability in the Active Young

What Have We Learned from Realignment Surgery?

Vicente Sanchis-Alfonso, Fermín Ordoño, Alfredo Subías-López, and Carmen Monserrat

Introduction

For many years, patellofemoral malalignment (PFM), an abnormality of patellar tracking that involves lateral displacement or lateral tilt of the patella (or both) in extension that reduces in flexion, was widely accepted as an explanation for the genesis of anterior knee pain and patellar instability, the most common knee complaints in clinical practice in young patients.[11,16,18,19,22,23,27] Moreover, this concept had a great influence on orthopedic surgeons, who developed several surgical procedures to "correct the malalignment," such as Insall's proximal realignment (IPR).[20] Currently, however, this concept is questioned by many, and is not universally accepted to account for the presence of anterior knee pain and/or patellar instability. In fact, the number of realignment surgeries has dropped dramatically in recent years, due to a reassessment of the paradigm of PFM. Despite a large body of literature on patellofemoral realignment procedures, little information is available on the in-depth long-term results of these surgical procedures.[1,2,8] It has been the practice in our institution to evaluate patients carefully with regular follow-up, scrutinizing their results so that we may learn from them and continually improve our techniques and outcomes.

The current retrospective clinical study was conducted to evaluate critically the long-term results of the operative treatment of "isolated symptomatic PFM," recalcitrant to conservative treatment, by IPR, in order to clarify the following points: (1) whether there is a relationship between the presence of PFM and the presence of anterior knee pain and/or patellar instability; (2) long-term response of vastus medialis obliquus (VMO) muscle fibers to increased resting length; and (3) incidence of patellofemoral arthrosis after IPR surgery.

Patients and Methods
Subjects

From 1991 through 1999, 59 IPRs were performed on 45 patients by the first author (V.S-A). To obtain a homogeneous population, we included in the study group only those cases with the following criteria: (1) PFM demonstrated with CT at 0° of knee flexion; (2) no previous knee surgery; (3) no associated intraarticular pathology (such as synovial plica, meniscal tears, ACL/PCL tears or osteoarthrosis) confirmed arthroscopically or by x-rays; and (4) IPR as an isolated surgical procedure. Moreover, we excluded patients involved in workman's compensation or other pending litigation claims and patients who had recurrent dislocation of the patella associated with Down syndrome. Sixteen of 45 surgical patients were excluded because they did not meet the aforementioned criteria or they were not available for follow-up.

Thus, only 40 IPRs (20 right and 20 left) performed on 29 patients composed the study group. There were 26 females and 3 males. The average age at the onset of symptoms was 16 (range 10–23 years). Onset of symptoms was secondary to a twisting injury while participating in sports in 16 cases (40%), and secondary to a fall onto the flexed knee in one case (2.5%). In 23 cases (57.5%), the onset of symptoms occurred spontaneously without injury. Surgery was performed after a mean of 24 months following onset of symptoms (range 2 months–11 years). The main motive that led the patient to surgery was disabling patellofemoral pain in 21 cases (52.5%) and patellar instability in 19 cases (47.5%). Therefore, two populations were analyzed in this study: "patellar pain patients with PFM" (group I) and "patellar instability patients with PFM" (group II). For the purposes of this paper, the term *patellar instability* is used to describe giving way as a result of the patella partially slipping out of the trochlea, and dislocation (complete displacement of the patella out of the trochlea). The average age of the patients at the time of surgery was 19 (range 11–26 years). Eleven patients (38%) were operated on both knees. The average follow-up after surgery was 8 years (range 5–13 years). This series had been evaluated clinically at medium-term (average follow-up after surgery: 3 years) (unpublished data). The average age of patients at the time of follow-up was 27 (range 21–36 years).

Diagnostic Criteria for Isolated Symptomatic PFM

We define patients with "isolated symptomatic PFM" as those with anterior knee pain, or patellar instability, with abnormalities of patellar tracking during the physical examination, verified with computed tomography (CT) at 0° and 30° of knee flexion, and no associated intra-articular pathology shown during arthroscopy.[28]

Patient Selection for IPR

The operation was indicated in young patients (even with open physis) with severe and persistent peripatellar pain and/or patellar instability (with or without recurrent dislocation of the patella), with Q angle < 20°, in which CT demonstrated PFM type 1 (subluxation without tilt) or 2 (subluxation with tilt), according to the classification of Schutzer and colleagues,[32] that produced significant disability for daily living activities (ADL), and that did not improve generally after a minimum of 6 months following standard nonoperative treatment.[25] Only in

three of our cases, the patient was operated on before 6 months after onset of symptoms because of severe instability with various episodes of falling to the ground. Nonoperative treatment includes physical therapy, medication, counseling, modification of activities, stopping certain activities, and most important, time. Generally, surgery should be considered as a last recourse after all conservative options have been exhausted.

Surgical Technique

A proximal realignment, as described by Insall,[19] was performed on all patients. A lateral retinacular release extending along the most distal fibers of the vastus lateralis (vastus lateralis obliquus), the lateral patellar edge, and the lateral edge of the patellar tendon was always performed before the medial imbrication. Medial capsular tightening was achieved by overlapping the medial flap on the patella; the medial flap extends from the upper edge of the VMO into the quadriceps tendon over the patella and above the patellar tendon. Realignment was effected by advancing the vastus medialis laterally and distally, which was held with several preliminary sutures. After realignment, the knee was moved through the range of motion, and the tracking of the patella in the femoral sulcus was assessed. The patella was determined to be centralized if it tracked entirely within the intercondylar sulcus, with no medial or lateral tilt and/or subluxation.

Follow-up Evaluation

We conducted comprehensive follow-up evaluation. All studies were performed by the same examiners, who were blinded to the clinical results.

The clinical results were rated according to the Cincinnati symptom rating scale,[5] Lysholm score,[21] Tegner activity level,[34] and Cincinnati patient perception scale of the overall condition of the knee.[5] We used the visual analog scale to report the severity of pain, which allows us to quantify numerically (numerical scale) the pain through a 10 cm bar with 1 cm gradations. Pain is rated from 0 to 10, with 0 representing the absence of pain and 10 indicating excruciating pain. Moreover, this permits us to quantify verbally the pain (verbal scale): light (0–3.3), moderate (3.3–6.6), and severe pain (6.6–10)[33].

Roentgenographic staging of patellofemoral osteoarthrosis was made in all the patients, except in 2 due to pregnancy, (37 knees) at the follow-up examination with the axial view x-rays at 45° flexion of the knee, using the method of Merchant.[24] Moreover, preoperative radiographs were reviewed in all the patients. Signs of retropatellar arthrosis were rated according to the Sperner classification: Stage 1: subchondral sclerosis, no osteophyte formation; Stage 2: osteophyte formation on the patella; Stage 3: patellofemoral joint space narrowing, marked osteophytes on the patella and femoral condyles; and Stage 4: gross narrowing or complete obliteration of joint space.[36] Osteoarthrosis in Stage 1 was excluded from this study, because it may vary among investigators due to its slight changes. Moreover, CT examinations at 0° of knee flexion at the long-term follow-up examination were made in all patients, except in 2 due to pregnancy, (37 knees) following a previously well-described technique, given that it is an acceptable way to detect subtle PFM.[25]

Finally, surface electromyographic (SEMG) analysis of amplitude and voluntary activity pattern of VMO and vastus lateralis muscle (VL) of both knees was made in all the patients operated on one knee, the contralateral knee being asymptomatic (12 patients, 24 knees). The contralateral asymptomatic knee was used as a control. Amplitude analyses were conducted to evaluate the magnitude and timing of muscle activity. Voluntary activity pattern was rated in four grades according to the classification of Buchthal.[6] Voluntary activity pattern measures in an indirect way the number of motor units, very useful when there is suspicion of muscle atrophy or hypertrophy. Electromyography data were collected with the Esaote Reporter® (Florence, Italy) electromyography system of 4 channels, with a program specifically designed for this study, with 2 channels fitted out, 5 seconds of sweep screen, filters of 100 Hz and 1 kHz, and 10 mV of amplitude. After skin preparation, which included shaving and cleaning with isopropyl alcohol, surface electrodes were placed on the muscle belly and tendinous attachment of both VMO and VL. A ground electrode was placed on the contralateral aspect of the thigh. We confirm optimal electrode placement by observation and palpation of the patient's quadriceps during isometric contraction with the knee extended. We evaluated the VMO and VL during five maximum voluntary isometric contractions with knee extension, of at least 2 seconds, following a previously well-

described technique.[16] The amplitude was obtained by calculating the average of the amplitudes of each of the 5 contractions. Between each pair of contractions enough time was left for the muscle to rest. All the patients were able to complete the test without problems or pain. In both knees we calculated SEMG ratios for VMO:VL function to assess muscle balance.

Statistical Analyses of Data

Statistical analysis was performed using the software SPSS version 10.0 (SPSS Inc., Chicago, Illinois) for Windows. Data are presented as mean ± SD. Descriptive statistics, Student's t-test, Chi-square test, Fisher's test and Pearson's correlation coefficient were used for the analysis. A P value < 0.05 was accepted as reflecting statistical significance. Finally, to determine if we had enough knees in this study to show a clinically significant difference, we performed power analyses.

Results
Clinical Results

At long-term follow-up, all the patients demonstrated improvement based on pain, instability, knee function, activity level, and subjective perception of the condition of her or his knee.

Group I (Patellar Pain Patients with PFM; 21 Knees)

Referring to pain, according to the Cincinnati symptom rating scale, preoperatively, 52.4% of the patients had severe pain, constant and not relieved, with ADL; 28.6% had moderate pain, frequent and limiting, with ADL; 9.5% had pain only with severe work/sports activities; 4.8% were able to do ADL without pain, but they had pain with light work/sports activities; and 4.8% had pain only with moderate work/sports activities. Postoperatively, at long-term follow-up, 42.9% of the patients had no pain; 23.8% had pain only with strenuous work/sports, but they were able to do moderate works/sports without pain; 23.8% had pain only with moderate work/sports; 5% had moderate pain with ADL; and 9.5% had pain with light work/sports. Concerning instability, according to the Cincinnati symptom rating scale, preoperatively 94.4% of the patients, suffered partial giving-way (partial knee collapse but no fall to the ground) and 5.6% total giving-way (knee collapse with actual falling to the ground).

Postoperatively, at long-term follow-up, 90.5% had no instability and 9.5% suffered giving-way.

According to Lysholm's score, preoperatively 71% of the knees were catalogued as poor and 29% as fair. Postoperatively, at long-term follow-up, the results were excellent in 8 cases (38%), good in 10 (47.6%), fair in one (4.7%), and poor in 2 (9.5%). The preoperative Lysholm score averaged 49.76 (SD, 19.94; range 12–76). The postoperative Lysholm score averaged 95.15 (SD, 4.76; range 88–100) at the medium-term follow-up. At long-term follow-up it averaged 89 (SD, 13.19; range 53–100). There was no statistically significant worsening when comparing the results at medium- and long-term follow-ups (p = 0.178; 1-ß = 55.2%). Tegner activity score improved from 0.73 ± 1.01 to 3.44 ± 1.01 at long-term follow-up.

Subjectively, according to the Cincinnati patient perception scale, preoperatively 60% of the knees were catalogued as fair (moderate limitations that affected ADL, no sports possible) and 40% as poor (significant limitations that affected ADL). Postoperatively, at long-term follow-up, 19% of the knees were catalogued as normal (the patient is able to do whatever he or she wishes with no problems), 57% as good (some limitations with sports, but the patient can participate), and 24% as fair.

Group II (Patellar Instability Patients with PFM; 19 Knees)

Referring to pain, according to the Cincinnati symptom rating scale, preoperatively, 61.1% of the patients had moderate pain, frequent and limiting, with ADL; 11.1% had severe pain constant and not relieved, with ADL; 5.6% had pain only with severe work/sports activities; 5.6% were able to do ADL without pain, but they had pain with light work/sports activities; and 5.6% had pain only with moderate work/sports activities. Postoperatively, at long-term follow-up, 68.4% of the patients had no pain; 15.8% had pain only with strenuous work/sports, but they were able to do moderate works/sports without pain; 10.5% had moderate pain with ADL; and 5.3% had pain only with moderate work/sports. Concerning instability, according to the Cincinnati symptom rating scale, preoperatively 83.3% of the patients suffered total giving-way and 16.7% partial giving-way. Postoperatively, at long-term follow-up, 94.7% had no instability and 5.3% suffered giving-way.

According to Lysholm's score, preoperatively 78% of the knees were catalogued as poor and 22% as fair. Postoperatively, at long-term follow-up, the results were excellent in 13 cases (68%), good in 4 (21%), fair in one (5%), and poor in one (5%). The preoperative Lysholm score averaged 47.56 (SD, 16.31; range 17–76). The postoperative Lysholm score averaged 96.63 (SD, 3.20; range 90–100) at the medium-term follow-up. At long-term follow-up it averaged 92.89 (SD, 11.05; range 54–100). There was no statistically significant worsening when comparing the results at medium- and long-term follow-ups (p = 0.256; 1-ß = 88.6%). Tegner activity score improved from 1.08 ± 1.19 to 4.36 ± 0.5 at long-term follow-up.

Subjectively, according to the Cincinnati patient perception scale, preoperatively 66.7% of the knees were catalogued as poor and 33.3% as fair. Postoperatively, at long-term follow-up, 42.1% of the knees were catalogued as normal (excellent), 47.4% as good, 5.3% as fair, and 5.3% as poor.

In only one knee (5.2%) a redislocation of the patella occurred spontaneously without traumatism 7 years after surgery; until then, this knee had an excellent result (Lysholm score of 95 points). Since then, the result was catalogued as poor (Lysholm score of 54 points). We had two cases (10.5%) of knee motion limitation, which required manipulation under general anesthesia with an excellent result at 6 and 8 years of follow-up (Lysholm scores 95 and 96 points).

There were no statistically significant differences at long-term follow-up of Lysholm scores in both groups (p = 0.321; 1-ß = 70.4%) with equal variances assumed (F [18, 20] = 0.565, p = 0.457).

Image Analyses

Postoperative CT at 0° of knee flexion, at long-term follow-up, demonstrated PFM type 1 or 2 according to the classification of Schutzer and colleagues[32] in 21 cases (56.75%). In the other 16 cases (43.24%), there was a satisfactory centralization of the patella in the femoral trochlea. Eighteen out of 21 cases (85.7%) that presented PFM had a satisfactory result (excellent or good), while the other 3 cases (14.3%) presented a poor result. Fourteen out of 16 cases (87.5%) that presented a satisfactory centralization of the patella had a satisfactory result, while the other 2 cases (12.5%) presented a fair result. There is no relation between the result (satisfactory vs. unsatisfactory) and the presence or no presence of PFM ($\chi^2 = 0.025$, p = 0.875) (Figures 2.1 and 2.2). In 12 patients, in whom the contralateral nonoperated knee was completely asymptomatic, we found objective PFM in 9 cases, and in 3 cases we found a satisfactory centralization.

Preoperatively, we found no radiographic degenerative changes in any case. Roentgenographic assessment, at long-term follow-up, revealed no detectable signs of retropatellar arthrosis in 34 (92%) out of 37 operated knees evaluated by x-rays. One patient had a narrowing of the femorpatellar joint gap (6 years of follow-up, Lysholm score 94 points); one patient had

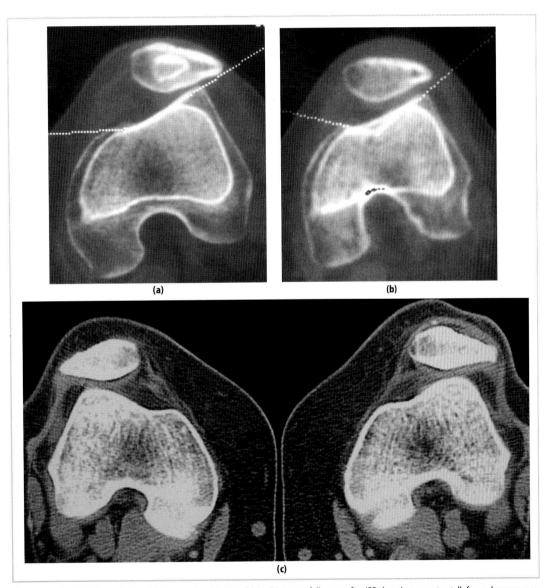

(a)

(b)

(c)

Figure 2.1. CT at 0° of knee flexion. **(a)** Preoperative CT: PFM. **(b)** At short-term follow-up after IPR there is a correct patellofemoral congruence. **(c)** At long-term follow-up (13 years after IPR) we can observe a bilateral asymptomatic PFM. (Part A is reproduced with permission from V Sanchis-Alfonso, E Roselló-Sastre, and V Martinez-SanJuan, Pathogenesis of anterior knee pain syndrome and functional patellofemoral instability in the active young: A review, *Am J Knee Surg* 1999; 12: 29–40.)

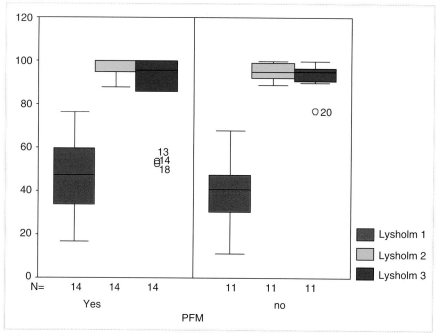

Figure 2.2. Lysholm scores of the patients with and without PFM. Lysholm 1 = Preoperative Lysholm score; Lysholm 2 = Lysholm score at medium-term follow-up; Lysholm 3 = Lysholm score at long-term follow-up.

marked osteophytes on the patella and femoral condyles with a narrow joint gap (12 years of follow-up, Lysholm score 91 points) (Figure 2.3); and one patient had marked osteophytes on the patella and femoral condyles without a narrow joint gap (6 years of follow-up, Lysholm score 96 points). In the last patient we found a severe

patellar chondropathy during surgery. In the three cases the contralateral asymptomatic knee had no osteoarthritic changes.

SEMG Analysis

We found in all the cases a normal voluntary activity pattern (grade IV according to the

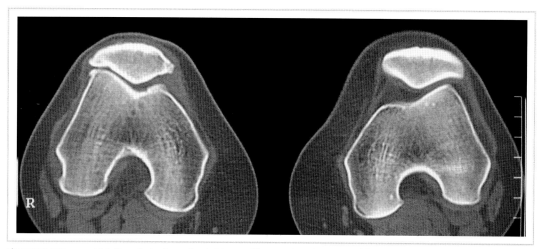

Figure 2.3. CT images at 0° of knee flexion from a female 36 years old operated on 12 years ago of the right knee with an Insall's proximal realignment. We can see osteophytes on the patella and femoral condyles with a visible narrowing of the patellofemoral joint gap (right knee). However, clinical result at 12-year follow-up was good. The left knee is asymptomatic despite the PFM.

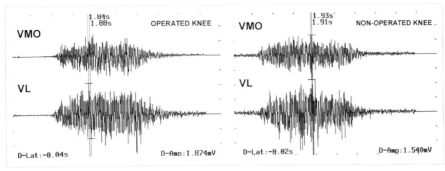

Figure 2.4. SEMG activity of the VMO of the operated knee and VMO of the contralateral asymptomatic nonoperated knee. SEMG activity of the VL of the operated knee and VL of the contralateral asymptomatic nonoperated knee.

classification of Buchthal[6]), in both VMO and VL (Figure 2.4). VMO amplitude of the operated knee averaged 1.30 ± 0.54. VMO amplitude of the nonoperated knee averaged 1.23 ± 0.53. We found no statistically significant differences between the amplitude of VMO of the operated knee, in comparison with the VMO of the contralateral asymptomatic knee (p = 0.506). VL amplitude of the operated knee averaged 1.27 ± 0.39. VL amplitude of the nonoperated knee averaged 1.41 ± 0.53. Neither have we found statistically significant differences between the amplitude of VL of the operated knee, in comparison with the VL of the contralateral asymptomatic knee (p = 0.189). The average VMO:VL ratio in the operated knee was 1.06 (range 0.51–1.96). The average VMO:VL ratio in the nonoperated knee was 0.9 (range 0.42–1.82). We found no statistically significant differences between the VMO:VL ratio of the operated knee, in com-

parison with the VMO:VL ratio of the contralateral asymptomatic knee (F [1,22] = 1.768; p = 0,1972) (Figure 2.5), although in the operated knee the muscle balance was better (Figure 2.6). We have found a linear correlation between the VMO and VL in the operated knee (Pearson's correlation coefficient = 0.592, p = 0.043). In contrast, we have not found a linear correlation between the VMO and VL in the nonoperated knee (Pearson's correlation coefficient = 0.550, p = 0.064).

Discussion

Patients with patellar symptoms can be divided into two groups: those with patellar instability and those with anterior knee pain. Instability has a clear biomechanical basis. In fact, over the past decade, attention began to be focused on the medial patellofemoral ligament (MPFL) as a restraint of lateral patellar translation, and the traditional approach of "realign" the quadriceps

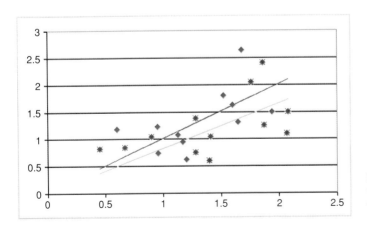

Figure 2.5. VMO:VL ratio of the operated knee (green [.1]line) vs. nonoperated knee (red line). Asterisk = nonoperated knee. Rhombus = operated knee.

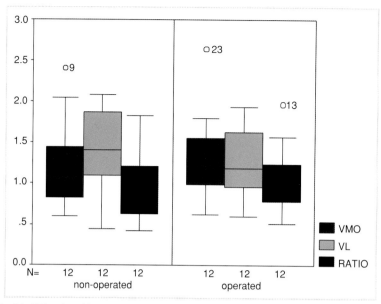

Figure 2.6. Amplitude of the VMO and VL of the operated knee and the contralateral asymptomatic nonoperated knee. VMO:VL ratio of the operated knee vs. nonoperated knee.

has been replaced by the reconstruction of the MPFL.[13] On the contrary, the causative mechanisms of patellar pain remain less well understood, in spite of its high prevalence. For many years, the PFM concept was widely accepted as an explanation for the genesis of anterior knee pain and patellar instability,[11,16,18,19,22,23,27] and influenced the way orthopedic surgeons evaluated and treated such patients. More recently, Scott Dye came up with the tissue homeostasis theory.[9] For this author, the loss of both osseous and soft tissue homeostasis is more important in the genesis of anterior knee pain than structural characteristics. In fact, patients with anterior knee pain often lack an easily identifiable structural abnormality to account for the symptoms.[9] Likewise, we have patients with no PFM who have recurrent patellar dislocations. Thus, the main objective of this paper is to reassess critically a concept from the 1970s, the PFM, based on our personal experience in IPR surgery.

The first goal of our study was to identify whether there is a relationship between the presence of PFM and the presence of anterior knee pain and/or patellar instability. A fact that could reflect the relationship between PFM and symptoms would be the diminishment or disappearance of symptoms with realignment surgery, as we have seen in a previous paper.[25] Moreover,

IPR, in our experience, provides a satisfactory centralization of the patella in the femoral trochlea, which is detected in postoperative CT scans performed between 3 and 6 months after surgical treatment.[25] Therefore, our satisfactory clinical results could be attributed to restoration of patellofemoral congruence. In this sense, Insall and colleagues[20] reported that nonsatisfactory results (by either persistent pain or instability) were related to the existence of postoperative residual malalignment, whereas if patellofemoral congruence was reestablished, the results were almost always good or excellent. In contrast, as shown by Wojtys and colleagues, there are authors who have failed to show objective improvements of malalignment after isolated lateral release, despite the fact that this procedure frequently lessens pain.[35]

Therefore, the resolution of pain or instability by realignment surgery, as we have seen in our series, does not necessarily mean that PFM caused theses symptoms. Some studies have implicated neural damage and hyperinnervation into the lateral retinaculum as a possible source of pain in this population.[15,26,29] In this way, we agree with Abraham and colleagues,[1] who suggested that pain relief after IPR may be attributed in part to denervation. Because the sensory innervation of the patella comes in large part from its superomedial aspect via branches of the saphenous nerve, some authors have postulated that operations on the medial side of the patella, such as IPR, work simply by further denervation of the patella.[16] Moreover, IPR would also eliminate the tensile forces that are produced in the retracted lateral retinaculum of patients with chronic lateral patellar subluxation during knee flexo-extension, which would stimulate free nerve endings; finally it would break the ischemia–hyperinnervation–pain circle.[14,29,30,31]

Interestingly, in the present study, we have found that the satisfactory centralization of the patella in the femoral trochlea, obtained at short-term follow-up,[25] is lost in the CT scans performed at long-term follow-up in almost 57% of the cases, and in spite of this, the vast majority of these patients presented satisfactory results at long-term. Therefore, we postulate that PFM could influence the tissue homeostasis negatively, and that realignment surgery could allow the restoring of joint homeostasis when nonoperative treatment of symptomatic PFM fails. Once we have achieved joint homeostasis, these PFM knees can exist happily within the envelope of function.

On the other hand, in our series, 12 patients presented with unilateral symptoms. In 9 of them the contralateral asymptomatic knee presented a PFM and only in 3 cases was there a satisfactory centralization of the patella into the femoral trochlea. That is, there is a poor relationship between malaligment and symptoms.

In conclusion, we have observed that not all PFM knees show symptoms. Moreover, we have found that there is no relation between the result of IPR (satisfactory vs. nonsatisfactory) and the presence or absence of PFM at long-term follow-up. Therefore, PFM is not a sufficient condition for the onset of symptoms. As a consequence of our findings, it is mandatory to reassess the concept of PFM in the genesis of anterior knee pain and patellar instability.

It has been stated that the VMO is responsible for patellar stability, but we have not found convincing evidence in the literature for this belief; and, as ligaments are the joint stabilizers, this premise would appear to be faulty. In theory, the VMO resists lateral patellar motion, either by active contraction or by passive muscle resistance. In this way, in Farahmand's study,[10] lateral patellar force-displacement behavior was not affected by simulated muscle forces at any flexion angle from 15 to 75°. Regarding resisting lateral patellar displacement, the orientation of the VMO varies greatly during knee flexion. The VMO's line of pull most efficiently resists lateral patellar motion when the knee is in deep flexion, at which time trochlear containment of the patella is independent of soft tissues influences.[3,10,17] The question is: How can we explain our satisfactory results with IPR regarding instability? It seems likely that operations that advance the VMO, such as IPR, include tightening of the underlying MPFL, and it would be responsible for the success of the surgical technique. In this sense, we must note that the VMO tendon becomes confluent with the MPFL in the region of patellar attachment.[12] Therefore, it would be more logical to protect the VMO and address the ligament deficiency surgically as needed.

Advancement of the VMO to increase passive stiffness would have unpredictable effects, because the long-term response of VMO muscle fibers to increased resting length is unknown. We have used SEMG to record muscle action potentials with skin surface electrodes. This is, to our knowledge, the first report specifically addressing long-term response of VMO muscle fibers to increased resting length. We have not found differences between the amplitude of VMO of the operated knee, in comparison with the VMO of the contralateral asymptomatic knee. Neither have we found differences between the amplitude of VL of the operated knee, in comparison with the VL of the contralateral asymptomatic knee. Moreover, we have found VMO:VL ratios within the limits of normality.[7] EMG relationship for each muscle could be problematic if the relationships demonstrate nonlinearity, but this was not the case in our patients. In this sense we have found a linear correlation between VMO and VL in the operated knee. Therefore, IPR does not provoke an imbalance in the patellofemoral joint. However, we must remember that SEMG VMO:VL activity of each knee of unilaterally symptomatic patients was similar to each other but different from that in knees of healthy subjects.[16] Finally, we found no deficit of the voluntary activity pattern of VMO. Therefore, we can conclude that advancement of VMO has no deleterious effects on VMO from the SEMG point of view.

Muscle activity results in compressive patellofemoral joint forces. It is possible that the generation of high joint reaction forces may be partially responsible for the arthrosis that can occur after realignment surgery.[4,8] Crosby and Insall have not found late osteoarthritis after soft-tissue corrections without movement of the tibial tubercle.[8] However, Zeichen and colleagues[36] have found patellofemoral osteoarthrosis in 36.8% of the patients at medium-term follow-up after IPR. We have found retropatellar arthrosis in only 3 knees (8%). Furthermore, clinical results are not comparable with degenerative changes presented at long-term follow-up.

Conclusions

This study is not intended to advocate for a particular surgical technique, but it does provide insight into improving our understanding of the pathophysiology of anterior knee pain syndrome. Our objectives were: to identify a relationship, or lack of one, between the presence of PFM and the presence of anterior knee pain and/or patellar instability; to analyze the long-term response of VMO muscle fibers to increased resting length; and to determine the incidence of patellofemoral arthrosis after IPR surgery. Our findings indicate (1) that not all PFM knees show symptoms; that is, PFM is not a sufficient condition for the onset of symptoms, at least in postoperative patients; (2) that the advancement of VMO has no deleterious effects on VMO; and (3) that IPR does not predispose to retropatellar arthrosis.

Acknowledgments

The authors gratefully acknowledge the invaluable assistance of Professor Jesús Basulto from the University of Sevilla, Spain, with the statistical analysis, and Paco Ferriz for his technical assistance in CT studies.

References

1. Abraham, E, E Washington, and TL Huang. Insall proximal realignment for disorders of the patella. *Clin Orthop* 1989; 248: 61–65.
2. Aglietti, P, R Buzzi, P De Biase et al. Surgical treatment of recurrent dislocation of the patella. *Clin Orthop* 1994; 308: 8–17.
3. Ahmed, AM, and NA Duncan. Correlation of patellar tracking pattern with trochlear and retropatellar surface topographies. *J Biomech Eng* 2000; 122: 652–660.
4. Arnbjornsson, A, N Egund, and O Rydling. The natural history of recurrent dislocation of the patella: Long-term results of conservative and operative treatment. *J Bone Joint Surg* 1992; 74-B: 140–142.
5. Barber-Westin, SD, FR Noyes, and JW McCloskey. Rigorous statistical reliability, validity and responsiveness testing of the Cincinnati knee rating system in 350 subjects with uninjured, injured, or anterior cruciate ligament-reconstructed knees. *Am J Sports Med* 1999; 27: 402–416.
6. Buchthal, F. *An Introduction to Electromyography*. Glydendal: Scandinavian University Books, 1957.
7. Cerny, K. Vastus medialis oblique/vastus lateralis muscle activity ratios for selected exercises in persons with and without patellofemoral pain syndrome. *Phys Ther* 1995; 75: 672–683.
8. Crosby, EB, and Insall. Recurrent dislocation of the patella: Relation of treatment to osteoarthritis. *J Bone Joint Surg* 1976; 58-A: 9–13.
9. Dye, SF, HU Staubli, RM Biedert et al. The mosaic of pathophysiology causing patellofemoral pain: Therapeutic implications. *Oper Tech Sports Med* 1999; 7: 46–54.
10. Farahmand, F, and MN Tahmasbi, and AA Amis. Lateral force-displacement behaviour of the human patella and its variation with knee flexion: A biomechanical study in vitro. *J Biomech* 1998; 31: 1147–1152.
11. Ficat, P, C Ficat, and A Bailleux. Syndrome d`hyperpression externe de la rotule (S.H.P.E.). *Rev Chir Orthop* 1975; 61: 39.
12. Fithian, DC, E Nomura, and E Arendt. Anatomy of patellar dislocation. *Oper Tech Sports Med* 2001; 9: 102–111.
13. Fithian, DC, EW Paxton, and AB Cohen. Indications in the treatment of patellar instability. *J Knee Surg* 2004; 17: 47–56.
14. Fulkerson, JP. The etiology of patellofemoral pain in young active patients: A prospective study. *Clin Orthop* 1983; 179: 129–133.
15. Fulkerson, JP, R Tennant, and JS Jaivin. Histologic evidence of retinacular nerve injury associated with patellofemoral malalignment. *Clin Orthop* 1985; 197: 196–205.
16. Grelsamer, RP, and J McConnell, eds. *The Patella: A Team Approach*. Gaithersburg, MD: Aspen, 1998.
17. Heegaard, J, PF Leyvraz, and A Van Kampen. Influence of soft structures on patellar three-dimensional tracking. *Clin Orthop* 1994; 299: 235–243.
18. Hughston, JC. Subluxation of the patella. *J Bone Joint Surg* 1968; 50-A: 1003–1026.
19. Insall, JN. "Chondromalacia Patellae": Patellar Malalignment Syndrome. *Orthop Clin North Am* 1979; 10: 117–127.
20. Insall, J, PG Bullough, and AH Burnstein. Proximal "tube" realignment of the patella for chondromalacia patellae. *Clin Orthop* 1979; 144: 63–69.
21. Lysholm, J, and J Gillquist. Evaluation of knee ligament surgery results with special emphasis on use of a scoring scale. *Am J Sports Med* 1982; 10: 150–154.
22. Merchant, AC, RL Mercer, and RH Jacobsen. Roentgenographic analysis of patellofemoral congruence. *J Bone Joint Surg* 1974; 56-A: 1391–1396.
23. Merchant, AC, and RL Mercer. Lateral release of the patella: A preliminary report. *Clin Orthop* 1974; 103: 40.
24. Merchant, AC. Radiography of the patellofemoral joint. *Oper Tech Sports Med* 1999; 7: 59–64.
25. Sanchis-Alfonso, V, E Gastaldi-Orquín, and V Martinez-SanJuan. Usefulness of computed tomography in evaluating the patellofemoral joint before and after Insall's realignment: Correlation with short-term clinical results. *Am J Knee Surg* 1994; 7: 65–72.
26. Sanchis-Alfonso, V, E Roselló-Sastre, C Monteagudo-Castro et al. Quantitative analysis of nerve changes in the lateral retinaculum in patients with isolated symp-

tomatic patellofemoral malalignment: A preliminary study. *Am J Sports Med* 1998; 26: 703–709.

27. Sanchis-Alfonso, V, E Roselló-Sastre, and V Martinez-SanJuan. Pathogenesis of anterior knee pain syndrome and functional patellofemoral instability in the active young: A review. *Am J Knee Surg* 1999; 12: 29–40.

28. Sanchis-Alfonso, V, and E Roselló-Sastre. Immuno-histochemical analysis for neural markers of the lateral retinaculum in patients with isolated symptomatic patellofemoral malalignment: A neuroanatomic basis for anterior knee pain in the active young patient. *Am J Sports Med* 2000; 28: 725–731.

29. Sanchis-Alfonso, V, E Roselló-Sastre, and F Revert. Neural growth factor expression in the lateral retinaculum in painful patellofemoral malalignment. *Acta Orthop Scand* 2001; 72: 146–149.

30. Sanchis-Alfonso, V, and E Roselló-Sastre. Anterior knee pain in the young patient: What causes the pain? "Neural model." *Acta Orthop Scand* 2003; 74: 697–703.

31. Sanchis-Alfonso, V, E Roselló-Sastre, F Revert et al. Histologic retinacular changes associated with ischemia in painful patellofemoral malalignment. *Orthopedics* 2005; 28: 593–599.

32. Schutzer, SF, GR Ramsby, and JP Fulkerson. The evaluation of patellofemoral pain using computerized tomography: A preliminary study. *Clin Orthop* 1986; 204: 286–293.

33. Scott, J, and EC Huskisson. Graphic representation of pain. *Pain* 1976; 2: 175–184.

34. Tegner, Y, and J Lysholm. Rating systems in the evaluation of knee ligament injuries. *Clin Orthop* 1985; 198: 43–49.

35. Wojtys, EM, DN Beaman, RA Glover et al. Innervation of the human knee joint by substance-P fibers. *Arthroscopy* 1990; 6: 254–263.

36. Zeichen, J, P Lobenhoffer, T Gerich et al. Medium-term results of the operative treatment of recurrent patellar dislocation by Insall proximal realignment. *Knee Surg Sports Traumatol Arthrosc* 1999; 7: 173–176.

3

Neuroanatomical Bases for Anterior Knee Pain in the Young Patient: "Neural Model"

Vicente Sanchis-Alfonso, Esther Roselló-Sastre, Juan Saus-Mas, and Fernando Revert-Ros

Introduction

Despite an abundance of clinical and basic science research, anterior knee pain syndrome remains, according to John Insall, an orthopedic enigma ("Black Hole of Orthopedics"). The numerous treatment regimes that exist for anterior knee pain highlights the lack of knowledge regarding the etiology of the pain. At present, no theory provides a comprehensive explanation of the true nature of this pathological condition or how to hasten its resolution in a safe and reliable way. This chapter synthesizes our research on anterior knee pain pathophysiology. Based on our studies, we have developed what we call the "Neural Model" as an explanation for the genesis of anterior knee pain in the young patient.[57] This topic is clinically relevant because patient management will be greatly simplified when we understand what is the cause for the anterior knee pain in the young patient.

We are fully aware that anterior knee pain cannot be imputed to one single factor, but rather a multiplicity of factors are involved. Peripheral neurological signals resulting in perceived pain can only come from innervated structures. Articular cartilage has no nerve endings. However, the infrapatellar fat pad, subchondral bone, the quadriceps tendon, the patellar ligament, the synovium, and the medial and lateral retinaculum all have a rich nerve supply, and each of these structures, individually or in combination, could be a potential source of nociceptive output resulting in the perception of pain at any given moment.[9,14,15,17,18,19,20,29,41,50,52,53,54,55,56,58,66,67] One way to shed some light on the etiology of pain is the histological study of these anatomical structures.

"Neural Model" in the Genesis of Anterior Knee Pain

Our studies on anterior knee pain pathophysiology have been focused on the lateral retinaculum retrieved during patellofemoral realignment surgery for "isolated symptomatic patellofemoral malalignment" (PFM) because there is clinical support to think that this anatomical structure plays a key role in the genesis of anterior knee pain in the young patient.[9,18,20,50,51,54,55,58,67] We define the term "isolated symptomatic PFM" as anterior knee pain or patellar instability, or both, with abnormalities of patellar tracking during physical examination verified with CT scans at 0° of knee flexion, but with no associated intra-articular abnormality demonstrated arthroscopically.[54] According to Fulkerson,[17] in patients with PFM there is an adaptative shortening of the lateral retinaculum as a consequence of the lateral displacement of the patella. With knee flexion, the patella migrates medially into the femoral trochlea,[49] which produces a recurrent stretching on the shortened lateral retinaculum that may cause nerve changes such as neuromas and neural myxoid degeneration.[17]

Morphologic Neural Changes into the Lateral Retinaculum

Some studies have implicated neural damage into the lateral retinaculum as a possible source of pain in the young patient. In 1985, Fulkerson and colleagues[18] described nerve damage (demyelination and fibrosis) in the lateral retinaculum of patients with intractable patellofemoral pain requiring lateral retinacular release or realignment of the patellofemoral joint. The changes observed by these authors in the retinacular nerves resembled the histopathologic picture of Morton's interdigital neuroma. Later, in 1991, Mori and colleagues[41] published a paper in which they analyzed histologically the lateral retinaculum of 35 knees of 22 patients suffering from anterior knee pain. They found severe degenerative neuropathy in 9 knees, moderate change in 9, and slight in 11; the remaining 6 knees were normal. Like these authors, we[50,58] have also observed in many cases, into the lateral retinaculum, chronic degenerative nonspecific changes in nerve fibers, with myxoid degeneration of the endoneurium, retraction of the axonal compo-

nent, and perineural fibrosis (Figure 3.1). Likewise, a smaller group of specimens presented nerve fibers mimicking amputation neuromas seen in other parts of the body[50,58] (Figure 3.1). However, we have found no inflammatory component associated with vascular or nerve structures that could explain the presence of pain in these patients, except for a population of mast cells immersed in the fibrous bands surrounding vessels (Figure 3.2). Regarding neuromas, we have seen a clear relationship between their presence and anterior knee pain.[50,54,58] In contrast, we have found no relationship between neural myxoid degeneration and anterior knee pain.[50,54]

Nerve damage occurs diffusely in the affected retinaculum, and therefore one must consider the possibility of multiple neurological sequelae in the peripatellar region, including altered proprioceptive innervation.[18] This is in agreement with the clinical study of Jerosch and Prymka in 1996,[28] which revealed a highly significant reduction in knee proprioception after patella dislocation, explained by the damage of neuro-proprioceptive fibers.[28,65] Current research

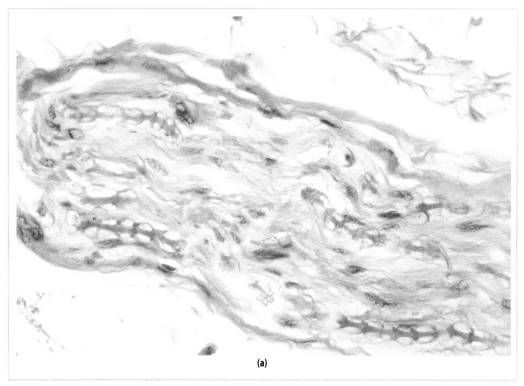

(a)

Figure 3.1. Histological features of a normal nerve. **(a)** a nerve with neural myxoid degeneration

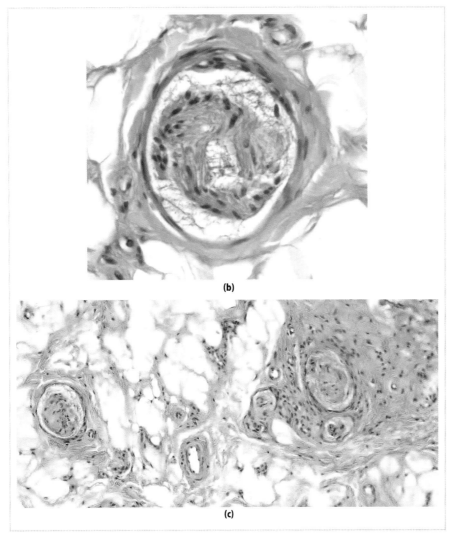

Figure 3.1. *(continued)* **(b)**, and a tissular neuroma **(c)** in the lateral retinaculum. (Hematoxylin-Eosin stain.) (Parts B and C are reproduced with permission from Sanchis-Alfonso, V, E Roselló-Sastre, C Monteagudo-Castro et al., Quantitative analysis of nerve changes in the lateral retinaculum in patients with isolated symptomatic patellofemoral malalignment: A preliminary study. *Am J Sports Med* 1998; 26: 703–709.)

shows the importance of proprioceptive information from joint mechanoreceptors for proper knee function. Connective tissues, in addition to their mechanical function, play an important role in transmitting specific somatosensory afferent signals to the spinal and cerebral regulatory systems. Thus, the giving-way in patients with patellofemoral pain can be explained, at least in part, because of the alteration or loss of joint afferent information concerning proprioception due to the nerve damage of ascendant proprioception pathway or decrease of healthy nerve fibers capable of transmitting proprioceptory stimuli.[50] In conclusion, it seems likely that, to a certain degree, the instability depends not only on mechanical factors (such as overuse, quadriceps angle increase, patella alta, soft tissue dysplasia, and patellar and trochlear dysplasia) but also on neural factors (proprioceptive deficit both in the sense of position and in slowing or diminution of stabilizing and protective reflexes).[19,21,28,65]

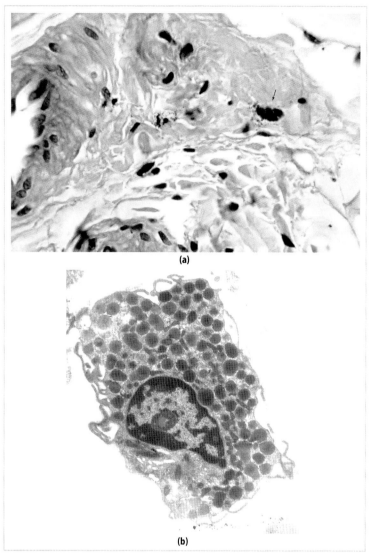

Figure 3.2. Mast cells are abundant in the stroma (arrow), mainly in a perivascular disposition. Some of them show a degranulation process (activated mast cells) **(a)**. (Giemsa stain.) Ultrastructural image of a mast cell of the lateral retinaculum with its cytoplasm full of chemotactic granules, (TEM) **(b)**. (Part A is reproduced with permission from Sanchis-Alfonso, V, and E Roselló-Sastre, Immunohistochemical analysis for neural markers of the lateral retinaculum in patients with isolated symptomatic patellofemoral malalignment: A neuroanatomic basis for anterior knee pain in the active young patient. *Am J Sports Med* 2000; 28: 725–731.)

Relationship Between Hyperinnervation into the Lateral Retinaculum and Anterior Knee Pain: Immunohistochemical Analysis for Neural Markers

Our studies have implicated hyperinnervation into the lateral retinaculum as a possible source of anterior knee pain in the young patient.[50,58] Thus, we found an increase in the number of nerves in the lateral retinaculum of patients with painful PFM, there being higher values in those with severe pain compared with those with moderate or light pain.[58] Moreover, we have seen that the lateral retinaculum of the patients with pain as the predominant symptom showed a higher innervation pattern than the medial retinaculum or the lateral retinaculum of patients with patellar instability.[54] This nerve ingrowth consisted of myelinated (specifically immunoreactive to S-100 protein) and unmyelinated nerve fibers (specifically immunoreactive to neurofilament protein [NF]) (Figure 3.3) with a predominant nociceptive component.[54]

The nociceptive properties of at least some of these nerves are evidenced by their substance P (SP) immunoreactivity. SP, which is found in primary sensory neurons and C fibers (slow-chronic pain pathway), is involved in the neurotransmission pathways of nociceptive signals.[3,5,6,7,12,16,23,31,32,33,45,67] SP was detected in the axons of big nerve fibers, in free nerve endings, and in the vessel walls in some patients with pain as predominant symptom[54] (Figure 3.4). Nociceptive fibers, that is, neural fibers with intra-axonal SP, were in a lower number than NF fibers, indicating that not all the tiny perivascular or interstitial nerves were nociceptive.[54]

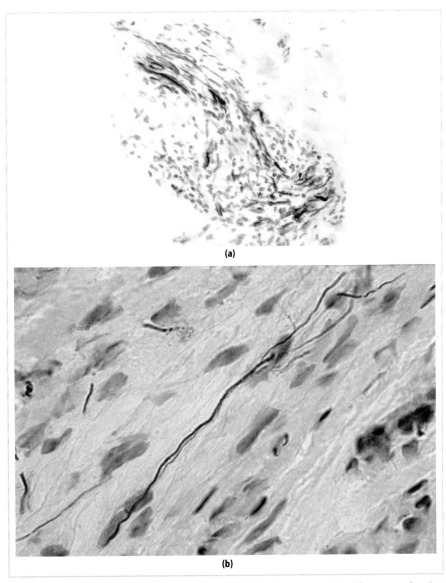

(a)

(b)

Figure 3.3. An increased innervation is evident in the connective tissue, showing microneuromas **(a)** and free nerve endings immersed in the stroma **(b)**

(continued)

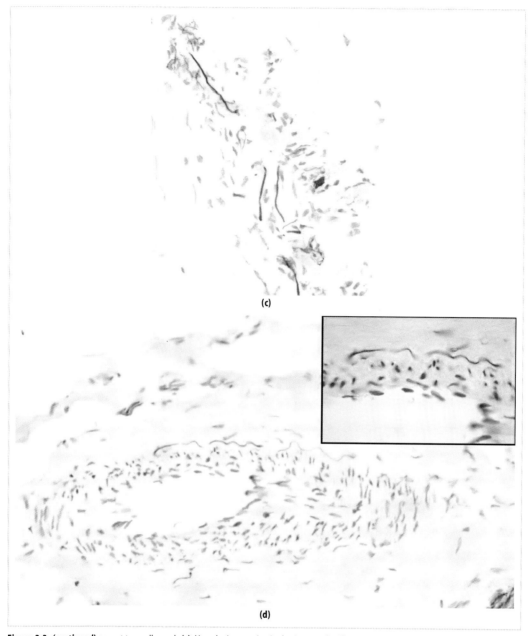

Figure 3.3. *(continued)* or next to small vessels **(c)**. Vascular innervation is also increased with tiny axons arranged like a necklace in the adventitia **(d)**. (Immunohistochemistry for Neurofilaments. Frozen sections.) (Reproduced with permission from Sanchis-Alfonso, V, and E Roselló-Sastre, Immunohistochemical analysis for neural markers of the lateral retinaculum in patients with isolated symptomatic patellofemoral malalignment: A neuroanatomic basis for anterior knee pain in the active young patient. *Am J Sports Med* 2000; 28: 725–731.)

Interestingly, our finding that SP-fibers were more abundant in the lateral retinaculum than in its medial counterpart reinforce the role of the lateral retinaculum as a main source of pain in these patients.[54] Moreover, we have observed that the number of these nociceptive fibers was higher in PFM patients suffering from pain as main symptom than in those with instability as predominant symptom (with little or no pain between instability episodes).[54]

Nerve ingrowth is mostly located within and around vessels[50,54,58] (Figure 3.5). Thus, we have seen, into the lateral retinaculum of patients with painful PFM, S-100 positive fibers in the adventitial and within the muscular layer of medium and small arteries, resembling a necklace. S-100 protein is a good marker when studying nerves, because of its ability to identify Schwann cells that accompany the axons in their myelinated part. It is well known that myelinated fibers lose their myelin sheath before entering into the muscular arterial wall, but this was not the case in our patients. Since we were studying by S-100 immunostaining only the myelinated fibers, and the myelin sheath is supposed to be lost before the nerve enters the muscular arterial wall, we were surprised by the identification of S-100-positive fibers within the muscular layer of

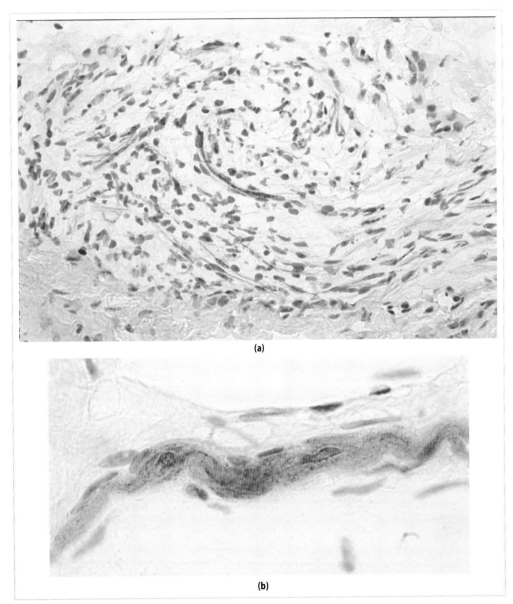

(a)

(b)

Figure 3.4. Neuromas are rich in nociceptive axons, as can be demonstrated studying substance P **(a)**. Substance P is present in the axons of the nerves and in the free nerve endings with a granular pattern **(b)**, and

(continued)

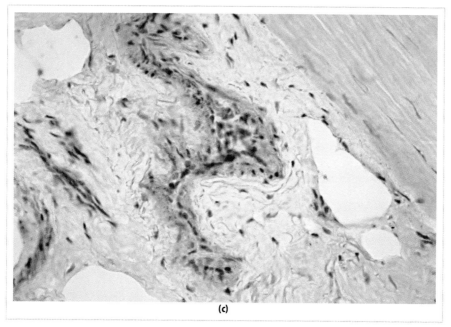

(c)

Figure 3.4. *(continued)* can be observed in the vessel walls in some patients with a painful clinic **(c)**. (Immunohistochemistry for Substance P. Frozen sections.) (Parts A and B are reproduced with permission from Sanchis-Alfonso, V, and E Roselló-Sastre, Immunohistochemical analysis for neural markers of the lateral retinaculum in patients with isolated symptomatic patellofemoral malalignment: A neuroanatomic basis for anterior knee pain in the active young patient. *Am J Sports Med* 2000; 28: 725–731.)

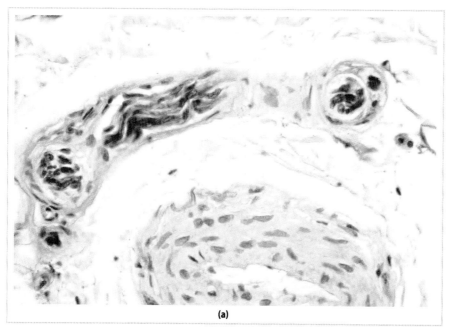

(a)

Figure 3.5. An increase in periadventitial innervation is detectable in our patients expressed as a rich vascular network made up of tiny myelinated fibers that, from the arterial adventitia, enter into the outer muscular layer, conforming a necklace **(a & b)**. Transversal section **(c)** and

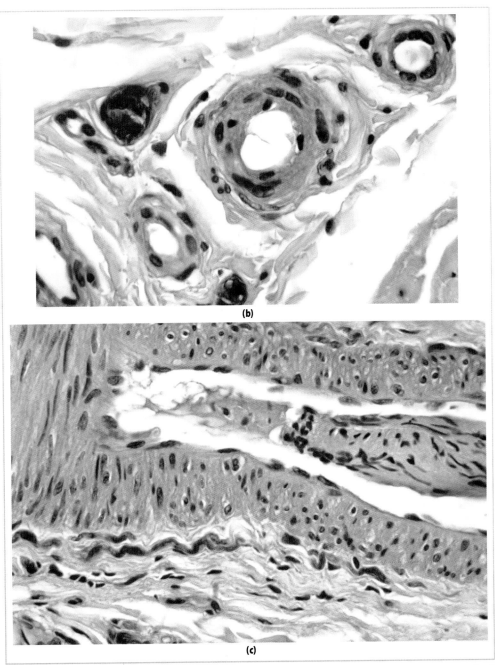

(b)

(c)

(continued)

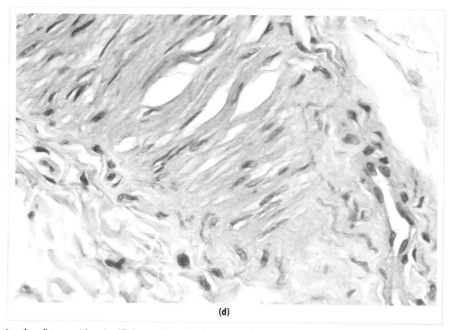

(d)

Figure 3.5. *(continued)* tangential section **(d)**. (Immunohistochemistry for protein S-100.) (Reproduced with permission from Sanchis-Alfonso, V, E Roselló-Sastre, C Monteagudo-Castro et al., Quantitative analysis of nerve changes in the lateral retinaculum in patients with isolated symptomatic patellofemoral malalignment: A preliminary study. *Am J Sports Med* 1998; 26: 703–709.)

medium and small arteries. Therefore, our findings may be considered as an increase in vascular innervation. We have demonstrated that vascular innervation was more prominent (94%) in patients with severe pain, whereas we found this type of hyperinnervation in only 30% of the patients with light or moderate pain.[58] Our findings are in agreement with the statement of Byers, who postulated in 1968 that the mechanism of pain in the osteoid osteoma could be generated and transmitted by vascular pressure-sensitive autonomic nerves.[10]

In reviewing the literature, we have seen that hyperinnervation is also a factor implicated in the pathophysiology of pain in other orthopedic abnormalities such as chronic back pain and jumper's knee.[12,16,52] On the other hand, pain has also been related with vascular innervation in some pathologies as is the case in osteoid osteoma,[24] where the authors found an increase in perivascular innervation in all their cases, postulating that pain was more related with this innervation than with the release of prostaglandin E2. Grönblad and colleagues[22] have also found similar findings in the lumbar pain of the facet syndrome. Finally, Alfredson and colleagues[4] related pain in Achilles tendinosis with vasculo-neural ingrowth.

We have demonstrated that hyperinnervation is associated with the release of neural growth factor (NGF), a polypeptide that stimulates axonogenesis.[55] NGF adopted a granular pattern in the cytoplasm of Schwann cells of the thick nerve fibers and in the muscular wall of the arterial vessels and the amount of staining for this neurotrophin was related with increased perivascular innervation[54] (Figure 3.6). NGF has two biologically active precursors: a long form of approximately 34 kD of molecular weight and a short form of 27 kD.[13] We have found in the lateral retinaculum of patients with painful PFM the 34 kD precursor. The fact that some of the nerve fibers of the lateral retinaculum express NGF means that these nerve fibers must still be in a proliferative phase.[54] As expected, we found that NGF is higher in patients with pain that in those with instability as the main symptom[55] (Figure 3.7). Gigante and colleagues[20] have also found NGF and TrkA expression into the lateral retinaculum of patients with PFM, but not in patients with jumper's knee or meniscal tears. TrkA (the NGF receptor) plays a crucial role in pain sensation.

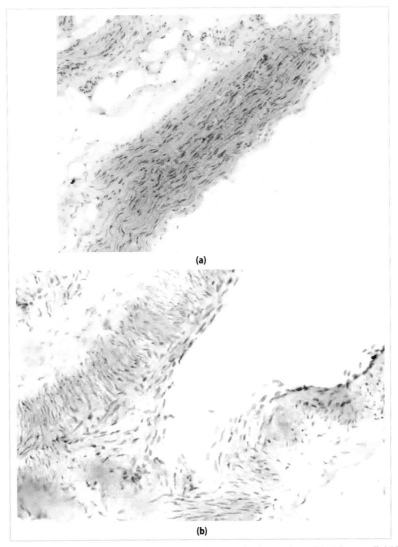

Figure 3.6. NGF is present in thick nerves into the axons in a granular distribution and in the cytoplasm of the Schwann cells **(a)** but is also detected in the vessel wall, after its release by the nerves **(b)**. (Immunohistochemistry for NGF. Frozen sections.) (Reproduced with permission from Sanchis-Alfonso, V, E Roselló-Sastre, and F Revert, Neural growth factor expression in the lateral retinaculum in painful patellofemoral malalignment. *Acta Orthop Scand* 2001; 72: 146–149.)

However, NGF is related not only to neural proliferation in vessels and perivascular tissue but also to the release of neuroceptive transmitters, such as substance P.[37] We postulate that both mechanisms are involved in the pathogenesis of pain in isolated symptomatic PFM. Thus, we suggest that two pathobiological mechanisms may lead to symptomatic PFM: (1) pain as the main symptom, with detectable levels of NGF that cause hyperinnervation and stimulus of SP release, and (2) instability as the predominant symptom, with lower levels of local NGF release,

less neural proliferation, and less nociceptive stimulus.[55] This means that there must be other factors acting on a PFM to conduct it versus pain or instability as the main symptom. In other words, symptoms appear to be related to multiple factors with variable clinical expression, and our imperfect understanding of these factors may explain the all-too-frequent failure to achieve adequate symptom relief with the use of realignment procedures. The question is: Which are the mechanisms that stimulate NGF release in these patients? We hypothesize that periodic

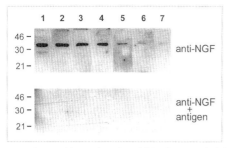

Figure 3.7. Immunoblotting detection of NGF, showing a thick band located at the level of NGF precursor in patients with pain (cases 1 to 4) and absence or a very thin band in the patients with instability as the main symptom (cases 5 to 7). The numbers at the left indicate molecular mass in kD. (Reproduced with permission from Sanchis-Alfonso, V, E Roselló-Sastre, and F Revert, Neural growth factor expression in the lateral retinaculum in painful patellofemoral malalignment. *Acta Orthop Scand* 2001; 72: 146–149.)

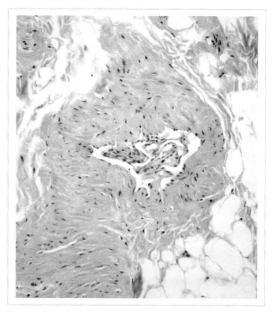

Figure 3.8. Arterial vessel in the retinacular tissue can show a prominent and irregular endothelium and thick muscular walls or even an irregular reduction of the vascular lumen. (Hematoxylin-Eosin stain.)

short episodes of ischemia could be the primary mechanism of NGF release, hyperinnervation, and therefore could be implicated in pain, in most of the cases of young patients with anterior knee pain syndrome.[51]

Role of Hypoxia in the Genesis of Anterior Knee Pain

According to some authors NGF synthesis can be induced by ischemia.[1,35,68] Moreover, it has been shown that NGF stimulates neural sprouting and hastens neural proliferation in vessel walls,[26,30] and it is just this pattern of hyperinnervation that is seen in the lateral retinaculum of patients with painful PFM.[50,54,58] Similar changes have been studied in animal models and are present in the coronary innervation of patients with myocardial infarcts and brain ischemia.[1,30,35] Thus, we hypothesize that short episodes of tissular ischemia, due to a mechanism of vascular torsion or vascular bending, may be the main problem in painful PFM.[51,54,55,58] Vascular bending could be induced mechanically by medial traction over the retracted lateral retinaculum, due to PFM, with knee flexion.

Although vascular bending has not yet experimentally been proved in animal models, we have demonstrated histological retinacular changes associated with hypoxia in painful PFM.[58] In this way, we find lesions that can lead to tissular anoxia such as arterial vessels with obliterated lumina and thick muscular walls (Figure 3.8),[51,58] and in addition we find other lesions that are a consequence of ischemia such as infarcted foci of the connective tissue

(Figure 3.9), myxoid stromal degeneration (Figure 3.10), and ultrastructural findings related with anoxia (degenerated fibroblasts with autophagic intracytoplasmic vacuoles [Figure 3.11], endothelial cells with reduplication of the basal lamina, young vessels with endothelial cells containing active nuclei and conspicuous nucleoli, and neural sprouting[34,48,51,58,61] [Figure 3.12]). In Figure 3.12C we can see the phenomenon of neural sprouting: After axonal damage has been established due to ischemia, the distal end of the axon degenerates and subsequent regeneration occurs in the swollen end of the proximal axon. The neuronal body is able to produce new microtubules and microfilaments that arrive at the swollen end of the proximal axon and induce neural sprouting. Schwann cells try to surround and engulf the new axons, giving a typical image of neural regeneration. We ought to bear in mind that, at the experimental level, it has been found that neural sprouting finishes when NGF infusion ends.[26]

Another phenomenon related with ischemia is angiogenesis, given that chronic ischemia leads to VEGF-release, inducing hypervascularization in order to satisfy the needs of the tissue.[60] We have performed a quantitative analysis of vascularization into the lateral retinaculum

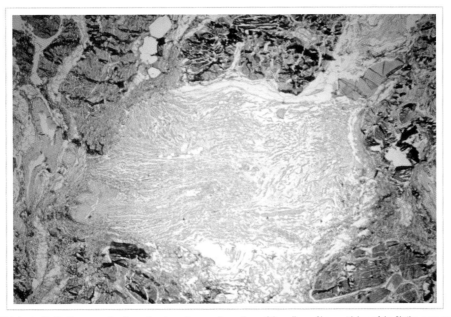

Figure 3.9. Infarcted foci in the connective tissue showing a degenerative pattern of the collagen fibers, with loss of the fibrilar component and accumulation of myxoid material in the interstitium. (Masson's Trichrome stain.) (Reproduced with permission from Sanchis-Alfonso, V, and E Roselló-Sastre, Proliferación neural e isquemia. *Rev Patol Rodilla* 1998; 3: 60–63.)

excised at the time of surgical patellofemoral realignments using a panvascular marker, anti-Factor VIII-related antigen.[58] Factor VIII is one of the three functional components of the antihemophilic factor and is synthesized by endothelial cells of blood vessels; hence it is considered as a specific marker for endothelial cells.[42] Thus, we found an increase in the number of vessels in the lateral retinaculum of patients with painful PFM, there being higher values in the severe pain group compared with those of moderate or light pain.[58] Moreover, as expected, we found a positive linear correlation between number of vessels and number of nerves.[58]

Tissular ischemia induces vascular endothelial growth factor (VEGF) release by fibroblasts, synovial cells, mast cells, or even endothelial cells.[36,40,43,69] Following these principles, we performed a study of VEGF expression into the lateral retinaculum of patients with PFM by immunohistochemistry and immunoblot.[58] VEGF is a potent hypoxia-inducible angiogenic factor that causes hypervascularization.[8,25,27,36,38,40,47,60,64] VEGF release begins 8 hours after hypoxia and the peptide disappears in 24 hours if the ischemic crisis is over.[25] Therefore, VEGF positivity reflects

that, at this moment, we face an ischemic process, or better said, we are between 8 and 24 hours from the onset of the transitory ischemic episode. However, given the fact that the average life of VEGF is very short, its negativity has no significance regarding the presence or absence of a transitory ischemic process.

Although this process has been well documented in joints affected by rheumatoid arthritis and osteoarthritis,[8,27,43,46,69] it has never been documented in PFM until our study.[58] In our series, VEGF production was seen in stromal fibroblasts, vessel walls, certain endothelial cells, and even nerve fibers, as much in axons as in perineurium[58] (Figure 3.13). We complemented immunohistochemistry to identify and locate VEGF with immunoblotting so as to detect even minimal expression of VEGF. Our immunohistochemical findings were confirmed by immunoblot analysis. VEGF levels were higher in patients with severe pain than in those with light-to-moderate pain, whereas the protein was barely detectable in two cases with light pain[58] (Figure 3.14). VEGF expression is absent in normal joints[27] although inflammatory processes can stimulate its release.[8,27,46] In such cases, synovial hypoxia secondary to articular

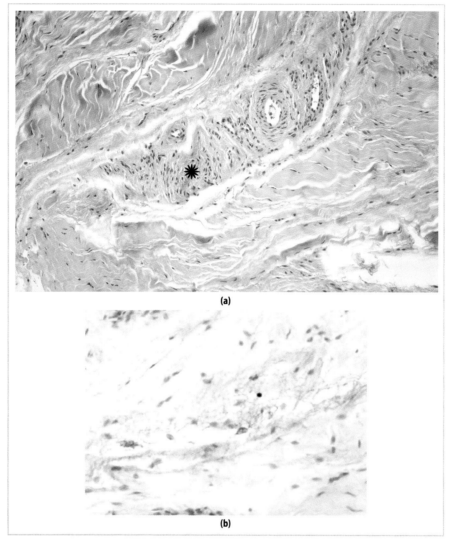

Figure 3.10. A focus of myxoid stromal degeneration (asterisk) in the middle of the fibrous retinacular tissue is seen next to a "hot vascular spot" **(a)**. Detail from the myxoid material (asterisk) **(b)**. (Hematoxylin-Eosin stain.)

inflammation is supposed to trigger VEGF production.[27] However, we have not observed inflammatory changes into the lateral retinaculum in our cases. Furthermore, it has been reported that peripheral nervous system hypoxia can simultaneously trigger VEGF and NGF synthesis via neurons[11] inflammatory or stromal cells.[1,35,68] VEGF induces hypervascularization and NGF induces hyperinnervation. Both facts have been observed in our cases.[58]

Limitations of Our Studies: In Criticism of Our Results

We are fully aware of the limitations of our histological studies. First, the number of lateral retinaculae samples is small, given that only a few patients undergo surgery. Second we do not have a genuine normal control group because biopsy to obtain samples of normal lateral retinaculum in live age-matched healthy persons is not possible for ethical reasons. In our first paper we used

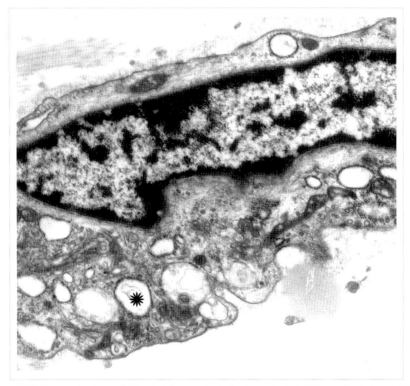

Figure 3.11. Degenerative changes in fibroblasts (increased autophagic vacuoles [asterisk]) secondary to hypoxia (TEM).

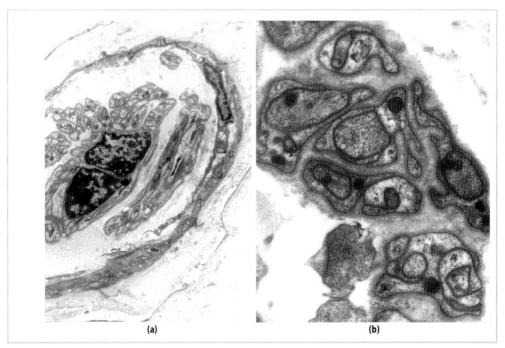

(a)   (b)

Figure 3.12. Neural sprouting is detected ultrastructurally as a bunch of tiny axons immersed in the Schwann cell cytoplasm **(a)**. Detail **(b)**.

(*continued*)

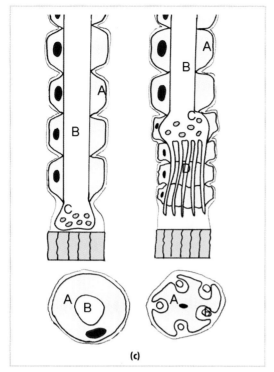

Figure 3.12. *(continued)* Comparative image with the scheme of a normal nerve ending (left) and damaged nerve ending with neural sprouting (right) **(c)**. A: Schwann cell, B: Axon, C: End bulb, and D: New axon sprouts.

as control group the lateral retinaculum of a newborn infant who died of hyaline membrane disease.[50] In the next study we used the lateral retinaculum of patients operated on for jumper's knee or meniscal tears, and the medial retinaculum of patients with symptomatic PFM.[54] In our last papers the study group consisted of patients with pain as the predominant symptom (given that the objective of theses reports was the study of the etiology of pain), and patients with instability as the primary symptom with low or no pain between instability episodes comprised the control group,[55,58] and we used the visual analog scale to report the severity of pain. Third, a further potential problem is the difficulty in quantifying the pain, given its subjectivity. However, we believe that using previously validated pain reporting techniques is appropriate. Finally, we have not yet designed an idoneous experimental model to prove our hypothesis.

Histological Findings in Chronic Tendinopathy: In Defense of Our Results

Our histological results are in agreement with those of Messner and colleagues[39] in experimen-

tally induced Achilles tendinosis. Their histo-logical evaluation of tendinosis showed hyperinnervation, hypervascularization, and increased immunoreactivity for substance P. In addition, Alfredson and colleagues[4] found vasculo-neural ingrowth in the structurally changed part of the chronic painful Achilles tendinosis tendons that possibly can explain the pain suffered for these patients. Thus, in our experience we[52] found neovascularization and hyperinnervation with nerve fibers ingrowth showing a histological pattern of neural sprouting, with vascular hyperinnervation and stromal neuromatous changes in chronic patellar tendinosis. We must remember that Achilles tendinosis and patellar tendinosis are a consequence of repetitive overloading of the tendon, that is to say microtraumas, and related to activity duration and intensity, a mechanism similar to symptomatic PFM. Therefore, the results of these studies lend credence to the validity of our histological results.

Authors' Proposed Anterior Knee Pain Pathophysiology

We hypothesize that short and repetitive episodes of tissular ischemia, due maybe to a mechanism of vascular torsion or vascular bending, which could be induced by a medial traction over a retracted lateral retinaculum, could trigger release of NGF and VEGF on PFM. Once NGF is present in the tissues, it induces hyperinnervation, attraction of mastocytes, and substance P release by free nerve endings.[37] In addition, VEGF induces hypervascularization and plays a role increasing neural proliferation.

Free nerve endings are slowly adapting receptors that mediate nociception. These receptors are activated in response to deformation of tissues resulting from abnormal tensile and compressive forces generated during flexo-extension of the knee, or in response to the stimulus of chemical agents such as histamine, bradykinin, prostaglandins, and leukotrienes.[31,62,63] Therefore, SP is released from peripheral endings of nociceptive afferents as a result of noxious chemical or mechanical stimulation. The nociceptive information relayed by these free nerve endings is responsible, at least in part, for the anterior knee pain.

Once SP is liberated on the connective tissue, the neuropeptide induces as well the release of prostaglandin E2, one of the biochemical agents known to stimulate nociceptors.[3] The activation of nociceptive pathways by prostaglandins

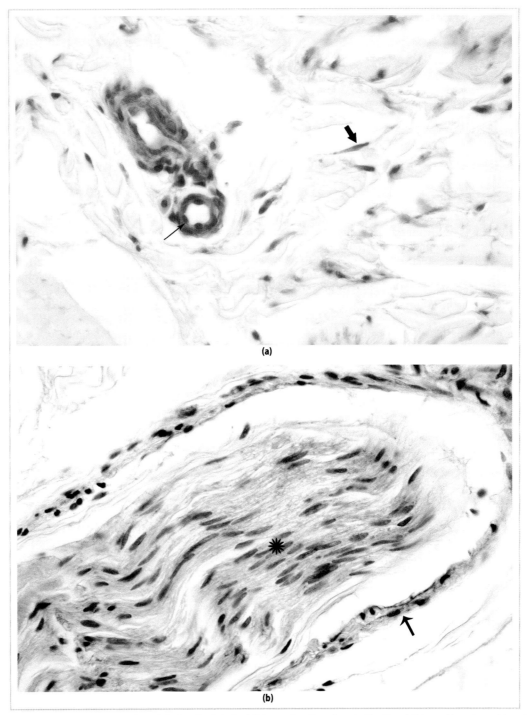

(a)

(b)

Figure 3.13. VEGF is present in small vessels (wall and endothelium) (thin arrow) and in perivascular fibroblasts (thick arrow) in patients with moderate-severe pain **(a)**. Some cases have VEGF expression even in the perineural shift (thin arrow) and inside the axons (asterisk) **(b)**. (Immunohistochemistry for VEGF.)

the jump follows a previous run.[38] As jumping is a repetitive gesture, it is understandable how damaging it can become for the player's knee. For instance, a player of the NBA is supposed to jump at least 70 times per match.[39] The heavy weight and great height of the basketball players are additionally negative factors. On the other hand, during running the impact forces against the ground reach 2 to 3 times the body weight.[9] This has a cumulative effect along the training and competition periods, without forgetting the sport practice by adolescents in physical education classes, which on its own or associated to other predisposing factors, can cause the onset of the symptoms. These sportive movements are inevitable and form part of the sport itself, but they can be mitigated.

Importance of Footwear, Ground Surface, and Personal Technique in the Origin and Prevention of the Lesions

The human body has some natural systems of shock absorption to protect itself from the effect derived from jumping and running: soft heel tissue, pronation of the hindfoot, ankle dorsiflexion, flexion of the knee, menisci, articular cartilage, and flexion of the hip.[8,35] As pointed out by Gross and Nelson,[21] the series of articular movements on landing from a vertical jump starts with the distal joints to end in the proximal ones (metatarsophalangeal, midtarsal, subtalar, ankle, knee, and hip joints). The knee and the hip have a first-rate role in the process of shock absorption after a jump, whereas the foot pronation (subtalar joint) is the main shock absorber when running.[35] However, this knee flexion, with a positive effect as shock absorber, shows a negative effect also as it increases the PFJR force, as will be seen in the next section. On the other hand, the total strength of the impact suffered by the organism depends not only on the applied force, but also on the time that force is being applied. It is considered a good technique of dissipation or absorption of the impact when the force is distributed along a certain time. Shock absorption can be incremented by using these natural mechanisms (i.e., good sport technique, speed of the fall) or using external materials (i.e., appropriate footwear and adequate playing surface). In this way, prevention of the lesions related to overuse or diminution of the negative impact on the knee of certain

inevitable stresses like running and jumping is probably possible.

Footwear can contribute to reducing the reaction force after impact in three fundamental ways: (1) increasing the natural shock-absorbing mechanisms (appropriate heel insole to increase heel fat shock-absorbing role and a strong heel stiffener to prevent hyperpronation), (2) supplementing the aforesaid mechanisms (good-quality sole materials, air chambers, and insoles), and (3) avoiding limiting the natural shock-absorbing mechanisms like heel dorsiflexion (boot-type footwear increases the charges transmitted to the muscular skeletal system by limiting ankle mobility, as opposed to the shoe-type footwear). Overlooking these norms in sport footwear will increase the impact stresses when jumping and running and therefore it will produce an overload of the knee and will favor the development of overload chronic lesions. Having the ankle supported (boot-type footwear) diminishes the efficiency when running and swivelling, very frequent gestures in handball, and so this type of footwear is not advised for this sport.[46] Finally, having the sole empty at mid-foot level would allow a certain independence of movement between the fore and the hindfoot, diminishing shoe rigidity. This would favor the mobility of the midtarsal joint (natural shock-absorbing system).

Excessive adherence of shoe to playing surface is another lesion-producing factor. On the other hand, lack of this adherence can, as well, be the cause of lesions. In handball, for instance, it is necessary to have a good adherence between shoe and court as there are frequent changes in direction and breaking movements in this sport.[46] When practiced in a pavilion, sports shoes with "caramel soles," called thus because of their aspect, are used. These soles have a great parquet adherence; this increases the performance, but they are not advisable because this adherence can provoke a knee lesion. It has been said that a pattern under the head of the first metatarsal should be added to the specific sole pattern to facilitate the turn over this zone, diminishing the overload on the knee joint, and in this way counteracting the adherence of the sole to the playing surface. An excessive adherence can provoke lesions. For instance, rhythmic gymnastics on a mat should be practiced barefooted or with slippers, as normal sports shoes could provoke a severe knee lesion due to (a type of nociceptor),[31] and would break the ischemia–hyperinnervation–pain circle.

We suggest proprioceptive neuromuscular training as a beneficial aspect of rehabilitation programs following realignment knee surgery to improve function and knee proprioception and therefore decrease the risk of reinjury. Moreover, the fact that the instability is due in part to proprioceptive deficit may explain that McConnell taping or bracing can considerably improve stability, in spite of their doubtful biomechanical efficacy by increasing proprioceptive feedback.

Future Directions

If the "neural model" of anterior knee pain proves to have a certain validity, it would lead in many cases to therapeutic recommendations to alleviate pain more effectively and safely than the attempts to correct "malalignment." Thus, a selective pharmaceutical approach (e.g., drug inhibitors of synthesis and release of SP, such as capsaicin, or SP receptor antagonists) could be of special interest in the treatment of pain in these patients, in combination or as an alternative to surgery. Finally, if we demonstrate that regional anoxia plays a key role in the genesis of pain, topical periferic vasorelaxant drugs (for preventing vasospasm) could also be of special interest in the treatment of pain in these patients.

Conclusions

The observations reported here provide a neuroanatomic basis for anterior knee pain syndrome in the young patient and support the clinical observation that the lateral retinaculum may have a key role in the origin of this pain. Our findings, however, do not preclude the possibility of pain arising in other anatomical structures.

We hypothesize that periodic short episodes of ischemia could be implicated in the pathogenesis of anterior knee pain by triggering neural proliferation of nociceptive axons (SP positive nerves), mainly in a perivascular location. Moreover, we believe that instability in patients with anterior knee pain syndrome can be explained, at least in part, because of the damage of nerves of the lateral retinaculum that can be related with proprioception.

References

1. Abe, T, DA Morgan, and DD Gutterman. Protective role of nerve growth factor against postischemic dysfunction of sympathetic coronary innervation. *Circulation* 1997; 95: 213–220.

2. Abraham, E, E Washington, and TL Huang. Insall proximal realignment for disorders of the patella. *Clin Orthop* 1989; 248: 61–65.

3. Ahmed, M, J Bergstrom, H Lundblad et al. Sensory nerves in the interface membrane of aseptic loose hip prostheses. *J Bone Joint Surg* 1998; 80-B: 151–155.

4. Alfredson, H, L Ohberg, and S Forsgren. Is vasculo-neural ingrowth the cause of pain in chronic Achilles tendinosis? An investigation using ultrasonography and colour Doppler, immunohistochemistry, and diagnostic injections. *Knee Surg Sports Traumatol Arthrosc* 2003; 11: 334–338.

5. Ashton, IK, BA Ashton, SJ Gibson et al. Morphological basis for back pain: the demonstration of nerve fibers and neuropeptides in the lumbar facet joint capsule but not in ligamentum flavum. *J Orthop Res* 1992; 10: 72–78.

6. Ashton, IK, S Roberts, and DC Jaffray. Neuropeptides in the human intervertebral disc. *J Orthop Res* 1994; 12: 186–192.

7. Ashton, IK, DA Walsh, JM Polak et al. Substance P in intervertebral discs: Binding sites on vascular endothelium of the human annulus fibrosus. *Acta Orthop Scand* 1994; 65: 635–639.

8. Berse, B, JA Hunt, RJ Diegel et al. Hypoxia augments cytokine-induced vascular endothelial growth factor secretion by human synovial fibroblasts. *Clin Exp Immunol* 1999; 115: 176–182.

9. Biedert, RM, and V Sanchis-Alfonso. Sources of anterior knee pain. *Clin Sports Med* 2002; 21: 335–347.

10. Byers, PD. Solitary benign osteoblastic lesions of bone: Osteoid osteoma and benign osteoblastoma. *Cancer* 1968; 22: 43–57.

11. Calzà, L, L Giardino, A Giuliani et al. Nerve growth factor control of neuronal expression of angiogenetic and vasoactive factors. *Proc Natl Acad Sci USA* 2001; 98: 4160–4165.

12. Coppes, MH, E Marani, RT Thomeer et al. Innervation of "painful" lumbar discs. *Spine* 1997; 22: 2342–2349.

13. Dicou, E, B Pflug, M Magazin et al. Two peptides derived from the nerve growth factor precursor are biologically active. *J Cell Biol* 1997; 136: 389–398.

14. Dye, SF, GL Vaupel, and CC Dye. Conscious neurosensory mapping of the internal structures of the human knee without intra-articular anesthesia. *Am J Sports Med* 1998; 26: 773–777.

15. Dye, SF, HU Staubli, RM Biedert et al. The mosaic of pathophysiology causing patellofemoral pain: Therapeutic implications. *Oper Tech Sports Med* 1999; 7: 46–54.

16. Freemont, AJ, TE Peacock, P Goupille et al. Nerve ingrowth into diseased intervertebral disc in chronic back pain. *Lancet* 1997; 350: 178–181.

17. Fulkerson, JP. The etiology of patellofemoral pain in young active patients: A prospective study. *Clin Orthop* 1983; 179:129–133.

18. Fulkerson, JP, R Tennant, JS Jaivin et al. Histologic evidence of retinacular nerve injury associated with patellofemoral malalignment. *Clin Orthop* 1985; 197: 196–205.

19. Fulkerson, JP, and DS Hungerford. *Disorders of the Patellofemoral Joint*. Baltimore: Williams & Wilkins, 1990.

20. Gigante, A, C Bevilacqua, A Ricevuto et al. Biological aspects in patello-femoral malalignment. *Eleventh Congress European Society of Sports Traumatology, Knee Surgery and Arthroscopy, Book of Abstracts*, Athens, 5–8 May, 2004: 218.

21. Grelsamer, RP, and J McConnell. The Patella: A Team Approach. Gaithersburg, MD: Aspen, 1998.
22. Grönblad, M, O Korkala, YT Konttinen et al. Silver impregnation and immunohistochemical study of nerves in lumbar facet joint plical tissue. *Spine* 1991; 16: 34–38.
23. Grönblad, M, JN Weinstein, and S Santavirta. Immunohistochemical observations on spinal tissue innervation: A review of hypothetical mechanisms of back pain. *Acta Orthop Scand* 1991; 62: 614–622.
24. Hasegawa, T, T Hirose, R Sakamoto et al. Mechanism of pain in osteoid osteomas: An immunohistochemical study. *Histopathology* 1993; 22: 487–491.
25. Hayashi, T, M Sakurai, K Abe et al. Expression of angiogenic factors in rabbit spinal cord after transient ischaemia. *Neuropathol Appl Neurobiol* 1999; 25: 63–71.
26. Isaacson, LG, and KA Crutcher. The duration of sprouted cerebrovascular axons following intracranial infusion of nerve growth factor. *Exp Neurol* 1995; 13: 174–179.
27. Jackson, JR, JAL Minton, ML Ho et al. Expression of vascular endothelial growth factor in synovial fibroblasts is induced by hypoxia and interleukin 1a. *J Rheumatol* 1997; 24: 1253–1259.
28. Jerosch, J, and M Prymka. Knee joint propioception in patients with posttraumatic recurrent patella dislocation. *Knee Surg, Sports Traumatol, Arthrosc* 1996; 4: 14–18.
29. Kasim, N, and JP Fulkerson. Resection of clinically localized segments of painful retinaculum in the treatment of selected patients with anterior knee pain. *Am J Sports Med* 2000; 28: 811–814.
30. Kawaja, MD. Sympathetic and sensory innervation of the extracerebral vasculature: Roles for p75NTR neuronal expression and nerve growth factor. *J Neurosci Res* 1998; 52: 295–306.
31. Kocher, MS, FH Fu, and ChD Harner. Neuropathophysiology. In Fu, FH, ChD Harner, KG Vince, eds., *Knee Surgery.* Baltimore: Williams and Wilkins, 1994, pp. 231–249.
32. Konttinen, YT, M Grönblad, I Antti-Poika et al. Neuroimmunohistochemical analysis of peridiscal nociceptive neural elements. *Spine* 1990; 15: 383–386.
33. Korkala, O, M Grönblad, P Liesi et al. Immunohistochemical demonstration of nociceptors in the ligamentous structures of the lumbar spine. *Spine* 1985; 10: 156–157.
34. Kraushaar, BS, and RP Nirschl. Tendinosis of the elbow (tennis elbow). *J Bone Joint Surg* 1999; 81-A: 259–278.
35. Lee, TH, H Kato, K Kogure et al. Temporal profile of nerve growth factor-like immunoreactivity after transient focal cerebral ischemia in rats. *Brain Res* 1996; 713: 199–210.
36. Liu, Y, SR Cox, T Morita et al. Hypoxia regulates vascular endothelial growth factor gene expression in endothelial cells: Identification of a 5° enhancer. *Circ Res* 1995; 77: 638–643.
37. Malcangio, M, NE Garrett, S Cruwys et al. Nerve growth factor- and neurotrophin-3-induced changes in nociceptive threshold and the release of substance P from the rat isolated spinal cord. *J Neurosci* 1997; 17: 8459–8467.
38. Marti, HJ, M Bernaudin, A Bellail et al. Hypoxia-induced vascular endothelial growth factor expression precedes neovascularization after cerebral ischemia. *Am J Pathol* 2000; 156: 965–976.
39. Messner, K, Y Wei, B Andersson et al. Rat model of Achilles tendon disorder: A pilot study. *Cells Tissues Organs* 1999; 165: 30–39.

40. Minchenko, A, T Bauer, S Salceda et al. Hypoxic stimulation of vascular endothelial growth factor expression in vitro and in vivo. *Lab Invest* 1994; 71: 374–379.
41. Mori, Y, A Fujimoto, H Okumo et al. Lateral retinaculum release in adolescent patellofemoral disorders: Its relationship to peripheral nerve injury in the lateral retinaculum. *Bull Hosp Jt Dis Orthop Inst* 1991; 51: 218–229.
42. Mukai, K, J Rosai, and WH Burgdorf. Localization of factor VIII-related antigen in vascular endothelial cells using an immunoperoxidase method. *Am J Surg Pathol* 1980; 4: 273–276.
43. Nagashima, M, S Yoshino, T Ishiwata et al. Role of vascular endothelial growth factor in angiogenesis of rheumatoid arthritis. *J Rheumatol* 1995; 22: 1624–1630.
44. Nilsson, G, K Forsberg-Nilsson, Z Xiang et al. Human mast cells express functional TrkA and are a source of nerve growth factor. *Eur J Immunol* 1997; 27: 2295–2301.
45. Palmgren, T, M Grönblad, J Virri, et al. Immunohistochemical demonstration of sensory and autonomic nerve terminals in herniated lumbar disc tissue. *Spine* 1996; 21: 1301–1306.
46. Pufe, T, W Petersen, B Tillmann et al. The splice variants VEGF121 and VEGF189 of the angiogenic peptide vascular endothelial growth factor are expressed in osteoarthritic cartilage. *Arthritis Rheum* 2001; 44: 1082–1088.
47. Richard, DE, E Berra, and J Pouyssegur. Angiogenesis: How a tumor adapts to hypoxia. *Biochem Biophys Res Commun* 1999; 266: 718–722.
48. Richardson, EP, and U DeGirolami. *Pathology of the Peripheral Nerve.* Philadelphia: W.B. Saunders, 1995.
49. Sanchis-Alfonso, V, E Gastaldi-Orquín, and V Martinez-SanJuan. Usefulness of computed tomography in evaluating the patellofemoral joint before and after Insall's realignment: Correlation with short-term clinical results. *Am J Knee Surg* 1994; 7: 65–72.
50. Sanchis-Alfonso, V, E Roselló-Sastre, C Monteagudo-Castro et al. Quantitative analysis of nerve changes in the lateral retinaculum in patients with isolated symptomatic patellofemoral malalignment: A preliminary study. *Am J Sports Med* 1998; 26: 703–709.
51. Sanchis-Alfonso, V, and E Roselló-Sastre. Proliferación neural e isquemia. *Rev Patol Rodilla* 1998; 3: 60–63.
52. Sanchis-Alfonso, V, E Roselló-Sastre, and A Subías-López. Mechanisms of pain in jumper's knee: A histological and immunohistochemical study. *J Bone Joint Surg* 1999; 81-B (SUPP I): 82.
53. Sanchis-Alfonso, V, E Roselló-Sastre, and V Martinez-SanJuan. Pathogenesis of anterior knee pain syndrome and functional patellofemoral instability in the active young: A review. *Am J Knee Surg* 1999; 12: 29–40.
54. Sanchis-Alfonso, V, and E Roselló-Sastre. Immunohistochemical analysis for neural markers of the lateral retinaculum in patients with isolated symptomatic patellofemoral malalignment: A neuroanatomic basis for anterior knee pain in the active young patient. *Am J Sports Med* 2000; 28: 725–731.
55. Sanchis-Alfonso, V, E Roselló-Sastre, and F Revert. Neural growth factor expression in the lateral retinaculum in painful patellofemoral malalignment. *Acta Orthop Scand* 2001; 72: 146–149.
56. Sanchis-Alfonso, V, E Roselló-Sastre, and A Subías-López. Neuroanatomic basis for pain in patellar tendinosis ("jumper's knee"): A neuroimmunohistochemical study. *Am J Knee Surg* 2001; 14: 174–177.

57. Sanchis-Alfonso, V, and E Roselló-Sastre. Anterior knee pain in the young patient: What causes the pain? "Neural model." *Acta Orthop Scand* 2003; 74: 697–703.

58. Sanchis-Alfonso, V, E Roselló-Sastre, F Revert, et al. Histologic retinacular changes associated with ischemia in painful patellofemoral malalignment. *Orthopedics* (in press).

59. Sherman, BE, and RA Chole. A mechanism for sympathectomy-induced bone resorption in the middle ear. *Otolaryngol Head Neck Surg* 1995; 113: 569–581.

60. Shweiki, D, A Itin, D Soffer et al. Vascular endothelial growth factor induced by hypoxia may mediate hypoxia-initiated angiogenesis. *Nature* 1992; 359: 843–845.

61. Society for Ultrastructural Pathology. *Handbook of Diagnostic Electron Microscopy for Pathologists-in-Training.* New York-Tokyo: Igaku-Shoin Medical Publishers Committee, 1995.

62. Soifer, TB, HJ Levy, FM Soifer et al. Neurohistology of the subacromial space. *Arthroscopy* 1996; 12: 182–186.

63. Solomonow, M, and R D'Ambrosia. Neural reflex arcs and muscle control of knee stability and motion. In Scott, WN, ed., *Ligament and Extensor Mechanism Injuries of the Knee: Diagnosis and Treatment.* St. Louis: Mosby-Year Book, 1991, pp. 389–400.

64. Steinbrech, DS, BJ Mehrara, PB Saadeh et al. Hypoxia regulates VEGF expression and cellular proliferation by osteoblasts in vitro. *Plast Reconstr Surg* 1999; 104: 738–747.

65. Wilson, AS, and HB Lee. Hypothesis relevant to defective position sense in a damaged knee. *J Neurol Neurosurg Psychiatry* 1986; 49: 1462–1463.

66. Witonski, D, and M Wagrowska-Danielewicz. Distribution of substance-P nerve fibers in the knee joint in patients with anterior knee pain syndrome. *Knee Surg Sports Traumatol Arthrosc* 1999; 7: 177–183.

67. Wojtys, EM, DN Beaman, RA Glover, and D Janda. Innervation of the human knee joint by substance-P fibers. *Arthroscopy* 1990; 6: 254–263.

68. Woolf, CJ, A Allchorne, B Safieh-Garabedian et al. Cytokines, nerve growth factor and inflammatory hyperalgesia: The contribution of tumour necrosis factor alpha. *Br J Pharmacol* 1997; 121: 417–424.

69. Yamada, T, M Sawatsubashi, H Yakushiji et al. Localization of vascular endothelial growth factor in synovial membrane mast cells: Examination with "multi-labelling subtraction immunostaining." *Virchows Arch* 1998; 433: 567–570.

4

Biomechanical Bases for Anterior Knee Pain and Patellar Instability in the Young Patient

Vicente Sanchis-Alfonso, Jaime M. Prat-Pastor,
Carlos M. Atienza-Vicente, Carlos Puig-Abbs,
and Mario Comín-Clavijo

Introduction

The mechanical theory has received more attention than the neural hypothesis in orthopedic bibliography.[2,12-20,23,25,27-29,36,42,48-50,60,61] Subchondral bone overload, with the consequent increment of the subchondral intraosseous pressure, is a direct result of patellofemoral malalignment (PFM). Subchondral bone overload can also be increased when the knee, with or without malalignment, is subject to an overuse or to a direct or indirect traumatism, as is very frequently seen in the practice of sports. Indeed, 49% of the patients in our surgical series suffered an indirect traumatism during sport activities before the onset of symptoms, and 5% of them suffered a direct hit.[50] Furthermore, certain attitudes that are necessary to adopt in some sports (inherently) can contribute on the one hand to the increase of the subchondral bone overload due to the increment of the patellofemoral joint reaction (PFJR) force, and on the other hand to the increment of the Q angle.

Sport is an important agent in the pathogenesis of the anterior knee pain syndrome and in the functional patellar instability as seen by the fact that 73% of our operated patients (unpublished data) used to play energetic sports (volleyball, basketball, handball, football, rhythmic gymnastics, or hockey) of level I (4–7 days a week of practice) or level II (1–3 days a week of practice) before the symptoms started. In addition to this, the degree of pain was related to the patient's level of activity. It is worth remembering the undoubted relation between sport activities and the articular overuse concept. Overuse is defined in general terms as a repetitive microtrauma of a sufficient degree to overcome the regeneration capacity of the tissues.[43] In all types of tissues, the microtraumatism, provoked by the application of repetitive tensions, produces microlesions in the collagen fibers, in addition to direct or indirect effects on the vascular supply. Additional factors in the genesis of the overuse syndromes include using the wrong techniques, training inadequately (including overtraining), and not employing the right equipment.

Reaction Forces Generated by the Impacts Produced While Running and Jumping

Running, jumping, turning, and swivelling form part of a great many energetic sports as mentioned before. Out of these, jumping is the main culprit in the origin of chronic lesions of the knee. Furthermore, jumping is one of the principal causes of the patellar tendinopathy ("jumper's knee"), which is the typical example of overuse knee lesion, and in 49% of our cases it was linked to a symptomatic PFM (unpublished data). The reaction forces generated when jumping from the standing position, transmitted through the musculoskeletal system from feet to head, can be up to four times the weight of the player, and up to nine times when the jump follows a previous run.[38] As jumping is a repetitive gesture, it is understandable how damaging it can become for the player's knee. For instance, a player of the NBA is supposed to jump at least 70 times per match.[39] The heavy weight and great height of the basketball players are additionally negative factors. On the other hand, during running the impact forces against the ground reach 2 to 3 times the body weight.[9] This has a cumulative effect along the training and competition periods, without forgetting the sport practice by adolescents in physical education classes, which on its own or associated to other predisposing factors, can cause the onset of the symptoms. These sportive movements are inevitable and form part of the sport itself, but they can be mitigated.

Importance of Footwear, Ground Surface, and Personal Technique in the Origin and Prevention of the Lesions

The human body has some natural systems of shock absorption to protect itself from the effect derived from jumping and running: soft heel tissue, pronation of the hindfoot, ankle dorsiflexion, flexion of the knee, menisci, articular cartilage, and flexion of the hip.[8,35] As pointed out by Gross and Nelson,[21] the series of articular movements on landing from a vertical jump starts with the distal joints to end in the proximal ones (metatarsophalangeal, midtarsal, subtalar, ankle, knee, and hip joints). The knee and the hip have a first-rate role in the process of shock absorption after a jump, whereas the foot pronation (subtalar joint) is the main shock absorber when running.[35] However, this knee flexion, with a positive effect as shock absorber, shows a negative effect also as it increases the PFJR force, as will be seen in the next section. On the other hand, the total strength of the impact suffered by the organism depends not only on the applied force, but also on the time that force is being applied. It is considered a good technique of dissipation or absorption of the impact when the force is distributed along a certain time. Shock absorption can be incremented by using these natural mechanisms (i.e., good sport technique, speed of the fall) or using external materials (i.e., appropriate footwear and adequate playing surface). In this way, prevention of the lesions related to overuse or diminution of the negative impact on the knee of certain

inevitable stresses like running and jumping is probably possible.

Footwear can contribute to reducing the reaction force after impact in three fundamental ways: (1) increasing the natural shock-absorbing mechanisms (appropriate heel insole to increase heel fat shock-absorbing role and a strong heel stiffener to prevent hyperpronation), (2) supplementing the aforesaid mechanisms (good-quality sole materials, air chambers, and insoles), and (3) avoiding limiting the natural shock-absorbing mechanisms like heel dorsiflexion (boot-type footwear increases the charges transmitted to the muscular skeletal system by limiting ankle mobility, as opposed to the shoe-type footwear). Overlooking these norms in sport footwear will increase the impact stresses when jumping and running and therefore it will produce an overload of the knee and will favor the development of overload chronic lesions. Having the ankle supported (boot-type footwear) diminishes the efficiency when running and swivelling, very frequent gestures in handball, and so this type of footwear is not advised for this sport.[46] Finally, having the sole empty at mid-foot level would allow a certain independence of movement between the fore and the hindfoot, diminishing shoe rigidity. This would favor the mobility of the midtarsal joint (natural shock-absorbing system).

Excessive adherence of shoe to playing surface is another lesion-producing factor. On the other hand, lack of this adherence can, as well, be the cause of lesions. In handball, for instance, it is necessary to have a good adherence between shoe and court as there are frequent changes in direction and breaking movements in this sport.[46] When practiced in a pavilion, sports shoes with "caramel soles," called thus because of their aspect, are used. These soles have a great parquet adherence; this increases the performance, but they are not advisable because this adherence can provoke a knee lesion. It has been said that a pattern under the head of the first metatarsal should be added to the specific sole pattern to facilitate the turn over this zone, diminishing the overload on the knee joint, and in this way counteracting the adherence of the sole to the playing surface. An excessive adherence can provoke lesions. For instance, rhythmic gymnastics on a mat should be practiced barefooted or with slippers, as normal sports shoes could provoke a severe knee lesion due to the excessive adherence of the shoe to the mat (avoidable technical error). This happened to one of our patients who was a gymnastics teacher.

Finally, outwearing sports shoes is a negative factor, as the adherence and shock-absorbing mechanisms have lost their efficiency (avoidable factor).[9,10] Possibly the wearing too long of this type of shoe is related to their high price and for this reason some athletes opt for funny and dangerous solutions, for example, soaking the soles of their shoes in Coca-Cola, Reflex, honey, lacquer, or something that the handball players call "stick," a resin that they put on their hands to prevent the ball from slipping. The final aim is to increase the adherence of the shoe to the court.

Relating to the playing surface, a high percentage of amateur sportsmen and -women in our media play and train on hard surfaces. For instance, more than half of the handball players in the Valencian Community train and play on hard surfaces, cement or asphalt, during more than half of their sports time.[9] This situation repeats itself with basketball, which is the most popular sport in our media.[10] These hard surfaces favor the development of overload lesions due to the fact that the reaction forces after the impacts provoked by jumping and running are very high. Ideally, they should train and play over parquet or synthetic materials with a high shock-absorbing capacity. The problem is the lack of properly fitted sports pavilions.

Patellofemoral Joint Reaction Force: Patellofemoral Contact Areas

Different pathologies can vary the physiological patellofemoral contact surface, but generally speaking a reduction of the reaction force in the patellofemoral joint (PFJ) is associated with pain lessening. It is therefore necessary to determine the value that such a reaction force can reach at each sport movement and for each rehabilitation exercise, or at least to determine what knee positions are associated with maximal values of these reaction forces.

Isolating the knee joint, in a schematic way, as can be seen in Figure 4.1A, can show that the forces acting on the PFJ, on extension of the knee, are the quadriceps muscular force (F_Q), the force transmitted to the patellar tendon (F_{PT}), and the reaction force generated upon the PFJ (F_{PFJR}). Supposing, in a simple way, that the force transmitted to the patellar tendon and

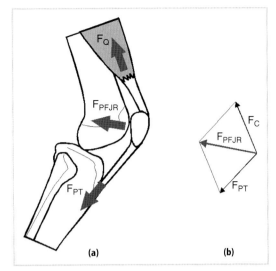

Figure 4.1. Simplified scheme of the forces acting on the patellofemoral joint (**a**). Graphic calculation of the PFJR force (**b**). F_Q: force upon quadriceps; F_{PT}: force transmitted to the patellar tendon; F_{PFJR}: reaction force on the patellofemoral joint.

the one exerted by the quadriceps are equal (this hypothesis is more inexact the higher the degrees of flexion), the PFJR force can be determined graphically as can be seen in Figure 4.1B.

Using the graphic method it is easy to see that for a determined quadriceps muscle force, the PFJR force increases as the angle of flexion of the knee does, therefore being minimal at complete extension[2,15,19,28,42,61,64] (Figure 4.2A). For example, for a quadriceps force of 1.000 N (approximately 100 kg) and a flexion of 5°, the PFJR force nears 60 kg, whereas if the flexion goes up to 90° the reaction force increases to values around 130 kg (Figure 4.2A). This would increase for further flexion values. The patellar articular cartilage is one of the thickest in the body, which is very useful to withstand these great compressive loads. In numerous sports, the repetitive and maintained knee flexion positions are frequent, producing increases in the PFJR forces and subjecting the patellar cartilage to a maximal risk despite its thickness (Figure 4.2B).

It is necessary to apply the concept of moment (product of a force and the distance from its line of action to a point) to estimate the quadriceps extension force that has to apply in determined positions (Figure 4.3). The flexion moment due to external forces (in the figure the 60 kg of body weight) has to be balanced by an extensor moment, which, in a simplified way,

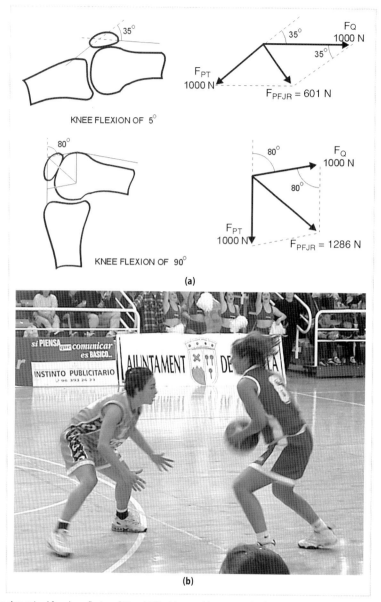

Figure 4.2. PFJR force determined for a knee flexion of 5° and 90° with a quadriceps muscular force of 1000N **(a)**. The reaction force increases as the knee flexion increases. Positions of maintained knee flexion are frequent in sports **(b)**. (Part B is reproduced with permission of Promo Sport.)

can be supposed to be due only to the quadriceps. The flexion moment is calculated multiplying the force that bends the joint (body weight) by the distance of its line of action (the line that passes through the center of gravity) to the center of rotational movement (which coincides with the point of joint contact between the femur and the tibia). In the same way, the extensor moment will be equal to the quadriceps force multiplied by the distance of its line of action

(roughly the medial line of the patella) to the center of rotation. In an approximate way, for a position like the one depicted in Figure 4.3A with a flexion of 45°, the distance from the body weight action line to the center of the joint is 5 cm and coincides with the distance of the line of action of the extensor force to the same center. Therefore, the extensor force should also coincide with the body weight force. If knee flexion increases to 115° (Figure 4.3B), the distance of

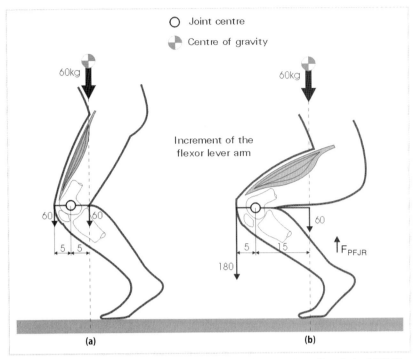

Figure 4.3. Body weight line of action and quadriceps extension force applied to different positions of knee flexion (**a&b**). Effect of the increment of the flexor lever arm on the reaction force in the patellofemoral joint (F_{PFJR}). (Units of force Kg and distance cm.)

the body weight action line to the joint center increases threefold (15 cm), and so, for the same body weight, the extensor force ought to augment in the same proportion reaching a value of 180 kg. It has to be considered that the increase in quadriceps force when the flexion augments is even greater when it becomes contact force in the PFJ. For a given quadriceps force the increase in reaction force is a little more than one and a half times the former when passing from 45° to 115° of flexion; therefore, while quadriceps force increases threefold, reaction force does it more than four and a half times.

From these simple mechanical considerations it becomes clear the enormous importance of the position, during extensor exercises, upon the patellofemoral reaction force, which is directly related to the joint pain.

Reilly and Martens[45] have calculated that the reaction force at the PFJ during walking is 0.5 times the body weight. Climbing up stairs increases the loads 3.3 times the body weight and full flexions of the knee goes up to 7 to 8 times the body weight. Certain activities of daily life are responsible for the increase in the PFJR

force. This would be the reason why climbing up stairs, squatting, bicycle riding, and sitting for a time with the knees bent, like in the cinema or in a car, provoke pain in the group of patients we are studying. Bandi[18] undertook the same work as Reilly and Martens, adding the effect of hip flexion on the final results of PFJR force (Figure 4.4). This author found that the PFJR force while squatting was only 3.8 times the body weight. So, one way of reducing the PFJR force would be to associate a hip flexion, as this approximates the line of action of the body weight to the knee.

Summarizing, the PFJR force not only increases with knee flexion due to the resultant force increment, but also because the flexor lever arm, which requires a quadriceps response, increases in length. As a general rule, it is not advisable to bend the knees excessively when they are under strain (e.g., supplementary weight [Figure 4.5], speed, short breaking distance, etc.). It becomes clear that, with a good personal and a good training technique, it is possible to partly lessen the bad effect of the PFJR force. Additionally, we can understand how loss of weight, obviously when the patient is

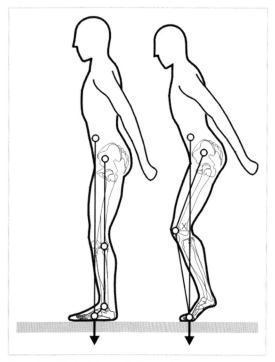

Figure 4.4. Effect of the hip flexion on the reaction force at the patellofemoral joint.

overweight, is a fundamental part in the treatment of this type of patients. Obesity is a main factor in the overloading of the PFJ and cannot be overlooked in the treatment.

Another important factor to study is PFJ contact stress (pressure) (reaction force/contact surface). Eisenhart-Rothe and colleagues[14] have analyzed the three-dimensional kinematic and contact area of the PFJ of healthy volunteers by 3D image postprocessing. During knee flexion (30°–90°), patellofemoral contact areas increased significantly in size (134 mm^2 vs. 205 mm^2) (Figure 4.6). Therefore, for healthy persons during knee flexion an increase of the reaction force shows to be related to a bigger contact surface and a moderate increase in PFJ pressures. Contrarily, contact stress (pressure) at the PFJ increases in the PFM during knee flexion in the same or bigger proportion as a consequence of patellofemoral contact area decrease (Figure 4.7). Brechter and Powers[6] have studied the patellofemoral stress during walking in persons with and without patellofemoral pain. On the average, PFJ stress was significantly greater in subjects with PFP compared with control subjects during level walking. The observed increase in PFJ stress in the PFP group was

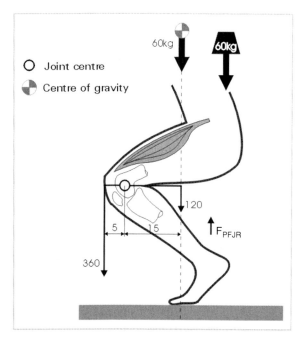

Figure 4.5. Effect of the complementary weights (60 Kg) on the PFJR force (F_{PFJR}). (Units of force Kg and distance cm.)

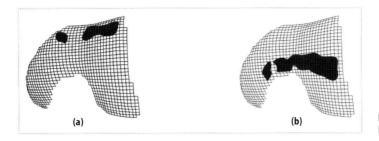

Figure 4.6. Patellofemoral contact areas at 30° of knee flexion **(a)** and 90° of knee flexion **(b)**.

attributed to a significant reduction in PFJ contact area, as the PFJR forces were similar between these to groups.

Hamstring and triceps sural contractures can have an indirect effect in the patellofemoral dynamics as they increase the reaction force at the PFJ, as these contractures produce a maintained flexion of the knee. Lastly a quadriceps contracture directly increases the contact pressure between patella and femur.

In a similar way, anterior knee pain after intra-articular reconstruction of the anterior cruciate ligament (ACL) with a bone-patellar tendon-bone autograft is related more to a maintained flexion contracture of the knee, and therefore, to an increment of the reaction force of the PFJ, than to the actual graft harvesting.[31,51,53] Because of this, regaining full hyperextension of the knee early after ACL surgery is advisable, as it is clear that it does not affect negatively knee stability in the long-term.[53] An unstable knee is better tolerated by the patient than a stable one with a permanent flexion deformity. The latter is one of the causes of anterior knee pain. Anterior knee pain after ACL surgery has been also related to the patellar tendon pretibial adhesions that produce an increase in the PFJR force (Figure 4.8).[1]

Q Angle and Valgus Vector

The Q angle implies the existence of a vector pointing laterally with contraction of the quadriceps, called the valgus vector (Figure 4.9A), which favors not only the lateral subluxation of the patella, counteracted by the medial patellofemoral ligament, but also an increase of the traction tensions at the insertion of the patellar tendon in the lower patellar pole. This Q angle increases when there is hip anteversion, external tibial torsion, genu valgum, tightness of the fascia lata and of the iliotibial band, gluteus medius weakness, and pronated feet. Women have wider pelvis (gynecoid pelvis), which conditions a bigger knee valgus with the consequent

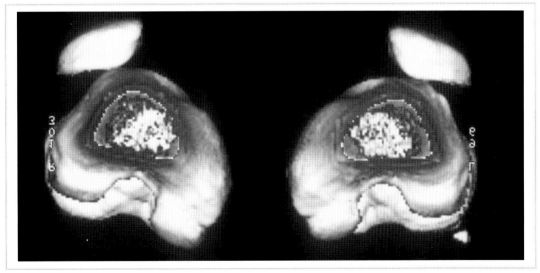

Figure 4.7. Tridimensional CT scan showing the diminution of the patellofemoral contact area in PFM.

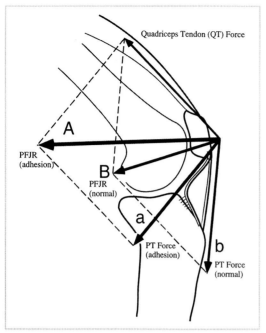

Figure 4.8. PFJR force (F_{PFJR}) in a knee with patellar tendon adhesions to the proximal tibial surface. (Reproduced with permission from Ahmad, CS, SD Kwak, GA Ateshian et al., *Effects of patellar tendon adhesion to the anterior tibia on knee mechanics, Am J Sports Med* 1998; 26: 715–724.)

pronation of the feet and a bigger Q angle. This angle is also increased in certain attitudes practiced in sports (Figure 4.9B). As the knee starts to flex, the tibia derotates, diminishing the Q angle and the valgus vector. From 20° or 30° of flexion, resistance to lateral subluxation is mainly provided by the lateral femoral condyle.

Out of all these factors, pronated foot is one of the most important in the etiology of patellofemoral pain[60] (Table 4.1). Pronated foot should not be confused with flat foot, as it is not

Table 4.1. Etiology of pronation

Intrinsic causes
　Forefoot varus
　Hindfoot varus
　Tibial varus

Extrinsic causes
　Flexibility deficit (triceps sural, hip flexors, iliotibial tract, hip rotators and hamstrings).
　Resistance deficit (ankle inversion, hip rotators, gluteus medius and/or lumbar quadratus).
　Leg length discrepancy.

From Wallace, LA and MF Sullivan (ref. 60).

necessary for the foot to be flat to suffer an excessive pronation. Pronation is not a position; it is a function. An excessive pronation leads to[44,60] (1) an increase in the Q angle; (2) an anterior displacement of the proximal tibia, with the consequent flexion of the knee and because of this an increase in the PFJR force; (3) an increase of the impact forces that reach the knee joint, due to the calcaneal eversion, which is, therefore, unable to increase its eversion (we must remember that calcaneal eversion constitutes an important shock-absorbing mechanism, to lessen the impact forces when jumping or running); and (4) an internal tibial rotation that affects the PFJ dynamics. Leg length discrepancy is one of the causes of pronated feet. It would be logical to correct it as part of the conservative treatment, although up to now there are no studies relating to leg length discrepancy and anterior knee pain.[44] All this justifies the occasional utility of orthopedic insoles in the treatment of anterior knee pain (Figure 4.10).

These factors could explain the frequent association between jumper's knee and symptomatic PFM that we have found in our series. Therefore, in this group of patients it is necessary to carry on a complete physical examination, not only of the knee but of the whole limb, with special attention dedicated to the foot structures. The association between hip anteversion, in-facing patellae, external tibial torsion, pronated feet (positive Helbing sign [medial arching of the Achilles tendon]), and bayonet sign is known in the orthopedic bibliography as "miserable malalignment syndrome."[61]

Relation Between Morphotype and Extensor Mechanism Pathology

Lower limb possibilities of malalignment in the different spatial planes are: (1) frontal plane (*genu valgum* and *genu varum*); (2) sagittal plane (*genu recurvatum* and *genu flexum*); and (3) transversal plane (femoral and tibial torsion).

Valgus knees (*genu valgum*) show the tibial tuberosity further lateral than normal and following this an increase in the Q angle that will be even bigger when there is external tibial torsion.[59] In *genu varum* the tibial tuberosity is placed more medial than in normal knees and it provokes not only an important overload in the medial compartment of the knee, but also a moderate overload in the medial region of the patellofemoral joint.[59]

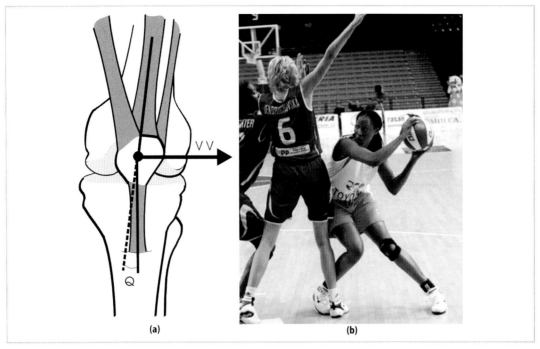

Figure 4.9. Q angle and valgus vector (VV). The Q angle imposes a valgus vector in the last degrees of extension **(a)**. In many sport positions knee valgus is strained, which increases the Q angle and the valgus vector **(b)**. (Part B is reproduced with permission of ROS CASARES/JACOBO PAYA.)

Genu recurvatum is frequently associated with patella alta. This type of knee, more frequent in women, shows a higher incidence of recurrent dislocation of the patella, especially when it is associated with *genu valgum* and external tibial torsion.[59] In addition to this, *genu recurvatum* is frequently associated with anterior knee pain.[59] *Genu flexum* is also associated with anterior knee pain as it increases the PFJR force.

An external tibial torsion produces lateral tilt, lateral rotation, and lateral displacement of the patella.[58] On the other hand, an internal tibial

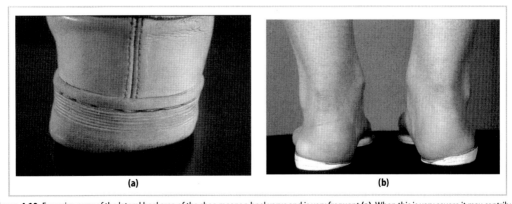

Figure 4.10. Excessive wear of the lateral heel area of the shoe means a heel varus and is very frequent **(a)**. When this is very severe it may contribute to the production of lateral knee pain. In this situation treatment with orthopedic insoles is fundamental **(b)**.

torsion causes medial tilt, medial rotation, and medial displacement of the patella.[58]

Such deformities as increased femoral anteversion or internal femoral torsion are closely related to patellofemoral pathology.[33] Both produce an increase of the quadricipital angle, which causes excessive lateral displacement of the patella when the muscle contracts. This leads to an excess of the tension on the medial patellofemoral ligament (MPFL) as well as of the stresses on the lateral side of the patella and the trochlea. Initially this induces pain and later it provokes instability, chondromalacia and patellofemoral osteoarthrosis.[33] Pain provokes inhibition atrophy of the quadriceps, which aggravates the symptoms. Quadriceps exercises occasionally provoke an overcharge of the knee joint that increases the pain and the inhibition of the muscle, in the end paradoxically causing greater atrophy.

Kijowski and colleagues[33] observed statistically significant changes in the contact area and in the contact pressure of the PFJ with femur rotation. Internal rotation of the femur (e.g., secondary to an excessive femoral anteversion) induces an increase in the contact area and pressure at the lateral side of the PFJ and a decrease of both at the medial side of the same joint. Obviously, external rotation produces the opposite effects. In addition to this, these authors proved that internal rotation of the femur up to 30° produces a statistically significant increase of the MPFL tension when the knee is at 30° of flexion. These alterations could be partially responsible for the frequency of patellofemoral pathology in people with an abnormal rotational femoral alignment.

Swimming as an Example of Pain by Overuse

To highlight the importance of excessive valgus and PFJR force in the pathology we are dealing with, we will look at swimming.[47] Knee pain in this sport is a paradigm of pain by overuse, as in this competitive sport there is no weight-bearing or contact. In freestyle, backstroke, and butterfly there is a knee flexion associated with every kick, with a repetitive contraction of the quadriceps that can lead to an anterior knee pain caused by a patellofemoral cumulative overcharge (Figure 4.11). In addition to this, when pushing against the wall when starting and turning a strong contraction of quadriceps with the knee in high flexion takes place with an increment of the PFJR force (Figure 4.11). Another cause for this pain could be an increase in valgus alignment and external tibial torsion, which are both normal components of the breaststroke kick (Figure 4.12).

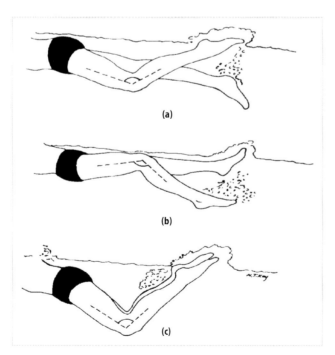

Figure 4.11. Flexion of the knee in freestyle **(a)**, backstroke **(b)**, and butterfly **(c)**. Degree of flexion associated with each impulse. (Reprinted from Rodeo, SA, Knee pain in competitive swimming, *Clin Sports Med* 1999; 18: 379–387 with permission from Elsevier.)

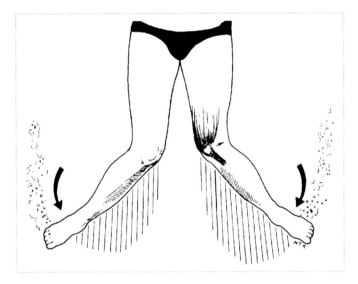

Figure 4.12. Position of the lower limbs in breast stroke. (Reprinted from Rodeo, SA, Knee pain in competitive swimming, *Clin Sports Med* 1999; 18: 379–387 with permission from Elsevier.)

Impingement Mechanism Between the Inferior Pole of the Patella and the Posterior Surface of the Proximal Third of the Patellar Tendon

Maintained and repetitive hyperflexion knee positions are often present in sports (Figure 4.13). These positions would favor the impingement of the inferior pole of the patella against the posterior surface of the patellar tendon proximal third. This is the pathogenic theory of the patellar tendinopathy (jumper's knee) proposed by some authors.[30] In fact, the maneuver that is demonstrative of the jumper's knee is in fact a reproduction of the impingement mechanism (Figure 4.13D).

Anatomical Factors Associated with Patellar Pain and Instability: Anatomical Predisposing Anomalies; Imbalance as an Alternative to Malalignment

The aforementioned factors as well as other predisposing anatomical factors, such as insufficiency of the vastus medialis obliquus (VMO) muscle, a lax medial retinaculum, patellar dysplasia, trochlear dysplasia (congenital flattening of the lateral femoral condyle), patella alta, and generalized ligamentous laxity (Figure 4.14), contribute to start or aggravate the patellar pain and instability.[11-16,19,20,24,28,36,42,49,54,61] These fac-

tors contribute to create what could be called "knee at risk" or favorable environment for the development of the anterior knee pain syndrome and patellar functional instability. One isolated factor might be insignificant, but when there are many associated factors these are cumulative. The association of these factors varies among patients, and it provokes a great variety of symptoms. That is why there are many types of clinical presentation.

Among all these anatomical factors possibly the main one is the insufficiency of the VMO, for this muscle has an essential role in the dynamic stabilization of the patella, opposing its lateral displacement during the first degrees of flexion. The fibers of the VMO exert a force that actively displaces the patella medially during the first degrees of knee flexion. The electrical activity of the VMO fibers is twice as much as the rest of the quadriceps.[34] An imbalance of this 2:1 proportion can lead to a lateral patellar displacement at knee extension caused by traction of the vastus lateralis. In this sense, patellar tilt and a high patellofemoral congruence angle could be considered a measurable expression of the quadricipital dysplasia. This VMO insufficiency could be secondary to a high insertion (congenitally) or to a disuse atrophy (acquired). Floyd and colleagues[17] suggest that many cases of recurrent dislocation of the patella are caused by a primary muscular defect (abundance of abnormal muscular fibers, type 2C). On the other hand, Robert Teitge, distinguished

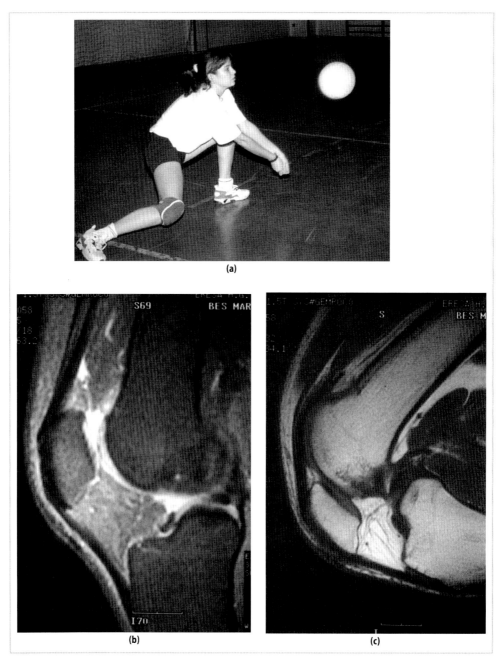

Figure 4.13. Volleyball player with her left knee in a maintained hyperflexion position (increase of the PFJR force) **(a)**. The right knee is forced into excessive valgus and, eventually, will sustain an indirect or direct traumatism **(a)**. Functional study of the knee by MRI in a patient suffering from right jumper's knee **(b&c)**. On flexion of the knee the inferior patellar pole impinges on the patellar tendon posterior aspect in its proximal end **(b:** Sagittal FSE PDW Fat Sat MR image; **c:** Sagittal SE T1W MR image with knee flexion). The patient referred severe pain in the knee after any position with maintained hyperflexion. He had problems with daily living activities like driving a car.

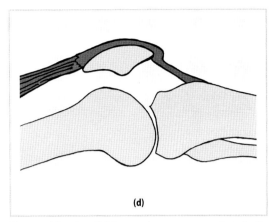

(d)

Figure 4.13 *(continued)* Scheme to show maneuver to palpate the distal polo of the patella and the proximal patellar tendon. With this maneuver impingement of the patellar inferior pole on the patellar tendon is produced **(d)**.

member of the International Patellofemoral Study Group, does not believe that VMO is responsible for patellar stability.[56] In his opinion, patellar stability depends on the geometry of bone and ligaments, the MPFL being the main one, whereas the medial meniscopatellar ligament has only a secondary role.[56] This way of thinking coincides with that of many other authors (see Chapters 5 and 20).

The medial retinacular laxity can be secondary to its tear after a dislocation or to an elonga-

tion secondary to a tense lateral retinaculum, chronic effusion, or recurrent external subluxation of the patella.

Dejour and colleagues[12] believe that the trochlear dysplasia (Figure 4.15) is the distinctive finding in the objective patellar instability, and the high frequency of bilateral cases (92.5%) makes them think that it is a constitutional anomaly.

Insall and colleagues[24] and Blackburn and Peel[5] have highlighted the role that patella alta plays in the patellar instability, which is logical thinking considering that this patella has a longer stretch outside the femoral trochlea on flexion and extension of the knee and therefore is less stable than a normal patella. Moreover, knees with patella alta show an increase in the PFJR force.[2] Patellar tilt and patella alta are present in both knees in more than 90% of the cases with objective patellar instability, even when one of them is asymptomatic.[12] This finding highlights the fact that patellar tilt and patella alta are not a consequence of the dislocation, but of a constitutional anomaly: the quadricipital dysplasia. Ward and Powers[62] have studied the influence of patella alta on PFJ stress during normal and fast walking. Persons with patella alta demonstrated greater calculated patellofemoral stress during fast walking. This

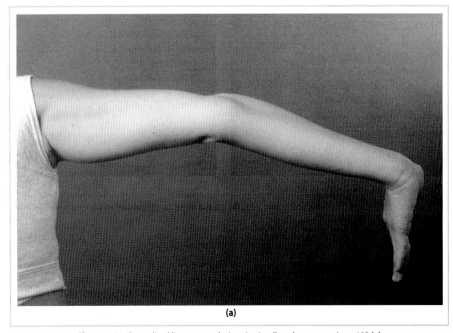

(a)

Figure 4.14. Generalized ligamentous laxity criteria: elbow hyperextension >10° **(a)**,

(continued)

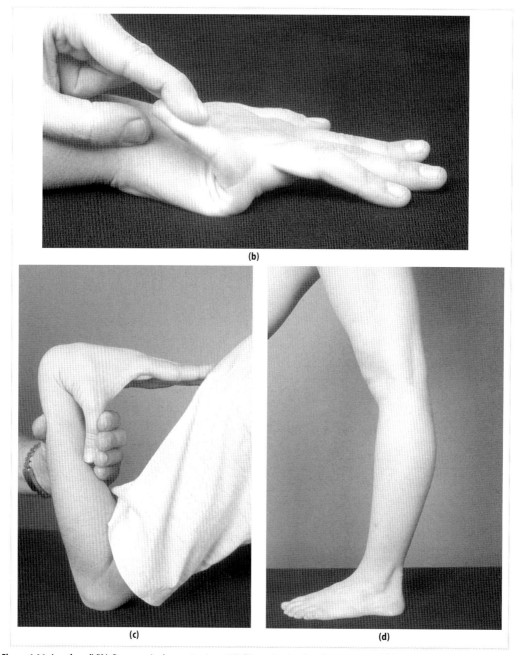

Figure 4.14. *(continued)* fifth finger passive hyperextension >90° **(b)**, passive thumb to forearm contact **(c)**, knee hyperextension >10° **(d)**,

was the result of reductions in contact area as joint reaction forces were similar between groups.

Finally, generalized ligamentous laxity[11,54] has to be taken into account especially because of its clinical consequences related to the association between acute patellar dislocation and chondral lesion. Stanitski[54] studied the relationship between joint hypermobility and chondral lesion after an acute patellar dislocation and found that the chondral lesion was 2.5 times more frequent in the patients without joint

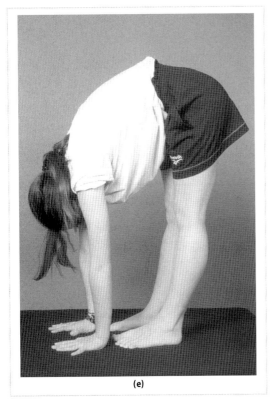

Figure 4.14. *(continued)* palms in contact with the ground with knees extended **(e)**. Ligamentous laxity exists when the patient can do three or more of these tests.

hypermobility than in the ones that showed generalized ligamentous laxity.

Mechanism of Pain Production According to the Mechanical Theory

The patellar articular cartilage lesion is the result of the application of tangential forces on the PFJ or of compression forces that do not disperse in an adequate way on the patellar articular surface. As we have mentioned before, the increase of the compression force is produced during activities that require an increase of the knee flexion, or as a consequence of a direct trauma, situations that happen frequently in sport practice or everyday life (falls, traffic accidents) given the protective function of the patella.

As a consequence of the direct or indirect traumatisms that the patella suffers without malalignment, but more so with it, the lesion of the articular cartilage is produced, which frees the araquidonic acid, which could initiate a series of biochemical changes leading to the liberation of catepsin with the consequent progressive degradation of the articular cartilage, probably mediated by the prostaglandins.[19] Furthermore, the prostaglandin E provokes bone resorption, which induces an internal bone remodeling (intense bone metabolism) that can cause a painful patella. The intra-articular

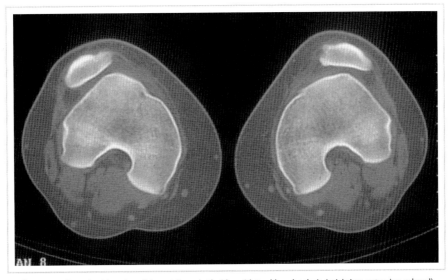

Figure 4.15. Lateral subluxation of the patella on both sides with trochlear dysplasia (axial view, extension, relaxed).

presence of the degradation products of the cartilage produces a chemical synovitis ("gunk synovitis"[42]) that could explain the popliteal pain that sometimes accompanies the anterior knee pain syndrome. The hypothesis of the chemical synovitis is favored by the clinical finding that a simple arthroscopic lavage could improve the pain in these patients. On the other hand, the abnormal pressure transmitted to the subchondral bone due to the softening of the patellar articular cartilage stimulates the subchondral nerves and the remodeling of the subchondral bone. These phenomena could constitute another mechanism of pain production. Therefore, the patella itself could be the main source of pain in some patients.

It is then clear to see the overlapping of the mechanical and neural theories. Furthermore the intraoseous hypertension secondary to the microscopic stress fractures caused by the alteration of the load transmission to the subchondral bone, which follows the articular cartilage failure, could also be another cause of anterior knee pain.[22] Brill[7] observed, nevertheless, that gammagraphies are not often positive in young sports players who suffer from anterior knee pain. This could be due to the fact that the cause of their anterior knee pain lies fundamentally in the peripatellar tissues and in the patellar tendon. This coincides with our clinical observations. A positive gammagraphic result would then be an objective clue for the indication of a decompression surgery (e.g., anteromedial transfer of the tibial tubercle by Fulkerson).

Finally the pain threshold in the subchondral bone could be surpassed, even with an intact cartilage, under an excessive stress or under a strong force (sport or direct trauma) or else under a normal stress applied on a knee with PFM.

Clinical Relevance

Because of the complexity and variability in the pathogenesis of the clinical entity we are now studying, it is easy to understand how difficult it is to establish the most appropriate treatment for each individual case. More than 100 surgical treatments have been described with different percentages of success, which reflects a problematic situation from the point of view of the pathogenesis, diagnostics, and treatment.[3,12,15,19,26,28,29,41,42,48,49,52,57,61,63] Therefore, it is fundamental to identify the pathological factor responsible for the clinical manifestations of each patient in order to select the most effective

treatment based on clinical findings ("made to measure" treatment). This policy will give us the most satisfactory results.

Given the aspects treated in this chapter and in the previous one, the importance of the following elements in the treatment of the clinical picture is easily understandable: (1) when the symptoms appear on stopping the sport activity; (2) treatment for pain and for tissue normalization (galvanic or continuous current, iontophoresis, diadynamic currents, Travert currents, transcutaneous electric stimulation (TENS), pulsating ultrasound, phonophoresis, cryotherapy, technique of deep transverse friction or technique by Cyriax); (3) stretching exercises (hamstrings, quadriceps, iliotibial tract, gastrocnemius, and lateral retinaculum); (4) strengthening of quadriceps (with special attention to the VMO), gluteus medius, and posterior tibial muscle; (5) proprioception exercises; and (6) knee braces, functional bandages, and foot insoles.

Some of the aspects that, if they are overlooked or unknown, may lead to erroneous treatments and iatrogenic problems will be analyzed next.

How Should the Quadriceps Muscle Be Strengthened? Closed versus Open Kinetic Chain Exercises; Eccentric versus Concentric Phase Exercises

At present the best exercises to strengthen the quadriceps in patients with patellofemoral dysfunction in the intermediate and advanced phases of the treatment are the techniques of closed kinetic chain (mini-squatting, lateral step [Figure 4.16], bicycling with a high saddle, etc.) in the last degrees of extension (from 0° to 30°), as the joint is subject to the minimal pressures (stresses).[49] Furthermore, the strengthening of the VMO is favored if the mini-squatting is associated to an adduction of the hips, which can be achieved with the use of a balloon. The clinical experience shows that patients with PFJ problems seem to tolerate best the exercises of leg press (closed kinetic chain) through the functional mobility range (less contact pressure [force times area] upon the PFJ), but they tend to present an increase of the symptoms during the leg extension exercises in open kinetic chain against resistance, in the functional mobility range (greater contact pressure [force times area] upon the PFJ).[55] Additionally, many patients without

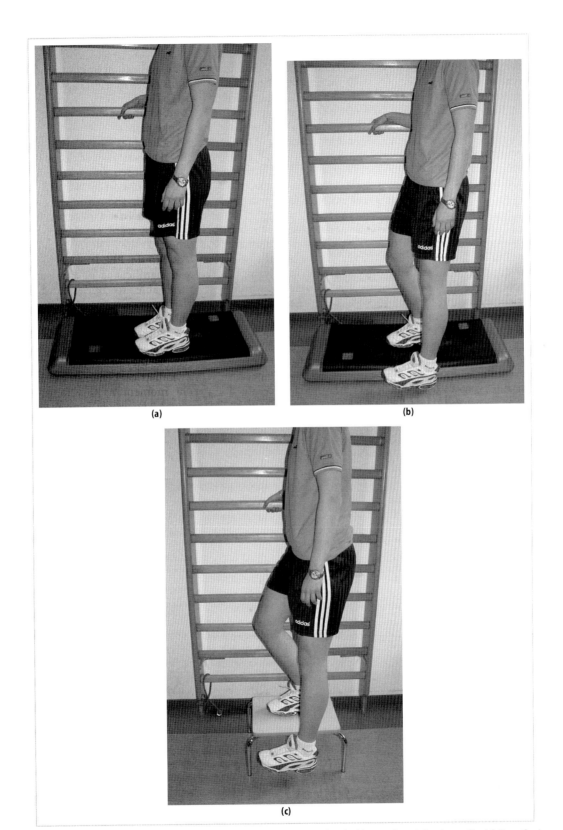

Figure 4.16. Exercises for quadriceps (of the right leg) in closed kinetic chain (lateral step) with eccentric work. Starting position **(a)**. Strengthening position **(b)**. Strengthening position with a higher step **(c)**.

problems in the PFJ develop symptoms after this last type of exercise.[55] Our philosophy should be to regain the muscular resistance along a painless arc of flexion. In the process of rehabilitation pain is the best guide. The expression "lack of pain, lack of progress" is not applicable to the rehabilitation of the extensor mechanism.

The eccentric isotonic exercises (Figure 4.17) constitute a vital part in the muscular strengthening program as a weakness of the muscles in the eccentric phase could increment the reaction forces in the PFJ.[37] It has been demonstrated that patients with anterior knee pain and patellar instability develop a larger torsional moment in the quadriceps concentric contraction than in the eccentric one.[4] On the contrary, the isotonic exercises against resistance in the concentric phase should be prohibited (this would mean condemnation to the "electric chair" for the knee). It is important to point out that there could be risk of lesions when doing the eccentric work with maximal loads, for which we advise doing this type of exercise with less than maximal and progressively controlled loads, always following the golden rule of absence of pain.

Summarizing, the indication or contraindication of the different types of exercises seems to be mainly related to the contact pressure generated in the PFJ and to the major or minor friction that can provoke pain.

Steinkamp and colleagues[55] have studied the different mechanical effects of quadriceps rehabilitation exercises in closed and open kinetic chains. As this is very important we will deal with the subject in detail. The parameters used to show the differences between these two types of rehabilitation therapy were: (1) the articular moment in the knee; (2) the PFJR force; and (3) the pressure (stress) in the PFJ. It is worth analyzing the clinical significance of these three parameters to be able to understand the obtained results.

The articular moment of the knee flexo-extension movement is the total of all the forces that favor knee joint flexion or extension movements, which, because they act at different distances from the geometrical center of the knee, create a different moment in this joint. For instance, if we hang a 2 kg weight from the knee joint in a sitting individual with the knee in

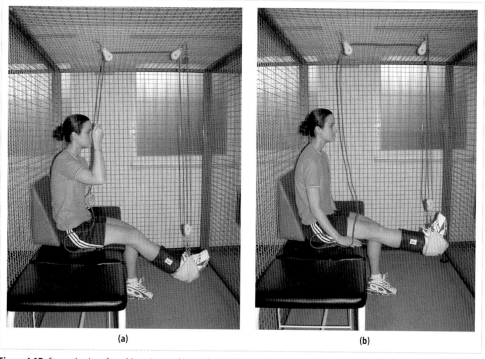

(a)   (b)

Figure 4.17. Strengthening of quadriceps in open kinetic chain with eccentric work. Patient sitting down (in Rocher cage). With the help of pulleys the patient extends the limb **(a)**. After that she flexes the knee, exercising the quadriceps in eccentric phase **(b)**.

extension, the generated moment in the knee (flexion moment, as this weight would tend to flex the knee) would be bigger than the one generated by hanging the same weight at the center of the leg (shin), as in this case the force is the same (2 kg) but the flexion moment generated in the knee (force × distance to the center of the knee) is smaller. Therefore, depending on the magnitude and direction of the acting force and on the distance to the geometrical center of the knee, the flexion moments (they tend to flex the knee) or extension moments can vary according to the exercise. As the main function of quadriceps is to extend the knee, the bigger the flexor moment generated, the bigger the muscular activity that the quadriceps muscle will have to perform to oppose this flexion force.

The reaction force in the PFJ corresponds to a much simpler concept and refers to the global force in a perpendicular direction between the femoral and patellar articular surfaces in each one of the angles of flexion of the joint, as we have mentioned before. It seems logical to suppose that more pain will be produced in this

joint as the reaction forces increase on any movement of the knee. Articular pressure can make the results vary as we will see next.

The stress (pressure) in the PFJ tells us about the distribution of the global reaction force in this joint (reaction force/contact surface). Therefore, the smaller the contact surface, the bigger will be the pressures in the joint. In spite of being completely different from a mechanical point of view, we could compare this to the explanation of the articular moment. With reference to the pressures, we have to talk about the values of the reaction force magnitude and of the contact surface, and we have to realize, paradoxically, that with a small reaction force and reduced contact surfaces higher pressures can be produced than with bigger reaction forces acting on wide contact surfaces. In a similar way to what was explained about the reaction forces, the presence of high stresses (pressures) while doing rehabilitation exercises will be associated with an increase in the articular pain.

In Figure 4.18 the three parameters (moment, reaction force, and pressures) are analyzed in

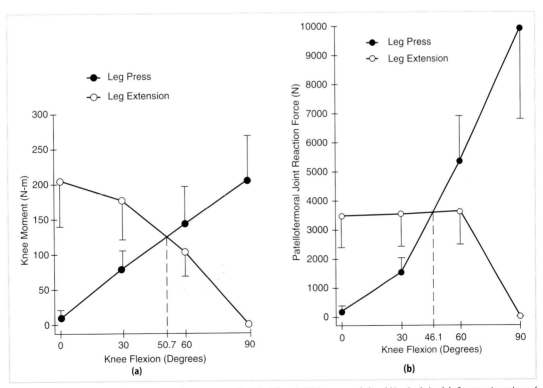

Figure 4.18. Comparative values of the articular moment at 0°, 30°, 60°, and 90° in open and closed kinetic chains **(a)**. Comparative values of the PFJR force at 0°, 30°, 60°, and 90° in open and closed kinetic chains **(b)**.

(continued)

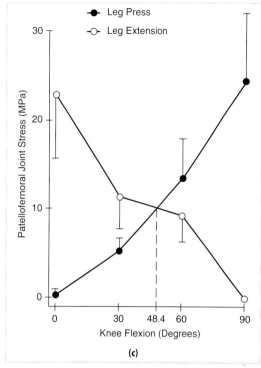

Figure 4.18. *(continued)* Comparative values of the pressures at 0°, 30°, 60°, and 90° in open and closed kinetic chains **(c)**. (Reproduced with permission from Steinkamp, LA, MF Dillingham, MD Markel et al., Biomechanical considerations in patellofemoral joint rehabilitation, *Am J Sports Med* 1993; 21: 438–444).

different amounts of knee flexion and with the two rehabilitation methods proposed. It is clear that the exercises in closed kinetic chain have a minimum in complete extension and a maximum in flexion of 90°. In a similar way the exercises in open kinetic chain show a minimum at 90° and a maximum in extension, which coincides with the intuitive appreciation that maximal relaxation of the quadriceps happens at 90° of flexion. Analyzing Figure 18 it becomes clear that the rehabilitation graphics in open and closed kinetic chains cross at one point, which corresponds with a definite flexion angle (50.7° [articular moment], 46.1° [reaction force], and 48.4° [pressure]). These intersecting values indicate that below them, the closed kinetic chain exercises provoke smaller moment, lesser reaction forces, and smaller pressure in the PFJ and due to that, they are less harmful for the patient. Nevertheless, once over these intersecting values, the open chain exercises are the ones with smaller moment, reaction forces, and pressure. Notwithstanding this, as the articular

range between 0° and 50° is more common in daily life than the range between 50° and 90°, the authors of the paper point out the convenience of rehabilitation exercises in closed chain. They also stress that these findings coincide with the clinical fact that the closed kinetic chain exercises at the physiological mobility range are less painful.

Finally, the conclusions are applicable to a comparison between two exercises performed in some determined positions and therefore only valid for the comparison of these two conditions. They are not applicable to a general comparison of the open versus closed kinetic chain exercises, as any modification of the positions and conditions in which the exercises take place would alter the obtained results, thus being able to obtain opposite results when varying the mechanical conditions in which they take place (position of the patient, suspension of weights, angle of the inclined surface).

Conclusions

The anterior knee pain syndrome and functional patellar instability in the active young person is one of the most complex knee disorders, with a multiple factor and highly variable pathogenesis, with intermingling mechanical and neurological factors. Probably the neural factor is the cause of the well-established symptoms in patients with certain mechanical anomalies and a knee overuse.

The word *overuse* is closely linked to sport, which is one of the most popular activities nowadays. In addition to favoring personal relationships, sport is a source of physical and mental health. It is amusing, relaxing, it encourages a sense of discipline, fellowship, team spirit, and will to excel. Therefore we ought to encourage it and support those who practice it. But sport can be the cause of lesions, and it is the orthopedic surgeon's duty not only to diagnose and heal them, but also to play an active role in the education of the patient to prevent them. This prevention implies detecting persons and risk situations and taking an active part in the education of the sportsplayer by means of teaching healthy habits (e.g., training of the proprioception). It could be said that the sport lesions are not accidental ones, as many of them can be prevented. If the doctor, the physiotherapist, the physical trainer, and the administration do not cooperate in this prevention, the practice of sport should not be encouraged.

Taking into account that overuse, training errors, and specific patterns of mobility in each sport can be important factors in the appearance of the symptoms, it is then easy to understand that reeducating the patient is necessary for the success of treatment and the prevention of relapses. To achieve these ends it is necessary to analyze the gait and video-analyze how the patient practices the sport. Any treatment program overlooking reeducation (training of brain "software," altering the expectations and the life style) will fail in the long run. In addition to that, the surgeon, the patient, and his family should judge whether it is convenient for the patient himself to continue practicing the same sport at the same level as before the onset of the symptoms. One has to be realistic when counseling the patient's return to sport. We have to keep in mind that not everyone is fit to practice a sport, for instance, people who show important biomechanical alterations in the alignment of the lower limbs.

References

1. Ahmad, CS, SD Kwak, GA Ateshian et al. Effects of patellar tendon adhesion to the anterior tibia on knee mechanics. *Am J Sports Med* 1998; 26: 715–724.
2. Amis, AA, and F Farahmand. Biomechanics of the knee extensor mechanism. *Knee* 1996; 3: 73–81.
3. Bellemens, J, F Cauwenberghs, E Witvrouw et al. Anteromedial tibial tubercle transfer in patients with chronic anterior knee pain and subluxation-type patellar malalignment. *Am J Sports Med* 1997; 25: 375–381.
4. Bennett, JG, and WT Stauber. Evaluation and treatment of anterior knee pain using eccentric exercise. *Med Sci Sports Exerc* 1986; 18: 526–530.
5. Blackburne, JS, and TE Peel. A new method of measuring patellar height. *J Bone Joint Surg* 1977; 59-B: 241–242.
6. Brechter, JH, and CM Powers. Patellofemoral stress during walking in persons with and without patellofemoral pain. *Med Sci Sports Exerc* 2002; 34: 1582–1593.
7. Brill, D. Sports nuclear medicine: Bone imaging for lower extremity pain in athletes. *Clin Nucl Med* 1984; 8: 101–116.
8. Brizuela, G, S Llana, AC García et al. Calzado para el baloncesto: Su efecto sobre la amortiguación del impacto y el rendimiento. *Biomecánica* 1995; 4: 146–151.
9. Brizuela, G, S Llana, and R Ferrandis. Aspectos epidemiológicos del balonmano y su relación con el calzado. *Arch Med Dep* 1996; 54: 267–274.
10. Brizuela, G, R Ferrandis, and S Llana. Aspectos epidemiológicos del calzado para baloncesto. *Arch Med Dep* 1996; 55: 391–396.
11. Carter, C, and R Sweetnam. Familial joint laxity and recurrent dislocation of the patella. *J Bone Joint Surg* 1958; 40-B: 664–667.
12. Dejour, H, G Walch, L Nove-Josserand et al. Factors of patellar instability: An anatomic radiographic study. *Knee Surg Sports Traumatol Arthrosc* 1994; 2: 19–26.
13. Eifert-Mangine, M, and JT Bilbo. Conservative management of patellofemoral chondrosis. In Mangine, RE, ed., *Clinics in Physical Therapy: Physical Therapy of the Knee,* 2nd ed. New York: Churchill Livingstone, 1995, pp. 113–142.
14. Eisenhart-Rothe, R, M Siebert, C Bringmann et al. A new in vivo technique for determination of 3D kinematics and contact areas of the patello-femoral and tibio-femoral joint. *J Biomech* 2004; 37: 927–934.
15. Ficat, P, and D Hungerford. *Disorders of the Patellofemoral Joint.* Baltimore: Williams & Wilkins, 1977.
16. Fithian, DC, DK Mishra, PF Balen et al. Instrumented measurement of patellar mobility. *Am J Sports Med* 1995; 23: 607–615.
17. Floyd, A, P Phillips, MR Khan et al. Recurrent dislocation of the patella: Histochemical and electromyographic evidence of primary muscular pathology. *J Bone Joint Surg* 1987; 69-B: 790–793.
18. Fu, FH, MJ Seel, and RA Berger. Patellofemoral biomechanics. In Fox, JM, and W Del Pizzo, eds., *The Patellofemoral Joint.* New York: McGraw-Hill, 1993, pp. 49–62.
19. Fulkerson, JP, and DS Hungerford. *Disorders of the Patellofemoral Joint.* Baltimore: Williams & Wilkins, 1990.
20. Fulkerson, JP, and KP Shea. Current concepts review: Disorders of patellofemoral alignment. *J Bone Joint Surg* 1990; 72-A: 1424–1429.
21. Gross, TS, and RC Nelson. The shock attenuation role of the ankle during landing from a vertical jump. *Med Sci Sports Excerc* 1988; 20: 506–514.
22. Gruber, MA. The conservative treatment of chondromalacia patellae. *Orthop Clin North Am* 1979; 10: 105–115.
23. Guzzanti, V, A Gigante, A Di Lazzaro et al. Patellofemoral malalignment in adolescents: Computerized tomographic assessment with or without quadriceps contraction. *Am J Sports Med* 1994; 22: 55–60.
24. Insall, J, V Goldberg, and E Salvati. Recurrent dislocation and the high-riding patella. *Clin Orthop* 1972; 88: 67–69.
25. Insall, J. "Chondromalacia patellae": Patellar malalignment syndrome. *Orthop Clin North Am* 1979; 10: 117–127.
26. Insall, J, PG Bullough, and AH Burnstein. Proximal "tube" realignment of the patella for chondromalacia patellae. *Clin Orthop* 1979; 144: 63–69.
27. Insall, J, P Aglietti, and A Tria. Patellar pain and incongruence. *Clin Orthop* 1983; 176: 225–232.
28. Insall, J. *Surgery of the Knee.* New York: Churchill Livingstone, 1993.
29. Johnson, LL. *Arthroscopic Surgery: Principles and Practice.* St. Louis: C.V. Mosby, 1986.
30. Johnson, DP, ChJ Wakeley, and I Watt. Magnetic resonance imaging of patellar tendonitis. *J Bone Joint Surg* 1996; 78-B: 452–457.
31. Kartus, J, L Magnusson, S Stener et al. Complications following arthroscopic anterior cruciate ligament reconstruction: A 2–5-year follow-up of 604 patients with special emphasis on anterior knee pain. *Knee Surg Sports Traumatol Arthrosc* 1999; 7: 2–8.
32. Kibler, WB, and TJ Chandler. Sport-specific conditioning. *Am J Sports Med* 1994; 22: 424–432.

33. Kijowski, R, D Plagens, SJ Shaeh et al. The effects of rotational deformities of the femur on contact pressure and contact area in the patellofemoral joint and on strain in the medial patellofemoral ligament. Presented at the *Annual Meeting of the International Patellofemoral Study Group*, Napa Valley, San Francisco, CA, September 1999.

34. Lieb, FJ, and J Perry. Quadriceps function: An EMG study under isometric conditions. *J Bone Joint Surg* 1971; 53-A: 749–758.

35. Llana, S, and G Brizuela. Estudio biomecánico de los impactos en los saltos. *Biomecánica* 1996; 5: 103–107.

36. Mäenpää, H, and MUK Lehto. Patellar dislocation has predisposing factors: A roentgenographic study on lateral and tangential views in patients and healthy controls. *Knee Surg Sports Traumatol Arthrosc* 1996; 4: 212–216.

37. Maunder, T. Conservative treatment of patellofemoral joint problems. *Knee* 1996; 3: 104.

38. McClay, Y, J Robinson, T Andriacchi et al. A profile of ground reaction forces in professional basketball. *J Appl Biomech* 1994; 10: 222–236.

39. McClay, Y, Robinson, T Andriacchi et al. A kinematic profile of skills in professional basketball players. *J Appl Biomech* 1994, 10: 205–221.

40. McNeil, R. *Aquatic Therapy*, 2nd ed. Abingdon: Aquatic Therapy Services, 1988.

41. O'Neill, DB. Open lateral retinacular lengthening compared with arthroscopic release: A prospective, randomized outcome study. *J Bone Joint Surg* 1997; 79-A: 1759–1769.

42. Pickett, JC, and EL Radin. *Chondromalacia of the Patella*. Baltimore: Williams and Wilkins, 1983.

43. Pitner, MA. Pathophysiology of overuse injuries in the hand and wrist. *Hand Clin* 1990; 6: 355–364.

44. Post, WR. Clinical evaluation of patients with patellofemoral disorders. *Arthroscopy* 1999; 15: 841–851.

45. Reilly, DT, and M Martens. Experimental analysis of quadriceps muscle force and patellofemoral joint reaction force for various activities. *Acta Orthop Scand* 1972; 43: 126–137.

46. Robinson, JR, EC Frederick, and LB Cooper. Systematic ankle stabilization and the effect on performance. *Med Sci Sports Exerc* 1986; 18: 625–628.

47. Rodeo, SA. Knee pain in competitive swimming. *Clin Sports Med* 1999; 18: 379–387.

48. Sanchis-Alfonso, V, E Gastaldi-Orquin, and V Martinez-SanJuan. Usefulness of computed tomography in evaluating the patellofemoral joint before and after Insall's realignment: Correlation with short-term clinical results. *Am J Knee Surg* 1994; 7: 65–72.

49. Sanchis-Alfonso, V. Cirugía de la rodilla: Conceptos actuales y controversias. Madrid: Editorial Médica Panamericana, 1995.

50. Sanchis-Alfonso, V, E Roselló-Sastre, and V Martinez-SanJuan. Pathogenesis of anterior knee pain syndrome and functional patellofemoral instability in the active young: A review. *Am J Knee Surg* 1999; 12:29–40.

51. Sanchis-Alfonso, V, A Subías-López, C Monteagudo-Castro et al. Healing of patellar tendon donor defect created after patellar tendon autograft harvesting: A long-term histological evaluation in the lamb model. *Knee Surg Sports Traumatol Arthrosc* 1999; 7: 340–348.

52. Scuderi, G, F Cuomo, and WN Scott. Lateral release and proximal realignment for patellar subluxation and dislocation. *J Bone Joint Surg* 1988; 70-A: 856–861.

53. Shelbourne, KD, and RV Trumper. Preventing anterior knee pain after anterior cruciate ligament reconstruction. *Am J Sports Med* 1997; 25: 41–47.

54. Stanitski, CL. Articular hypermobility and chondral injury in patients with acute patellar dislocation. *Am J Sports Med* 1995; 23: 146–150.

55. Steinkamp, LA, MF Dillingham, MD Markel et al. Biomechanical considerations in patellofemoral joint rehabilitation. *Am J Sports Med* 1993; 21: 438–444.

56. Teitge, RA. Treatment of complications of patellofemoral joint surgery. *Oper Tech Sports Med* 1994; 2: 317–334.

57. Trillat, A, H Dejour, and A Couette. Diagnostic et traitement des subluxations récidivantes de la rotule. *Rev Chir Orthop* 1964; 50: 813–824.

58. Van Kampen, A, and R Huiskes. The three dimensional tracking pattern of the human patella. *J Ortho Res* 1990; 8: 372–382.

59. Vilarrubias, JM. Patología del aparato extensor de la rodilla. Barcelona: Editorial JIMS, 1986.

60. Wallace, LA, and MF Sullivan. Foot alignment and knee pathology. In Mangine, RE, ed., *Clinics in Physical Therapy: Physical Therapy of the Knee,* 2nd ed. New York: Churchill Livingstone, 1995, pp. 87–110.

61. Walsh, WM. Patellofemoral joint. In DeLee, JC, and D Drez, eds., *Orthopaedic Sports Medicine: Principles and Practice*. Philadelphia: W.B. Saunders, 1994, pp. 1163–1248.

62. Ward, SR, and CM Powers. The influence of patella alta on patellofemoral joint stress during normal and fast walking. *Clin Biomech* 2004; 19: 1040–1047.

63. Weiker, GT, and KP Black. The anterior femoral osteotomy for patellofemoral instability. *Am J Knee Surg* 1997; 10: 221–227.

64. Wirhed, R. Habilidad atlética y anatomía del movimiento. Barcelona: Edika-Med, 1989.

5

Anatomy of Patellar Dislocation

Donald C. Fithian and Eiki Nomura

Abstract

Acute patellar dislocation is a common injury that can lead to disabling knee pain and/or recurrent instability. In the past 10 years, research has begun to focus on the injuries associated with acute patellar dislocation, and the specific contributions the injured structures make to patellar stability in intact knees. The implication is that injury to specific structures may have important consequences in converting a previously asymptomatic, though perhaps abnormal, patellofemoral joint into one that is painful and/or unstable. These studies have been intended to improve the precision of surgical treatment for patellar instability, and their results are driving refinements in our surgical indications as well as technique.

Introduction

Patellar dislocation can lead to disabling sequelae such as pain and recurrent instability, particularly in young athletes.[1-7] In recognition of its importance, more than 100 different procedures have been described for the treatment or prevention of recurrent patellar instability after the initial dislocation.[8,9] But surgical treatment has not been uniformly successful.[10-20] The wide array of surgical approaches suggests general uncertainty among authors about the most appropriate treatment. Widespread reports of mixed results[9,13,19-27] or outright failure[11,12] of surgical treatment suggest that such uncertainty is justified. Perhaps we've been missing something.

Despite the enormous volume of literature on patellofemoral instability and anterior knee pain, there was until recently little attention given to the structures that are injured during patellar dislocation, and the contributions these injured structures make in controlling patellar motion in the intact knee. Since the early 1990s, some investigators have focused on the individual components of the knee extensor mechanism that limit lateral patellar motion.[28-35] In vivo studies of the surgical pathology[36-43] and magnetic resonance (MR) imaging studies[36,41-44] have reported the pathoanatomy of the primary dislocation with specific attention to injuries within structures thought to play a role in controlling lateral patellar displacement. The importance of these lines of research is that they have focused attention on (1) the pathological anatomy of the initial dislocation event, and (2) the specific components of the extensor mechanism that limit lateral patellar displacement in the normal knee. This represents a novel approach to the clinical problem of the unstable patella, which holds promise for new therapeutic approaches that may enhance our understanding and treatment of this challenging problem. The purpose of this article is to bring the results and implications of this body of research into perspective within the context of the prevailing literature on patellar dislocation.

Normal Limits of Lateral Patellar Motion

Two components of the knee extensor apparatus primarily affect the limits of passive mediolateral patellar motion, as depicted in Figure 5.1. These components are: (1) bony constraint due to congruity between the patella and the femoral trochlea,[45,46] and (2) soft tissue tethers. The combination of articular buttress and soft tissue tension determines the limits of passive patellar displacement.

Studying the complex articular geometry of the patellofemoral joint between 30 and 100 degrees of knee flexion, Ahmed[29] reported that mediolateral patellar translation was controlled by the passive restraint provided by the topographic interaction of the patellofemoral contacting surfaces. In particular, patellar medial-lateral translation was controlled by the trochlear topography, while retropatellar topography also had a significant role in the control of patellar rotations ("tilt" and "spin"). Heegard[28] observed that constraint within the femoral groove dominated over the stabilizing effect of the soft-tissues through most of the range of motion in normal cadaver knees. At full extension, however, when there was little or no contact between patella and femur, the influence of the retinacula was greatest relative to that of the trochlea.[28] Figures 5.1 and 5.2 show the patellofemoral relationships at various angles of flexion. The differences between the intact and dissected knee kinematics suggested that patellar motion was controlled by the transverse soft-tissue structures near extension, and by the patellofemoral joint geometry during further flexion.[28]

Farahmand[34] measured the patellar lateral force-displacement behavior at a range of knee flexion angles and extensor muscle loads in normal human cadaver specimens. They reported that a 5 mm lateral patellar displacement required a constant displacing force (i.e., the patella had constant lateral stability) up to 60 degrees knee flexion, with a significant increase in the force at 90 degrees knee flexion. In a related study Farahmand[35] measured the trochlear depth and sulcus angle throughout the range of patellofemoral contact, and reported that the trochlear groove did not deepen with progressive knee flexion. These studies suggest that, with respect to the limits of mediolateral patellar motion in normal human knees, the trochlear shape assumes a dominant role at an early stage of knee flexion, and simulated muscle forces do not greatly enhance the constraint provided by the passive stabilizers.[34]

The anatomy of the medial and anterior knee structures has been described in detail by Warren and Marshall,[47] Kaplan,[48] Reider,[49] and Terry.[50] Warren and Marshall delineated a three-layered arrangement of tissue planes. Layer 1 includes the superficial medial retinaculum (SMR), which courses from the anteromedial tibia and extends proximally to blend with fibers of the superficial medial retinaculum over the distal patella. The medial patellotibial ligament (MPTL) is an obliquely oriented band of fibers coursing from the anteromedial tibia and blending with the fibers of the retinaculum to insert on the medial border of the patella.[31,32,50] Warren and Marshall considered the medial patellofemoral ligament (MPFL), along with the superficial medial collateral ligament (MCL), to be part of layer 2.[47] The MPFL courses from the medial femoral epicondyle,[30,40,47-49] adductor tubercle,[31,50] anterior to the medial femoral epicondyle[51] or superoposterior to the medial femoral epicondyle,[52,53] to the superomedial two-thirds of the patella. As the MPFL extends anteriorly, its fibers fuse with the undersurface of the vastus medialis tendon as shown in Figure 5.3.[49,53] Layer 3 includes the medial patellomeniscal ligament (MPML), a condensation of fibers along the medial border of the infrapatellar fat pad,[32] which inserts on the inferomedial one-third of the patella, distal to the MPFL insertion.[31,32]

The reported size and robustness of the MPFL varies considerably among anatomical cadaver studies. Reider could not even identify the medial patellofemoral ligament in some specimens.[49] Conlan found it to be variable, representing a distinct structure in 29 of 33 fresh frozen cadaver knees.[31] In 2 of 25 knees that were tested for patellar mobility, the ligament was not grossly palpable. Both these knees demonstrated greater than average lateral mobility. In a study of 9 fresh frozen cadavers, Desio et al. reported that the medial patellofemoral ligament was identified in all specimens, though its size was variable.[32] In a second study of fresh frozen human cadaver knees reported by the same group, the MPFL again was present in all specimens.[33] Hautamaa et al.[30] reported a sequential cutting and repair study where in all cases there was a palpable band running along undersurface of the distal

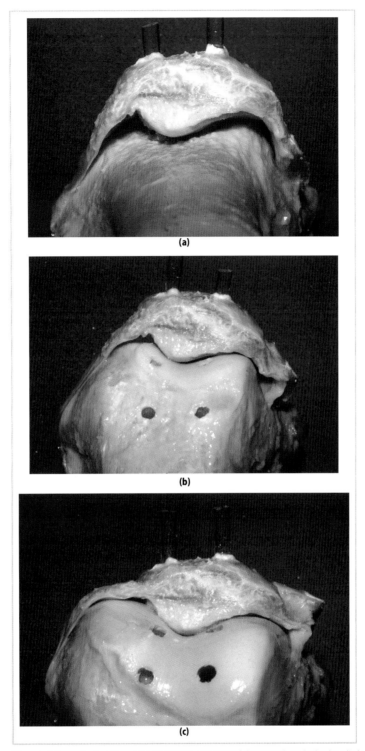

Figure 5.1. Axial view of the patellofemoral articulation at **(a)** 0˚, **(b)** 60˚, and **(c)** 120˚ flexion with a 1 kg load applied to the quadriceps. (From Nomura, E, Y Horiuchi, and M Kihara, Medial patellofemoral ligament restraint in lateral patellar translation and reconstruction, *Knee* 2000; 7(2): 121–127.)

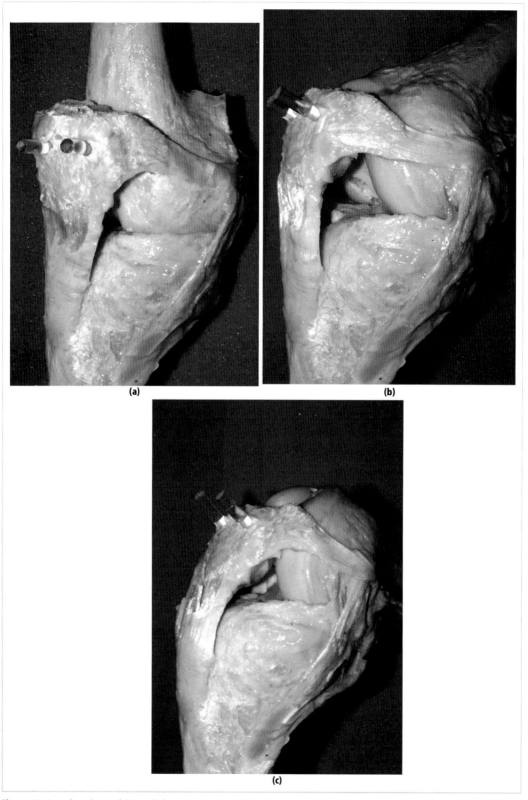

Figure 5.2. Anterolateral view of the patellofemoral articulation at **(a)** 0˚, **(b)** 60˚, and **(c)** 120˚ flexion with a 1 kg load applied to the quadriceps. (From Nomura, E, T Fujikawa, T Takeda et al., Anatomical study of the medial patellofemoral ligament, *Orthop Surg Suppl* 1992; 22: 2–5.)

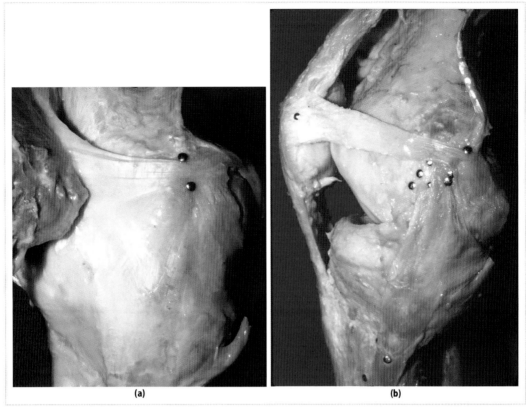

(a)   (b)

Figure 5.3. Macroscopic observation of the MPFL. When the VMO is reflected, the **(a)** MPFL can be seen. **(b)** With VMO resected the full course of the MPFL is seen. Two pins are placed at the femoral attachment. (From Nomura, E, T Fujikawa, T Takeda et al., Anatomical study of the medial patellofemoral ligament, *Orthop Surg Suppl* 1992; 22: 2–5.)

vastus medialis obliquus (VMO), attaching to both the medial femoral epicondyle and the proximal two-thirds of the patella.[30] These fibers represent the MPFL, which is distinguishable from the tendon of the VMO as it courses between the femoral epicondyle and the patella, without interposition of muscle fibers. Nomura[53] observed in 2 of 30 knees that the MPFL inserted not directly into the medial border of the patella, but into the medial aspect of the quadriceps tendon immediately proximal to its insertion at the patella. Nomura reported the dimensions of the MPFL in detail along its length, and described the relationship of the MPFL to the VMO tendon.[53] Measurement points and dimensions are summarized in Figures 5.4 and 5.5. Figure 5.6 shows the relationship of the MPFL to the VMO as they approach their respective insertions, viewed from the femoral perspective.

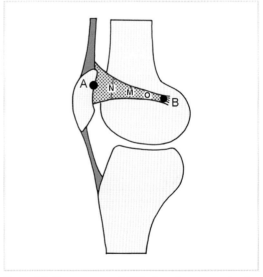

Figure 5.4. Nomura measured MPFL dimensions at several points along its length. Points N,M,O divide length AB into quarters. (From Nomura, E, T Fujikawa, T Takeda et al., Anatomical study of the medial patellofemoral ligament, *Orthop Surg Suppl* 1992; 22: 2–5.)

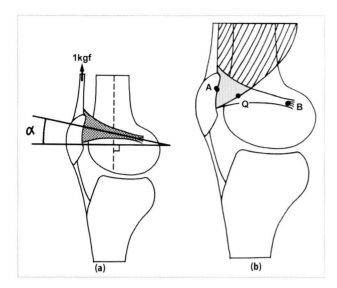

Figure 5.5. (a) The axis of the MPFL deviates proximally from a line drawn perpendicular to the femoral axis. **(b)** The VMO tendon becomes confluent with the MPFL in the region from Q to a. (From Nomura, E, T Fujikawa, T Takeda et al., Anatomical study of the medial patellofemoral ligament, *Orthop Surg Suppl* 1992; 22: 2–5.)

The contribution of specific medial retinacular structures to restraint against lateral patellar displacement has been studied in normal cadaver knees using sequential cutting methods.[30-32,52] Ligamentous retinacular structures that may be relevant to lateral patellar instability include: (1) the superficial medial patellar retinaculum (MPR),[49] (2) the medial patellotibial ligament (MPTL),[50] (3) the medial patellomeniscal ligament (MPML),[30-32] and (4) the medial patellofemoral ligament (MPFL).[30-33,49,52] These studies have consistently shown that the MPFL is the primary ligamentous restraint against lateral patellar displacement.

Nomura[52] studied the anatomy and contributions of the medial patellofemoral ligament (MPFL) and superficial medial retinaculum in restraining lateral patellar displacement using 10 fresh frozen human knee specimens. Lateral shift ratios were measured during the application of a 10 N laterally directed force with the knee in 20–120 degrees of flexion. Isolated sectioning of the MPFL greatly increased lateral displacement in the range of knee flexion studied, and isolated MPFL reconstruction restored patellar displacement to within normal limits.[52]

In selective cutting studies of human cadaver medial retinacular tissues, the MPFL has consistently been shown to provide the primary restraint against lateral patellar displacement. Conlan reported the MPFL contributed 53% of the restraining force against lateral patellar displacement.[31] In Desio's study, the MPFL contributed an average of 60 ± 13% (range 41% to 80%) of the restraining force against lateral patellar displacement in cadaver knees.[32] Interestingly, Desio et al. reported that isolated

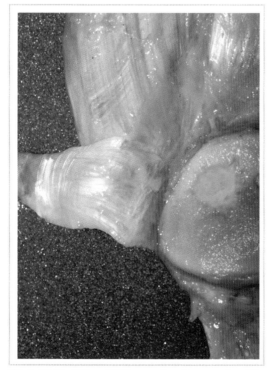

Figure 5.6. The MPFL and VMO as seen from the perspective of the femur. (From Nomura, E, T Fujikawa, T Takeda et al., Anatomical study of the medial patellofemoral ligament, *Orthop Surg Suppl* 1992; 22: 2–5.)

lateral release actually reduced resistance to lateral displacement.[32] Hautamaa observed that isolated section of the MPFL increased lateral patellar displacement 50% over that in intact knees.[30] Repair of the MPFL alone restored lateral mobility to within normal values.[30,52] Repair of more superficial retinacular tissues, as typically seen with "medial reefing," was neither necessary nor sufficient to restore stability.[30,52]

Although the vastus medialis obliquus (VMO)[8,54,55] is oriented to resist lateral patellar motion either by active contraction or by passive muscle resistance, the effect of muscle forces on patellar motion limits has not been defined clearly. With respect to resisting lateral patellar displacement, the orientation of the VMO varies greatly during knee flexion, as shown in Figure 5.7. As shown in the figures, the VMO's line of pull most efficiently resists lateral patellar motion when the knee is in deep flexion, at which time, by all accounts, trochlear containment of the patella is quite independent of soft tissue influences.[28,29,34] In Farahmand's study, lateral patellar force-displacement behavior was not affected by variations in simulated

muscle forces at any flexion angle from 15 to 75 degrees.[34]

It is worth noting that these cadaver studies were performed in normal knees, where bony geometry would in fact be expected to dominate over all soft tissue influences at all positions except early flexion.[28] On the other hand, in Hautamaa's study, which was performed at 30 degrees of knee flexion, the application of as little as 5 lb load to the central slip of the quadriceps tendon caused a measurable reduction in patellar displacement in response to medially or laterally directed 5 lb force.[30] As in other articulations, the magnitude and direction of joint compressive forces affect patellofemoral kinematics. This is particularly true during active muscle contraction. Powers et al.[56] have shown that appropriate anatomical modeling of muscle forces affects patellofemoral contact pressures. Muscle activity can affect patellar motion either by increasing joint reaction force or by generating net medializing or lateralizing force vectors within the patellofemoral joint. Therefore, depending on whether the muscle forces tend

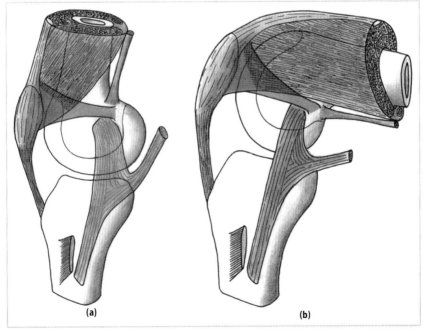

(a)   (b)

Figure 5.7. (a) Schematic drawing of the relationships between the VMO and the MPFL. **(b)** The vastus medialis overlies the distal one-third of the MPFL. (From Nomura, E, T Fujikawa, T Takeda et al., Anatomical study of the medial patellofemoral ligament, *Orthop Surg Suppl* 1992; 22: 2–5.) Its angle of pull relative to the MPFL fibers changes dramatically as the knee is flexed.

(continued)

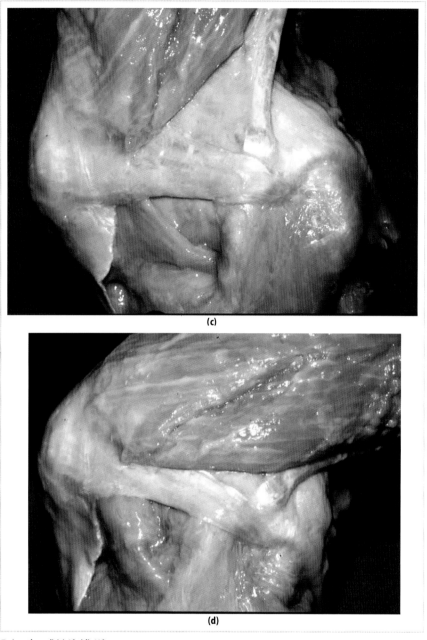

Figure 5.7. *(continued)* **(c)** 0°, **(d)** 60°,

to reduce or displace the patella with respect to the trochlea, muscle activity has an inconsistent effect on patellar kinematics.[57] If quadriceps activation reduces the patella, it prevents medial or lateral displacement and protects against dislocation; if quadriceps activation displaces the patella from the trochlea, it can cause dislocation if the passive medial restraints (ligaments) and lateral trochlear buttress fail to contain the patella.

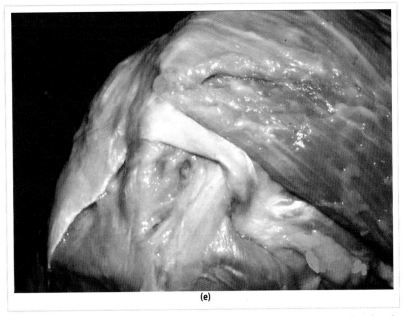

Figure 5.7. *(continued)* **(e)** 120°. (From Nomura, E, Y Horiuchi, and M Kihara, Medial patellofemoral ligament restraint in lateral patellar translation and reconstruction, *Knee* 2000; 7(2): 121–127.)

Even when muscles are aligned so as to center the patella in the trochlea, they must be activated in order to do so. While it is possible that passive muscle tension in the vastus medialis obliquus (VMO) resists lateral patellar displacement, this possibility has not been studied. Muscles are designed to do work; for them to do the work of passive stabilizers is inefficient. Muscle activity requires effort and results in compressive joint forces in order to compensate for ligamentous laxity. It is possible that the generation of high joint reaction forces may be partially responsible for the arthrosis that can occur after realignment surgery for recurrent patellar dislocation.[12,13] Advancement of the VMO in order to increase passive stiffness would have unpredictable effects because the long-term response of VMO muscle fibers to increased resting length is unknown.

In summary, muscle contraction can have inconsistent and unpredictable effects on joint mobility; it can either cause or prevent abnormal joint motions depending on the magnitude and direction of the resultant muscle force relative to the ligament deficiency.[58,59] Since muscle forces can reduce the apparent limits of joint motion by increasing joint contact force and reducing shear compliance, care must be taken when examining a joint for instability that the muscles are relaxed.[60-62] Alternatively, muscle forces that displace a joint in the direction of its pathologic laxity will result in subluxation.[58] The alignment of the extensor mechanism determines whether quadriceps contraction will tend to reduce the patella in the trochlea or displace it from the trochlea. However, the normal patella cannot be dislocated because the passive restraints prevent it from being displaced from the trochlea.[30,63,64] There exists no evidence that any amount of malalignment will cause dislocation unless the passive stabilizers are damaged. On the other hand, a hypermobile patella is unstable using Noyes's definition,[65] even if the muscles are realigned to eliminate lateralizing forces. Using this definition of patellar instability, excessive passive laxity is the essential element in instability of the patellofemoral joint, and the role of extensor alignment and muscle forces is not clear.

Anatomical Features of Acute Patellar Dislocators: The "Patella at Risk"

It has long been appreciated that there are anatomical features that seem to be characteristic of patellar instability.[66-68] Several of these features can, either alone or in combination, reduce "containment" of the patella within the trochlear groove, thus predisposing the patella to dislocation. A knee with one or more of these abnormalities may therefore be characterized as possessing a "patella at risk" for dislocation. In fact, Heywood[69] noted that the mechanism in such knees was rarely traumatic. Cash[70] and others[5,71] have noted an association between what have been called "dysplastic features" and the risk of redislocation after primary patellar dislocation, although Larsen[72] reported such a preponderance of dysplastic features among their study population that they were unable to demonstrate a specific association between most abnormalities and the risk of recurrent dislocation.

The typical "morphotype"[73] of the patellar dislocator has been characterized extensively as an adolescent female[74,75] with ligamentous laxity and multiple developmental anomalies[71,76] including patella alta,[72,76] trochlear dysplasia,[77] and rotational and angular bony malalignment.[27,78,79] Trochlear dysplasia and patella alta, which reduce the "containment" of the patella within the femoral trochlea at any given flexion angle compared to the normal knee, contribute directly to the risk of recurrent patellar dislocation by reducing the relative height of the lateral trochlear buttress.

First described by Albee in 1915,[66] and reported on axial views by Brattstrom in 1964,[67] dysplasia of the femoral sulcus is widely felt to be the most critical anatomical abnormality predisposing individuals to lateral patellar dislocation because the patella is not securely contained within the trochlea.[72,80-84] This situation puts the remaining patellar stabilizers at a disadvantage and increases their susceptibility to failure, which would produce a subluxation or dislocation.

Patella alta also is strongly associated with patellar dislocation.[2,68,72,76,85-94] A high-riding patella may be produced by spastic neuromuscular disorders such as cerebral palsy,[95] but in most cases of patellar instability it is idiopathic.[88] In patients with patella alta, Geenen reported that little trauma was required to produce a dislocation.[96] It was his opinion that patella alta was the only significant contributing factor in patellar dislocation because a high-riding patella does not engage the trochlea in time to control the rotational and lateralizing forces produced by weightbearing activities.[96] Hvid[97]

and more recently Nietosvaara[80] have shown evidence that patella alta may contribute to dysplasia of the trochlea because of altered patellofemoral mechanics during skeletal development. Whatever its effect on trochlear development, a patella such as the one shown in Figure 5.8 can be viewed as balanced on the convexity of the femoral shaft for a good part of early knee flexion. In such a knee, the medial soft tissue restraints are virtually alone in establishing the limits of lateral patellar displacement, and surely are at risk of sudden or gradual failure.

Dejour[77] defined the "crossing sign" as an intersection of the deepest part of the femoral groove with the most prominent aspect of the lateral femoral trochlear facet when viewed from a strict lateral projection on plain radiographs. This finding had high diagnostic value for the presence of patellar instability. The eminence represented the overhang of the trochlear end line in relation to the anterior cortex of the femur, which takes the shape of a beak or bump at the junction of the groove and the anterior femoral cortex. Dejour et al.[98] compared radiographs and computed tomography (CT) scans of knees with "objective" patellar instability, contralateral asymptomatic knees, and control knees. Four relevant factors were identified in

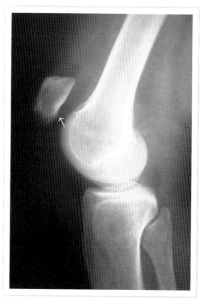

Figure 5.8. Lateral radiograph taken after reduction of a lateral patellar dislocation. Note that even at the moderate degree of flexion shown, the patella has barely entered the trochlear groove.

knees with symptomatic patellar instability: (1) trochlear dysplasia (85%), as defined by the crossing sign (96%) and quantitatively expressed by the trochlear bump, pathological above 3 mm or more (66%), and the trochlear depth, pathologic at 4 mm or less; (2) "quadriceps dysplasia" (83%), which they defined as present when the patellar tilt in extension was more than 20° on the CT scans; (3) patella alta (Caton-Deschamps) index greater than or equal to 1.2 (24%); and (4) tibial tuberosity-trochlear groove (TT-TG) distance, which they defined as pathological when greater than or equal to 20 mm (56%). The factors appeared in only 3% to 6.5% of the control knees. Like many other authors before and since, they concluded from these data that the etiology of patellar instability is multifactorial.

Because the patella is a sesamoid bone, its position and rotation are widely used to indicate the condition of the surrounding soft tissues. Extensor mechanism malalignment is a poorly defined abnormality of patellar position or rotation described on static radiographs that is often reported in the setting of patellar instability. It has been studied using axial views[45,68,99-105] and lateral views.[57,78,106,107] While it must be acknowledged that there is more to patellofemoral mechanics than bony architecture, it is doubtful that malalignment as measured in these studies offers specific evidence or clear indications as to the pathologic anatomy involved. It has already been shown that the subchondral bone does not accurately reflect the topography of the articular surface.[80,108,109] Given the limitations of radiographs, it is quite possible that they are equally imprecise in defining the condition of the ligaments and muscles around the patella. Patellar tilt and lateral subluxation, the two most frequently observed abnormalities, are caused by imbalance in the soft tissues.[98] But these effects can be produced by muscle imbalance,[8,79,92,98,110] medial laxity,[111] by lateral tightness,[104] by degenerative wear of the lateral patellar cartilage,[104,112] or a combination. Thus, the finding of tilt or lateral subluxation is ambiguous and offers only a vague suggestion as to the pathologic anatomy of the soft tissues.

Soft tissue dysplasias are seen more commonly among patellar dislocators than among normal subjects.[76,107,113-116] Ligamentous hyperlaxity, which has been described in patients with patellar instability,[69,76,113,117,118] can reduce the ability of the medial ligamentous tethers to resist lateral patellar displacement. Dysplasia of soft tissues can contribute directly to patellar dislocation if it results in hyperlaxity of the ligaments responsible for preventing lateral patellar displacement.[69,113] Muscular weakness or imbalance has been associated with patellar instability.[8,74,119] It is not known whether it is developmental[107] or the result of dislocations.[36,44,59,64,79,120] Whether primary muscular dysplasia is directly responsible for patellar dislocation has not been conclusively shown. But muscular imbalance can produce a dislocation in a knee where the passive patellar restraints are already deficient.

Familial history of patellar dislocations has been reported to increase the risk of failed surgical stabilization.[10] Reportedly, at least some of the anatomical factors that contribute to patellar instability are heritable.[116,121,122]

Patho-Anatomy of Patellar Dislocation

For a quarter century, the group at Duke University[36,43,51,59,123] has written that acute lateral patellar dislocation may result in specific medial retinacular injuries, and that the location and extent of the injuries should be documented as a part of thorough management.[59] Medial retinacular tenderness and bloody effusion have been used by numerous authors to document that a patellar dislocation has occurred.[1,4,5,37,38,59,72,124] In a retrospective series of 55 patients who underwent surgery for acute primary patellar dislocation, Vanionpää et al. reported that medial retinaculum was ruptured in 54 and stretched in 1 patient.[37]

MR imaging has enhanced the accuracy of noninvasive methods for documenting retinacular injury.[33,36,41-44] Comparison studies evaluating the diagnostic accuracy of MR imaging for identifying complete retinacular injuries have shown 95–100% agreement between preoperative MR films and the findings at surgical exploration.[33,36,42]

In his report on the surgical pathology of acute dislocation, Vanionpää did not specify the precise location of the rupture. O'Donoghue thought that the majority of cases involved avulsion of the medial retinaculum from the patella.[125] Sargent shared this view.[126] In contrast, Avikainen reported that 14 of 14 patients who underwent surgical exploration for acute patellar dislocation had avulsion of the MPFL from its femoral attachment.[40] Sallay reported a retrospective study of MR imaging and early surgical exploration and repair.[36] The study sample included 23 patients collected over a 5-year period who had presented with acute primary (first-time) patellar dislocation. Preoperative MR revealed a tear of the MPFL at the adductor tubercle in 87% of cases. Remote (parapatellar) injury, indicated by increased MR signal, was noted as well in 43% of knees, though only one patient appeared to have a complete rupture at that location. Arthroscopic evaluation was unrevealing in the majority of cases, with only three knees showing subsynovial hemorrhage in the medial gutter near the adductor tubercle. Open surgical dissection revealed avulsion of the MPFL from the adductor tubercle in 94% of knees.

Marangi reported a prospective series of 56 patients who underwent MR imaging for primary acute lateral patellar dislocation.[44] Sixty-three percent of patients had evidence of medial retinacular injury. Approximately half of all complete retinacular ruptures (27% of injured knees) were noted near the patellar insertion of the MPFL. Nine percent had complete rupture of the MPFL at the adductor tubercle. Importantly, retinacular injury commonly was noted at more than one location along the course of the MPFL (Figure 5.9). Because this imaging study

was part of a larger natural history study of patellar dislocation, surgical exploration was not performed. This weakens the conclusions because the MR findings were not confirmed by direct anatomical inspection.

Burks reported a simulation of patellar dislocation using normal cadaver knees that directly compared MR and gross anatomical findings.[33] Ten fresh-frozen cadaver knees underwent lateral patellar translation equal to 135% of the patellar width. They performed MR imaging, then dissected the medial structures to determine where ligamentous injuries had occurred, and correlated the surgical findings with the MR images. The MPFL was injured in 8 of 10 knees. The location of injury varied, but the most frequent site of injury was at the femoral attachment of the MPFL. The MPML also was avulsed from the inferomedial patella in 8 of 10 specimens. MR images showed MPFL injury in 6 of 10 knees: 2 at the femur, 3 at the patella, and 1 at both the patella and the femur. The authors felt that MR evidence of retinacular injury or avulsion fracture along the medial border of the patella represented injury to the insertion of the MPML, whereas retinacular injury near the femoral attachment of the retinaculum represented injury to the MPFL.

Nomura[41] evaluated the remnants of the medial patellofemoral ligament (MPFL) of 67 knees of 64 patients, 18 with acute patellar dislocation and 49 with chronic patellar dislocation. The MPFL injuries of the acute cases could be classified into 2 groups: an avulsion tear type and an in-substance tear type. The chronic cases fell into 3 groups: those with loose femoral attachment (9 knees), those with scar tissue formation or abnormal scar branch formation (29 knees), and those with no evidence or continuity of the ligament (absent type) (11 knees). The authors concluded that incompetence of the MPFL was a major factor in the occurrence of recurrent patellar dislocation and/or an unstable patella following acute patellar dislocation in their study sample.[41]

Clearly, retinacular injury is evident following the primary dislocation event in most cases where the retinaculum is inspected, and the injury frequently involves the MPFL. The evidence presented above suggests strongly that residual laxity of the ligament is primarily responsible for patellar instability after the initial dislocation event. Injury to the MPFL may occur at more than one location along its length during the dislocation.[33,36,44] The question arises

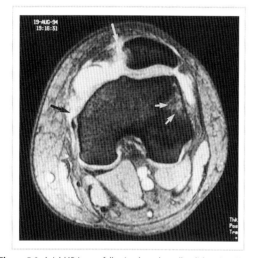

Figure 5.9. Axial MR image following lateral patellar dislocation. Note complete discontinuity of signal in the area of the MPFL (indicative of complete rupture) both at the medial femoral epicondyle (black arrow) and at the medial border of the patella (long white arrow). Lateral condylar marrow edema is also seen (short white arrows).

as to whether the ligament must be repaired at the site of injury for it to function normally. It has not been determined whether a rupture of the MPFL results, after healing, merely in lengthening of the ligament, as in MCL injuries,[127] or in a completely incompetent ligament, as in ACL injuries. Because of its close proximity and anatomical similarities to the MCL, we have hypothesized that the MPFL will heal at an increase length, and that in late repairs (after recovery from the initial dislocation) it may simply be shortened to its correct length in order to restore patellar stability. On the other hand, if acute operative repair is undertaken, failure to identify any and all locations of disruption can jeopardize the success of the repair. In such cases, the entire ligament would need to be inspected, and all sites of injury repaired. Preoperative MR imaging would be of value, as would arthroscopy. Both the MPFL and the MPML lie in the deep layer of the medial retinaculum as it inserts into the patella, and both have been shown to contribute significantly in limiting lateral patellar displacement. The goal of any surgical repair should be to restore these structures to their pre-injury status.

Obviously, the documentation of significant retinacular injury in a large number of first-time dislocators has implications for the risk of recurrent dislocation. Garth,[38] Ahmad,[39] Sallay,[36] Sargent,[126] and Vanionpää[128] have all reported satisfactory results after acute repair of the injured retinaculum. Nevertheless, some natural history studies have seemed to suggest that the absence of retinacular injury, a less traumatic mechanism of injury, and familial history of patellar instability predicted a higher risk of redislocation.[6,10] It may be that the anatomical predisposition is the most important factor in predicting recurrence after the initial dislocation event. But it may be that specific structures, when injured, also play a role in recurrent instability. It remains to be seen how important that role is.

Summary and Future Directions

Patella dislocation often occurs in knees with an identifiable anatomic predisposition. Yet the initial dislocation event itself often results in injury to the medial ligaments responsible for restraining the patella. The central question for the immediate future is: What anatomical features play major roles in determining the risk of primary dislocation and recurrent instability? Note that these are not the same thing. Though many clinical studies combine primary and recurrent dislocators, it is not clear that the two groups represent the same population. The authors believe that failure to distinguish between them is partly responsible for the confusion that remains about patellofemoral instability.

Other areas of particular interest at this time include the biology of MPFL healing and studies comparing the surgical pathology of primary and recurrent dislocations. It is not known how the location of MPFL injury affects its healing potential, and longitudinal studies have not been published showing tissue healing over time after dislocation.

Finally, prospective clinical trials are needed to narrow the range of surgical approaches and compare their success rates in specific clinical scenarios. The anatomical concepts presented in this paper provide principles that could be used to design such studies.

Acknowledgments
The authors wish to thank the members of the International Patellofemoral Study Group, whose collaboration inspires and informs our work.

References
1. Nietosvaara, Y, K Aalto, and PE Kallio. Acute patellar dislocation in children: incidence and associated osteochondral fractures. *J Pediatr Orthop* 1994; 14(4):513–515.
2. Atkin, DM, DC Fithian, KS Marangi et al. Characteristics of patients with primary acute lateral patellar dislocation and their recovery within the first 6 months of injury [in process citation]. *Am J Sports Med* 2000; 28(4): 472–479.
3. Levy, AS, MJ Wetzler, M Lewars et al. Knee injuries in women collegiate rugby players. *Am J Sports Med* 1997; 25(3): 360–362.
4. Cofield, RH, and RS Bryan. Acute dislocation of the patella: Results of conservative treatment. *J Trauma* 1977; 17(7): 526–531.
5. Hawkins, RJ, RH Bell, and G Anisette. Acute patellar dislocations: The natural history. *Am J Sports Med* 1986; 14(2): 117–120.
6. Maenpaa, H, H Huhtala, and MU Lehto. Recurrence after patellar dislocation. Redislocation in 37/75 patients followed for 6–24 years. *Acta Orthop Scand* 1997; 68(5): 424–426.
7. Dandy, DJ. Recurrent subluxation of the patella on extension of the knee. *J Bone Joint Surg [Br]* 1971; 53(3): 483–487.
8. Hughston, JC. Subluxation of the patella. *J Bone Joint Surg [Am]* 1968; 50(5): 1003–1026.
9. Madigan, R, HA Wissinger, and WF Donaldson. Preliminary experience with a method of quadricepsplasty in recurrent subluxation of the patella. *J Bone Joint Surg [Am]* 1975; 57(5): 600–607.

10. Maenpaa, H, and MU Lehto. Surgery in acute patellar dislocation: Evaluation of the effect of injury mechanism and family occurrence on the outcome of treatment. *Br J Sports Med* 1995; 29(4): 239–241.

11. Nikku, R, Y Nietosvaara, PE Kallio et al. Operative versus closed treatment of primary dislocation of the patella: Similar 2-year results in 125 randomized patients [see comments]. *Acta Orthop Scand* 1997; 68(5): 419–423.

12. Arnbjornsson, A, N Egund, O Rydling et al. The natural history of recurrent dislocation of the patella: Long-term results of conservative and operative treatment. *J Bone Joint Surg [Br]* 1992; 74(1): 140–142.

13. Crosby, EB, and J Insall. Recurrent dislocation of the patella: Relation of treatment to osteoarthritis. *J Bone Joint Surg [Am]* 1976; 58(1): 9–13.

14. Wall, JJ. Compartment syndrome as a complication of the Hauser procedure. *J Bone Joint Surg [Am]* 1979; 61(2): 185–191.

15. Barbari, S, TS Raugstad, N Lichtenberg et al. The Hauser operation for patellar dislocation: 3-32-year results in 63 knees. *Acta Orthop Scand* 1990; 61(1): 32–35.

16. Juliusson, R, and G Markhede. A modified Hauser procedure for recurrent dislocation of the patella: A long-term follow-up study with special reference to osteoarthritis. *Arch Orthop Trauma Surg* 1984; 103(1): 42–46.

17. Hampson, WG, and P Hill. Late results of transfer of the tibial tubercle for recurrent dislocation of the patella. *J Bone Joint Surg [Br]* 1975; 57(2): 209–213.

18. Lanier, BE. Stuck medial patella: Unusual complication of a Hauser-Hughston patellar-shaving procedure. *NY State J Med* 1977; 77(12): 1955–1957.

19. DeCesare, WF. Late results of Hauser procedure for recurrent dislocation of the patella. *Clin Orthop* 1979(140): 137–144.

20. Chrisman, OD, GA Snook, and TC Wilson. A long-term prospective study of the Hauser and Roux-Goldthwait procedures for recurrent patellar dislocation. *Clin Orthop* 1979(144): 27–30.

21. Brown, DE, AH Alexander, and DM Lichtman. The Elmslie-Trillat procedure: Evaluation in patellar dislocation and subluxation. *Am J Sports Med* 1984; 12(2): 104–109.

22. Cartier, P, C Cistac, and D Maulaz. Results of surgical treatment of patellar disequilibrium: Apropos of 311 cases. *Acta Orthop Belg* 1989; 55(3): 395–409.

23. Cox, JS. Evaluation of the Roux-Elmslie-Trillat procedure for knee extensor realignment. *Am J Sports Med* 1982; 10(5): 303–310.

24. Fielding, JW, WA Liebler, ND Krishne Urs et al. Tibial tubercle transfer: A long-range follow-up study. *Clin Orthop* 1979(144): p. 43–44.

25. Larsen, E, and JE Varmarken. Recurrent dislocation of the patella: Two principles of treatment prospectively studied. *Acta Orthop Belg* 1988; 54(4): 434–438.

26. Morshuis, WJ, PW Pavlov, and KP de Rooy. Anteromedialization of the tibial tuberosity in the treatment of patellofemoral pain and malalignment. *Clin Orthop* 1990(255): 242–250.

27. Trillat, A, H DeJour, and A Couette. Diagnostic et traitement des subluxations recidivantes de la rotule. *Rev Chir Orthop (Paris)* 1964; 50: 813-824.

28. Heegaard, J, PF Leyvraz, A Van Kampen et al. Influence of soft structures on patellar three-dimensional tracking. *Clin Orthop* 1994(299): 235–243.

29. Ahmed, AM, and NA Duncan. Correlation of patellar tracking pattern with trochlear and retropatellar surface topographies. *J Biomech Eng* 2000; 122(6): 652–660.

30. Hautamaa, PV, DC Fithian, KR Kaufman et al. Medial soft tissue restraints in lateral patellar instability and repair. *Clin Orthop* 1998(349): 174–182.

31. Conlan, T, WP Garth, Jr., and JE Lemons. Evaluation of the medial soft-tissue restraints of the extensor mechanism of the knee. *J Bone Joint Surg Am* 1993; 75(5): 682–693.

32. Desio, SM, RT Burks, and KN Bachus. Soft tissue restraints to lateral patellar translation in the human knee. *Am J Sports Med* 1998; 26(1): 59–65.

33. Burks, RT, SM Desio, KN Bachus et al. Biomechanical evaluation of lateral patellar dislocations. *Am J Knee Surg* 1998; 11(1): 24–31.

34. Farahmand, F, MN Tahmasbi, and AA Amis. Lateral force-displacement behaviour of the human patella and its variation with knee flexion: A biomechanical study in vitro. *J Biomech* 1998; 31(12): 1147–1152.

35. Farahmand, F, W Senavongse, and AA Amis. Quantitative study of the quadriceps muscles and trochlear groove geometry related to instability of the patellofemoral joint. *J Orthop Res* 1998; 16(1): 136–143.

36. Sallay, PI, J Poggi, KP Speer et al. Acute dislocation of the patella: A correlative pathoanatomic study. *Am J Sports Med* 1996: 24(1): 52–60.

37. Vainionpaa, S, E Laasonen, H Patiala et al. Acute dislocation of the patella: Clinical, radiographic and operative findings in 64 consecutive cases. *Acta Orthop Scand* 1986; 57(4): 331–333.

38. Garth, WP Jr., DG DiChristina, and G Holt. Delayed proximal repair and distal realignment after patellar dislocation. *Clin Orthop* 2000(377): 132–144.

39. Ahmad, CS, BE Stein, D Matuz et al. Immediate surgical repair of the medial patellar stabilizers for acute patellar dislocation: A review of eight cases. *Am J Sports Med* 2000; 28(6): 804–810.

40. Avikainen, VJ, RK Nikku, and TK Seppanen-Lehmonen. Adductor magnus tenodesis for patellar dislocation: Technique and preliminary results. *Clin Orthop* 1993(297): 12–16.

41. Nomura, E. Classification of lesions of the medial patello-femoral ligament in patellar dislocation. *Int Orthop* 1999; 23(5): 260–263.

42. Kirsch, MD, SW Fitzgerald, H Friedman et al. Transient lateral patellar dislocation: diagnosis with MR imaging. *AJR Am J Roentgenol* 1993; 161(1): 109–113.

43. Spritzer, CE, DL Courneya, DL Burk Jr. et al. Medial retinacular complex injury in acute patellar dislocation: MR findings and surgical implications. *AJR Am J Roentgenol* 1997; 168(1): 117–122.

44. Marangi, K, LM White, J Brossmann et al. *Magnetic Resonance Imaging of the Knee Following Acute Lateral Patellar Dislocation,* 63rd Annual Meeting of the American Academy of Orthopaedic Surgeons, Atlanta, GA, February 22–26, 1996.

45. Merchant, AC, RL Mercer, RH Jacobsen et al. Roentgenographic analysis of patellofemoral congruence. *J Bone Joint Surg [Am]* 1974; 56(7): 1391–1396.

46. Willems, S, R Litt, A Albassir et al. Comparative study of a series of normal knees and a series of knees with patellar instability. *Acta Orthop Belg* 1989; 55(3): 339–345.

47. Warren, LF, and JL Marshall. The supporting structures and layers on the medial side of the knee: An anatomical analysis. *J Bone Joint Surg [Am]* 1979; 61(1): 56–62.

48. Kaplan, EB. Factors responsible for the stability of the knee joint. *Bull Hosp Joint Dis* 1957; 18: 51–59.

49. Reider, B, JL Marshall, B Koslin et al. The anterior aspect of the knee joint. *J Bone Joint Surg [Am]* 1981; 63(3): 351–356.

50. Terry, GC. The anatomy of the extensor mechanism. *Clin Sports Med* 1989; 8(2): 163–177.

51. Feller, JA, JA Feagin Jr., and WE Garrett Jr. The medial patellofemoral ligament revisited: An anatomical study. *Knee Surg Sports Traumatol Arthrosc* 1993; 1(3–4): 184–186.

52. Nomura, E, Y Horiuchi, and M Kihara. Medial patellofemoral ligament restraint in lateral patellar translation and reconstruction. *Knee* 2000; 7(2): 121–127.

53. Nomura, E, T Fujikawa, T Takeda et al. Anatomical study of the medial patellofemoral ligament. *Orthop Surg Suppl* 1992; 22: 2–5.

54. Lieb, FJ, and J Perry. Quadriceps function: An anatomical and mechanical study using amputated limbs. *J Bone Joint Surg Am* 1968; 50(8): 1535–1548.

55. Scharf, W, R Weinstrabl, and W Firbas. Anatomic studies of the extensor system of the knee joint and its clinical relevance. *Unfallchirurg* 1986; 89(10): 456–462.

56. Powers, CM, JC Lilley, and TQ Lee. The effects of axial and multi-plane loading of the extensor mechanism on the patellofemoral joint. *Clin Biomech (Bristol, Avon)* 1998; 13: 616–624.

57. Maldague, B, and J Malghem. Significance of the radiograph of the knee profile in the detection of patellar instability: Preliminary report. *Rev Chir Orthop Reparatrice Appar Mot* 1985; 71(Suppl 2): 5–13.

58. Daniel, DM, J Lawler, LL Malcom et al. The quadriceps anterior cruciate interaction. *J Bone Joint Surg* 1982.

59. Bassett, FH. Acute dislocation of the patella, osteochondral fractures, and injuries to the extensor mechanism of the knee. In *Amer Acad Orth Surg Instr Course Lect* 1976; *Amer Acad Orth Surg*: Rosemont: 40–49.

60. Shoemaker, SC, and DM Daniel. The limits of knee motion: In vitro studies. In Daniel, DM, WH Akeson, and JJ O'Connor, eds., *Knee Ligaments: Structure, Function, Injury, and Repair.* New York: Raven Press, 1990, pp. 153–161.

61. Daniel, DM. Assessing the limits of knee motion. *Am J Sports Med* 1991; 19(2): 139–147.

62. Daniel, DM. Diagnosis of a ligament injury. In Daniel, DM, WA Akeson, and JJ O'Connor, eds., *Knee Ligaments: Structure, Function, Injury, and Repair.* New York: Raven Press, 1990, pp. 3–10.

63. Teitge, RA, WW Faerber, P Des Madryl et al. Stress radiographs of the patellofemoral joint. *J Bone Joint Surg Am* 1996; 78(2): 193–203.

64. Fithian, DC, DK Mishra, PF Balen et al. Instrumented measurement of patellar mobility. *Am J Sports Med* 1995; 23(5): 607–615.

65. Noyes, FR, ES Grood, and PA Torzilli. Current concepts review: The definitions of terms for motion and position of the knee and injuries of the ligaments [see comments]. *J Bone Joint Surg [Am]* 1989; 71(3): 46–72.

66. Albee, RH. The bone graft wedge in the treatment of habitual dislocation of the patella. *Med Record* 1915; 88: 257–259.

67. Brattstrom, H. Shape of the intercondylar groove normally and in recurrent dislocation of patella: A clinical and x-ray anatomical investigation. *Acta Orth Scand Suppl* 1964; 68: 134–148.

68. Wiberg, G. Roentgenographic and anatomic studies on the patellofemoral joint: With special reference to chondromalacia patella. *Acta Orthop Scand* 1941; 12: 319–410.

69. Heywood, AWB. Recurrent dislocation of the patella: a study of its pathology and treatment in 106 knees. *J Bone Joint Surg Br* 1961; 43: 508–517.

70. Cash, JD, and JC Hughston. Treatment of acute patellar dislocation. *Am J Sports Med* 1988; 16(3): 244–249.

71. Maenpaa, H, and MU Lehto. Patellar dislocation has predisposing factors: A roentgenographic study on lateral and tangential views in patients and healthy controls. *Knee Surg Sports Traumatol Arthrosc* 1996; 4(4): 212–216.

72. Larsen, E, and F Lauridsen, Conservative treatment of patellar dislocations: Influence of evident factors on the tendency to redislocation and the therapeutic result. *Clin Orthop* 1982(171): 131–136.

73. Lerat, JL. Morphotypes of patellar instability. *Rev Chir Orthop Reparatrice Appar Mot* 1982; 68(1): 50–52.

74. Floyd, A, P Phillips, MR Khan et al. Recurrent dislocation of the patella: Histochemical and electromyographic evidence of primary muscle pathology. *J Bone Joint Surg [Br]* 1987; 69(5): 790–793.

75. MacNab, I. Recurrent dislocation of the patella. *J Bone Joint Surg Br* 1952; 34: 957–967.

76. Runow, A. The dislocating patella: Etiology and prognosis in relation to generalized joint laxity and anatomy of the patellar articulation. *Acta Orthop Scand Suppl* 1983; 201: 1–53.

77. Dejour, H, G Walch, P Neyret et al. Dysplasia of the femoral trochlea. *Rev Chir Orthop Reparatrice Appar Mot* 1990; 76(1): 45–54.

78. Murray, TF, JY Dupont, and JP Fulkerson. Axial and lateral radiographs in evaluating patellofemoral malalignment. *Am J Sports Med* 1999; 27(5): 580–584.

79. Insall, J, PG Bullough, and AH Burstein. Proximal "tube" realignment of the patella for chondromalacia patellae. *Clin Orthop* 1979(144): 63–69.

80. Nietosvaara, Y, and K Aalto. The cartilaginous femoral sulcus in children with patellar dislocation: An ultrasonographic study. *J Pediatr Orthop* 1997; 17(1): 50–53.

81. Jacobsen, K, and P Metz. Occult traumatic dislocation of the patella. *J Trauma* 1976; 16(10): 829–835.

82. Kujala, UM, K Osterman, M Kormano et al. Patellofemoral relationships in recurrent patellar dislocation. *J Bone Joint Surg [Br]* 1989; 71(5): 788–792.

83. Schutzer, SF, GR Ramsby, and JP Fulkerson. Computed tomographic classification of patellofemoral pain patients. *Orthop Clin North Am* 1986; 17(2): 235–248.

84. Buard, J, J Benoit, A Lortat-Jacob et al. The depth of the patellar groove of the femur (author's trans.). *Rev Chir Orthop Reparatrice Appar Mot* 1981; 67(8): 721–729.

85. Simmons, E Jr., and JC Cameron. Patella alta and recurrent dislocation of the patella. *Clin Orthop* 1992(274): 265–269.

86. Leung, YF, YL Wai, and YC Leung. Patella alta in southern China: A new method of measurement. *Int Orthop* 1996; 20(5): 305–310.

87. Lancourt, JE, and JA Cristini. Patella alta and patella infera: Their etiological role in patellar dislocation, chondromalacia, and apophysitis of the tibial tubercle. *J Bone Joint Surg [Am]* 1975; 57(8): 1112–1115.

88. Caton, J, A Mironneau, G Walch et al. Idiopathic high patella in adolescents. Apropos of 61 surgical cases. *Rev Chir Orthop Reparatrice Appar Mot* 1990; 76(4): 253–260.

89. Glimet, T. Course of recurrent dislocation of the patella, patellar syndrome without dislocation and femoropatellar osteoarthritis. *Ann Radiol (Paris)* 1993; 36(3): 215–219.

90. Insall, J, V Goldberg, and E Salvati. Recurrent dislocation and the high-riding patella. *Clin Orthop* 1972; 88: 67–69.

91. Blackburne, JS, and TE Peel. A new method of measuring patellar height. *J Bone Joint Surg Br* 1977; 59(2): 241–242.

92. Bernageau, J, D Goutallier, J Debeyre et al. New exploration technic of the patellofemoral joint: Relaxed axial quadriceps and contracted quadriceps. *Rev Chir Orthop Reparatrice Appar Mot* 1975; 61(Suppl 2): 286–290.

93. Kimberlin, GE. Radiological assessment of the patellofemoral articulation and subluxation of the patella. *Radiol Technol* 1973; 45(3): 129–137.

94. Norman, O, N Egund, L Ekelund et al. The vertical position of the patella. *Acta Orthop Scand* 1983; 54(6): 908–913.

95. Aparicio, G, JC Abril, J Albinana et al. Patellar height ratios in children: An interobserver study of three methods. *J Pediatr Orthop B* 1999; 8(1): 29–32.

96. Geenen, E, G Molenaers, and M Martens. Patella alta in patellofemoral instability. *Acta Orthop Belg* 1989; 55(3): 387–393.

97. Hvid, I, LI Andersen, and H Schmidt. Patellar height and femoral trochlear development. *Acta Orthop Scand* 1983; 54(1): 91–93.

98. Dejour, H, G Walch, L Nove-Josserand et al. Factors of patellar instability: An anatomic radiographic study. *Knee Surg Sports Traumatol Arthrosc* 1994; 2(1): 19–26.

99. Guzzanti, V, A Gigante, A Di Lazzaro et al. Patellofemoral malalignment in adolescents: Computerized tomographic assessment with or without quadriceps contraction. *Am J Sports Med* 1994; 22(1): 55–60.

100. Shelbourne, KD, DA Porter, and W Rozzi. Use of a modified Elmslie-Trillat procedure to improve abnormal patellar congruence angle. *Am J Sports Med* 1994; 22(3): 318–323.

101. Malghem, J, and B Maldague. Patellofemoral joint: 30 degrees axial radiograph with lateral rotation of the leg. *Radiology* 1989; 170(2): 566–567.

102. Dixon, AM. Demonstration of lateral patellar subluxation: The 30 degrees LR projection lateral rotation. *Radiogr Today* 1991; 57(647): 20–21.

103. Morscher, E. Indications and possibilities of patella wedge osteotomy. *Orthopade* 1985; 14(4): 261–265.

104. Schutzer, SF, GR Ramsby, and JP Fulkerson. The evaluation of patellofemoral pain using computerized tomography: A preliminary study. *Clin Orthop* 1986(204): 286–293.

105. Somer, T, and B Bokorov. The axial image of the femoropatellar joint. *Med Pregl* 1985; 38(5–6): 283–287.

106. Moller, BN, B Krebs, and AG Jurik. Patellofemoral incongruence in chondromalacia and instability of the patella. *Acta Orthop Scand* 1986; 57(3): 232–234.

107. Nove-Josserand, L, and D Dejour. Quadriceps dysplasia and patellar tilt in objective patellar instability. *Rev Chir Orthop Reparatrice Appar Mot* 1995; 81(6): 497–504.

108. Staubli, HU, U Durrenmatt, B Porcellini et al. Anatomy and surface geometry of the patellofemoral joint in the axial plane. *J Bone Joint Surg Br* 1999; 81(3): 452–458.

109. Nietosvaara, Y. The femoral sulcus in children: An ultrasonographic study. *J Bone Joint Surg Br* 1994; 76(5): 807–809.

110. Delgado-Martinez, AD, C Estrada, EC Rodriguez-Merchan et al. CT scanning of the patellofemoral joint: The quadriceps relaxed or contracted? *Int Orthop* 1996; 20(3): 159–162.

111. Arendt, E, Personal Communication 1996.

112. Ficat, RP, J Philippe, and DS Hungerford. Chondromalacia patellae: A system of classification. *Clin Orthop* 1979(144): 55–62.

113. Stanitski, CL. Articular hypermobility and chondral injury in patients with acute patellar dislocation. *Am J Sports Med* 1995; 23(2): 146–150.

114. Gunn, DR. Contracture of the quadriceps muscle: A discussion on the etiology and relationship to recurrent dislocation of the patella. *J Bone Joint Surg Br* 1964; 46: 492–497.

115. Jeffreys, TE. Recurrent dislocation of the patella due to abnormal attachment of the ilio-tibial tract. *J Bone Joint Surg Br* 1963; 45: 740–743.

116. Beighton, PH, and FT Horan. Dominant inheritance in familial generalised articular hypermobility. *J Bone Joint Surg Br* 1970; 52(1): 145–147.

117. Carter, C, and R Sweetnam. Familial joint laxity and recurrent dislocation of the patella. *J Bone Joint Surg Br* 1958; 40: 664–667.

118. Ahstrom, JP Jr. Osteochondral fracture in the knee joint associated with hypermobility and dislocation of the patella: Report of eighteen cases. *J Bone Joint Surg [Am]* 1965; 47(8): 1491–1502.

119. Mariani, PP, and I Caruso. An electromyographic investigation of subluxation of the patella. *J Bone Joint Surg Br* 1979; 61-B(2): 169–171.

120. Fox, TA. Dysplasia of the quadriceps mechanism: Hypoplasia of the vastus medialis muscle as related to the hypermobile patella syndrome. *Surg Clin North Am* 1975; 55: 199–226.

121. Miller, GF. Familial recurrent dislocation of the patella. *J Bone Joint Surg [Br]* 1978; 60-B(2): 203–204.

122. Rouvillain, JL, N Piquion, A Lepage-Lezin et al. A familial form of bilateral recurrent dislocation of the patella with major trochlea dysplasia. *Rev Chir Orthop Reparatrice Appar Mot* 1998; 84(3): 285–291.

123. Boden, BP, AW Pearsall, WE Garrett Jr. et al. Patellofemoral instability: Evaluation and management. *J Am Acad Orthop Surg* 1997; 5(1): 47–57.

124. Maenpaa, H, and MU Lehto. Patellar dislocation: The long-term results of nonoperative management in 100 patients. *Am J Sports Med* 1997; 25(2): 213–217.

125. O'Donoghue, DH. *Treatment of Injuries to Athletes*, 3rd ed. Philadelphia: Saunders, 1976, pp. 600–617.

126. Sargent, JR, and WA Teipner. Medial patellar retinacular repair for acute and recurrent dislocation of the patella-a preliminary report. *J Bone Joint Surg [Am]* 1971; 53: 386.

127. Murphy, PG, CB Frank, and DA Hart. The cell biology of ligaments and ligament healing. In Jackson, DW, ed., *The Anterior Cruciate Ligament: Current and Future Concepts*. New York: Raven Press, 1993, pp. 165–177.

128. Vainionpaa, S, E Laasonen, T Silvennoinen et al. Acute dislocation of the patella: A prospective review of operative treatment. *J Bone Joint Surg [Br]* 1990; 72(3): 366–369.

6

Evaluation of the Patient with Anterior Knee Pain and Patellar Instability

Vicente Sanchis-Alfonso, Carlos Puig-Abbs, and Vicente Martínez-Sanjuan

Introduction

When dealing with patients suffering from anterior knee pain and patellar instability a thorough anamnesis and a complete and careful physical examination are the main means to reach a correct diagnosis and once this done, start the most appropriate treatment. Imaging studies only help to confirm the diagnosis or to complement the data obtained by the history and examination of the patient. This chapter provides an overview of the most important aspects of the history, physical examination, emotional and psychiatric evaluation, imaging studies, and arthroscopic evaluation. Obviously, if the etiology of patellofemoral pain and patellar instability is multifactorial, then the evaluation must also consider all the different factors.

History

The first diagnostic step is a thorough history. This is the main clue for an exact diagnosis. For instance, absence of a traumatic episode or presence of bilateral symptoms should lead toward patellofemoral pathology and against meniscal derangement in the young patient; on the contrary, the presence of effusion suggests intra-articular pathology (e.g., meniscal rupture, pathologic plicae, osteochondral or chondral loose bodies, synovial pathology, peripatellar synovitis) rather than a peripatellar condition. A small effusion, however, may be present with patellofemoral syndrome.

However, poliarthralgiae are not a part of the pathology we are now dealing with.

Patients with patellar symptoms can be divided into two groups: those with anterior knee pain and those with patellar instability. We must determine if the main complaint is pain or instability. It is common to have symptoms in both knees that may change from one knee to the other over time. This is a tip-off of a patellofemoral problem.

Generally, the onset of symptoms is insidious, without traumatism, reflecting an overuse condition or an underlying malalignment. Overuse can be the result of a new activity or of the increase in time, frequency, or intensity of a previous work or sport activity. In these cases, history should be oriented to determine which supraphysiological loading activity or activities are of importance in the origin of anterior knee symptoms. Identification and rigorous control of the activities associated with the initiation and persistence of symptoms is crucial for the treatment success. For example, patients with left anterior knee pain should avoid driving a car with a clutch for prolonged periods of time because it aggravates the symptoms. In these cases patient education is crucial to prevent recurrence. In other cases, symptoms can be secondary to a direct (e.g., automobile accident in which the anterior knee strikes the dashboard ["dashboard knee"]) or indirect (internal rotation of the femur on an externally rotated tibia in a flexed and valgus knee position) knee traumatism.

Pain is often described as dull with occasional episodes of acute sharp pain. Pain rarely is constant and asymptomatic periods are frequent. It is difficult for the patient with anterior knee pain to pinpoint the area of pain, placing his or her hand over the anterior aspect of the knee when we ask them to locate the pain. However, the pain can also be medial, lateral, or popliteal. Generally, patients have multiple painful sites with different pain intensity. Pain related to extensor mechanism is typically exacerbated by physical activity, descending stairs (which requires eccentric quadriceps contraction), or after prolonged sitting, for instance during a long trip by car or prolonged sitting in a cinema ("movie sign" or "theater sign"), and improves by extending the knee. A constant and severe pain far out of proportion to physical findings must make us think of psychological issues or reflex sympathetic dystrophy (RSD) even when the classic vasomotor findings are absent.[25] Finally, constant burning pain indicates a neuromatous origin.

One must not forget the possibility of pain secondary to a posterior cruciate ligament (PCL) deficiency when there has been a knee traumatism. This is a well-known cause for anterior knee pain, given that PCL tears increase patellofemoral joint reaction force by posterior displacement of the tibial tuberosity.[25] It is also important to examine the integrity of the anterior cruciate ligament (ACL) as anterior knee pain is present in 20–27% of patients with ACL chronic insufficiency.[25]

Regarding instability, "giving-way" episodes due to ACL or meniscal tears are brought about by rotational activities, whereas giving-way episodes related to patellofemoral problems are associated to activities that do not imply rotational strains,[11] and are a consequence of a sudden reflex inhibition and/or atrophy of the quadriceps muscle.

Patients sometimes report locking of the knee, which usually is only a catching sensation, but they are able to actively unlock the knee and therefore this type of locking should not be mixed up with the one experienced by patients with meniscal lesions. Another symptom is the crepitus, which should not be mistaken from the snapping sensation more consistent with a pathologic plica.

Physical Examination

The second diagnostic step is a complete and careful physical examination. Its primary goal is to locate the painful zone, and reproduce the symptoms (pain and/or instability). The location of pain can indicate which structure is injured, which is extremely helpful to make the diagnosis and plan the treatment. Both legs should be examined.

The lateral retinaculum ought to be felt and assessed carefully. Tenderness somewhere over the lateral retinaculum, especially where the retinaculum inserts into the patella, is a very frequent finding (90%) in patients with anterior knee pain.[9] We perform the patellar glide test (Figure 6.1) to evaluate lateral retinacular tightness. This test is performed with the knee flexed 30°, and the quadriceps relaxed. The patella is divided into four longitudinal quadrants. The patella is displaced in a medial direction. A medial translation of one quadrant or less is suggestive of excessive lateral tightness.[25] With this test pain is elicited over the lateral retinaculum. Patellar tilt test can also detect a tight lateral retinaculum, and should always be carried out (Figure 6.2). In a normal knee, the patella can be lifted from its lateral edge farther than the transepicondylar axis, with a fully extended knee. On the contrary, a patellar tilt of 0° or less indicates a tight lateral retinaculum. Lateral retinacular tightness is very common in patients with anterior knee pain, and it is the hallmark of the excessive lateral pressure syndrome

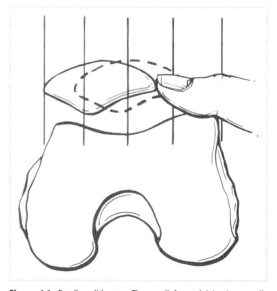

Figure 6.1. Patellar glide test. The patellofemoral joint is mentally divided into quadrants and patellar mobility is assessed in both directions. (Reprinted from DeLee and Drez, eds., *Orthopaedic Sports Medicine: Principles and Practice*, p. 1179, 1994 with permission from Elsevier.)

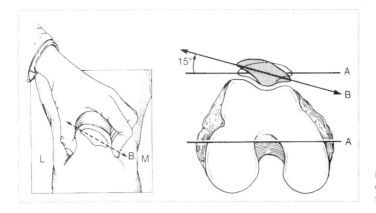

Figure 6.2. Patellar tilt test. (Reprinted from Scuderi, Giles R, ed., *The Patella*, p. 79, 1995 with permission from Springer-Verlag.)

described by Ficat.[8] In those cases with anterior knee pain after ACL reconstruction we passively "tilt" the inferior pole of the patella away from the anterior tibial cortex to rule out pretibial patellar tendon adhesions (see Chapter 18).

Axial compression test of the patella (or patellar grind test) should be part of the systematic examination as it elicits anterior knee pain originated in the patellofemoral articular surfaces (patellar and/or trochlear subchondral bone). We also perform the sustained knee flexion test, which when positive (appearance of pain) means that the patella is the origin of the pain, and it is caused by an increase of the intraosseous pressure.[14] To perform the axial compression test (Figure 6.3) we compress the patella against the trochlea with the palm of the hand at various angles of knee flexion. In addition, this test allows us to determine the location of the lesion in the patellar articular cartilage. With knee flexion, the femoropatellar contact zone is displaced proximally in the patella and distally in the femur. Thus, proximal lesions will yield pain and crepitation at approximately 90° of knee flexion. On the contrary, distal lesions are tender in the early degrees of knee flexion. For the sustained knee flexion test, the patient lies supine on a couch with his or her knee

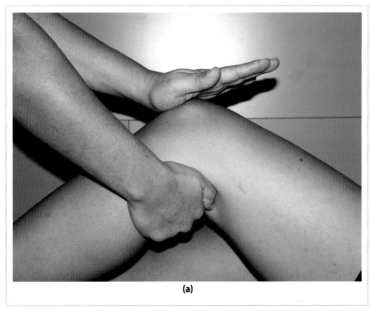

(a)

Figure 6.3. Axial compression patellar test.

(*continued*)

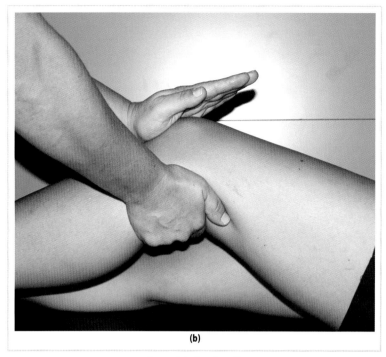

(b)

Figure 6.3. *(continued)*

extended and relaxed. The knee is then flexed fully and kept firmly in a sustained flexion for up to 45 seconds. The test is positive if the patient complains of increasing pain after a pain-free interlude of 15 to 30 seconds.

Allen and colleagues[1] have found, in patients referred with anterior knee pain, a significant association between proximal patellar tendinosis and abnormal patellar tracking. Therefore, in order to discard patellar tendinopathy, palpation of the inferior pole of the patella ought to be carried out in all cases (Figure 6.4). To perform this test we press downward on the proximal patella, with which the inferior pole of the

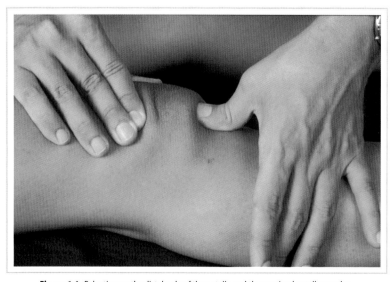

Figure 6.4. Palpation on the distal pole of the patella and the proximal patellar tendon.

patella tilts anteriorly. This maneuver lets us palpate the proximal patellar tendon attachment. However, quite often there is a mild tenderness at the attachment of the patellar tendon at the inferior pole of the patella in sportsplaying subjects. Thus, only moderate and severe tenderness is to be valued. Moreover, Hoffa's fat pad should always be felt as it can be a source of pain as well.[12] Finally, existing scars should be palpated and Tinel's sign performed to detect neuromas. Injecting a local anesthetic will confirm this diagnosis by immediate relief of pain (see Chapter 23).

In the second place, patellar instability ought to be tested. It is extremely important that the surgeon should assess in what direction the instability takes place. We must note that not all instability is in a lateral direction; some patellae have medial instability and some patients suffer from multidirectional instability.

Generally, the most frequent direction of instability is lateral. Fairbanks patellar apprehension test (Figure 6.5), when positive (pain and muscle defensive contraction on lateral patellar displacement with 20° to 30° of knee flexion), indicates that lateral patellar instability is an important part of the patient's problem. This test may be so positive that the patient withdraws the leg rapidly when the examiner approaches the knee with his or her hand, preventing thus any contact, or he or she grabs the examiner's arm.

In order to evaluate instability we also perform the patellar glide test. A medial or lateral displacement of the patella greater than or equal to 3 quadrants, with the patellar glide test, is consistent with incompetent lateral or medial restraints[25] (Figure 6.6).

Medial patellar instability is much less frequent than lateral patellar instability, but should be suspected especially in patients who remain symptomatic after unnecessary or excessive realignment surgery or lateral retinacular release (see Chapters 21 and 22). Our primary method for diagnosis of medial patellar subluxation is the Fulkerson's relocation test[10] (Figure 6.7). To perform this test we hold the patella slightly in a medial direction with the knee extended. Then, we flex the knee while letting go the patella, which causes the patella to go into the femoral trochlea. In patients with medial subluxation this test reproduces the patient's symptom. If this test is positive, we should put an appropriate brace (e.g., Trupull brace, DJ Orthopedics, Vista, California) that should diminish or eliminate the symptoms. This is another way to confirm our diagnosis before indicating a surgical treatment.

It is very important to assess the flexibility of quadriceps, hamstring, and gastrocnemius muscles and that of the iliotibial band, as the pathology under scrutiny is often associated to a decrease in flexibility of these structures. Tightness of these structures indicates the need

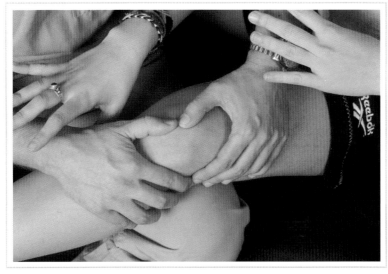

Figure 6.5. Patellar apprehension test.

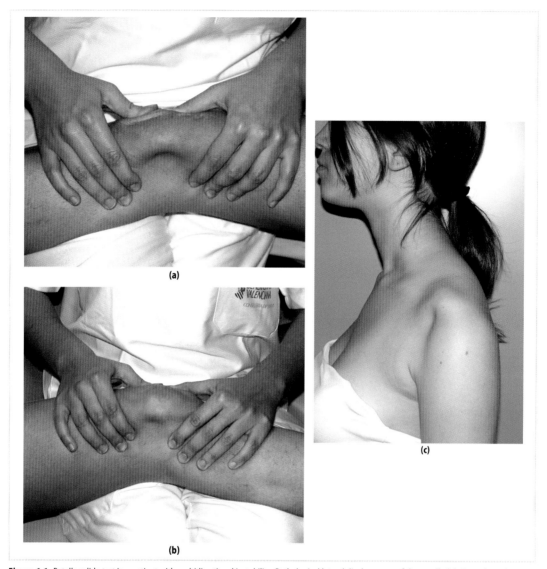

(a)

(b)

(c)

Figure 6.6. Patellar glide test in a patient with multidirectional instability. Pathological lateral displacement of the patella **(a)**. Contralateral asymptomatic knee **(b)**. We have seen an image **(a)** similar to the sulcus sign observed in patients with multidirectional instability of the shoulder **(c)**.

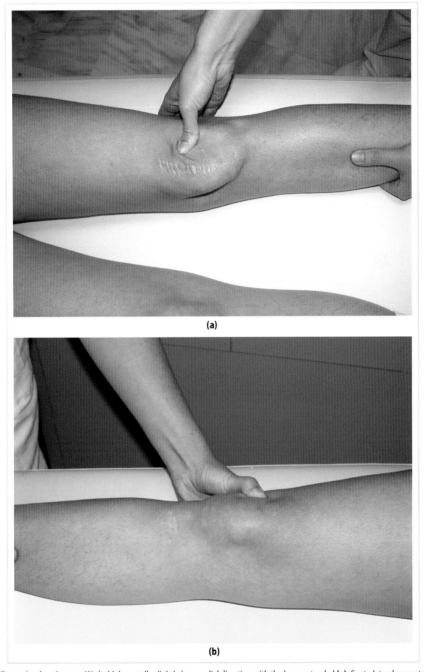

Figure 6.7. Fulkerson's relocation test. We hold the patella slightly in a medial direction with the knee extended **(a)**. Contralateral asymptomatic knee **(b)**.

(continued)

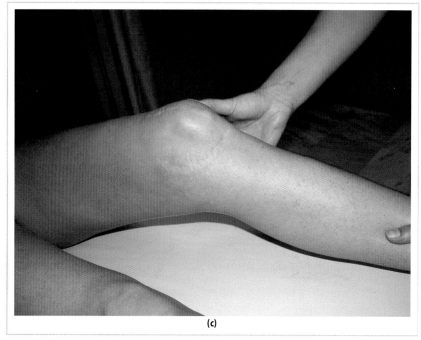

(c)

Figure 6.7. *(continued)* Then, we flex the knee while letting go the patella, which causes the patella to go into the femoral trochlea **(c)**.

for specific stretching exercises and possible modification of training.

To test quadriceps flexibility the patient lies prone and the knee is passively flexed with one hand while stabilizing the pelvis with the other hand to prevent compensatory hip flexion (Figure 6.8). We can measure the quadriceps tightness as degrees of prone knee flexion. Suggestions of quadriceps retraction are:[34] (1)

asymmetry, that is to say, a different flexion of one knee as compared to the other, (2) feeling of tightness in the anterior aspect of the thigh, and (3) elevation of the pelvis due to flexion of the hip. It is important to assess quadriceps contracture as this can increase in a direct way the contact pressure between patella and femur.

To test hamstring flexibility the patient lies supine with the hip at 90° of flexion. The patient

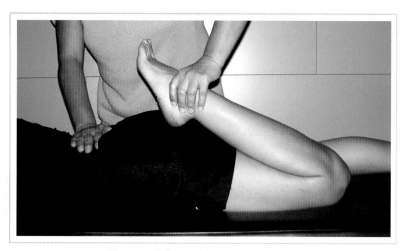

Figure 6.8. Evaluation of the quadriceps flexibility.

is then asked to straighten his or her knee (Figure 6.9). If complete extension is not possible, there is a hamstring contracture, and its amount is measured by the popliteal angle. Most young athletic individuals have popliteal angles between 160 and 180 degrees.[25] Hamstring tightness implies an increase in the quadriceps force necessary to extend the knee, which augments the patellofemoral joint reaction (PFJR) force. Hamstring tightness could also be associated with spondylolisthesis.

We evaluate gastrocnemius tightness performing a passive ankle dorsiflexion with the knee extended and the foot in slight inversion (Figure 6.10). Normally this should reach 15° from the neutral position.[34] This test also serves to rule out lumbar radiculopathy or a herniated nucleus pulposus manifesting itself as an anterior knee pain (referred pain). Tightness of the gastrocnemius, in the same way as hamstrings tightness, increases the PFJR force, producing a maintained flexed position of the knee. Moreover, limited ankle dorsiflexion results in increased subtalar joint pronation that causes an increment of tibial internal rotation that has deleterious effects on patellofemoral biomechanics.[25]

The iliotibial band (ITB) is often tight in patients who have patellofemoral pain. This causes lateral patellar displacement and tilt as well as weakness of the medial patellar retinaculum. We use the Ober's test to assess ITB flexibility

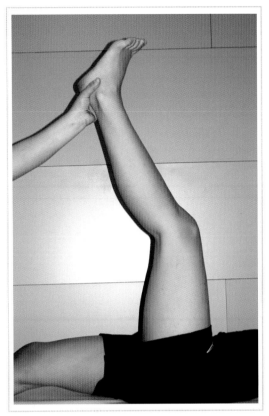

Figure 6.9. Evaluation of the hamstrings flexibility.

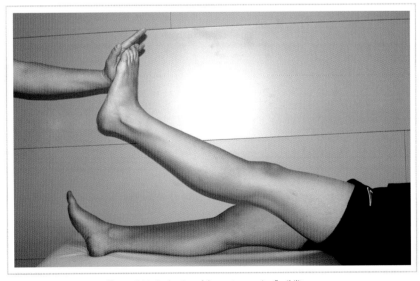

Figure 6.10. Evaluation of the gastrocnemius flexibility.

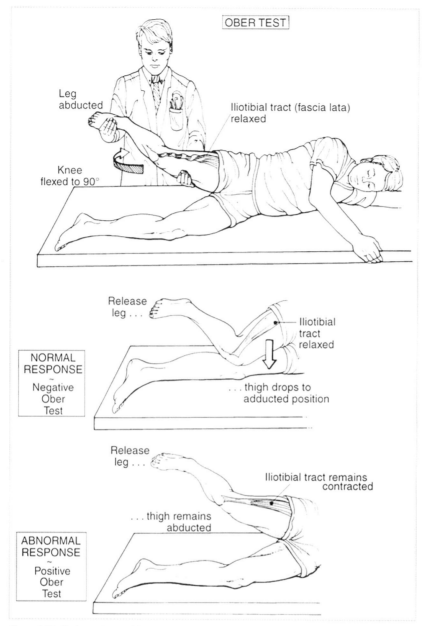

Figure 6.11. Ober's test. (Reprinted from Scuderi, Gilles R, ed., *The Patella*, p. 80, 1995 with permission from Springer-Verlag.)

(Figure 6.11). To perform this test, the patient lies on the side opposite the affected leg with the hip and knee of the bottom leg fully flexed to eliminate the lumbar lordosis. Then, the examiner flexes the involved knee and hip 90° each. After that, he abducts passively the involved hip as far as possible and extends the thigh so that it is in line with the rest of the body (neutral position), which places the ITB on maximal stretch. Palpation of the ITB just proximal to the lateral femoral condyle during maximal stretch will cause severe pain in patients who have excessive ITB tightness. At this position, we ask the patient to relax, and then the thigh is adducted passively. If the thigh remains suspended off the table, the test is positive (shortened ITB). If the thigh drops into an adducted position, the test is negative (normal ITB).

As we have seen, patients suffering from patellofemoral problems usually show a flexibility deficit, but some may have a hypermobility. It is, therefore, important to evaluate the presence of ligament laxity, as is shown in Chapter 4. Thus, patellar dislocation is six times more frequent in hypermobile patients in comparison with age-matched controls.[26] Furthermore, articular injuries during patellar dislocation are less frequent in hypermobile patients.[26,31] In addition to this, these patients may show an excessive skin laxity (Figure 6.12). The presence of Ehlers-Danlos syndrome should be ruled out due to the serious systemic complications that may be present.

It is very important to evaluate quadriceps atrophy. When the quadriceps is weak, it fails in its role of shock absorber, and therefore patellofemoral loads increase.[25] This could explain the pain while descending stairs. Patients with anterior knee pain syndrome usually have a visible and palpable atrophy of the vastus medialis obliquus (VMO) muscle. In 1984, Spencer and colleagues[30] published a study designed to elucidate the role of knee effusion in producing the reflex inhibition and subsequent atrophy of the quadriceps. They found that VMO inhibition is produced with approximately 20–30 ml of intra-articular fluid.[30] This may result in dynamic malalignment, which might explain the possibility of anterior knee pain after surgery for a meniscal or ligamentous injury. Thus, control of effusion is essential for adequate rehabilitation.

Patellar tracking should be examined using the "J" sign (Figure 6.13). With the patient seated on the examination table with the legs

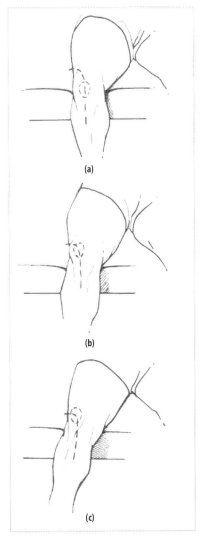

Figure 6.13. The "J" sign. When the knee is extended from 90 **(a)** to 0° **(c)** the patella describes an inverted J-shaped course. (Reprinted from DeLee and Drez, eds., *Orthopaedic Sports Medicine: Principles and Practice*, p. 1174, 1994 with permission from Elsevier.)

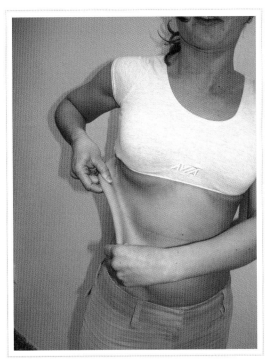

Figure 6.12. Skin laxity in Ehlers-Danlos syndrome.

hanging over the side and the knees flexed 90°, he or she is asked to extend the knee actively to a fully extended position. Normally, the patella follows a straight line as the knee is extended. However, as the knee is extended the patella runs proximally and laterally describing an inverted "J" when patellofemoral malalignment (PFM) is present.

As stated in Chapter 4, examination of the feet is essential, as pronated feet (Figure 6.14) have an important role in the origin of anterior knee pain.

Moreover, leg-length measurement is also important because leg-length discrepancy may be associated with anterior knee pain in the short leg.[25]

Anomalies of the normal knee alignment (genu varum, genu valgum, genu flexum, and genu recurvatum) and rotational abnormalities of the femur and tibia have to be taken into account, as is shown in Chapters 4, 10, and 11.

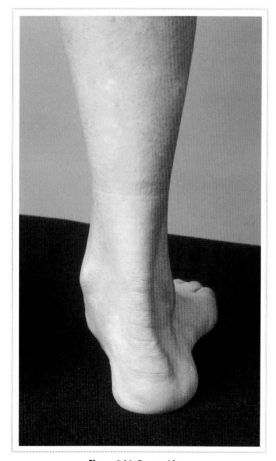

Figure 6.14. Pronated foot.

In this context, increased femoral anteversion and internal torsion are closely related to patellofemoral pathology.[20] An increased range of the internal over the external rotation by 30° or more indicates femoral anteversion.[18] Increase in femoral anteversion and internal femoral torsion cause an increase in the quadricipital angle, which produces a greater lateral displacement of the patella on quadriceps contraction. This leads to an increase in the medial patellofemoral ligament tension, as well as in the stresses upon the lateral side of the patella and the trochlea. This is initially the cause of pain and, later on, of instability, chondromalacia, and patellofemoral osteoarthrosis.[20] The pain itself causes quadriceps atrophy, which makes symptoms worse. Quadriceps exercises prescribed by the doctor often produce an overload upon the damaged joint, which increases quadriceps inhibition, and paradoxically are the cause of greater atrophy. On the other hand, if the hip mobility is limited and painful, this may indicate the presence of hip pathology (e.g., Perthes disease, slipped capital femoral epiphysis, or osteoarthrosis of the hip) manifesting itself as an anterior knee pain. Therefore, it is very important to evaluate patient's hips to rule out referred pain to the knee. The physician must consider the possibility of referred pain, from the hip or lumbar spine, when no tenderness is elicited about the knee itself. Moreover, a hip flexion contracture (Figure 6.15) must be ruled out because it results in increased knee flexion when walking, and therefore in increased PFJR force.[25]

Finally, the evaluation of the stability of the knee ligaments (i.e., Lachman test, pivot shift, and posterior drawer maneuvers) is very important to identify factors that may contribute to anterior knee pain and instability in the young patient.

Emotional and Psychiatric Evaluation

We must rule out an organic cause of anterior knee pain before saying the patient has psychosocial problems or he or she is malingering. Furthermore, we must not forget that patients with psychogenic pain can also have an organic cause associated.

There are patients who report false symptoms (e.g., attributable to secondary gain in a work compensation or medical-legal case). The difficulty

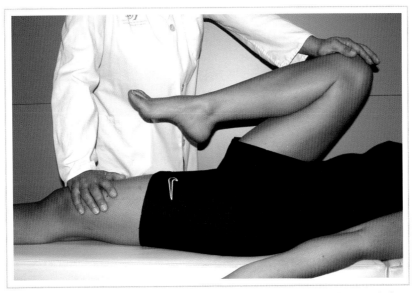

Figure 6.15. Evaluation of hip flexion contracture by flexing the contralateral hip completely. If the ipsilateral hip cannot lie flat on the table, hip flexion contracture is present.

lies in the fact that whereas in patients suffering from objective structured lesions (e.g., ACL or meniscus rupture) these are easily detected, patients with patellofemoral pain syndrome very often do not show any identifiable structural abnormality. Psychological assessment is indeed very important for patients who have undergone several surgical procedures.

Thomee and colleagues[33] evaluated how patients with patellofemoral pain syndrome experienced their pain, what coping strategies they used for the pain, and their degree of well-being. They concluded that the way patients with patellofemoral pain syndrome experience their pain, the coping strategies they use for their pain, and their degree of well-being were all in agreement with other patient groups who have chronic pain reported in the literature. However, the high scores reported for the catastrophizing coping strategy could indicate that these patients might have a more negative outlook on their pain and their prognosis than other groups of patients reported in the orthopedic literature. In some cases, there is a moderate elevation in hysteria and hypochondriasis, an unconscious strategy to cope with emotional conflict or control oversolicitous parents.[16] Carlsson and colleagues[3] found greater depression, hostility, and passive attitude in patients with long-term patellofemoral pain compared with healthy controls, matched for gender and age. Finally, Andrish has observed that anterior knee pain in some teenage females may represent a somatization of physical or sexual abuse.[5]

Therefore, it is essential to assess the emotional status of the patient. A long-lasting knee pain or an established instability with frequent falls, in the absence of a definite diagnosis by the treating doctor, can become a very stressing situation for the patient. For instance, in our series, one lady with a chronic ACL rupture and frequent falling-down episodes, who had been treated somewhere else for patellofemoral instability for two years, developed a hysteric blindness that required psychiatric treatment. Moreover, the patient's response to the problem and whether the associated depression is part of the orthopedic problem are also well worth assessing. We must find out whether we are dealing with a hostile, passive, or a "proper" patient. It is essential to analyze the patient's behavior as well as to observe whether it is the patient or his or her mother who "calls the shots."

Finally, it is worth keeping in mind the existence of the genupath.[15] The whole life and being of these persons centers around their knee symptoms, which become chronic and the cause of their failures in their private life and work commitments. With patience and persistence they can convince the orthopedic surgeon to perform a series of procedures, each one more drastic than the last. Self-mutilation can be suspected and in most some form of litigation is used to maintain their lifestyle. Orthopedic surgeons must be on their guard, as these patients will deliberately induce them to erroneous diagnosis and inappropriate surgical procedures, when what they need is psychiatric treatment. A rule to be always followed is never to operate on subjective symptoms alone. To give undue attention to isolated clinical data, instead of evaluating the whole picture, can lead to important diagnostic errors.[17] This will prevent making unnecessary mistaken operative indications and their disastrous consequences.

Psychological Pain versus Pain Due to Reflex Sympathetic Dystrophy: Objective Assessment

A constant and severe pain far out of proportion to physical findings must make us think of psychological issues or RSD. One way of differentiating them is performing a differential sympathetic block.[12] This has three components: (1) injection of saline, (2) injection of just enough anesthetic to block the sympathetic nerves (10 cc of 0.25% procaine), and (3) injection of added anesthetic to block the sensory and motor nerves. Patients who state that with the injection of saline their pain stops or those who have pain after their entire leg has been anesthetized are malingering. Patients who positively respond to the second injection have RSD. Finally, those who respond only to the third injection have nonneurogenic pain.

Imaging Studies

The methods of diagnosis by images are the second diagnostic step and they cannot replace the first step. Overlooking this rule can lead to diagnostic errors, followed by failed treatment and iatrogenic morbidity. A surgical indication should never be based solely on imaging techniques, as there is not a good correlation between clinical and image data. The image only confirms the clinical impression, but the history and physical examination are the fundamental elements in the evaluation of the patient with patellofemoral pain.

Nothing can replace the history and clinical examination.

Nowadays, there are two categories of imaging studies in patellofemoral pathology: structural imaging (radiographs, computed tomography [CT], and magnetic resonance imaging [MRI]) and metabolic imaging (technetium scintigraphy).

The majority of patients with patellofemoral pain only will require standard radiography (standing anteroposterior view, a true lateral view with the knee in 30° of flexion, and axial view with the knee in 30° of flexion). Generally, until thorough nonoperative management has failed, imaging studies beyond standard radiography are not indicated. Weightbearing anteroposterior projection allows one to evaluate varus, valgus, and joint space narrowing. The lateral view allows one to evaluate the patellar height: high-riding patella or patella alta (*alta* is Spanish) and low-riding patella or patella baja or infera (*baja* is Spanish and *infera* Latin). Moreover, a true lateral radiograph (overlapping of the posterior borders of the femoral condyles) allows one to assess trochlear dysplasia (defined by the crossing sign and quantitatively expressed by the trochlear bump and the trochlear depth) and patellar tilt.[2,4,12,22,32] Axial views can demonstrate patellofemoral maltracking (i.e., tilt, shift, or both) when this happens beyond 30° of knee flexion, sulcus angle, loss of joint space, subchondral sclerosis, and the shape of the patella. In addition to this, an axial view can detect intra-articular bodies or secondary clues of earlier dislocation episodes; for example, medial retinacular calcification is observed sometimes on the axial views and may occur in association with recurrent subluxation (Figure 6.16). Finally, standard radiography allows one to rule out associated and potentially serious bony conditions such as tumors or infections.

Adequate bony geometry and competent ligamentous structures are needed to produce stability of the patellofemoral joint. The osseous geometry can be seen in conventional x-ray plates, but the ligamentous tightness cannot. Unstable joints are generally congruent at rest, but stress can provoke an abnormal displacement. Axial stress radiographs[32] are useful to document hidden patellar instabilities, which could confirm clinical diagnosis. Stress radiographs can pinpoint lateral, medial, and multidirectional instabilities.

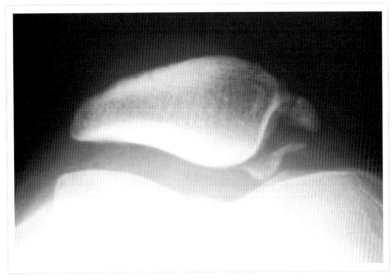

Figure 6.16. Merchant axial view, where two bony fragments are seen at the patellar medial border, sequelae from former dislocation episodes.

However, there are subtle cases of PFM, in fact the majority of them, which manifest themselves at the first degrees of knee flexion, in which the diagnosis is impossible by conventional radiology, since at 30° of knee flexion the patella relocates into the femoral trochlea, because with knee flexion the patella migrates medially and distally within the trochlear groove (Figure 6.17). CT allows us to evaluate patellar tracking from 0° to 30°. CT ought to be used after failure of conservative treatment and when realignment surgery is being considered.

By using CT scans in asymptomatic volunteers, we found that the patella is usually well-centered in the intercondylar groove in extension.[27] Schutzer and colleagues[28] identified three patterns of malalignment using CT imaging: type 1 includes patellar subluxation without tilt, type 2 is described as patellar subluxation with tilt, and type 3 is patellar tilt without subluxation. To assess patellar tilt we use the lateral patellofemoral angle (Figure 6.17). This angle is the result of the intersection of two lines: a line that runs across the apices of the femoral condyles and another line that is drawn along the articular surface of the lateral patellar facet. This angle is normal (negative for patellar tilt) when it opens laterally, and is considered as abnormal (positive for patellar tilt) when both lines are parallel or the angle opens medially (Figure 6.17).[7]

Furthermore, it is important to note that PFM in some cases is only a dynamic phenomenon, and in these cases CT at 0° of knee flexion with quadriceps contraction is the only way to identify PFM. A patellar subluxation with a relaxed quadriceps can remain unchanged, increase (Figure 6.17C), or decrease (phenomenon of dynamic reposition) with quadriceps contraction.[2] On the other hand, a patella well-centered with a relaxed quadriceps can subluxate laterally or medially with quadriceps contraction.[2] The comparison of static and dynamic CT scans gives important information and helps to determine the best treatment. Stress CT in extension with a relaxed quadriceps helps document objective instability.[2] If possible, comparison of the normal with the abnormal side is more important than the absolute amount of displacement.

Finally, CT scans can detect torsional anomalies of the lower limbs (e.g., increased femoral anteversion, internal femoral torsion, tibial torsion) (see Chapter 11).

Three-dimensional computed tomography (3D-CT) does not seem to bear any advantage over the conventional CT scans. 3D-CT not only shows a realistic volumetric representation of spatial relationships between the patella and femoral trochlea in the three spatial planes (sagittal, axial, and frontal) and visualization of

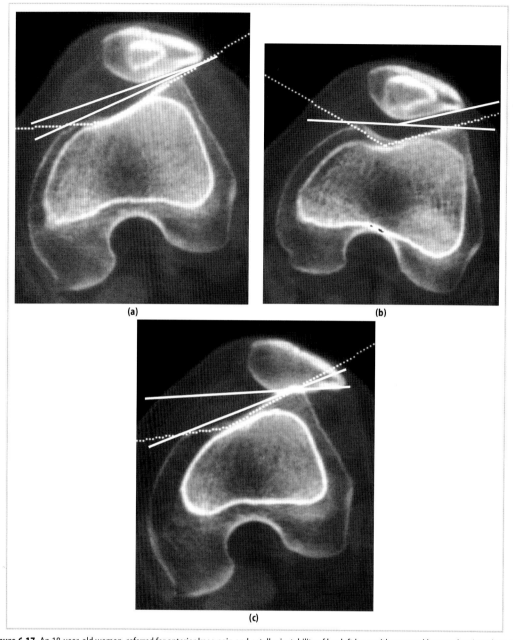

Figure 6.17. An 18-year-old woman, referred for anterior knee pain and patellar instability of her left knee with repeated haemarthrosis and severe giving-way with falling to the ground with activities of daily living. Conventional radiographs were normal and the patella was seen well-centered in the axial view of Merchant. CT shows PFM type 2 **(a)** with patellar relocated into the femoral trochlea at 30° **(b)**. With the contraction of the quadriceps increases subluxation and tilt **(c)**. (Reproduced with permission from Sanchis-Alfonso V, E Roselló-Sastre, and V Martinez-SanJuan, Pathogenesis of anterior knee pain syndrome and functional patellofemoral instability in the active young: A review, *Am J Knee Surg* 1999; 12: 29–40.)

the patellofemoral contact area in vivo,[19] but also shows with great fidelity the surface anatomy including size and location of the chondral lesions (Figure 6.18). However, its clinical utility is seriously hindered by the inability to show undersurface detail (Figure 6.18).

MRI is useful for evaluating moderate to severe patellar cartilage damage, although this structural damage may not necessarily be the cause of anterior knee pain. In addition, it also detects possible concomitant lesions that may worsen the symptoms or mimic patellofemoral

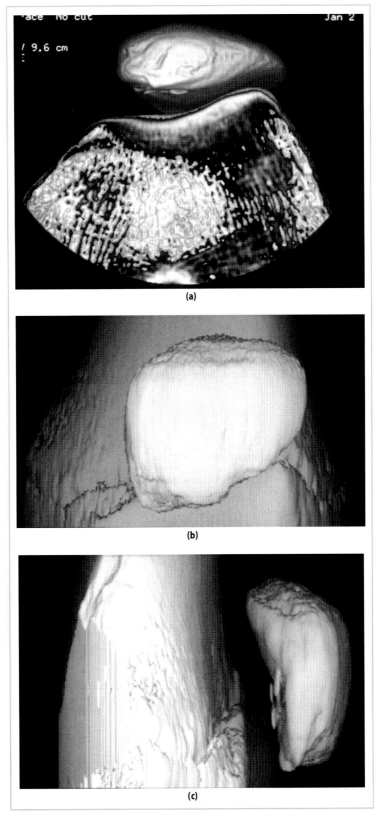

Figure 6.18. 3D-CT reconstruction of the patellofemoral joint. Axial plane showing degenerative changes of articular cartilage of the medial patellar facet **(a)**, frontal plane **(b)**, and sagittal plane **(c)**.

(*continued*)

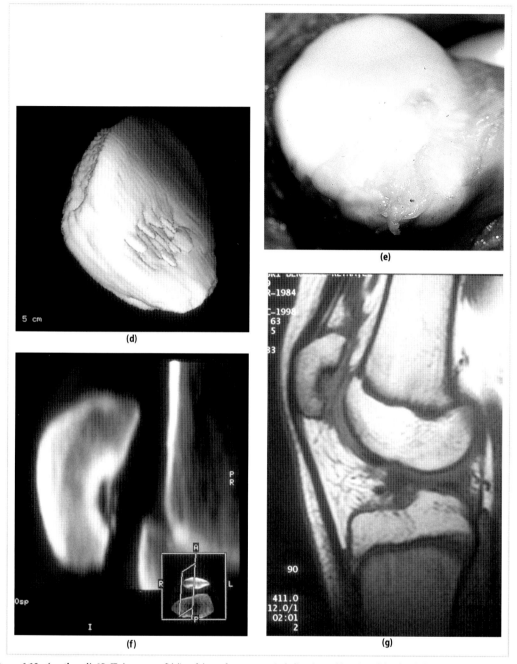

Figure 6.18. *(continued)* 3D-CT shows great fidelity of the surface anatomy including size and location of the chondral lesion **(d,e)**, although it is unable to show undersurface detail, which is clearly shown by conventional CT scans **(f)** or by MRI **(g)** [sagittal SE T1W MR image].)

syndrome. MRI also lets us detect patellar tracking abnormalities.[29,35] Grelsamer and Weinstein have found an excellent correlation between clinical and MRI tilt.[13] Tilt angles less than or equal to 10 degrees are found in patients without clinical tilt, and are considered as normal,

whereas tilt angles greater than 15 degrees are all found in subjects with clinical patellar tilt, and are considered as abnormal. In addition, MRI often shows low-grade effusions associated with symptomatic peripatellar synovitis, an underdiagnosed pathological condition of the knee.[5]

MRI plays a key role in the evaluation of the acute lateral patellar dislocation[7] confirming the clinical suspicion of patellar dislocation. The most frequent MRI signs[7] of acute lateral patellar dislocation are (Figure 6.19): contusions of the anterior portion of the lateral femoral condyle and of the medial patellae, osteochon-dral defects, intra-articular bodies, medial reti-nacular injuries, and joint effusions. Moreover, a concave impaction deformity at the inferome-dial patella, similar to the Hill-Sachs lesion of the humeral head that follows anterior disloca-tion of the glenohumeral joint, is a specific sign of previous patellar dislocation.[7] The precise

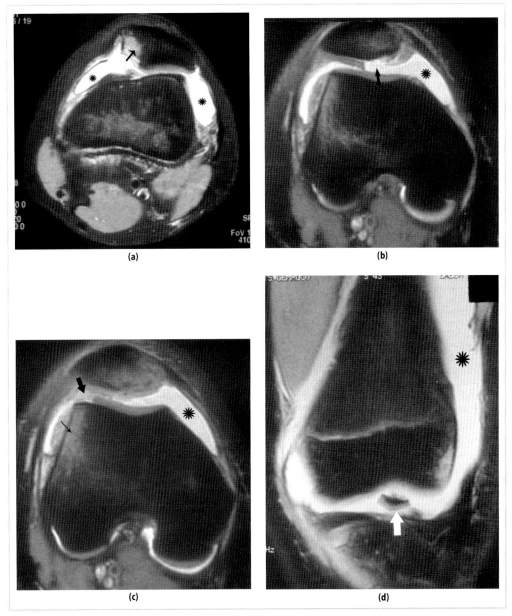

Figure 6.19. MRI signs of acute lateral patellar dislocation: contusions of the anterior portion of the lateral femoral condyle and of the medial patel-lae (black thin arrow), osteochondral defects (black thick arrow), intraarticular bodies (white thick arrow), and joint effusions (asterisk). **(a)** Axial FSE PDW Fat Sat MR image. **(b & c)** Axial FSE PDW Fat Sat MR images. **(d)** Coronal FSE PDW Fat Sat MR image.

delineation of the injury pattern is crucial in the surgical planning. In addition to all this, MRI is a good method to assess patellar tendinopathy.

Finally, bone scintigraphy using 99mTc methylene diphosphonate (99mTc-MDP), may be useful in selected cases. Dye and Boll[6] observed that about one-half of their patients with anterior knee pain presented increased patellar uptake in comparison with 4% of the control group. Biopsy demonstrated that this increased patellar uptake was secondary to the increased remodelling activity of bone. Bone scintigraphy can detect loss of osseus homeostasis, and often correlates well with the presence of patellar pain and its resolution.[5] According to Dye and Boll,[6] the bone scan commonly reverted to normal at an average time of 6.2 months (range 3–14 months), which is interpreted as restoration of osseous homeostasis. Scintigraphy may be especially useful in patients with injuries related to workers' compensation cases in which the physician wishes to establish objective findings. According to Lorberboym and colleagues,[21] single-photon emission computed tomography (SPECT) bone scintigraphy is highly sensitive for the diagnosis of patellofemoral abnormalities. For these authors, SPECT significantly improves the detection of maltracking of the patella and the ensuing increased lateral patellar compression syndrome. They conclude that this information could be used to treat patellofemoral problems more effectively.

Arthroscopic Evaluation

Once surgery is indicated, and before any realignment procedure is done, an arthroscopy should be performed. To inspect the patellofemoral joint the scope should be introduced through the superomedial portal. Arthroscopy is helpful in order to rule out any other unsuspected intra-articular pathology (e.g., synovial plicae, peripatellar synovitis, meniscus rupture) not obvious at the preoperative appraisal that may cause symptoms that mimic patellofemoral syndrome, and to evaluate patellar articular cartilage. Arthroscopy provides valuable information about articular cartilage breakdown location, extent, and pattern, which may help with future treatment decisions. Moreover, in order to establish a prognosis it is of great interest to ascertain the site of the chondral lesion. Pidoriano and colleagues[23] pointed out that after anteromedial transfer of the tibial tubercle better results were obtained in distal or lateral lesions than in proximal or medial ones. This may be due to the surgical displacement proximally and medially of the patellofemoral tracking area.

Arthroscopy, however, produces scanty information about patellar tracking. No realignment surgical procedure ought to be based entirely upon the arthroscopic analysis of the patellofemoral congruence, as many variable factors (intra-articular pressure, portal localization, contraction versus quadriceps relaxation, tourniquet and foot position) may lead to mistaken conclusions (i.e., impression of malalignment in patients who have normal alignment).[24]

Conclusion

There is no substitute for a thorough history and a complete and careful physical examination. The history and physical examination still remain the first step for making an accurate diagnosis of anterior knee pain and patellar instability above any technique of diagnostic image. Imaging studies are a second step and can never replace the former. Surgical indications should not be based only on methods of image diagnosis as there is a poor correlation between clinical and image data. Finally, arthroscopy should be used judiciously and no realignment surgery should be based solely on the arthroscopic analysis of the patellofemoral congruence.

References

1. Allen, GM, PG Tauro, and SJ Ostlere. Proximal patellar tendinosis and abnormalities of patellar tracking. *Skeletal Radiol* 1999; 28: 220–223.
2. Biedert, RM. *Patellofemoral Disorders: Diagnosis and Treatment.* John Wiley & Sons, Ltd., 2004.
3. Carlsson, AM, S Werner, CE Mattlar et al. Personality in patients with long-term patellofemoral pain syndrome. *Knee Surg Sports Traumatol Arthrosc* 1993; 1: 178–183.
4. Dejour, H, G Walch, L Nove-Josserand et al. Factors of patellar instability: An anatomic radiographic study. *Knee Surg Sports Traumatol Arthrosc* 1994; 2: 19–26.
5. Dye, SF. Reflections on patellofemoral disorders. In Biedert, RM, ed., *Patellofemoral Disorders: Diagnosis and Treatment.* John Wiley & Sons, Ltd., 2004, pp. 3–17.
6. Dye, SF, and DA Boll. Radionuclide imaging of the patellofemoral joint in young adults with anterior knee pain. *Orthop Clin North Am* 1986; 17: 249–262.
7. Elias, DA, LM White, and DC Fithian. Acute lateral patellar dislocation at MR imaging: Injury patterns of medial patellar soft-tissue restraints and osteochondral injuries of the inferomedial patella. *Radiology* 2002; 225: 736–743.
8. Ficat, P, C Ficat, and A Bailleux. External hypertension syndrome of the patella. Its significance in the recognition of arthrosis. *Rev Chir Orthop Reparatrice Appar Mot* 1975; 61: 39–59.

9. Fulkerson, JP. The etiology of patellofemoral pain in young, active patients: A prospective study. *Clin Orthop* 1983; 179: 129–133.

10. Fulkerson, JP. A clinical test for medial patella tracking. *Tech Orthop* 1997; 12: 165–169.

11. Gambardella, RA. Technical pitfalls of patellofemoral surgery. *Clin Sports Med* 1999; 18: 897–903.

12. Grelsamer, RP, and J McConnell. The patella: A team approach. Gaithersburg, MD: Aspen, 1998.

13. Grelsamer, R, and C Weinstein. Patellar tilt: An MRI study. *Tenth Congress European Society of Sports Traumatology, Knee Surgery and Arthroscopy*, Rome 23–27 April 2002, *Book of Abstracts*, p. 178.

14. Hejgaard, N, and CC Arnoldi. Osteotomy of the patella in the patellofemoral pain syndrome: The significance of increased intraosseous pressure during sustained knee flexion. *Int Orthop* 1987; 8: 189–194.

15. Jackson, AM. Anterior knee pain. *J Bone Joint Surg* 2001; 83-B: 937–948.

16. Johnson, LL. *Arthroscopic Surgery: Principles and Practice.* St. Louis: C.V. Mosby, 1986.

17. Johnson, LL, E van Dyk, JR Green et al. Clinical assessment of asymptomatic knees: Comparison of men and women. *Arthroscopy* 1998; 14: 347–359.

18. Kantaras, AT, J Selby, and DL Johnson. History and physical examination of the patellofemoral joint with patellar instability. *Oper Tech Sports Med* 2001; 9: 129–133.

19. Kawakubo, M, K Fujikawa, and H Matsumoto. Evaluation of patellofemoral joint congruence using three-dimensional computed tomography. *Knee* 1999; 6: 165–170.

20. Kijowski, R, D Plagens, SJ Shaeh et al. The effects of rotational deformities of the femur on contact pressure and contact area in the patellofemoral joint and on strain in the medial patellofemoral ligament. Presented at the *Annual Meeting of the International Patellofemoral Study Group,* Napa Valley, San Francisco, USA, September 1999.

21. Lorberboym, M, DB Ami, D Zin et al. Incremental diagnostic value of 99mTc methylene diphosphonate bone SPECT in patients with patellofemoral pain disorders. *Nucl Med Commun* 2003; 24: 403–410.

22. Merchant, AC. Radiography of the patellofemoral joint. *Oper Tech Sports Med* 1999; 7: 59–64.

23. Pidoriano, AJ, RN Weinstein, DA Buuck et al. Correlation of patellar articular lesions with results from anteromedial tibial tubercle transfer. *Am J Sports Med* 1997; 25: 533–537.

24. Pidoriano, AJ, and JP Fulkerson. Arthroscopy of the patellofemoral joint. *Clin Sports Med* 1997; 16: 17–28.

25. Post, WR. History and physical examination. In Fulkerson, JP, ed., *Disorders of the Patellofemoral Joint,* 4th ed. Philadelphia: Lippincott Williams & Wilkins, 2004, pp. 43–75.

26. Runow, A. The dislocating patella: Etiology and prognosis in relation to generalized joint laxity and anatomy of the patellar articulation. *Acta Orthop Scand Suppl* 1983: 201: 1–53.

27. Sanchis-Alfonso, V, E Gastaldi-Orquín, and V Martinez-SanJuan. Usefulness of computed tomography in evaluating the patellofemoral joint before and after Insall's realignment: Correlation with short-term clinical results. *Am J Knee Surg* 1994; 7: 65–72.

28. Schutzer, SF, GR Ramsby, and JP Fulkerson. Computed tomographic classification of patellofemoral pain patients. *Orthop Clin North Am* 1986; 17: 235–248.

29. Shellock, FG, JH Mink, AL Deutsch et al. Patellar tracking abnormalities: Clinical experience with kinematic MR imaging in 130 patients. *Radiology* 1989; 172: 799–804.

30. Spencer, JD, KC Hayes, and IJ Alexander. Knee joint effusion and quadriceps inhibition in man. *Arch Phys Med Rehabil* 1984; 65: 171–177.

31. Stanitski, CL. Articular hypermobility and chondral injury in patients with acute patellar dislocation. *Am J Sports Med* 1995; 23: 146–150.

32. Teitge, RA. Plain patellofemoral radiographs. *Oper Tech Sports Med* 2001; 9: 134–151.

33. Thomee, P, R Thomee, and J Karlsson. Patellofemoral pain syndrome: Pain, coping strategies and degree of well-being. *Scand J Med Sci Sports* 2002; 12: 276–281.

34. Walsh, WM. Patellofemoral joint. In DeLee, JC, and D Drez, eds., *Orthopaedic Sports Medicine: Principles and Practice.* Philadelphia: W.B. Saunders, 1994, pp. 1163–1248.

35. Witonski, D, and B Goraj. Patellar motion analyzed by kinematic and dynamic axial magnetic resonance imaging in patients with anterior knee pain syndrome. *Arch Orthop Trauma Surg* 1999; 119: 46–49.

7

Uncommon Causes of Anterior Knee Pain

Vicente Sanchis-Alfonso, Erik Montesinos-Berry, and
Francisco Aparisi-Rodriguez

Introduction

Anterior knee pain is a common symptom,
which may have a large variety of causes.
Although, patellofemoral malalignment (PFM)
is a potential cause of anterior knee pain in
young patients, not all malalignments are symptomatic. To think of anterior knee pain as somehow being necessarily tied to PFM is an
oversimplification that has positively stultified
progress toward better diagnosis and treatment
of patients with anterior knee pain syndrome.
PFM could be the single culprit for the pain but
it is also possible that it bears no relation whatsoever with the patient's complaint or that it is
only partly to blame for the problem. PFM can
exist without anterior knee pain, and anterior
knee pain can exist without PFM. There are
many causes of anterior knee pain, some of
them related to PFM and many more not related
to PFM. Likewise, we should bear in mind that
there are teenage patients with anterior knee
pain who lack evidence of organic pathology
(i.e., their condition is of a psychosomatic
nature[20]) and also patients who suffer from the
"malingering syndrome." In this chapter we
analyze uncommon causes of anterior knee
pain, emphasizing the fact that not all malaligments are symptomatic.

The question to be addressed is, therefore,
what factor is responsible for the patient's
symptoms? As with any other pathology, it is
necessary to make an accurate diagnosis before
embarking on a specific treatment plan. An
incorrect diagnosis may lead to inappropriate
or unnecessary surgical procedures, which can
cause morbidity and unnecessary expenses.
Moreover, an unsuitable treatment, resulting
from an incorrect diagnosis, may worsen the situation. The final result could be disastrous since
it may add to an already serious condition a
reflex sympathetic dystrophy or an iatrogenic
medial dislocation of the patella.

The goal of an orthopedic surgeon treating
patients with anterior knee pain is to precisely
determine the etiology of the pain since this is
the only way to come up with a "tailored
treatment."

Anterior Knee Pain Related to Patellofemoral Malalignment

There are some uncommon injuries (e.g., osteochondritis dissecans [OCD] of the patellofemoral
groove, or painful bipartite patella) that result
from PFM but that do not require specific treatment since healing is achieved by treating the
malalignment.

OCD of the patellofemoral groove is a very
rare cause of patellofemoral pain. Mori and colleagues[35] regard overuse and the excessive lateral pressure syndrome as factors involved in
the development of OCD of the patellofemoral
groove. These authors consider the isolated lateral retinacular release to be an effective treatment for these patients. In our own series, we
have two cases of OCD of the patellofemoral

groove associated with PFM that were treated with an Insall's proximal realignment, with satisfactory clinical results, leading to the healing of the osteochondral lesion, as shown by MRI (Figure 7.1).

Furthermore, the pain experienced by patients with a bipartite patella is, according to Mori and colleagues,[36] a result of excessive traction by the vastus lateralis and the lateral retinaculum on the superolateral bone fragment

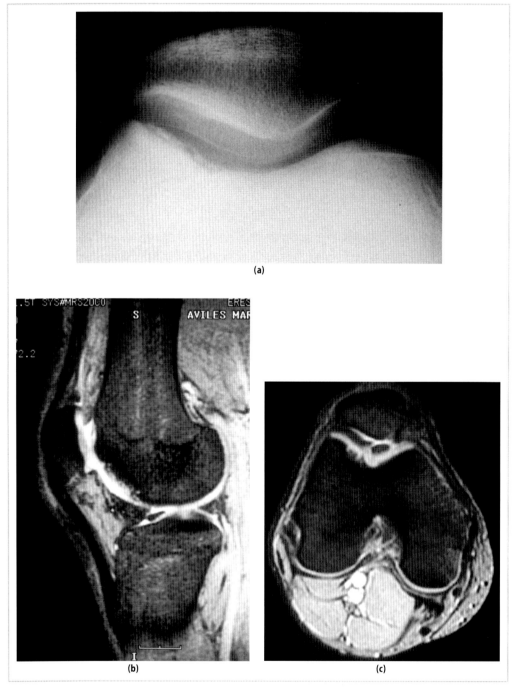

(a)

(b)

(c)

Figure 7.1. Osteochondritis dissecans of the patellofemoral groove in a patient with symptomatic PFM **(a–c)**. The MRI shows the chondral lesion healed a year and a half after realignment surgery **(d&e)**. (**b, c, d, e** – GrE T2* MR images.)

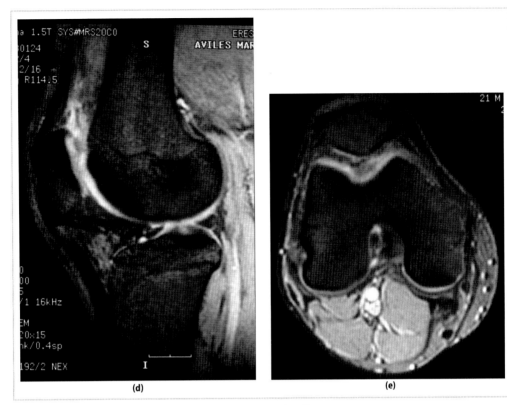

Figure 7.1. *(continued)*

(Figure 7.2). These authors have observed that a modified lateral retinacular release eliminates the anterior knee pain experienced by these patients and that, in 94% of cases, induces bony union between the superolateral fragment and the rest of the patella.

Anterior Knee Pain Not Related to Patellofemoral Malalignment

It should be remembered that the region of the knee is home to many infrequent lesions, some of them serious, which may mimic a symptomatic PFM but which bear no relation whatsoever to it. These lesions can cause confusion and hence lead to an incorrect diagnosis resulting in an erroneous treatment.

Within this group of infrequent lesions it is worth mentioning the following: intramuscular hemangioma of the vastus medialis obliquus muscle[12,44] (Figure 7.3), benign giant-cell tumor of the patellar tendon,[4] glomus tumor of Hoffa's fat pad,[17] Hoffa's fat pad disease,[10,32] localized pigmented villonodular synovitis[7,8,18,22,39,53] (Figure 7.4), hypertrophy of the synovium in the anteromedial joint compartment following minor trauma,[6] intra-articular hemangioma,[3,41] osteoid osteoma[15] (Figure 7.5), intra-articular ganglion[48,54] (Figure 7.6), deep cartilage defects of the patella,[28] double patella syndrome,[5] ossification of the patellar tendon,[30] symptomatic synovial plicae,[23,24,25,27] iliotibial friction band syndrome[42] (Figure 7.7), pes anserine bursitis and tendonitis,[42] semimembranous tendonitis,[42] medial collateral ligament bursitis,[42] popliteus tendonitis,[42] subluxation of the popliteus tendon,[31] proximal tibiofibular instability,[42] fabella syndrome,[42] occult localized osteonecrosis of the patella,[46] injuries to the infrapatellar branch of the saphenous nerve such as postsurgical neuromas or trauma,[40,52] saphenous nerve entrapment,[42] stress fractures in the region of the knee[34,38,51] (Figure 7.8), symptomatic oscicles in the anterior tuberosity of the tibia[45] (Figure 7.9), Osgood-Schlatter apophysitis, Sinding-Larsen-Johanssen apophysitis, pre-patellar bursitis ("housemaid's knee"), infrapatellar bursitis ("clergyman's knee"), infrapatellar contracture syndrome,[11] Cyclops syndrome[45] (Figure 7.10), infections,[1,9] and primary and metastatic tumors.[14,29,37]

We must remember that the clinical presentation of a musculoskeletal tumor may mimic that

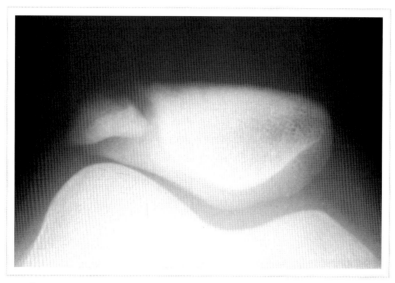

Figure 7.2. Bipartite patella of a volleyball player with excessive lateral pressure syndrome.

of an anterior knee pain syndrome. Moreover, a high proportion of primary aggressive benign or malignant bone tumors occur in the same age group than anterior knee pain syndrome, and have also a predilection for the knee. According to Muscolo and colleagues,[37] poor-quality radiographs and an unquestioned original diagnosis despite persistent symptoms seem to be the most frequent causes of an erroneous diagnosis, and therefore of an incorrect treatment. When a musculoskeletal tumor is initially misdiagnosed as a sports injury, its treatment may be adversely affected by the delay in diagnosis or by an inappropriate invasive procedure that can result in extension of the tumor and may close the door on a limb-salvage surgery.[37]

Moreover, a careful, thorough physical examination is very important to rule out referred pain arising from the lumbosacral spine (e.g., disc herniations, spondilolysthesis) and the hip (e.g., hip osteonecrosis, osteoid osteoma of the femoral neck, stress fractures of the femoral neck, slipped femoral epiphysis). Associated numbness or tingling suggests a lumbar

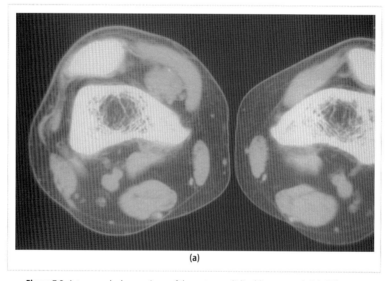

(a)

Figure 7.3. Intramuscular hemangioma of the vastus medialis obliquus muscle **(a)**. CT image.

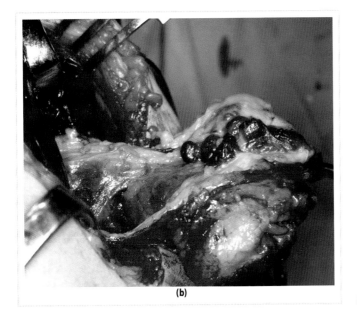

Figure 7.3. *(continued)* Macroscopic appearance (b).

problem. Referred pain from the hip usually affects the anterior aspect of the distal thigh and knee, and generally there is decreased internal rotation and pain on hip motion. For instance, a patient in our series who was being treated else-

where for an anterior knee pain syndrome and functional patellofemoral instability with "associated psychological factors" was in actual fact found to have a calcar osteoid osteoma. Once the tumoral lesion was addressed, both the

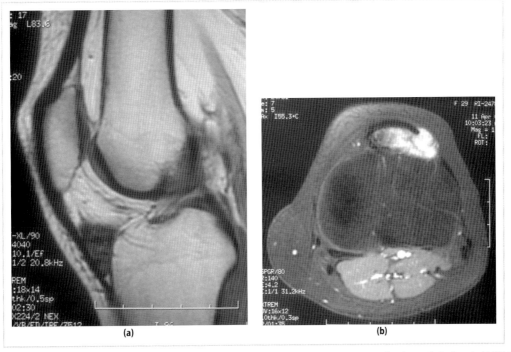

Figure 7.4. Localized pigmented villonodular synovitis of the Hoffa's fat pad. **(a)** Sagittal FSE T1W MR image. Hypointense lesion into the Hoffa's fat pad. **(b)** Axial GrE T1W + gd-DTPA. Heterogeneous enhancement lesion into the Hoffa's fat pad.

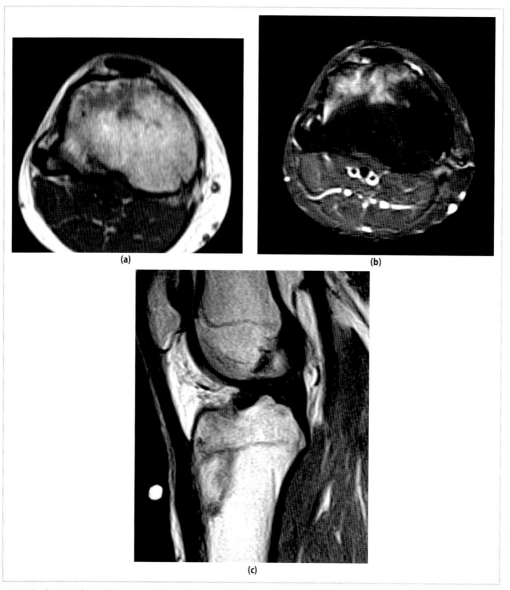

Figure 7.5. A subperiostial osteoid osteoma on the anterior aspect of the proximal end of the tibia is an extremely rare cause of anterior knee pain. Conventional x-rays were negative. Axial T1-weighted MR image **(a)**. Axial T2-weighted MR image (with fat suppression) **(b)**. Note a well-defined edematous area without significant extraosseous involvement. Sagittal T1-weighted MR image **(c)**.

patient's symptoms and large-scale quadriceps atrophy disappeared. Currently (9 years later), this patient is in a physically very demanding job, which he manages to do without any problem. In this case, the patient had knee pain resulting from a hip injury and instability was due to severe quadriceps atrophy.

Finally, we must note that in exceptional cases the source of the anterior knee pain may be in the posterior aspect of the knee[47] (see patient 1 under Case Histories). For instance, in Figure 7.11 we can see the case of a patient operated on five years ago with an Insall's proximal realignment of the right knee, who consulted

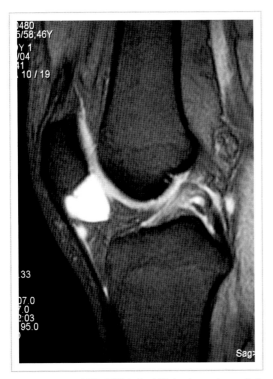

Figure 7.6. Sagittal FSE PDW Fat Sat MRI showing an intra-articular ganglion cyst into the Hoffa's fat pad.

for anterior right knee pain and functional patellofemoral instability. In the CT scan we can see a correct patellofemoral congruence of the right knee and an osteolytic area in the lateral

femoral condyle. MRI shows a mass in the popliteal aspect with bone involvement. Biopsy revealed a nonspecific chronic synovitis of the popliteal aspect. Symptoms of the anterior aspect of the knee disappeared after the resection of the lesion.

In conclusion, as a general rule, the more infrequent causes of anterior knee pain should be considered in the differential diagnosis of a painful knee when the treatment of the most frequent ones has proved ineffective.

Treat the Patient, Not the Image: Advances in Diagnostic Imaging Do Not Replace History and Physical Examination

In some cases, a distinction should be drawn between instabilities caused by an ACL tear and those caused by the patella. In our series there is a patient who was referred to us with knee instability secondary to indirect trauma caused by a skiing accident. The patient's MRI result was compatible with an ACL rupture (Figure 7.12). Clinical examination revealed a normal ACL, which was confirmed arthroscopically. What this patient really had was a symptomatic PFM, which was duly treated and cured. Another patient, referred to our department with knee pain and instability, previously diagnosed by CT-scan to have PFM, actually had an ACL rupture as well as a bucket handle tear of the medial meniscus

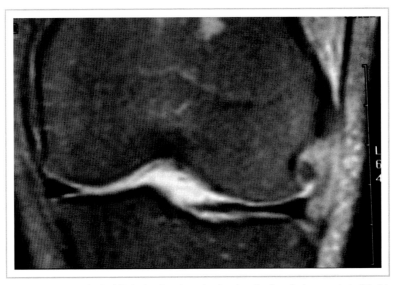

Figure 7.7. Coronal FSE PDW Fat Sat MRI. Iliotibial friction band syndrome in a female surfer. Note the bone exostosis of the lateral femoral condyle (arrow), which leads to an impingement on the iliotibial tract.

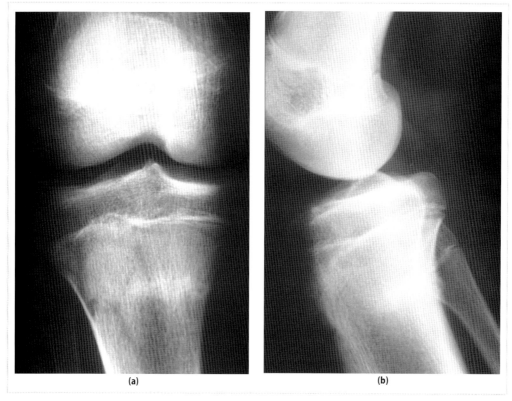

(a)   (b)

Figure 7.8. Stress fracture in the proximal tibia in a patient who consulted for anterior knee pain without traumatism.

(Figure 7.13). We should once more stress the importance of history and physical examination vis-à-vis the use of imaging techniques.

Regarding instability, it should be emphasized that giving-way episodes due to ACL tears are normally associated with activities involving turns, whereas giving-way episodes related to patellofemoral joint disorders are associated to activities that do not involve turns (i.e., straight movements such as walking or going down stairs). It should be remembered that quadriceps atrophy gives patients a feeling of instability, but this feeling appears without turning the knee. Obviously, clinically things tend to be more complicated since in cases of chronic ACL tears there is an associated quadriceps atrophy.

Moreover, we should remember that a "chondromalacia" can simulate a meniscal lesion, a fact already noted by Axhausen in 1922, resulting in the removal of normal menisci.[2] In this connection, Tapper and Hoover suspected that over 20%

of women who did badly after an open meniscectomy had a patellofemoral pathology.[50] Likewise, Insall[19] stated that patellofemoral pathology was the most common cause of meniscectomy failure in young patients, especially women. These young women who have undergone a meniscectomy often end up with severe osteoarthrosis (Figure 7.14). This confusion may be due to the fact that the region where patients with patellofemoral pathology feel their pain is normally the anteromedial aspect of the knee. Another possible explanation for this diagnostic confusion might lie in the fact that the patella and the anterior horns of both menisci are connected by Kaplan's ligaments (one medial and another lateral). Finally, unfortunately the diagnostic error may be due to an MRI false positive. On the other hand, in a young patient (unlike an elderly one) the lack of a history of trauma makes a diagnosis of meniscal rupture unlikely. However, a history of joint effusion would tilt the scales

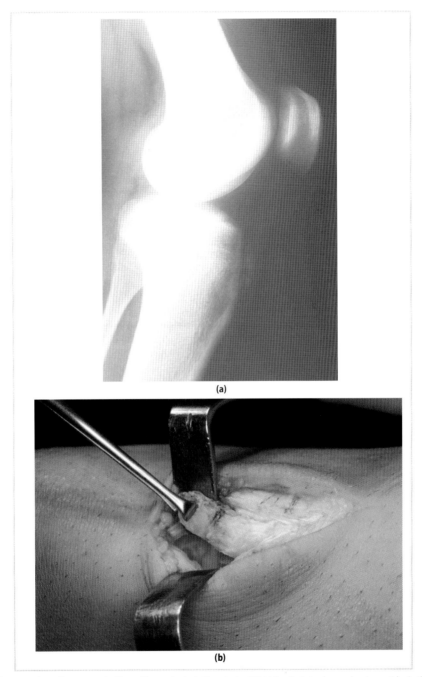

(a)

(b)

Figure 7.9. This is a patient who presented with swelling and pain in the anterior tibial tubercle. Lateral x-ray showing oscicles in the anterior tibial tubercle **(a)**. Excision of the oscicles via a transtendinous approach **(b)**.

toward a diagnosis of intra-articular pathology (e.g., meniscal rupture). To think of the sheer amount of menisci that have been needlessly sacrificed in patients with anterior knee pain syndrome! Obviously, this should nowadays be a thing of the past given the wide array of diagnostic techniques at our disposal. Nonetheless, in spite of all the diagnostic techniques available, the key factor remains the physical examination of the patient.[21]

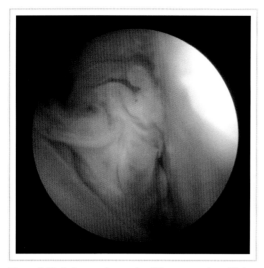

Figure 7.10. Cyclops syndrome after ACL reconstruction with bone-patellar tendon-bone 5 months ago.

It should be emphasized once again that we should treat patients, not x-rays, CT-scans, or MRI! Unfortunately, MRI seems to be taking the place of the clinical examination in assessing a painful joint, and this may lead to diagnostic confusion. This happens, for example, with the magic angle phenomenon, which can mislead us into diagnosing a patient without symptoms in the patellar tendon with patellar tendinopathy

(Figure 7.15). Nonetheless, MRI is obviously a very useful tool when it supplements physical examination since it can sometimes confirm a pathological condition in a patient involved in workman's compensation or other pending litigation claims (Figure 7.16).

Case Histories
Patient 1

A 49-year-old male was referred for severe anterior right knee pain with activities of daily living and during the night for about 8 months. The pain was vague, and the patient could not specifically locate it with one finger, sweeping his fingers along both sides of the quadriceps tendon, patella, and patellar tendon. Pain did not subside with rest, medication, or physical therapy, limiting significantly his activities of daily living (climbing stairs, squatting, and car driving). The patient underwent an endoscopic ACL reconstruction 1.5 years before using a four-bundled semitendinosus/gracilis graft fixed with bioabsorbable interferencial screws. The pain began 4 months after surgery after performing a squat of 140°, and it was progressing.

Physical Examination

Physical examination revealed peripatellar and retropatellar pain with positive compression patellar test and pain with passive medial patellar

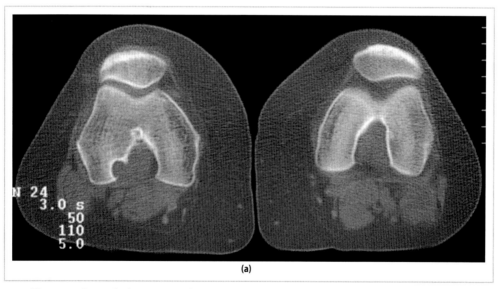

(a)

Figure 7.11. Nonspecific chronic synovitis of the popliteal aspect of the right knee. Axial CT scan at 0° of knee flexion **(a)**.

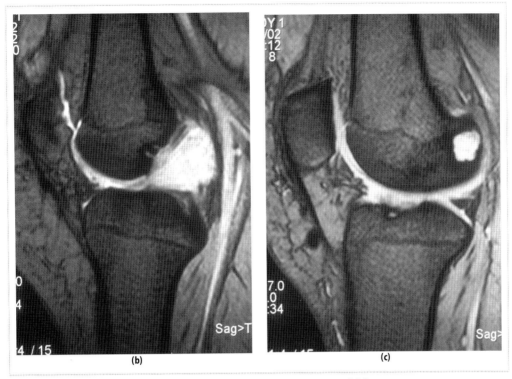

Figure 7.11. *(continued)* Sagittal GrE T2* MR images **(b&c)**.

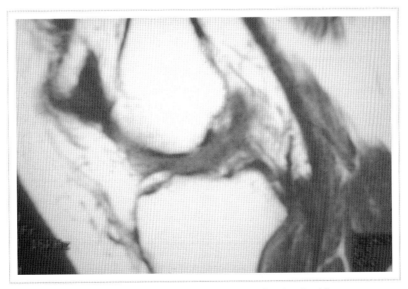

Figure 7.12. Sagittal SE T1W MR image. False positive detection of an ACL tear.

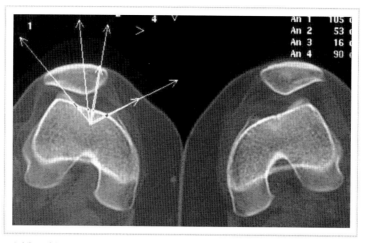

Figure 7.13. Asymptomatic bilateral PFM. CT-scan with the knees at 0° of flexion with a relaxed quadriceps. The patient's actual problem was a chronic rupture of the ACL and a bucket handle tear of the medial meniscus. The result of the physical examination of the extensor mechanism was negative for both knees. Two years after the CT-scan was performed, the results of the physical examination of the extensor mechanism were still negative. The importance of a physical examination cannot be underestimated.

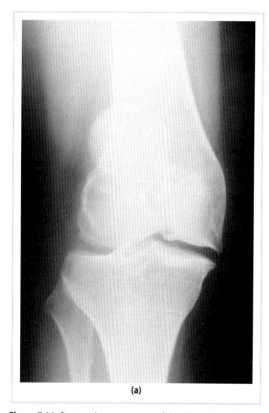

(a)

Figure 7.14. Post-meniscectomy osteoarthritis in a patient who had been mistakenly diagnosed with a rupture of the medial meniscus owing to a confusion between patellofemoral and meniscal pathologies **(a)**.

mobility, hypotrophy of the quadriceps, 5° lack of full active extension, a tight gastrocnemius, and calf pain that irradiated to the posterior aspect of the thigh. The remainder of the physical examination was completely normal.

Which Is the Source of the Anterior Knee Pain in Our Patient? Image Evaluation

This is the first question we must ask before proposing surgical treatment. To answer this question we performed a CT at 0° of knee flexion that revealed a patellar subluxation (Figure 7.17). Therefore, the most obvious reply to our question would be that the source of pain was in the anterior aspect of the knee. However, if we examine in depth the CT we can see an osteolytic area in the lateral femoral condyle and a structure that could correspond to the femoral interference screw (Figure 7.17). That is why we did an MRI that clearly showed a broken divergent femoral interference screw (Figure 7.18), as the surgery revealed (Figure 7.19). MRI tilt angle according to the method described by Grelsamer and Weinstein[16] was of 10°. These authors have found an excellent correlation between clinical and MRI tilt. Tilt angles less than or equal to 10°, as in our case, are found in patients without clinical tilt, and are considered as normal, whereas tilt angles greater than 15° are all found in subjects with

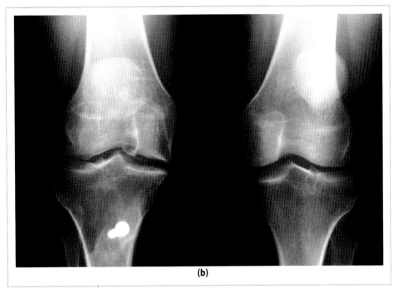

(b)

Figure 7.14. *(continued)* An extensor mechanism realignment surgery did away with the symptoms that led to the first operation **(b)**.

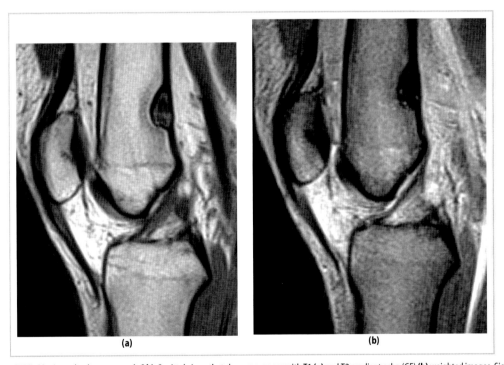

(a)   **(b)**

Figure 7.15. Magic angle phenomenon **(a&b)**. Sagittal views that show sequences with T1 **(a)** and T2 gradient echo (GE) **(b)** weighted images. Signal variations can be observed in the patellar tendon suggesting a structural alteration. If one looks at the image more closely, one notices that the signal variation follows the tendon's axis and that, in addition, there is no change whatsoever in its profile. This alteration corresponds to an imaging artifact arising from the magic angle phenomenon. This term covers the signal variations shown by certain structures when they are not aligned with the direction of the magnetic field (50°). This phenomenon is seen more often when the GE technique is used. This is therefore an example of a false positive.

(continued)

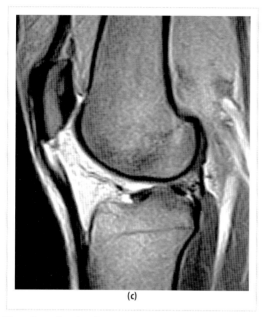

Figure 7.15. *(continued)* Typical MR image of a patellar tendinopathy, T2-weighted FSE image, sagittal plane **(c)**.

clinical patellar tilt, and are considered as abnormal. Therefore, the fact that in our patient the MRI tilt angle was 10°, is against the source of pain being in the anterior aspect of the knee. Consequently, we postulated that anterior knee pain was secondary to a severe femoral interference screw divergence. Now, we must note that a severe femoral screw divergence is not necessary accompanied by pain, neither in the anterior nor posterior aspects of the knee.

Treatment Plan

Based on our hypothesis we advised screw removal. Prior to surgery, we carried out an examination under general anesthesia that revealed that the knee was stable and the range of motion was complete. After that, we performed an arthroscopy that showed no abnormalities. Following arthroscopy, the patient was placed in the decubitus prone position and the femoral screw was removed through a Trickey's posterior approach. During surgery, we could see that the screw was incrusted into the lateral head of the gastrocnemius. Further, the screw was broken. The fact that the screw was broken reflects the

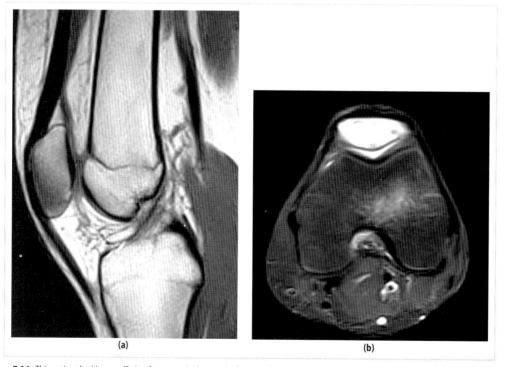

Figure 7.16. This patient had been suffering from anterior knee pain for several months caused by trauma from a car accident. Conventional x-rays did not show any pathological finding. However, MRI did. **(a)** Sagittal SE T1W MR image. **(b)** Axial FSE PDW Fat Sat MR image.

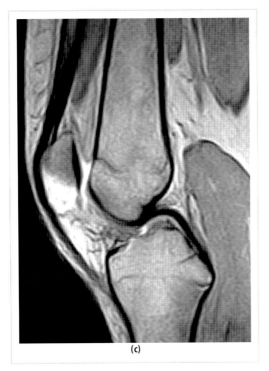

Figure 7.16. *(continued)* **(c)** Sagittal FSE T2W MR image.

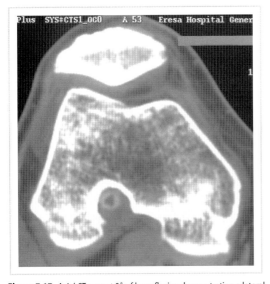

Figure 7.17. Axial CT scan at 0° of knee flexion demonstrating a lateral subluxation of the patella. Femoral screw (arrow). (Reprinted from Sanchis-Alfonso, V, and M Tintó-Pedrerol, Femoral interference screw divergence after anterior cruciate ligament reconstruction provoking severe anterior knee pain, *Arthroscopy* 2004; 20: 528–531, with permission from Arthroscopy Association of North America.)

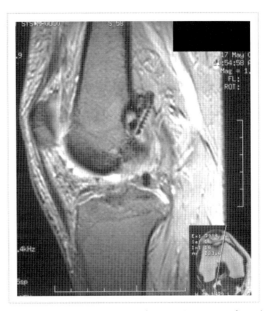

Figure 7.18. Sagittal GrE T2* MRI demonstrating a severe femoral screw/tunnel divergence. Moreover, you can note that the screw is broken (arrow). (Reprinted from Sanchis-Alfonso, V, and M Tintó-Pedrerol, Femoral interference screw divergence after anterior cruciate ligament reconstruction provoking severe anterior knee pain, *Arthroscopy* 2004; 20: 528–531, with permission from Arthroscopy Association of North America.)

existence of an important impingement between the screw and the surrounding soft tissues, specifically the lateral head of the gastrocnemius. We must note that the existence of impingement depends not only on the divergence in the sagittal plane, but also in the coronal plane. The fact that our patient was pain free after screw removal supports the hypothesis that the anterior knee pain source was in the posterior aspect of the knee.

How Can We Explain the Anterior Knee Pain in Our Patient, Basing Ourselves on the Proposed Hypothesis?

First, because of the increment of the patellofemoral joint reaction force (PFJR). This increment is secondary to the slight and maintained knee flexion, due to the contracture of the lateral head of the gastrocnemius caused by irritation caused by the femoral screw. Sachs and colleagues[43] first proposed the association between anterior knee pain with flexion contracture of the knee. Later, Shelbourne and Trumper emphasized the importance of obtaining full extension to reduce the incidence of anterior knee pain after ACL reconstruction.[49] The increment of the PFJR force contributes to

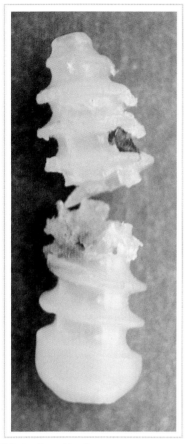

Figure 7.19. Broken femoral interference screw. (Reprinted from Sanchis-Alfonso, V, and M Tintó-Pedrerol, Femoral interference screw divergence after anterior cruciate ligament reconstruction provoking severe anterior knee pain, *Arthroscopy* 2004; 20: 528–531, with permission from Arthroscopy Association of North America.)

increasing overload of the subchondral bone of the patella, which could explain the positive compression patellar test documented in our patient.

Second, because of the increment of the valgus vector force at the knee. This increment is secondary to the increment in foot pronation of the subtalar joint due to the contracture of the lateral head of the gastrocnemius.[13,26,33] The increment of the valgus vector could explain pain with passive medial patellar mobility.

What Have We Learned from This Case?

The first lesson learned from this case is that although patellar subluxation is a potential cause of anterior knee pain, we must note that not all

malaligments are symptomatic. Hence, we must always rule out other causes of anterior knee pain that can resemble the symptoms of malalignment and lead to incorrect diagnosis and, consequently, incorrect treatment. The second lesson learned from this case is that anterior knee pain can arise in the posterior aspect of the knee.

Patient 2

An 18-year-old female presented in our outpatient clinic with a 1.5-year history of severe anterior left knee pain recalcitrant to conservative treatment. A joint effusion was aspirated twice at this interval of time, the obtained aspirate being yellowish. Moreover, the patient presented recurrent episodes of knee locking. There was no history of trauma. Pain was aggravated by forced knee flexion, by ascending stairs, squatting, and prolonged sitting with flexed knee. In the end, she had problems with activities of daily living.

Physical Examination

Physical examination revealed tenderness to palpation at the anteromedial aspect of the knee. Moreover, there was a precise painful area localized at the anteromedial aspect of the knee. There were no inflammatory signs, no localized swelling, no joint effusion, no palpable mass, and the meniscal and ligamentous tests were negative. The patella was painful when mobilized. The range of motion of the knee was normal.

Image Evaluation

Conventional radiography revealed no abnormalities. Because of the severity of the clinical symptoms contrasting with the paucity of the clinical examination, and the normality of routine x-rays, MRI was performed. MRI showed a well-demarcated and homogeneous solitary mass lesion within the infrapatellar Hoffa fat pad occupying the pretibial recess (Figure 7.20). MRI tilt angle according to the method described by Grelsamer and Weinstein[16] was of 20°.

Treatment Plan

Prior to resection of the lesion of the Hoffa fat pad a routine arthroscopy was performed using standard anterolateral and anteromedial portals under general anesthesia. We found an unexpected single yellowish-brown tumor-like ovoid mass, well encapsulated, in the anteromedial aspect of the left knee, just in front of the anterior horn of the medial meniscus (Figure 7.21A).

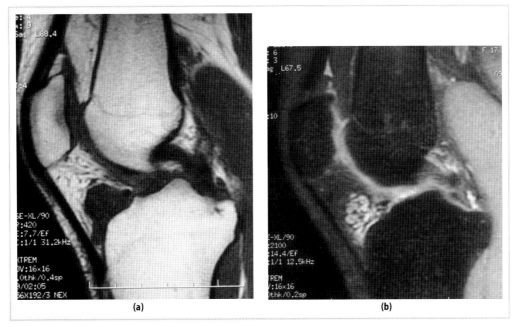

Figure 7.20. MRI. Sagittal plane FSE T1W, showing a rounded lesion involving the infrapatellar Hoffa's fat pad, isointense with skeletal muscle, displacing the intermeniscal ligament but without affecting either bone or the patellar tendon **(a)**. Oblique sagittal plane FSE PDW with Fat Sat, showing the same lesion as in Figure 7.20A **(b)**. The lesion appears hyperintense, of polycyclic appearance, and with hemosiderin and/or ferritin within the interior and at periphery. Likewise, no bone or tendon involvement is noted in this image.

A long pedicle attached the mass to the adjacent synovial membrane (Figure 7.21B). According to Huang and colleagues[18] the observation of a pedicle, as in our case, is relevant because torsion of this pedicle can produce acute knee pain. Moreover, there was a discrete involvement of the surrounding synovium with hypertrophic villous-like projections with brownish

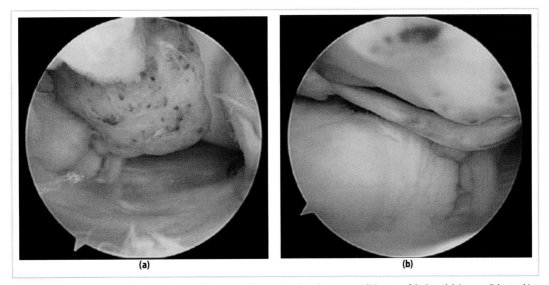

Figure 7.21. Arthroscopic view of the tumor. Tumor-like mass, well encapsulated, in the anteromedial aspect of the knee **(a)**. Long pedicle attaching the mass to adjacent synovium **(b)**.

(continued)

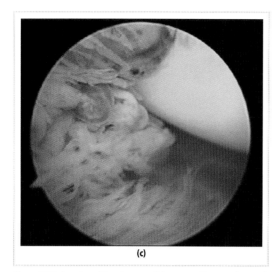

Figure 7.21. *(continued)* Involvement of the surrounding synovium with hypertrophic villous-like projections with brownish pigmentation **(c)**.

cells and a hyperplastic vascular pattern. The typical nodular proliferation of fibroblasts and macrophages was not present, nor were the giant cells.

The postoperative course was uneventful. The patient had a prompt and complete recovery of her symptoms and returned to her normal daily activities.

What Have We Learned from This Case?

The first lesson learned from this case is that MRI does not always allow us to detect synovial abnormalities, the arthroscopy being an important diagnostic and therapeutic tool. The second lesson learned from this case is that although patellar tilt is a potential cause of anterior knee pain, it is not always symptomatic. Hence, we must always rule out other causes of anterior knee pain that can resemble the symptoms of malalignment and lead to incorrect diagnosis and, consequently, incorrect treatment. Lastly, the presence of effusion is indicative of an intra-articular injury, a localized pigmented villonodular synovitis in our case, rather than retinacular injury.

pigmentation (Figure 7.21C). No other intra-articular abnormalities were noted. The intra-articular lesion was resected arthroscopically and easily removed through the medial portal, which had been previously enlarged with a surgical blade. The tumor was well-encapsulated and measured 1.5 cm long. After this, we performed an arthroscopic partial synovectomy of the surrounding synovitis with a motorized shaver introduced through the anteromedial portal. After arthroscopy, the solid tumor of the pretibial recess, the preoperative expected mass lesion, was removed through an anterior approach through the patellar tendon. The mass had a brownish aspect, well delimited and 3 cm in diameter.

Both nodules, and the surrounding synovium of the intra-articular mass, were submitted for histological study. Pathologists referred the intra-articular nodule to be a nodular form of a typical pigmented villonodular synovitis, with a proliferation of fibroblasts, giant cells, xanthomatous cells, and hemosiderin ladened macrophages. Similar histological features were observed in the surrounding synovium of the intra-articular mass. Nevertheless, the nodule localized in the Hoffa fat pad was considered as a nodular chronic nonspecific synovitis because, although it showed plenty of macrophages with hemosiderin deposits and xanthomatous changes, the stroma was myxoid, paucicellular, with small aggregates of lymph

References

1. Alexeeff, M, and MF Macnicol. Subacute patellar osteomyelitis. *Knee* 1995; 1: 237–239.
2. Axhausen, G. Zur Pathogenese der Artritis deformans. *Arch Orthop Unfallchir* 1922; 20: 1.
3. Bruns, J, G Eggers-Stroeder, D von Torklus. Synovial hemangioma: A rare benign synovial tumor. Report of four cases. *Knee Surg Sports Traumatol Arthrosc* 1994; 2: 186–189.
4. Carls, J, D Kohn, and H Maschek. Benign giant-cell tumor of the patellar ligament. *Arthroscopy* 1998; 14: 94–98.
5. Cipolla, M, G Cerullo, V Franco et al. The double patella syndrome. *Knee Surg Sports Traumatol Arthrosc* 1995; 3: 21–25.
6. Chow, JCY, M Hantes, and JB Houle. Hypertrophy of the synovium in the anteromedial aspect of the knee joint following trauma: an unusual cause of knee pain. *Arthroscopy* 2002; 18: 735–740.
7. Choi, NH. Localized pigmented villonodular synovitis involving the fat pad of the knee. *Am J Knee Surg* 2000; 13: 117–119.
8. Delcogliano, A, M Galli, A Menghi et al. Localized pigmented villonodular synovitis of the knee: Report of two cases of fat pad involvement. *Arthroscopy* 1998; 14: 527–531.
9. Dhillon, MS, C Rajasekhar, and ON Nagi. Tuberculosis of the patella: Report of a case and review of the literature. *Knee* 1995; 2: 53–56.
10. Duri, ZAA, PM Aichroth, and G Dowd. The fat pad: Clinical observations. *Am J Knee Surg* 1996; 9: 55–66.

11. Ellen, MI, HB Jackson, and SJ DiBiase. Uncommon causes of anterior knee pain: A case report of infrapatellar contracture syndrome. *Am J Phys Med Rehabil* 1999; 78: 376–380.

12. Elliot, AJ, and JP Fulkerson. Skeletal muscle hemangioma: A cause of unexplained pain about the knee. *Arthroscopy* 1989; 5: 269–273.

13. Eng, JJ, and MR Pierrynowski. Evaluation of soft foot orthotics in the treatment of patellofemoral pain syndrome. *Phys Ther* 1993; 73: 62–70.

14. Ferguson, PC, AM Griffin, and RS Bell. Primary patellar tumors. *Clin Orthop* 1997; 336: 199–204.

15. Georgoulis, AD, PN Soucacos, AE Beris et al. Osteoid osteoma in the differential diagnosis of persistent joint pain. *Knee Surg Sports Traumatol Arthrosc* 1995; 3: 125–128.

16. Grelsamer, R, and C Weinstein. Patellar tilt: An MRI study. *Tenth Congress European Society of Sports Traumatology, Knee Surgery and Arthroscopy, Book of Abstracts*, Rome, 23–27 April 2002, p. 178.

17. Hardy, Ph, GP Muller, C Got et al. Glomus tumor of the fat pad. *Arthroscopy* 1998; 14: 325–328.

18. Huang, GS, CH Lee, WP Chan et al. Localized nodular synovitis of the knee: MRI imaging appearance and clinical correlates in 21 patients. *Am J Radiol* 2003; 181: 539–543.

19. Insall, *J. Surgery of the Knee*. New York: Churchill Livingstone, 1984.

20. Johnson, LL. *Arthroscopic Surgery: Principles and Practice*. St. Louis: C.V. Mosby, 1986.

21. Khan, KM, BW Tress, WSC Hare et al. "Treat the patient, not the x-ray": Advances in diagnostic imaging do not replace the need for clinical interpretation [lead editorial]. *Clin J Sport Med* 1998; 8: 1–4.

22. Kim, SJ, NH Choi, and SC Lee. Tenosynovial giant-cell tumor in the knee joint. *Arthroscopy* 1995; 11: 213–215.

23. Kim, SJ, SJ Shin, and TY Koo. Arch type pathologic suprapatellar plica. *Arthroscopy* 2001; 17: 536–538.

24. Kim, SJ, JY Kim, and JW Lee. Pathologic infrapatellar plica. *Arthroscopy* 2002; E25.

25. Kim, SJ, JH Jeong, YM Cheon et al. MPP test in the diagnosis of medial patellar plica syndrome. *Arthroscopy* 2004; 20: 1101–1103.

26. Klingman, RE, SM Liaos, and KM Hardin. The effect of subtalar joint position on patellar glide position in subjects with excessive rearfoot pronation. *J Sports Phys Ther* 1997; 25: 185–191.

27. Kurosaka, M, S Yoshiya, M Yamada et al. Lateral synovial plica syndrome: A case report. *Am J Sports Med* 1992; 20:92–94.

28. Lorentzon, R, H Alfredson, and Ch Hildingsson. Treatment of deep cartilage defects of the patella with periosteal transplantation. *Knee Surg Sports Traumatol Arthrosc* 1998; 6:202–208.

29. Lundy, DW, AJ Aboulafia, JB Otis et al. Myxoid liposarcoma of the retropatellar fat pad. *Am J Orthop* 1997; 26: 287–289.

30. Matsumoto, H, M Kawakabo, T Otani et al. Extensive posttraumatic ossification of the patellar tendon. *J Bone Joint Surg* 1999; 81-B: 34–36.

31. McAllister, DR, and RD Parker. Bilateral subluxating popliteus tendons: A case report. *Am J Sports Med* 1999; 27: 376–379.

32. McConnell, J. Fat pad irritation: A mistaken patellar tendinitis. *Sport Health* 1991; 9: 7–9.

33. McConnell, J. Conservative management of patellofemoral problems. In Grelsamer, RP, and J MacConnell, eds., *The Patella: A Team Approach*. Gaithersburg, MD: Aspen, 1998, pp. 119–136.

34. Meister, K, and AM Jackson. Longitudinal stress fracture of the patella: An autolateral release. A case report. *Am J Knee Surg* 1994; 7: 49–52.

35. Mori, Y, M Kubo, J Shimokoube et al. Osteochondritis dissecans of the patellofemoral groove in athletes: Unusual cases of patellofemoral pain. *Knee Surg Sports Traumatol Arthrosc* 1994; 2: 242–244.

36. Mori, Y, H Okumo, H Iketani et al. Efficacy of lateral retinacular release for painful bipartite patella. *Am J Sports Med* 1995; 23: 13–18.

37. Muscolo, DL, MA Ayerza, A Makino et al. Tumors about the knee misdiagnosed as athletic injuries. *J Bone Joint Surg* 2003; 85-A: 1209–1214.

38. Orava, S, S Taimela, M Kvist et al. Diagnosis and treatment of stress fracture of the patella in athletes. *Knee Surg Sports Traumatol Arthrosc* 1996; 4: 206–211.

39. Palumbo, RC, LS Matthews, and JM Reuben. Localized pigmented villonodular synovitis of the patellar fat pad: A report of two cases. *Arthroscopy* 1994; 10: 400–403.

40. Pinar, H, M Özkan, D Akseki et al. Traumatic prepatellar neuroma: An unusual cause of anterior knee pain. *Knee Surg Sports Traumatol Arthrosc* 1996; 4: 154–156.

41. Pinar, H, M Bozkurt, L Baktiroglu et al. Intra-articular hemangioma of the knee with meniscal and bony attachment. *Arthroscopy* 1997; 13: 507–510.

42. Safran, MR, and FHn Fu. Uncommon causes of knee pain in the athlete. *Orthop Clin North Am* 1995; 26: 547–559.

43. Sachs, RA, DM Daniel, ML Stone et al. Patellofemoral problems after anterior cruciate ligament reconstruction. *Am J Sports Med* 1989; 17: 760–765.

44. Sanchis-Alfonso, V, CI Fernandez, C Sanchez et al. Hemangioma intramuscular (Aportación de 6 casos y revisión de la literatura). *Rev Esp de Cir Ost* 1990; 25: 367–378.

45. Sanchis-Alfonso, V. *Cirugía de la rodilla: Conceptos actuales y controversias*. Madrid: Editorial Médica Panamericana, 1995.

46. Sanchis-Alfonso, V, E Roselló-Sastre, V Martinez-SanJuan et al. Occult localized osteonecrosis of the patella: Case report. *Am J Knee Surg* 1997; 10: 166–170.

47. Sanchis-Alfonso, V, and M Tintó-Pedrerol. Femoral interference screw divergence after anterior cruciate ligament reconstruction provoking severe anterior knee pain. *Arthroscopy* 2004; 20: 528–531.

48. Schmitz, MC, B Schaefer, and J Bruns. A ganglion of the anterior horn of the medial meniscus invading the infrapatellar fat pad: Case report. *Knee Surg Sports Traumatol Arthrosc* 1996; 4: 97–99.

49. Shelbourne, KD, and RV Trumper. Preventing anterior knee pain after anterior cruciate ligament reconstruction. *Am J Sports Med* 1997; 25: 41–47.

50. Tapper, EM, and NW Hoover. Late results after meniscectomy. *J Bone Joint Surg* 1969; 51-A: 517–526.

51. Teitz, CC, and RM Harrington. Patellar stress fracture. *Am J Sports Med* 1992; 20: 761–765.

52. Tennent, TD, NC Birch, MJ Holmes et al. Knee pain and the infrapatellar branch of the saphenous nerve. *J R Soc Med* 1998; 91: 573–575.

53. Williams, AM, and PT Myers. Localized pigmented villonodular synovitis: A rare cause of locking of the knee. *Arthroscopy* 1997; 13: 515–516.

54. Yilmaz, E, L Karakurt, I Ozercan et al. A ganglion cyst that developed from the infrapatellar fat pad of the knee. *Arthroscopy* 2004; E14.

8

Risk Factors and Prevention of Anterior Knee Pain

Erik Witvrouw, Damien Van Tiggelen, and Tine Willems

Introduction

Anterior knee pain (AKP) is known as a very common problem in the sporting population.[1,5,15,16,30] Many of the patients with anterior knee pain need conservative treatment to be able to return to sport or their daily activities. On the other hand, because of this high incidence of anterior knee pain, prevention of this pathology has been an important goal for many sports medicine practitioners for some years. However, before a scientific approach in planning and carrying out prevention and treatment of anterior knee pain can be set up, a thorough understanding of the etiology of anterior knee pain seems essential. This understanding refers to information on why a particular individual develops anterior knee pain and another individual, exposed to more or less the same exercise load, does not. In addition, it seems important to understand why some patients benefit from a treatment program while others do not, or not as well. To answer these important issues risk factors for the development of anterior knee pain need to be identified.

General consensus exists about the fact that myriad factors may contribute to the development of anterior knee pain. Anterior knee pain can be considered as a multi-risk phenomenon with various risk factors interacting at a given time.[32] Risk factors are traditionally divided into two main categories: intrinsic (or internal) and extrinsic (or external) risk factors. The extrinsic risk factors relate to environmental variables,

for example, exercise load, exercise intensity, exercise type, amount of physical activity, equipment, weather conditions, and playing field conditions. In contrast, intrinsic risk factors relate to the individual physical and psychological characteristics such as age, joint instability, gender, muscle strength, muscle flexibility, conditioning, and so forth.

Focusing on injury prevention requires the use of a dynamic model that accounts for the multifactorial nature of anterior knee pain. One such model is described by Meeuwisse.[32] This model describes how multiple factors interact to produce an injury (Figure 8.1). It can be seen in this model that numerous intrinsic factors theoretically may predispose an individual to anterior knee pain. This model also shows very well the interaction of both intrinsic and extrinsic factors, in the way that the extrinsic risk factors act on the predisposed athlete from outside. Consequently, knowledge of both the intrinsic and extrinsic risk factors of anterior knee pain seems essential in our understanding of the etiology, and thus in creating prevention and conservative treatment programs.

The Role of Extrinsic Risk Factors in the Development of Anterior Knee Pain

The association between clinical overload (external risk factors) and the development of anterior knee pain is well known.[14,34] Recently,

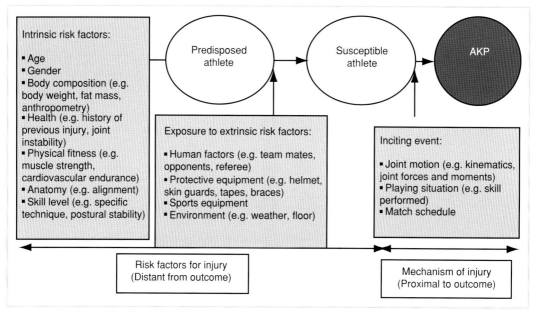

Figure 8.1. A dynamic, multifactorial model of sports injury etiology. (Adapted from Meeuwisse.[32])

Dye[11] stated that the function of the patellofemoral joint (and any other joint) could be characterized by a load/frequency distribution (the envelope of function) that defines a range of painless loading that is compatible with homeostasis of the joint tissues. If excessive loading is placed across the joint, loss of tissue homeostasis can occur, resulting in pain and other dysfunctions. Excessive loading on the PF joint can simply cause the source of loss of homeostasis. This supraphysiological loading can be a consequence of a single event (overload) or repetitive loading (overuse), but indicates the important association between extrinsic risk factors (amount of loading) and the etiology of anterior knee pain. An athlete who has sustained an overuse injury must have exceeded his or her limits in such way that the negative remodeling of the injured structure predominates over the repair process due to the stresses placed on the structure.[24] The goal of the conservative treatment is therefore to restore the homeostasis of the patellofemoral joint.[11] Repeated applied stresses below the tensile limit of a structure lead to a positive remodeling if sufficient time between stress applications is provided.[20,24] Consequently, this principle should be used in the construction of a conservative and a preventive program for anterior knee pain.

Importance and Identification of Intrinsic Risk Factors of Anterior Knee Pain

In the literature, several studies are available focusing on the relationship between the intrinsic risk factors and anterior knee pain. However, the majority of these studies are retrospective and/or lacking a control group. In the latter, it is impossible to deduce a causative relation between the examined intrinsic risk factors and anterior knee pain. Hence, to identify this causative relationship prospective studies are needed. Looking in the available literature, the amount of prospective research in the area of anterior knee pain focusing on the relationship between the intrinsic risk factors and anterior knee pain is very scarce.

The first prospective study focusing on the anterior knee pain and intrinsic risk factors was performed by Milgrom et al.[34] They prospectively examined 390 infantry recruits and revealed that an increased medial tibial intercondylar distance and an increased isometric strength of the quadriceps, tested at 85 degrees of knee flexion, had a statistically significant correlation with the incidence of anterior knee pain caused by overactivity. Recruits in that study who could generate higher patellofemoral contact forces because of stronger extensor muscle strength, or the presence of more genu varum, had a higher rate of anterior knee pain related to overactivity. The authors therefore concluded that anterior knee pain due to overactivity is caused by an overload of patellofemoral contact forces. In our own study[50] on 282 students in physical education we prospectively examined a broad variety of presumed intrinsic risk factors. Of this broad variety of parameters, only a shortened quadriceps muscle, an altered vastus medialis obliquus muscle reflex response time, a decreased explosive strength, and a hypermobile patella had a significant correlation with the incidence of anterior knee pain. Very conspicuous in this study was the finding that statistical analyses did not identify any of the clinically measured lower leg alignment characteristics (leg length difference, height, weight, Q angle, genu varum/valgum and recurvatum, foot alignment) as predisposing factors of anterior knee pain. This suggests that these parameters seem less important in the development of anterior knee pain, in contrast to what is frequently stated on the basis of theoretical models and/or retrospective studies. The results of our study are in agreement with the results of Milgrom et al.[34] in that they indicate that from a broad variety of parameters only a few contribute significantly to the development of anterior knee pain. In a recent prospective study on recreational runners[29] this conclusion was confirmed. Lun et al.[29] found that of the examined static biomechanical lower leg alignment parameters (genu varum/valgum and recurvatum, height, weight, leg length difference, Q angle, hip internal and external range of motion, ankle dorsiflexion and plantar flexion, rearfoot and forefoot valgus, standing longitudinal arch), only a smaller right ankle dorsiflexion ROM, a greater genu varum, and a greater left forefoot varus was significantly different between the runners who developed anterior knee pain and the uninjured runners. In a more recent prospective study in male military recruits Van Tiggelen et al.[47] identified a significant smaller peak torque at low concentric isokinetic speed as an intrinsic risk factor of AKP. This emphasizes the importance of the reinforcement of quadriceps strength in the treatment and prevention of AKP, as in other overuse injuries of the lower limb.[22]

Conclusions drawn on the basis of relatively few data should always be warranted. However, on the basis of the few existing prospective data

on anterior knee pain some trends can be identified. First, these studies have shown that clinically measured lower leg alignment characteristics such as leg length difference, height, weight, Q angle, genu varum/valgum and recurvatum, and foot alignment seem not to be very important in the development of anterior knee pain. This could be explained in different ways. First, it could be that these clinically measured parameters cannot be considered as intrinsic risk factors of anterior knee pain. Second, it could be that measuring these parameters clinically is not precise enough. For instance, small inter-individual differences, which might be important in the etiology of anterior knee pain, might not be identified since the measurement error is too large. Therefore, prospective studies should be set up using more precise measuring techniques (2- or 3-dimensional measurements in movement analysis labs). Third, it must be mentioned that all the available prospective studies were performed on a young sportive population (military recruits or students in physical education). This implies that this population is rather homogeneous and very select. Probably, measuring these parameters in the general population should give more inter-individual variation. In addition, subjects with large "abnormalities" in these clinically measured lower leg alignment characteristics could already have developed anterior knee pain and would therefore decide not to start such a physically demanding training program. Consequently, one must be very careful when applying these results to the general population of anterior knee pain patients. Clinical experience and retrospective data show us that patients with anterior knee pain show significantly more alterations of their lower leg alignment characteristics, compared to a control group. These findings let us believe that "large" deviations in lower leg alignment characteristics are probably important in the development of anterior knee pain. Yet, on the basis of the available studies it also seems that "small" deviations in lower leg alignment characteristics probably do not play a significant role in the genesis of anterior knee pain (unless the clinical measurements are not able to evaluate these small alterations with the necessary precision).

In contrast to the findings of the lower leg alignment characteristics, the prospective data on muscular characteristics show that the extensor muscle plays a vital role in the development of anterior knee pain. Lack of agreement between the different studies in the methods used to measure these muscular parameters limits the possibility of concluding which of the muscular parameters (strength, VMO/VL speed of contraction, flexibility) are more important than the others. However, today we can state that several muscular parameters are identified as intrinsic risk factors of anterior knee pain. Consequently, these parameters will probably play a vital role in the construction of a preventive and a conservative treatment program.

Constructing a Scientific Prevention Program for Anterior Knee Pain

Once intrinsic and extrinsic risk factors of anterior knee pain are identified, the next step in "the sequence of prevention" can be undertaken. Van Mechelen et al.[46] suggest a strategy of four stages that should be followed in order to scientifically have an impact on the incidence of anterior knee pain (prevention), and on the success rate of a conservative treatment program (Figure 8.2). After establishing the incidence and severity of anterior knee pain in the sports population (which has been done by several researchers), the risk factors and the mechanisms of the occurrence of anterior knee pain must be identified (cf. above). The next step is to introduce measures that are likely to reduce the risk of developing anterior knee pain. These measures should be based on the information about the intrinsic and extrinsic risk factors. However, as mentioned by Reider[43] after a correct identification of the risk factors, before a preventive program can be introduced it should be clear (1) whether the identified risk factors can be influenced, and (2) which program is best in altering these identified risk factors.

In order to examine this for anterior knee pain, we set up a randomized clinical trial to investigate which of the frequently used conservative programs (open versus closed kinetic chain programs) is best in altering the identified risk factors of anterior knee pain. Sixty patients with anterior knee pain were randomized into a 5-week program that consisted of only closed kinetic chain exercises or only open kinetic chain exercises. In this study the evaluation focused on those parameters that (1) were previously identified as intrinsic risk factors of anterior knee pain in prospective studies, and (2) can be influenced by a conservative program.

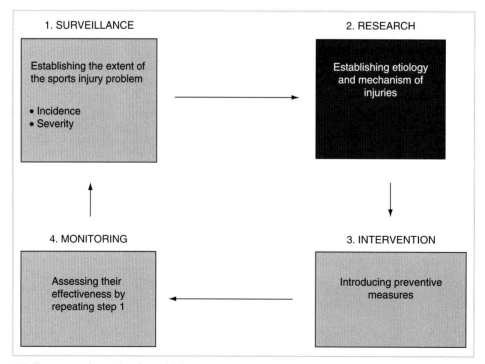

Figure 8.2. The sequence of prevention of sports injuries. (Adapted from Van Mechelen, with permission from Adis International, Wolters Kluwer Health).[46]

Only four parameters met these criteria at that time: namely muscle length of the quadriceps, explosive functional strength of the quadriceps (measured by the triple jump test), reflex response time of the VMO and VL, and mediolateral patellar mobility. Concerning the muscle-length measurements of the quadriceps, this study revealed significant increases in range of knee motion in both groups. However, since both training programs used the same stretching program, it was not surprising that no significant difference between both groups was observed (nor was it expected). The results of the study showed that only the closed kinetic chain group revealed a significant increase in explosive strength (jumping distance) during this study. This can be explained by the specificity of training, but favors the use of closed kinetic exercises for improving explosive functional strength. Looking at the reflex response times of VMO and VL in AKP patients, we found no significant alterations in this parameter either after an open or a closed kinetic chain program. This finding suggests that AKP patients still have an insufficient reflex response time of the VMO and VL after these training programs. Based on these findings we are making an attempt to state that if the primary objective of a conservative or preventive treatment protocol is to modify this neuromuscular parameter, the use of these two exercise programs is not to be advised. In addition, these findings emphasize the need for studies analyzing the effect of specifically designed "VMO timing" programs. Relating to the mediolateral patellar mobility, the study did not show any significant changes after a 5-week treatment period in any of the two exercise groups.

The next step in the sequence of prevention is to construct a prevention program on the basis of the research findings described above. Until today, no such studies have been set up. Only some studies have been undertaken to evaluate the effectiveness of preventive strategies in sports medicine in general, and lower limb injuries specifically. This research has generally revealed that strategies designed to prevent sports injuries can be effective. These studies generally examined the effectiveness of a multifactorial program consisting of different items like correction of training, sport-specific cardiovascular conditioning, strength training, flexibility, and proprioceptive exercises. Therefore it remains unclear which parts of the program

were effective and which were not. However, some studies have examined the effect of solitary regular ankle disc training as a preventive measure. Although these studies were not performed to evaluate its effect on the incidence of anterior knee pain, this training seems to be promising to prevent both ankle and traumatic knee injuries.[49]

Constructing a Prevention Program for Anterior Knee Pain
Influencing the Intrinsic Risk Factors of AKP by Exercises

On the basis of the available results in the literature we made an attempt to describe where the emphasis of a prevention program of anterior knee pain to influence intrinsic risk factors should lie.

First, some literature reveals that a decreased flexibility of the hamstrings and quadriceps can be considered as risk factors of AKP. Consequently, it can be concluded that stretching of the hamstring and quadriceps should be considered as an important aspect of a preventive (and conservative) treatment program in AKP patients, and should preferably be incorporated in these treatment programs.

Regarding the use of an open or closed kinetic chain exercise program it should be mentioned that these programs were not able to alter two of the four examined intrinsic risk factors. In addition, only the closed kinetic chain program was able to alter significantly the explosive strength. This seems to be an important issue since several investigators have found a strong association between quadriceps strength increase and locomotor function in patients with AKP.[41,45] Natri et al.[35] not only observed that this association was important in the short-term outcome, but identified a strong correlation between restoration of quadriceps muscle strength and the long-term (7-year) final outcome in AKP patients. This and the several clinical studies that show good-to-excellent results in AKP patients when emphasizing quadriceps strengthening point to the importance of a good functional quadriceps strength.[8] This implies that it can be stated that functional quadriceps strengthening should be an important aspect of a prevention program of AKP. The fact that a functional strength deficit, and not an analytical strength deficit, was identified as a risk factor of AKP leads us to conclude that the use of functional strength training as a

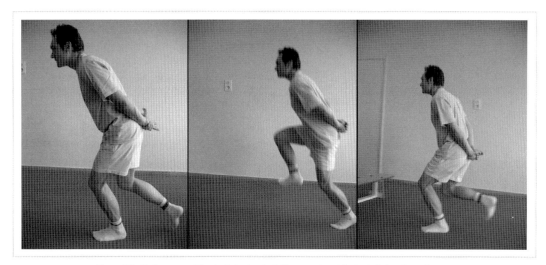

Figure 8.3. Performance of the single leg hop test. The arms stay at the back during the entire test.

preventive measure should be advised. To identify subjects with a low explosive strength we
advise the use of a single leg hop test or a triple
jump test (Figure 8.3).

Influencing the Intrinsic Risk Factors of AKP by External Devices

Using Foot Orthoses in the Prevention of AKP

Identification of Alterations in Foot Alignment in AKP

Lun et al.[29] identified forefoot varus as a potential risk factor of AKP in recreational runners.
On the basis of this prospective study, it is our
opinion that it is necessary to evaluate the foot
alignment of subjects in regard to a preventive
treatment approach. It has been shown that the
proper choice of adapted footwear has a positive
influence on all overuse injuries of the lower
limb by diminishing the deleterious impact
forces.[9,10,20,23,24]

Prior to describing the effect of foot orthoses,
it seems important to understand what is considered as a "normal" foot. According to
Livingston and Mandigo,[28] the subtalar joint
pronation accompanied by the eversion of the
calcaneum, knee flexion, and the internal rotation of the tibia play an important role in the
shock absorption at heel contact. The subtalar
joint continues to pronate until the end of the
footflat phase. Thereafter, the subtalar joint
starts to supinate combined with a knee exten-

sion and external rotation of the tibia. A delayed
subtalar supination and external rotation of the
tibial bone results in a compensatory reaction in
the knee joint and patellofemoral joint. For both
pes planus and pes cavus a higher risk of injury
has been reported among physically active
people.

Duffey et al.[10] demonstrated that as the foot
collides with the ground during the first 10% of
the support phase, the runner's weight, magnified by the acceleration of gravity, increases the
load on the lower extremity. Concurrently, the
support foot pronates, which serves to assist in
absorbing the shock impact. In their study, AKP
patients had 25% less pronation during this critical phase (5.1° versus 6.4°) although the maximum pronation and rearfoot motion was not
significantly different from a control group.
They hypothesize that this action might have
made a more rigid landing, thereby increasing
the shock to the lower limb and patellofemoral
joint. Duffey et al.[10] also recorded higher foot
arches in the AKP group, which is consistent
with the report of Cowan et al.[6] wherein an
increase of activity-related injuries correlates
with increased high arch height in army recruits.
Nigg et al.[38] demonstrated that the transfer of
foot inversion to internal leg rotation was found
to increase significantly with increasing arch
height.

Kaufmann et al.[26] performed a prospective
study on the effect of foot structure and range of
motion on AKP in approximately 140 recruits.

They did not find any significant differences in the foot structure or rearfoot motion. They evaluated static and dynamic values but only in a total range of motion. The different phases of the gait were not analyzed as in the study of Duffey et al.,[10] which might be the origin of these inconsistencies.

By evaluating other kinetic variables of the rearfoot, Messier et al.[33] did not find significant differences between runners with AKP and a control group regarding the rearfoot motion in their study. Regarding the literature on the relation between the rearfoot motion and AKP, many contradictions can be found. The methodological differences and the multifactorial nature of the conducted studies could explain parts of these discrepancies.

Effects of Foot Orthoses

The effects of foot orthoses have been biomechanically investigated through kinematics and pressure pattern of the foot. Orthoses have been reported to reduce maximum pronation velocity, time to maximal pronation, and total rearfoot motion during walking and running activities.[42] They also appear to limit the internal rotation of the tibia and the Q-angle at the patellofemoral joint. This latter effect will reduce the laterally directed resultant forces of the soft tissues and would theoretically reduce the contact pressure of the patella on the femoral condyles.[18]

Eng and Pierrynowski[13] studied the effect of soft foot orthotics on 3D lower-limb kinematics during walking and running activities. The analysis of 10 adolescent female subjects suffering from AKP and having a forefoot varus and calcaneal valgus greater than 6° showed small changes (1°–3°) in the transverse and frontal plane motion of the talocrural/subtalar joint and knee during both walking and running. These very small changes were sufficient to influence the symptoms of the subjects.[12]

According to several authors,[25,27,36,37] orthoses have no influence on the quadriceps muscle function (VMO-VL) but they contribute to the alignment of the patellofemoral joint by minor changes in the patellar position (medial glide). In a recently published study, Hertel et al.[21] contradict these earlier findings. During slow single-leg squat and lateral stepdown, the EMG recordings of the VM, VL, and gluteus medius muscle differed in the foot orthotic conditions. The most surprising finding in their study was

that all foot types react in the same, positive way to 4 different orthoses. These changes were not significant when performing explosive exercises like vertical jumps.

Sutlive et al.[44] conducted challenging research on the identification of AKP patients whose pain and symptoms improved after a combined program of orthoses and activity modification. Due to the multifactorial character of the impairment, not all AKP patients need orthoses. The identification of the risk factors in a primary prevention setting would be even more challenging.

We can conclude by assuming that the foot mechanics indirectly and subtly influences the patellofemoral joint although the exact mechanisms are not fully understood. AKP patients with altered foot alignment characteristics or running biomechanics might benefit from foot orthoses as demonstrated by some researchers. The use of orthoses as a preventive measure makes sense on a theoretical basis, but regarding the subtle biomechanical modifications caused by orthoses on AKP patients[13,18] it is doubtful that clear clinical guidelines could be fine-tuned. Striking is the finding that no prospective studies on the use of orthoses as preventive measure for AKP are yet performed. Therefore, today no substantial evidence exists on the preventive use of foot orthoses for AKP.

Patellofemoral Bracing

The malalignment of the patella and lower limb is widely accepted as an important etiological factor of AKP.[16] Despite the fact that prospective studies have minimized the importance of "minor" alterations in the clinically measured lower leg alignment characteristics, mediolateral patellar hyper mobility was identified as an intrinsic risk factor of AKP. Since this parameter seems to play an important role in the genesis of AKP, prevention programs should attempt to decrease this parameter in subjects with a hypermobile patella. Our study, however, failed to influence this characteristic after a 5-week training program with open or closed kinetic chain exercises. Interestingly, the function of patellofemoral knee braces is to improve the patellar tracking and maintain the patellofemoral alignment. Besides this mechanical function, some authors suggest other mechanisms (thermal effect, an increased sensory feedback, an altered circulation of the knee region) by which the brace may be effective.[4]

Preventive patellofemoral bracing may be viewed as a method to help maintain an ideal biomechanical environment in order to avoid irritation of the surrounding tissues.

To our knowledge, only two prospective studies have been published on the effectiveness of braces in the prevention of anterior knee pain.[2,48] BenGal et al.[2] studied the efficacy of the knee brace with supportive ring as a means of preventing AKPS in 60 young athletes. They found a significant reduction in the incidence of AKPS at the end of the study in the braced group compared to the control group. Van Tiggelen et al.[48] used a different brace: the On-Track (DJ-Orthopedics) dynamic patellofemoral brace (Figure 8.4). This brace consists of knee patches with Velcro (Velcro USA Inc., Manchester, NH) and a neoprene sleeve. The design of the brace is based on the correction of the position of the patella as described by McConnell.[30] The little plastic button (activator) foreseen to stimulate the vastus medialis obliquus (VMO) muscle was not used in this study. They performed their prospective study on 167 recruits (54 braced and 113 controls) undergoing basic military train-ing. A smaller number of recruits in the brace group appeared to develop anterior knee pain compared to the recruits in the control group (p = 0.02). Out of the 54 recruits in the brace group, 10 (18.5%) developed anterior knee pain during this study. In the control group (n = 113) 42 recruits (37%) developed anterior knee pain. Hence, the results of both studies seem to scientifically support the effectiveness of a knee brace in the prevention of AKP. Nonetheless, the mechanism by which bracing seems to influence the prevention or the treatment of AKP remains enigmatic.[41] In the literature, in addition to a pure mechanical mechanism,[39] an increased sensory feedback is proposed. By using the term "increased sensory feedback" an alteration in proprioception[3,31,40] and an altered muscular recruitment are proposed.[7,17,19,39] In a yet-unpublished report, we were interested in the long-term effects (6 weeks) of continuous brac-ing. In this study we analyzed, on an isokinetic device, the quadriceps muscle peak torque of the braced and non-braced recruits who didn't develop AKP in our previous study,[48] before and after the strenuous training in non-braced test

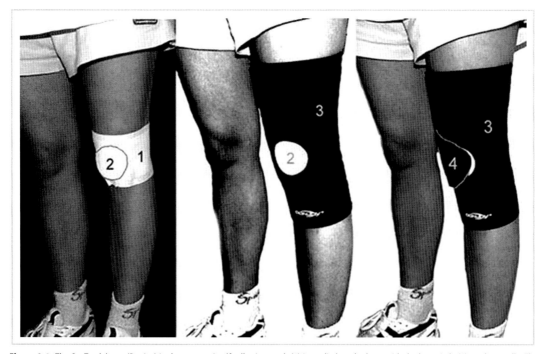

Figure 8.4. The On-Track brace (Donjoy) in three parts. A self-adhesive patch (1) is applied on the knee with the loop circle (2) on the patella. The neoprene cuff (3) is pulled onto the leg so the loop circle shows through the opening of the cuff. The hook circle (4) is attached to the loop circle on the patch. (Reproduced from reference 48 with kind permission of Springer Science+Business Media.)

conditions. After the 6-week vigorous basic military training program, we observed a significantly higher quadriceps peak torque in the braced group compared to the non-braced group. Since both groups showed equal strength prior to the basic military training program, the results suggest that 6 weeks of knee bracing has a positive effect on the quadriceps muscle strength. This suggests that besides the possible mechanical effect of bracing in controlling the mediolateral patellar mobility, knee bracing might prevent AKP by some way of facilitating muscular quadriceps activity.

Irrespective of the exact underlying mechanism of bracing, studies showed its significant preventive effect on the development of AKP during strenuous training. Therefore, the results of these studies support the use of prophylactic patellofemoral bracing in subjects undergoing vigorous activities. However, further research is needed to improve our insight in the underlying working mechanisms of prophylactic bracing on AKP.

Kneepads can also be used as a protective measure for AKP due to a direct blow (Figure 8.5). These are often used by athletes in volleyball, skating, and hockey, but also by plumbers, carpenters, welders, and even soldiers.

Conclusions

The etiopathogenic basis of AKP must be considered as multifactorial. Consequently, before any prevention program can be constructed, knowledge of the intrinsic and extrinsic risk factors of AKP is needed. The association between clinical overload of the patellofemoral joint (extrinsic risk factors) and AKP is well known. However, since only very few prospective studies are performed, the importance and identification of the different intrinsic risk factors of AKP remains enigmatic.

However, determination of these intrinsic risk factors of AKP is the first step in the sequence of injury prevention. Trying to interpret the few existing prospective and follow-up studies it seems clear that the quadriceps muscle can be considered as an important characteristic in the genesis of AKP. Consequently, training of this muscle seems the cornerstone in the prevention of AKP. Data on the quadriceps muscle seem to show that the flexibility and the functional strength are important. Accordingly, it can be postulated that stretching of the hamstring and quadriceps should be considered as

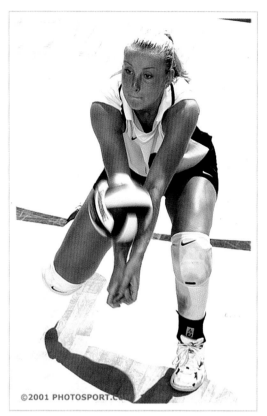

Figure 8.5. Kneepads can also be used as a protective measure for AKP due to a direct blow. Proper form combined with approved protective gear is essential in preventing injury (© 2001 PHOTOSPORT.COM with permission).

an important aspect of a preventive (and conservative) treatment program in AKP patients, and should preferably be incorporated in these treatment programs.

Concerning the muscle strength of the quadriceps, it seems that especially a lack of "functional" quadriceps strength is an important aspect in the development of AKP. This leads us to conclude that the use of functional strength training (closed kinetic chain exercises) as a preventive measure should be advised.

Striking, and not in agreement with common practice, these very few prospective data seem to indicate that clinically measured lower leg alignment characteristics such as leg length difference, height, weight, Q angle, genu varum/valgum and recurvatum seem not to be that important in the development of anterior knee pain.

Although some studies have shown the beneficial effect of the use of orthotics in the treatment of AKP, no prospective studies on the use of orthoses as preventive measure for AKP are yet performed. Therefore, today no substantial evidence exists on the preventive use of foot orthoses for AKP.

On the other hand, two prospective studies have shown that patellofemoral bracing does help to prevent AKP in subjects undergoing a strenuous training program. The exact underlying mechanism remains obscure, but one study showed that bracing is able to facilitate quadriceps strength.

However, it must be remembered that conclusions drawn in this chapter are based on the results of relatively few prospective data and should therefore always be warranted. Accordingly, it seems obvious that a lot of research is still needed before a scientific prevention program for AKP can be composed.

References

1. Almeida, SA, KM Williams, RA Shaffer, and SK Brodine. Epidemiological patterns of musculoskeletal injuries and physical training. *Med Sci Sports Exerc* 1999; Aug., 31(8): 1176–1182.
2. BenGal, S, J Lowe, G Mann, A Finsterbush, and Y Matan. The role of the knee brace in the prevention of anterior knee pain syndrome. *Am J Sports Med* 1997; Jan.–Feb., 25(1):118–122.
3. Birmingham, TB, JT Inglis, JF Kramer, and AA Vandervoort. Effect of a neoprene sleeve on knee joint kinesthesis: Influence of different testing procedures. *Med Sci Sports Exerc* 2000; 32: 304–308.
4. Cherf, J, and LE Paulos. Bracing for patellar instability. *Clin Sports Med* 1990; 9: 813–821.
5. Clement, DB, JE Taunton, GW Smart, and KL McNicol. A survey of overuse running injuries. *Phys Sports Med* 1981; 9: 47–58.
6. Cowan, DN, BH Jones, and JR Robinson. Foot morphologic characteristics and risk of exercise-related injury. *Arch Fam Ed* 1993; 2: 773–777.
7. Cowan, SM, KL Bennell, and PW Hodges. Therapeutic patellar taping changes the timing of vasti muscle activation in people with patellofemoral pain syndrome. *Clin J Sport Med*. 2002; Nov., 12(6): 339–347.
8. Crossley, K, K Bennell, S Green, S Cowan, and J McConnell. Physical therapy for patellofemoral pain: A randomized, double-blinded, placebo-controlled trial. *Am J Sports Med* 2002; Nov.–Dec., 30(6): 857–865.
9. Dixon, SJ, C Waterworth, CV Smith, and CM House. Biomechanical analysis of running in military boots with new and degraded insoles. *Med Sci Sports Exerc* 2003; Mar., 35(3): 472–479.
10. Duffey, MJ, DF Martin, DW Cannon, T Craven, and SP Messier. Etiologic factors associated with anterior knee pain in distance runners. *Med Sci Sports Exerc* 2000; 32(11): 1825–1832.
11. Dye, SF. Therapeutic implications of a tissue homeostasis approach to patellofemoral pain syndrome. *Sports Med Arthrosc Rev* 2001; 9: 306–311.
12. Eng, JJ, and MR Pierrynowski. Evaluation of soft foot orthotics in the treatment of patellofemoral pain syndrome. *Phys Ther* 1993; Feb., 73(2): 62–68; discussion 68–70.
13. Eng, JJ, and MR Pierrynowski. The effect of soft foot orthotics on three-dimensional lower-limb kinematics during walking and running. *Phys Ther* 1994; Sep., 74(9): 836–844.
14. Fairbank, JT, PB Pynsent, and JA Van Poortvliet. Mechanical factors in the incidence of knee pain in adolescents and young adults. *JBJS* 1984; 66B: 685–693.
15. Fulkerson, JP, and KP Shea. Current concepts review: Disorders of patellofemoral alignment. *J Bone Joint Surg Am* 1990; 72: 1424–1429.
16. Fulkerson, JP, and EA Arendt. Anterior Knee Pain in Females. *Clin Orthop Rel Res* 2000; 372: 69–73.
17. Gilleard, W, J McConnell, and D Parsons. The effect of patellar taping on the onset of vastus medialis obliquus and vastus lateralis muscle activity in persons with patellofemoral pain. *Phys Ther* 1998; 78: 25–32.
18. Gross, MT, and JL Foxworth. The role of foot orthoses as an intervention for patellofemoral pain. *JOSPT* 2003; 33(11): 661–670.
19. Gulling, LK, SM Lephart, DA Stone, JJ Irrgang, and DM Pincivero. The effect of patellar bracing on quadriceps EMG activity during isokinetic exercise. *Isokin Exerc Sci* 1996; 6: 133–138.
20. Hardin, EC, AJ van den Bogert, and J Hamill. Kinematic adaptations during running: Effects of footwear, surface, and duration. *Med Sci Sports Exerc* 2004; May, 36(5): 838–844.
21. Hertel, J, BR Sloss, and JE Earl. Effect of foot orthotics on quadriceps and gluteus medius electromyographic activity during selected exercises. *Arch Phys Med Rehabil* 2005; 86: 26–30.
22. Hoffman, JR, L Chapnik, A Shamis, U Givon, and B Davidson. The effect of leg strength on the incidence of lower extremity overuse injuries during military training. *Mil Med* 1999; 164(2): 153–156.
23. House, CM, C Waterworth, AJ Allsopp, and SJ Dixon. The influence of simulated wear upon the ability of insoles to reduce peak pressures during running when wearing military boots. *Gait & Posture* 2002; Dec., 16(3): 297–303.
24. Hreljac, A. Impact and overuse injuries in runners. *Med Sci Sports Exerc* 2004; May, 36(5): 845–849.
25. Hung, YJ, and MT Gross. Effect of foot position on electromyographic activity of the vastus medialis oblique and vastus lateralis during lower-extremity weight-bearing activities. *JOSPT* 1999; Feb., 29(2): 93–102; discussion 103–105.
26. Kaufman, KR, SK Brodine, RA Shaffer, CW Johnson, and TR Cullison. The effect of foot structure and range of motion on musculoskeletal overuse injuries. *Am J Sports Med* 1999; Sep.–Oct., 27(5): 585–593.
27. Klingman, RE. Foot pronation and patellofemoral joint function. *JOSPT* 1999; 29(7): 421.
28. Livingston, LA, and JL Mandigo. Bilateral rearfoot asymmetry and anterior knee pain syndrome. *JOSPT* 2003; 33: 48–55.
29. Lun, V, W Meeuwisse, P Stergiou, and D Stefanyshyn. Relation between running injury and static lower limb alignment in recreational runners. *Brit J Sports Med* 2004; 38: 576–580.

30. McConnell, J. The management of chondromalacia patellae: A long-term solution. *Australian J Physiother* 1986; 32: 215–223.
31. McNair, PJ, SN Stanley, and GR Strauss. Knee bracing: Effects on proprioception. *Arch Phys Med Rehabil* 1996; 77: 287–289.
32. Meeuwisse, WH. Assessing causation in sport injury: A multifactorial model. *Clin J Sports Med* 1994; 4: 166–170.
33. Messier, SP, SE Davis, WW Curl, RB Lowery, and RJ Pack. Etiologic factors associated with patellofemoral pain in runners. *Med Sci Sports Exerc* 1991; 23(9): 1008–1015.
34. Milgrom, C, A Finestone, N Shlamkovitch, M Giladi, and E Radin. Anterior knee pain caused by overactivity. *Clin Orthop Rel Res* 1996; 331: 256–260.
35. Natri, A, P Kannus, M Järvinen. Which factors predict the long-term outcome in chronic patellofemoral pain? *Med Sci Sports Exerc* 1998; 30: 1572–1577.
36. Nawoczenski, DA, and PM Ludewig. Electromyographic effects of foot orthotics on selected lower extremity muscles during running. *Arch Phys Med Rehabil* 1999; May, 80(5): 540–544.
37. Neptune, RR, IC Wright, and AJ van den Bogert. The influence of orthotic devices and vastus medialis strength and timing on patellofemoral loads during running. *Clin Biomech* (Bristol, Avon) 2000; Oct., 15(8): 611–618.
38. Nigg, BM, GK Cole, and W Nachbauer. Effects of arch height of the foot on angular motion of the lower extremities in running. *J. Biomech* 1993; 26: 909–916.
39. Parsons, D, and W Gilleard. The effect of patellar taping on quadriceps activity onset in the absence of pain. *J Appl Biomech* 1999; 15: 373–380.
40. Perlau, R, C Frank, and G Fick. The effect of elastic bandages on human knee proprioception in the uninjured population. *Am J Sports Med* 1995; 23: 251–255.
41. Powers, CM Rehabilitation of the patellofemoral joint disorders: A critical review. *JOSPT* 1998; 28(5): 345–354.
42. Razeghi, M, and ME Batt. Biomechanical analysis of the effect of orthotic shoe inserts: A review of the literature. *Sports Med* 2000; June, 29(6): 425–438.
43. Reider, B. An ounce of prevention. *Am J Sports Med* 2004; 32(6):1383–1384.
44. Sutlive, TG, SD Mitchell, SN Maxfield, CL McLean, JC Neumann, CR Swiecki, RC Hall, AC Bare, and TW Flynn. Identification of individuals with patellofemoral pain whose symptoms improved after a combined program of foot orthoses use and modified activity: a preliminary investigation. *Phys Ther* 2004; 84(1):49–61.
45. Thomee, R, J Augustsson, and J Karlsson. Patellofemoral pain syndrome: A review of current issues. *Sports Med* 1999; 28(4): 245–262.
46. Van Mechelen, W, H Hlobil, HCG Kemper et al. Incidence, aetiology and prevention of sports injuries: A review of concepts. *Sports Med* 1992; 14: 82–89.
47. Van Tiggelen, D, E Witvrouw, P Coorevits, JL Croisier, Ph Roget. Analysis of isokinetic parameters in the development of anterior knee pain syndrome: A prospective study in a military setting. *Isokin Exerc Sci* 2004; Dec., 12(4): 223–228.
48. Van Tiggelen, D, E Witvrouw, Ph Roget, D Cambier, L Danneels, and R Verdonk. Effect of bracing on the prevention of anterior knee pain: A prospective randomized study. *Knee Surg Sports Traumatol Arthrosc* 2004; Sep., 12(5): 434–439.
49. Wedderkopp, N, M Kaltoft, and B Lundgaard. Prevention of injuries in young female players in European team handball: A prospective intervention study. *Scand J Med Sci Sports* 1999; 9: 41–47.
50. Witvrouw. E, R Lysens, J Bellemans, D Cambier, and G Vanderstraeten. Intrinsic risk factors for the development of anterior knee pain in an athletic population: A two-year prospective study. *Am J Sports Med* 2000; July–Aug., 28(4): 480–489.

9

Conservative Treatment of Athletes with Anterior Knee Pain
Science: Classical and New Ideas
Suzanne Werner

Introduction

Anterior knee pain (AKP) is one of the most common knee disorders in physically active individuals.[27,32,91] The definition of AKP and the pathophysiological background are disputed. Despite several scientific studies through the years the reason for AKP is still unclear. Grana and Kriegshauser maintain that the cause of AKP is multifactorial.[48] Some authors mean that anatomical patella abnormalities could be causative factors (e.g., ref. 46), while others mean that it is an extensor mechanism disorder, resulting in patellar malalignment during flexion and extension of the knee joint.[45,50,57,113] Why this extensor mechanism disorder has developed is, however, not reported. There are also those authors maintaining that overuse is the most dominating reason for AKP, especially in youths.[32,110]

Symptoms

Typical symptoms are pain and/or problems during stair climbing, mostly when descending stairs and squatting as well as during prolonged sitting with flexed knees, the so-called movie sign.[40,91] AKP is often described as dull and aching with occasional episodes of acute sharp pain.[33] Giving way is another common symptom due to a sudden reflex inhibition of the quadriceps muscle often while performing some movement with the knee flexing or extending under load (e.g., during stair climbing). Patients sometimes report locking of the knee, which is usually only a catching sensation on an attempt to extend the knee joint under load. However, the AKP patients commonly are able to actively unlock the knee and therefore this type of locking should not be mixed up with the one experienced by patients with meniscal lesions.[40] A few AKP patients present with mild swelling due to synovial irritation.[40] The different symptoms in patients with AKP are frequently related to sports[1,36,45] and usually become aggravated by physical activity with knee loading characteristics.[59]

Patellar Pain versus Patellar Instability Problems

Some patients with AKP mostly complain of nonspecific knee pain localized peripatellarly, often anteromedially and/or retropatellarly,[1,36,45,59] while others complain of a feeling of patellar instability.[1,36,41] Patients that mostly complain of pain usually have a normal patellar mobility and they mainly report the symptoms to occur after physical activity, while those with patellar instability often present with a patellar hypermobility with noticeable tracking problems and they rather complain of knee problems during physical activity.[60] This means that the AKP patients should be divided into two treatment groups, one where the treatment mainly should be based on pain limitation and another one on stabilization of the patella.

Personality-Psychological Factors

Many authors have studied the relationship between personality and chronic pain (e.g., 13). Fritz et al. reported presence of psychological factors associated with knee pain in adolescence complaining of different types of knee pain.[37] Some studies on patients with AKP show a bad correlation between the patients clinical symptoms and the clinicians objective findings (e.g., 7). Jacobson and Flandry reported that some of the patients that came to visit the doctor for AKP problems at a Sport Medicine Clinic were having both chronic AKP and psychological problems.[60] Thomeé et al. studied the coping strategies for pain that AKP patients use.[111] They found that their degree of well-being is in agreement with other patient groups with chronic pain. However, some concerns could be raised in terms of the high scores that AKP patients reported for the coping strategy "catastrophizing."[111] Carlsson et al. used the Rorschach test and found elevations in psychological parameters such as hostility, dependency, and depression in AKP patients compared with healthy controls, matched for gender and age, as well as with three other reference groups.[14] However, these problems are not always evident for the patient him- or herself and their character may also vary.[14] In such cases a psychological evaluation is often advisable and therefore a collaboration with a pain clinic with psychological expertise may be beneficial.

Clinical Evaluation

The clinical examination establishes the diagnosis and tries to determine the underlying causative factors of the patient's symptoms and based on this the appropriate treatment program can be designed.[78,128] A thorough clinical examination is the key for optimal treatment of patients with AKP. This is because this category of patients presents with myriad symptoms and complaints. Since we still do not know the pathophysiological reason for AKP, we concentrate our treatment on the patient's symptoms and on the clinician's findings.

Risk Factors

A few studies on risk factors for AKP have been published. Milgrom et al. reported presence of genu varum and high isometric quadriceps strength to be risk factors for developing AKP.[82] Witvrouw et al. found that a shortened vastus medialis obliquus (VMO) reflex response time,

a decreased flexibility of the quadriceps muscle, an increased medial patellar mobility, and a reduction of vertical jump performance were significantly correlated with the incidence of AKP.[126]

History

It is important to obtain an accurate and thorough subjective history from the patient. Paying attention to this history will greatly aid the clinician in making an accurate assessment of the patient's condition and designing an appropriate treatment program.[4,15]

Differential Diagnosis

The careful objective evaluation must include screening to rule out other pathology than patellofemoral problems.[4] The differential diagnosis of AKP should primarily be based on localization of the pain. The patient with a "true" AKP syndrome is usually recognized by having a distinct palpable tenderness peripatellarly, mostly anteromedially and/or retropatellarly (e.g., 1, 36, 45, 59). We cannot rule out that patients complaining of retropatellar pain have pain due to other reasons than chondromalacia patellae, unless we examine this with arthroscopy or magnetic resonance imaging. However, chondromalacia patients usually present with the same variations of symptoms and findings as AKP patients without chondromalacia patellae. Nowadays both AKP patients with and without chondromalacia patellae are mainly receiving the same nonoperative treatment, based on each patient's symptoms and findings. Furthermore, tenderness in the lateral retinaculum, which might be tight,[120] and the insertion of the vastus lateralis (VL) is relatively common in patients with AKP.[38] Fairbank's sign, a passive movement of the patella laterally, is an apprehension test and a classical examination that can be used to differentiate AKP from two other diagnoses that should be treated differently, patellar subluxation and patellar dislocation. A positive Fairbank's sign is associated with a giving-way feeling of the patella laterally and tenderness at the medial margin of the patella.[36] When considering the possible differential diagnosis one should also be aware that the lumbar spine and the hip can refer symptoms to the knee.[78]

Alignment of the Lower Extremity

The clinical examination should consist of a careful control of the entire lower extremity. This should be performed in a standing position when determining the alignment of the lower extremity. Possible prevalence of increased internal femoral rotation that can be observed clinically, which often causes a squinting of the patella, and compensatory external tibial torsion should be noted as well as genu recurvatum, genu valgum, and hyperpronation of the subtalar joint (e.g., 15, 60, 78, 104). Furthermore, it is important to control the patient's foot position during weightbearing (e.g., walking and running), and check how his or her shoes, especially sport shoes, are worn.

Quadriceps Angle

Measurement of the quadriceps angle (Q-angle) belongs to the classical examination protocol in AKP patients, despite that the correlation between an increased Q-angle and the patient's symptoms can be questioned (e.g., 32). The Q-angle itself is not a reliable indicator of patellar alignment. However, it should be regarded as one bit of information, which might correlate with other clinical findings in order to understand a malalignment problem as fully as possible.[40] The measurement of the Q-angle has a good intra- and interreliability when performed with the patient in a supine position with relaxed quadriceps muscles[16] and the patella localized in the trochlea and approximately in 30° of knee flexion.[40] A normal Q-angle is reported to be 12° in males and 15° in females.[78]

Patellar Position

Assessing the orientation of the patella relative to the femur and controlling the patellar position within the patellofemoral joint should be done. An optimal patellar position is when the patella is parallel to the femur in the frontal and the sagittal planes, and when the patella is midway between the two condyles during 20° of knee flexion.[78] Possible anatomical variations such as patella alta, patella infera, tilted patella, and rotated patella should be checked for. One should be aware that a high-riding patella (patella alta) is reported to be a risk factor for patellar subluxation or dislocation,[58] while patients with patella infera rather seem to complain of patellar pain at the area of apex patellae. Tilted patella with a medial "opening," a lateral tilt, seems to be relatively common in AKP patients. The reason for this depends on tightness of the lateral retinaculum, which will tilt the patella so that the medial border of the patella is higher than the lateral border.[78] Furthermore, a

hypotrophy of the VMO may aid in creating lateral patellar tilt. There are some patients presenting with an externally rotated patella, when the inferior pole of the patella is sitting lateral to the long axis of the femur, indicating tightness of the lateral retinaculum. Very few patients present with the opposite, an internally rotated patella. The ideal patellar position is when the long axis of the femur is parallel to the long axis of the patella.[78]

Patellar Mobility

Patellar mobility should also be checked.[15,41,60,107] The "patellar tracking test" is performed by clinically observing patellar movement by manual resistance against concentric as well as eccentric open kinetic chain knee extension and during closed kinetic chain in knee loading conditions (e.g., single-leg squat). A number of patients complain mostly of patellar instability problems.[1,36,41] This patellar instability feeling is the second most common symptom in patients with imbalance of the muscles around the patellofemoral joint, which probably depends on a sudden inhibition of the quadriceps due to pain.[1] The patella can be unstable laterally, medially, or multidirectionally.[56,107,113] Clinically, those patients often have a hypermobile patella and an observable tracking disorder.[118] Assessment of patellar mobility belongs to a complete knee examination. Manually produced passive medial and lateral displacement is a reproducible method for checking passive patellar motion.[101] The patella is surrounded by a rather mobile structure, which means that in full extension the patella can be passively moved about 20 mm both laterally and medially.[36] However, as the knee flexes the patellar mobility decreases and it should be checked in a slight knee flexion (approximately 30° of knee flexion), when the patella has a better congruency in the patellofemoral joint. Osborne and Farquharson-Roberts suggest that a passive deviation of 10 mm as well laterally as medially should be diagnosed as a normal patellar mobility,[87] and this should be judged in the slightly flexed knee.

Quadriceps Muscle Strength

The quadriceps muscle is often weakened in patients with AKP.[119] Manual muscle testing performed as a side-to-side comparison gives a rough awareness of quadriceps strength. If possible, isokinetic measurement of the quadriceps torque is recommended. However, isokinetic testing must be used cautiously[39] and patients with patellar hypermobility should not be measured eccentrically during fast angular velocities (> 90°/s) due to risk of subluxation or even dislocation.[115] During the isokinetic measurements it is preferable to evaluate whether pain inhibition might interfere with the "true" result of muscle torques. This could nicely be done with twitch interpolation technique,[80] but also to some extent by evaluating possible pain with Borg's pain scale[9] or the visual analogue scale (VAS).[19,35,95]

Hamstring/Quadriceps Ratio

Imbalance between the hamstring and quadriceps muscles is frequently shown in patients with AKP. This usually depends on a weakened quadriceps muscle but a normal strength of the hamstrings, which subsequently results in a higher hamstring/quadriceps ratio compared to healthy subjects.[119] The hamstring/quadriceps ratio in patients with AKP is reported to be between 0.65 and 0.70, while the corresponding values in healthy subjects is about 0.50, when measurements have been performed with an isokinetic dynamometer, where torque values were corrected for gravitational force.[119]

Vastus Medialis versus Vastus Lateralis

Hypotrophy of the vastus medialis (VM) is common in AKP patients (e.g., 49, 75) and VM is the weakest and most vulnerable muscle of the extensor mechanism.[36] VL comprises the largest muscle mass and extensor power of the quadriceps muscle group. This is probably the reason why VM hypotrophy is a common finding in AKP patients,[15,49] and that the patients also often present with a reduced electromyography (EMG) activity of the VM in their symptomatic leg compared to their contralateral healthy leg (e.g., 15, 75). VMO:VL ratio has also been reported to be lower in AKP patients compared with healthy subjects.[11,17,83] The lower activity of VM and the higher activity of VL could lead to an imbalance between VM and VL.[75,92] Unbalanced actions of the quadriceps components are closely linked to patellar maltracking and AKP. During knee extension VM pulls the patella first medially and then proximally, while VL pulls the patella first proximally and then laterally. VMO pulls the patella mainly medially and vastus medialis longus (VML) more proximally.[71] It has also been reported that the onset of the VL contraction occurs before that of the VMO, indicating a difference in motor control

in AKP patients compared to asymptomatic controls.[21,22,24] Furthermore, it is postulated that the VMO needs time to develop force, relative to the VL, for optimal patellar tracking.[47] Since VL has a larger cross-sectional area than the VMO there is a tendency for the patella to track laterally. In a controlled laboratory EMG study maximum voluntary knee extensions during concentric as well as eccentric actions were evaluated in AKP patients and asymptomatic controls.[88] The result showed that the activation amplitude of the VMO and VL in AKP patients was mostly altered during eccentric contractions and differed significantly from the controls. The authors conclude that the activation amplitudes of the VMO and VL in AKP patients are consistent with a lateral tracking of the patella during eccentric contractions.[88] Furthermore, there are authors reporting that the time to activation often is disturbed in AKP patients.[114,125] Therefore, it is important to improve the onset of muscle activity of the VMO in many patients with AKP. Using EMG in a randomized double blind, placebo controlled trial Cowan et al. reported that at baseline the EMG onset of VL occurred prior to that of VMO in AKP patients.[24] Following a physical therapy intervention for six weeks there was a significant change in the time of onset of EMG of VMO compared to VL with the onsets occurring simultaneously. This change was also associated with a reduction in symptoms.[24] In another controlled study the same research group also showed that after six-treatment sessions of physical therapy over a six-week period the onset of VMO preceded VL in the eccentric phase and occurred at the same time in the concentric phase of a stair-stepping task.[21] Several authors maintain that the primary role of VMO is to enhance patellar stabilization within the patellofemoral joint and to prevent lateral patellar subluxation by pulling the patella medially during knee extension and flexion.[36,75,77,92,96] Portney et al. maintain that VM, especially VMO, is important for optimal patellar movement within the patellofemoral joint during knee extension.[92] Almost 50 years ago Brewerton,[12] followed by Lieb and Perry,[70] Martin and Londeree,[76] and Bose et al.,[10] reported VMO to be active during the full range of knee extension. Mariani et al. found the EMG activity of both VM and VL to be of similar degree and mostly pronounced during the last 30° of knee extension in healthy subjects.[75]

Recently, Werner found that the two vasti muscles, however, were active throughout the range of motion of 90°–10° of knee extension in healthy subjects. Furthermore, most healthy individuals present with higher EMG activity of the VL compared to VM, but there are also those that show higher EMG activity of the VM than VL and there is also a third group of healthy individuals that have about the same EMG activity of both vasti muscles (unpublished data). This means that it is important to check the muscle activity pattern between VM and VL of the patient's asymptomatic leg as well as his or her symptomatic leg when designing an optimal treatment protocol for patients with AKP. When bilateral problems exist, I suggest that one rely on the EMG activity pattern of the less symptomatic leg.

Flexibility

Soft tissue or muscle length is essential to musculoskeletal evaluation and has specific implications in patients with AKP. Smith et al. found poor hamstring and quadriceps flexibility to be correlated with AKP.[102] Tightness of the lateral muscle structures such as the tensor fascia lata and iliotibial band is associated with AKP.[28] All the above-mentioned muscle structures are relatively common and could have negative effects at the patellofemoral joint and should therefore be controlled. A tight iliotibial band will result in deviation of the patella laterally, lateral tracking and lateral tilting and usually also weakening of the medial retinaculum.[112] Tight hamstrings and gastrocnemius may lead to an increase in foot pronation of the subtalar joint resulting in an increased valgus vector force at the knee, which can cause AKP problems.[30,64,79] Dorsiflexion of the talocrural joint will also decrease if the gastrocnemius is tight,[79] indicating biomechanical limitations and possible knee problems during walking and running. Furthermore, AKP patients sometimes show tightness of the lateral retinaculum, which might lead to an "opening" of the patella on the medial side, a lateral patellar tilt.

Knee-Related Functional Performance Tests

Dynamic evaluation with knee-related functional performance tests could be preferably used to reproduce the patient's symptoms and to make comparisons before and after a treatment period. There are different types of pain provocation tests that comprise knee function.

Except for walking there are more stressful activities such as stair climbing (up and down), steps up and down on different heights, double-leg and single-leg squat and raise from a chair and sit down using one leg. These tests could be used to evaluate both quadriceps muscle function and the patient's subjective knee pain. Loudon et al. reported a good intrarater reliability of the following four functional performance tests: anteromedial lunge, step-down, single-leg press, and balance and reach.[73] Single-leg tests are very good indicators of controlling the extensor mechanism and thereby the patient's symptoms. Since the AKP patients often report symptoms during eccentric quadriceps work, walking downstairs is a good knee-related functional test for eccentric control of the quadriceps muscle. When the aim is to evaluate muscle function, those tests should be performed slowly, which makes it easier to observe possible patellar maltracking. However, those tests can also be evaluated according to the patient's subjective pain rating, which could be done by using Borg's pain scale[9] or the visual analogue scale.[19,35,95] Future research is needed to study intrarater reliability as well as interrater reliability, validity, and sensitivity of functional performance tests.[25]

Functional Knee Scores

During the last decade many knee-scoring systems for subjective evaluations have been utilized (e.g., 68). While signs such as effusion, muscle hypotrophy, and muscle tightness are identified by the examining clinician, a knee score is built on the patient's own subjective evaluation of his or her knee function. Each functional score should be tested for reproducibility, meaning that the score is reliable for repeated measurements under the same conditions. Furthermore, the most optimal functional score should be tested for validity or sensitivity and thereby tailored for a specific diagnosis.

A knee score for functional evaluation of patients with AKP should consist of different categories of symptoms that are common in these patients. The Werner functional knee score (Table 9.1) is modified from an earlier published version.[116] A test-retest of this score has revealed a very good reproducibility and to some extent we have also tested the sensitivity of the score, which reveals a good sensitivity to AKP patients (unpublished data). Fifty points at this particular knee score means lack of AKP, and subsequently

Table 9.1. Werner functional knee score for anterior knee pain

Please circle what usually applies to your knee problem(s):

Pain		Sitting with flexed knees > 30 min	
None	5	No problems	5
Slight & infrequent	3	Slightly impaired	4
Constant pain	0	Difficulties	2
Occurrence of pain		Unable	0
No activity-related pain	15	**Squatting**	
During or after running	12	No problems	5
After > 2 km walk	9	Slightly impaired	4
After < 2 km walk	6	Difficulties	2
During normal walk	3	Unable	0
During rest	0		
Feeling of patellar instability		**Walking upstairs**	
		No problems	5
Never	5	Slightly impaired	4
Sometimes	3	Difficulties	2
Frequently	0	Unable	0
Arretations-Catching		**Walking downstairs**	
Never	5	No problems	5
Sometimes	3	Slightly impaired	4
Frequently	0	Difficulties	2
		Unable	0
Sum of points: _____			

Table 9.2. Werner functional knee score for anterior knee pain following ACL reconstruction

Please circle what usually applies to your knee problem(s):

Pain		Sitting with flexed knees > 30 min	
None	5	No problems	5
Slight & infrequent	3	Slightly impaired	4
Constant pain	0	Difficulties	2
Occurrence of pain		Unable	0
No activity-related pain	15	**Squatting**	
During or after running	12	No problems	5
After > 2 km walk	9	Slightly impaired	4
After < 2 km walk	6	Difficulties	2
During normal walk	3	Unable	0
During rest	0		
Kneeling		**Walking upstairs**	
No problems	5	No problems	5
Slightly impaired	4	Slightly impaired	4
Difficulties	2	Difficulties	2
Unable	0	Unable	0
Arretations -Catching		**Walking downstairs**	
Never	5	No problems	5
Sometimes	3	Slightly impaired	4
Frequently	0	Difficulties	2
		Unable	0
Sum of points: _____			

0 means maximal knee problems. Due to the good reliability and sensitivity results we can recommend the use of the Werner functional knee score for evaluating patients with AKP syndrome.

In order to investigate a possible prevalence of AKP following anterior cruciate ligament reconstruction, we have modified the above-mentioned functional knee score and tailored it for anterior cruciate ligament reconstructed patients (Table 9.2). This score has shown a good reproducibility when tested three times in the same group of subjects. Furthermore, it has been shown to be most sensitive for patients with anterior cruciate ligament injuries (to be published).

Treatment

Nowadays most orthopedic surgeons agree that patients with AKP and without any malalignment should be treated nonoperatively.[27,41,62,104] Only if a careful long-term physical therapy program has failed one might consider surgery.[31,45] The treatment protocol should be based on findings from the patient's history, clinical examination, and functional assessment.[123,128] A comprehensive treatment approach is often required to treat AKP patients successfully. When designing a treatment program it is important to realize that each patient is specific and will present with different symptoms and signs, which makes it necessary to have a flexible treatment approach.[4] A thorough evaluation and assessment will reveal each patient's unique set of clinical signs, and the treatment protocol should be tailored to that patient.

Patient education is one of the key factors in the management of AKP. The patient must have a clear understanding of why the symptoms have occurred and what needs to be done to reduce the symptoms. Therefore, the patient should be informed already from the very start that the treatment period sometimes can last several months. This is due to the gradually progressive treatment protocol, often including a combination of different methods, that is needed to restore good muscle activity and muscle strength, improve balance and coordination, and end up in a normal knee functional movement pattern.

The cause of AKP varies between patients. Each patient is unique, which means that the same treatment in different patients may lead to different effects. Therefore it is important with a thorough clinical examination based on control of patellar mobility, muscle function, and each patient's specific functional problem. Furthermore, the patient's history should be included in order to design an individual treatment program based on each patient's specific symptoms and findings.

If patellar hypermobility exists, the patella could initially be supported by a patellar stabilizing brace or patellar taping during the physical therapy treatment. However, it is of most importance to check in what direction the patella is hypermobile, laterally, medially, or both. I recommend either taping or bracing in patients with a lateral or a medial hypermobility, and bracing in patients with both a lateral and medial hypermobility. The external patella supports, irrespective of what type, bracing or taping, should then gradually be removed when the patient improves and his or her symptoms are reduced. This means that the last step in the rehabilitation protocol will be to remove the patient's patella support during dynamic heavy knee loading exercises, which put great demands on stability of the patella.

Toward the end of the treatment period it is recommended to stimulate the patient either to return to some kind of sport/physical activity or to start with a suitable regular physical exercise, where long walks could be an alternative. The reason for this is that the improved muscle function and balance that have been gained through the rehabilitation need to be maintained by physical exercises. We have found that patients who started or continued with some kind of physical training following a treatment program were the ones with good long-term results of knee function.[116,117]

Extensor Mechanism: Quadriceps Strengthening

Several authors have emphasized the importance of quadriceps training in patients with AKP in order to improve the extensor mechanism (e.g., 41, 59, 104). Powers et al. reported functional ability to be associated with increased ability to generate quadriceps muscle torque.[94] However, the main objective is to strengthen the VM,[18] since appropriate timing and intensity of VMO activation relative to VL has been promoted as a key aspect in patients with AKP.[124,125]

Therefore, the balance between VMO and VL should be restored before starting to train the entire quadriceps muscle group.

Training of Vastus Medialis Obliquus

Muscular hypotrophy and a reduced and/or delayed EMG activity of the VM is very common in patients with AKP (e.g., 18, 49, 75). This will often result in an imbalance between the VM and the VL. Therefore, the initial treatment should consist of restoring the function of VMO in an attempt to enhance patellar stabilization.[8,17,36,75,77,103] The VMO is a stabilizing muscle, which means that endurance training is the ultimate goal and therefore the patient should increase the number of repetitions rather than load.[97] The importance of this initial stage of treatment is further magnified by the fact that the rate of strength development for the VM has been shown to be slower than for the VL and the rectus femoris,[36,48,70] which might create the potential for patellar tracking dysfunction and the accompanying knee problems.

In the literature there have been many suggestions to improve the VM by different exercises. Hanten and Schulthies reported significantly greater activity of the VM compared to VL by performing isometric hip adduction exercises.[51] Later Karst and Jewett performed a similar study, where they combined straight leg raises with hip adduction, but they could not repeat the beneficial results from Hanten and Schulthies and therefore suggest isometric quadriceps exercises without hip adduction.[63] Laprade et al. also studied EMG activity of VM and VL during different exercises and they did not find a greater recruitment of the VM compared with VL during hip adduction or a combination of hip adduction and knee extension.[67] Nor could Cerny find increased activity of the VM over that of VL in commonly prescribed exercises.[17] Only terminal knee extension with the hip medially rotated resulted in a somewhat higher VM/VL activity.[17] Sczepanski et al. suggested isokinetic concentric knee extension exercises at 120°/s angular velocity within 60°–85° of knee flexion in order to selectively activate the VMO and improve the balance between the two vasti muscles.[98] McConnell suggested patellar taping with a medial glide in order to prevent lateral tracking of the patella.[77] With the patella taped the patient is instructed to tighten the medial portion of the quadriceps by isometrically contracting the hip adductors.[77] This exercise should be performed in a weightbearing position, walk-stance with the symptomatic leg forward and the knee flexed to 30°.[77] Activation of adductor magnus has been reported to improve the contraction of the VMO during weightbearing.[54]

However, transcutaneous electrical muscle stimulation is the optimal way proven to selectively contract and improve the function of VM.[116] Steadman proposed electrical muscle stimulation of VM in order to keep the patella in a proper position within the patellofemoral joint.[104] With the help of computer tomography Werner et al. reported a significantly increased area of the VM after transcutaneous electrical stimulation of this muscle, while the VL was unchanged.[116] Two-thirds of those patients also improved from a functional point of view directly after 10 weeks of daily electrical stimulation, and at the follow-ups 1 year and 3.5 years later the same patients still were improved.[116] Those patients have also been followed prospectively on average 13 years later and more than half of the patients reported to be symptom-free (unpublished data). The rest of the patients reported to have minor AKP occurring mostly during physical activities such as running. Only one-fourth of the patients have received another type of treatment during those years. Today three-fourths of those patients are physically active, whereas the remaining one-fourth is not, mainly depending on lack of interest in sporting activities.

Isometric Training

Reports from earlier studies suggested isometric quadriceps exercises or training in a short arc motion toward the end of knee extension in order to decrease the knee pain by a reduced patellofemoral compression.[122,129] Based on the amount of electrical muscle activity Boucher et al.[11] and Signorile et al.[100] recently reported that the most effective angle for isometric quadriceps training would be with the knee at 90° of flexion and the foot held in a neutral position. However, isometric exercises are time consuming, since one mostly gains strength at a fixed position (knee joint angle).[72,130] Furthermore, isometric training does not improve functional performance and could therefore be questioned in AKP patients, since their knee problems most often result in a quadriceps mechanism disorder, which very likely should be treated during functional exercises. Therefore, in my opinion isometric quadriceps training is indicated only in patients who

present with such a severe pain inhibition that they are not able to perform dynamic exercises. Fortunately, these AKP patients are rare.

Isokinetic Training

During the last decade isokinetic quadriceps training has been suggested as a possible treatment for quadriceps strengthening.[6,55,91,117] The term "isokinetic" is defined as a dynamic muscular contraction, when the velocity of the movement is controlled and maintained constant by a special device.[109] Isokinetic training therefore provides optimal loading of the muscles and allows muscular performance at different velocities.[2] There are less compressive forces on the joint surfaces during high angular velocity. This means that isokinetic training at high angular velocity ($\geq 120°/s$) should be preferred in AKP patients during concentric actions. However, eccentric actions are more difficult to perform due to unfamiliarity with the decelerating type of movement and problems coordinating the different portions of the quadriceps muscles during decelerated knee extensions.[117,119] My suggestion is, therefore, that patients with AKP should perform isokinetic eccentric contractions at 90°/s or lower angular velocities. After improvement of muscle coordination some patients might be able to increase the angular velocity. There is a need for eccentric training particularly among AKP patients[119] and it should be pointed out that isokinetic quadriceps training is an outstanding method in order to improve eccentric muscle torque and should therefore be included in the rehabilitation protocol (if possible). However, those patients that show maltracking of the patella at the patellar tracking test should not perform isokinetic training at high angular velocities during eccentric action due to risk of possible patellar subluxation or even dislocation.[115] The advantage with isokinetic training in AKP patients is, except for rapid muscular effect and also a possibility of specific eccentric loading, training without body weightbearing and the exercise can be adjusted to possible knee pain and therefore diminish the risk for overload. However, there are also other exercises of a more functional character that improve the eccentric muscle strength (e.g., walking downstairs and stepping or jumping down from a height).

Closed and Open Kinetic Chain Training

Quadriceps can be strengthened during closed kinetic chain (CKC) as well as open kinetic chain (OKC) exercises. Palmitier et al. suggest that rehabilitation in a weightbearing position such as during CKC exercises may have a greater carryover to functional activities, as lower extremity function in daily weightbearing activities involves multiple muscle groups acting in synergy.[89] Stiene et al. found CKC to be more effective than OKC exercises in restoring perceived function in patients with AKP syndrome.[106] However, their CKC exercises, lateral step-ups, retro step-ups, double-leg squats, and StairMaster exercises are solely performed at the final knee extension and in my opinion quadriceps performance should be improved during the entire range of knee flexion. Souza and Gross reported greater VMO/VL ratio during step-up/step-down exercises.[103] This might suggest that the stabilizing function of the VMO is increased during CKC exercises. McConnell advocates performing CKC exercises with the hip in external rotation to improve VMO activity.[77] In conflict with this, Ninos et al. could not demonstrate any difference in either VMO or VL with the hip externally rotated.[85] However, for optimal functional quadriceps performance my suggestion is that the quadriceps muscle group should be strengthened during CKC as well as OKC. This is also in agreement with other authors (e.g., 52, 127). In order to reduce the patellofemoral joint reaction forces CKC exercises, such as leg press and step exercises, should be trained during the last 30° of knee extension, while OKC exercises, such as sitting knee extensions, should rather be trained between 90° and 40° of knee flexion.[29,105]

Stretching

A number of patients with AKP show tightness mostly of the iliotibial band and other lateral muscle structures, the quadriceps muscle, and sometimes also of the hamstrings and the gastrocnemius. Most of the stretching procedures could be performed by the patients themselves; therefore they should be instructed in how to stretch their tight muscle structures. The lateral retinaculum might also be tight, which could interfere with a normal patellar tracking, and should therefore be treated with medial patellar glide. With the patient in a sidelying position on the opposite side with the symptomatic knee in approximately 30° of knee flexion, the clinician moves the patella medially, tilts the medial border of the patella posteriorly, and stretches the lateral retinaculum.[79] Friction and massage of the

lateral retinacular tissue can also be recommended in order to improve a tight lateral retinaculum.

Balance and Coordination Training

AKP patients often have a reduced balance of their lower extremities, measured as postural sway, of their symptomatic as well as their asymptomatic leg (unpublished data). This indicates that balance and coordination training should be included in the treatment program. Physical training causes changes within the nervous system that leads to improved coordination between muscle groups and practice will result in automatics, which indicates a change and improvement in the motor program.[92,99] When the activity and the function of VM have improved, balance and coordination training of the lower extremity should be started. Balance and coordination exercises should preferably be performed during knee loading conditions and with slightly flexed knees in order to try to direct the training to the knee joint.

Knee-Related Functional Training

When the quadriceps muscle has improved and a good balance exists within the extensor mechanism, functional training with gradual increase of knee loading exercises could begin. The patient should practice slowly stepping on and off a step with adequate pelvic control. Initially a small step height should be used and the patient is recommended to train in front of a mirror to be able to observe muscle function. The pelvis must remain parallel with the floor, and the hip, knee, and foot should be aligned.[79] There is a wide variation of functional knee loading exercises that make different heavy demands upon the knee (e.g., walking, jogging, running, stair climbing, jumping, and bicycling).

Sport-Specific Exercises

Those athletic patients that have improved, that is, have good quadriceps strength, good muscle flexibility, and a proper movement pattern during functional heavy knee loading activities performed without pain or swelling, are encouraged to start sport-specific training.

Bracing and Taping

Supportive devices such as patellar stabilizing braces and patellar taping are aimed at improving patellar tracking problems.[34,74,90] Some authors suggest that AKP patients should be treated with patellar stabilizing orthoses,[53,59,74,84] although there is no evidence of any major alteration of patellar tracking.[40] Palumbo reported decreased symptoms in 92% when a patella stabilizing brace was used in AKP patients.[90] Sega et al. reported that an orthosis with a medial support gave a good pain reduction in patients with patellar instability.[99] We have found improvements in balance of the lower extremity, when patients with patellar hypermobility were supported with brace; that is, patients with a lateral patellar hypermobility improved when the patella had a lateral support and patients with a medial patellar hypermobility improved when the patella had a medial support (unpublished data). In military recruits with AKP Finestone et al. reported better response without a brace or with a simple sleeve compared with the use of a brace during physical exercise.[33] BenGal et al. performed a prospective investigation of the efficacy of knee brace on preventing AKP in young healthy subjects undergoing strenuous physical training.[5] Their data indicate that the use of a brace with a silicon patellar support ring might be effective to prevent the development of AKP in individuals participating in intensive physical exercise.[5]

Other authors recommend an elastic strap or taping in order to improve patellar tracking and thereby reduce patellar instability problems.[77,99] McConnell reported a success rate of 92% maintaining that patellar taping with a medial glide technique can modify patellar tracking and therefore act as pain relief.[77] Gilleard et al. found that the onset of VMO activity occurred earlier, when the patella was taped compared to untaped, during step-up and step-down tasks, while the activity of VL was unchanged during the step-up task and delayed during the step-down task with taping.[44] Gerrard reported a pain-free success rate of 96% after only five treatments using the McConnell taping technique.[43] Bockrath et al.[8] studied the effect of patella taping on patellar position (Merchant's x-ray view) and knee pain (VAS). They found a reduced perceived pain during a step-down task, when the patella was taped according to McConnell, but no significant changes occurred in patellar position.[8] Using a radiographic technique in a partial weightbearing position with the knee flexed 40° Larsen et al. indicated that the McConnell medial glide taping technique was effective in significantly moving the patella medially.[69] However, the taping was ineffective in maintaining this patellar position after a 15-minute

exercise program, including forward sprint, side shuffling, back peddling, figure-eight running, and mini-squats.[69] Powers et al. studied the effect of patellar taping according to McConnell on functional outcomes.[93] With the patella taped they reported an average pain reduction of 78% using the VAS. No significant differences were found in gait velocity or cadence between taped and untaped trials. A small increase in stride length during ascending a ramp was the only significant effect that improved with taping. However, patellar taping also resulted in a small increase in loading response knee flexion, which the authors believe demonstrates more willingness to load the knee joint.[93] Whether this finding depends on patellar taping or the effect of reduced pain is, however, not known. Kowall et al. performed a prospective study comparing two similar groups of anterior knee pain patients that were treated during four weeks. Both groups received the same physical therapy program, one group with the patella taped and the other group without taping. Both groups improved; however, no beneficial effect of adding patellar taping was found.[66] In contrast, Whittingham et al. reported that a combination of patellar taping and exercise was superior to exercise alone in terms of reduction of knee pain and improved knee function.[121] In another EMG study AKP patients and asymptomatic controls performed a stair-stepping task during three experimental conditions, therapeutic patellar tape, placebo tape, and no tape.[23] They reported that therapeutic patellar tape was found to alter the temporal characteristics of VMO and VL activation in AKP patients, whereas placebo tape had no effect. No change of onset of VMO and VL with either placebo or therapeutic tape was found in asymptomatic controls. The authors conclude that the use of patellar taping is an adjunct to rehabilitation of AKP patients.[23] Christou reported increased VMO activity and decreased VL activity in AKP patients when the patella was taped medially.[20] The benefits of patellar taping are not due to a change in patellar position but rather are due to enhanced support of the patellofemoral ligaments and/or pain modulation via cutaneous stimulation.[20] Werner et al. reported that patients with patellar hypermobility (≥ 15 mm deviation laterally or medially) improved their quadriceps muscle torque and agonist EMG activity during isokinetic knee extensions, when the patella was stabilized by taping, while patients with a normal patellar mobility did not benefit from taping.[118] However, we also found that in order to optimize the treatment for supporting the patella with tape, it is important to check the direction of the patient's patellar hypermobility, which can be laterally, medially, or both.[118] Furthermore, in order to control whether the patient needs a patellar support, orthosis, or taping, it is important to check patellar tracking within the patellofemoral joint during both concentric and eccentric knee extension ("patellar tracking" test). In my opinion patellar taping can be recommended only if patellar hypermobility exists and as a temporary treatment to facilitate physical therapy exercises, especially quadriceps training.

Foot orthotics to control excessive pronation of the subtalar joint have also been advocated to improve patellar tracking and lead to a decrease in AKP.[30,64,112] D'Amico and Rubin found that foot orthotics could reduce the Q-angle and therefore suggested that this foot-knee relationship might be an indication for using foot orthotics in AKP patients with malalignment.[26]

Furthermore, footwear should be closely evaluated for quality and fit, and the use of arch supports should be considered.[61]

Appendix: A Step-by-Step Treatment Protocol for AKP Patients
Phase 1
Goals

Reduce pain and swelling, improve VMO:VL balance and thereby patellar tracking, improve flexibility, restore normal gait, and decrease loading of the patellofemoral joint.

Treatment

- Cryotherapy – after the physical therapy exercise and daily activities, which exacerbate symptoms, to reduce pain and edema.[65,81]
- Transcutaneous electrical stimulation of VMO to restore the function of VMO and improve VMO:VL balance (Figure 9.1). This could be done according to our specific protocol (Table 9.3).

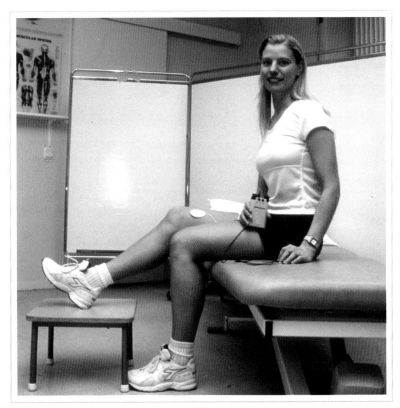

Figure 9.1. Transcutaneous electrical stimulation of VMO.

Table 9.3. Transcutaneous electrical stimulation protocol of VMO in patients with anterior knee pain syndrome

Keep the knee joint in approximately 30° of knee flexion. Stimulate passively without any activation of the quadriceps muscle.

Stimulation type	Constant pulse
Pulse width	300 μs
Frequency	40 Hz
Rise time	4 sec
On time	18 sec
Fall time	2 sec
Off time	25 sec

- Flexibility training. Stretching of tight muscle structures, usually the tensor fascia lata and the iliotibial band (Figure 9.2), the quadriceps, in particular rectus femoris (Figure 9.3), the

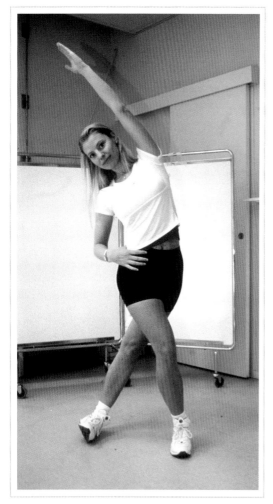

Figure 9.2. Stretching of lateral muscle structures, the tensor fascia lata and the iliotibial band.

hamstrings (Figure 9.4), and the gastrocnemius. Tight lateral retinaculum can, except for stretching, be treated with medial patellar glide, friction and massage.

- If gait has been altered, the patient should be instructed in proper gait mechanics, which preferably could be done in front of a mirror.
- Instruct the patient to change postural habits, such as standing in genu recurvatum.
- If patellar hypermobility exists, it is recommended either to tape the patella or to use a patellar stabilizing brace during the physical therapy exercises. However, patellar-supporting devices should only be used temporarily until exercises and functional activities can be performed without knee pain.
- If increased pronation of the subtalar joint exists, treat the patient with foot orthotics or arch taping. Foot orthotics can be used temporarily or may be needed indefinitely to improve patellar tracking and alignment of the lower extremity.
- Check the patient's shoe wear, in particular sport shoes, and if needed suggest shock-absorptive shoes.
- Modify daily activity level to temporarily reduce the load on the patellofemoral joint.

Phase 2

Goals:

Improve balance of the lower extremity, increase quadriceps strength, and restore good knee function.

Treatment, add

- Balance and coordination training with gradual increase of difficulty and loading on the patellofemoral joint. In order to try to mainly train the knee joint stabilizers I suggest that these exercises should be performed in a standing position with a slightly flexed knee joint. Balance training on a balance board can initially be performed standing on one leg with addition of electrical stimulation of VMO to facilitate a proper balance between VMO and VL (Figure 9.5). When good muscle control is achieved the patient can continue the balance exercise standing on one leg without electrical muscle stimulation (Figure 9.6) or standing on both legs on two balance boards (Figure 9.7).
- Stationary bicycle training with a high seat aimed to reduce a big knee flexion angle and thereby compression forces within the patellofemoral joint (Figure 9.8).[86] This type

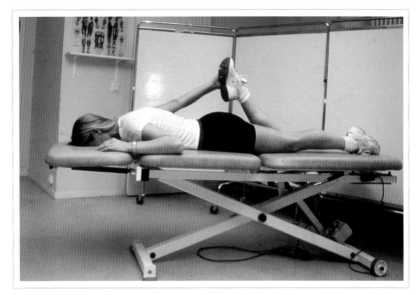

Figure 9.3. Stretching of rectus femoris.

of exercise might improve both physical conditioning and thigh muscle strength.
- Functional knee exercises. Start with shallow squats, and proceed with deeper ones. Squatting can initially be performed with addition of electrical stimulation of VMO to improve the

VMO:VL balance (Figure 9.9). Stepping down can also be started with addition of electrical muscle stimulation (Figure 9.10), and gradually be performed without (Figure 9.11).
- Quadriceps strengthening is recommended to be started when a good balance between VMO

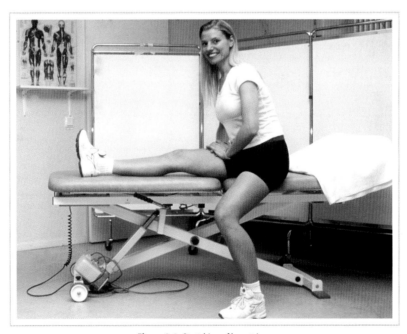

Figure 9.4. Stretching of hamstrings.

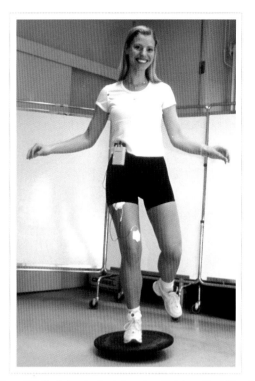

Figure 9.5. Single-leg standing balance board training with addition of electrical stimulation of VMO.

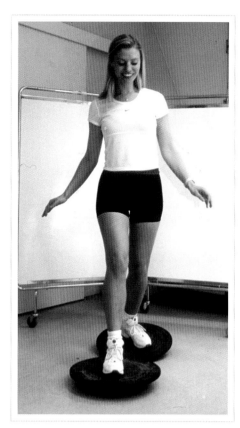

Figure 9.7. Balance board training standing on two legs on two balance boards.

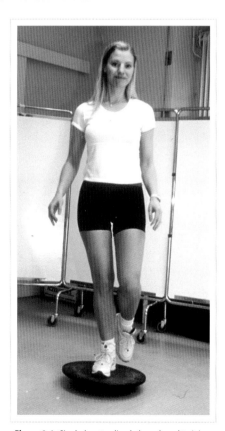

Figure 9.6. Single-leg standing balance board training.

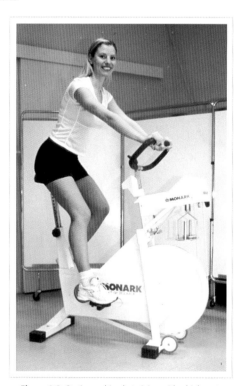

Figure 9.8. Stationary bicycle training with a high seat.

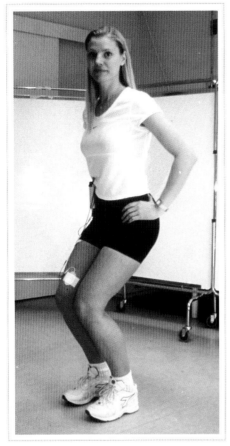

Figure 9.9. Squatting with addition of electrical stimulation of VMO.

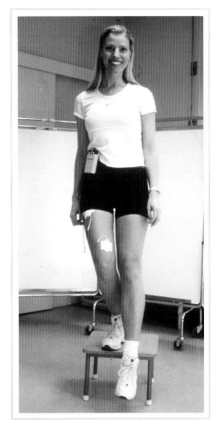

Figure 9.10. Stepping-down with addition of electrical stimulation of VMO.

and VL exists. Closed kinetic chain exercises should be performed during terminal knee extension, approximately between 30° and 0° of knee flexion, and open kinetic chain between approximately 90° and 40° of knee flexion. Isokinetic training should preferably be performed at 120°/s or higher during concentric actions and at 90°/s or lower during eccentric actions (Figure 9.12).

Phase 3

Goal

Return to previous physical activity level.

Treatment, add

- Functional training with a gradual increase of knee loading activities can begin after improved

quadriceps strength. Walking, jogging, and different types of jumping exercises are recommended during this phase. However, proceeding to a higher knee loading activity or exercise should only be allowed if there is no knee pain and no swelling.

- Sport-specific exercises with a gradual increase of intensity can start as soon as the athletic patient is pain free, and has a good muscle function and a proper movement pattern during functional knee exercises.

- It is recommended to give the patient individual guidelines for physical activity and exercises regarding, for example, number of repetitions, duration, intensity, and frequency.

- Patient education is also recommended in order to try to prevent recurrence of knee symptoms.

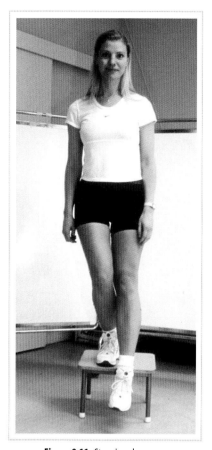

Figure 9.11. Stepping-down.

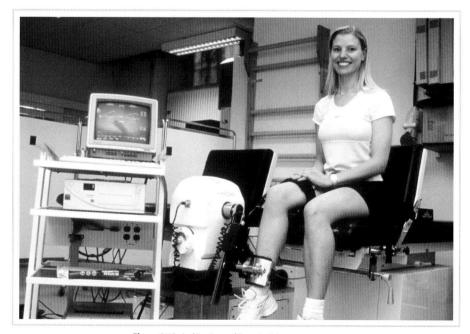

Figure 9.12. Isokinetic quadriceps training.

References

1. Aglietti, P, R Buzzi, and A Pisaneschi. Patella pain. *J Sports Trauma Rel Res* 1990; 12: 131–150.
2. Baltzopoulos, V, and DA Brodie. Isokinetic dynamometry: Applications and limitations. *Sports Med* 1989; 8: 101–116.
3. Bandy, WD, and JM Irion. The effect of time on static stretch on the flexibility of the hamstring muscles. *Phys Ther* 1994; 74(9): 845–852.
4. Beckman, M, R Craig, and RC Lehman. Rehabilitation of patellofemoral dysfunction in the athlete. *Clin Sports Med* 1989; 8(4): 841–860.
5. BenGal, S, J Lowe, G Mann, A Finsterbush, and Y Matan. The role of the knee brace in the prevention of anterior knee pain syndrome. *Am J Sports Med* 1997; 25(1): 118–122.
6. Bennett, JG, and WT Stauber. Evaluation and treatment of anterior knee pain using eccentric exercise. *Med Sci Sports Exerc* 1986; 18: 526–530.
7. Bentley, G, and G Dowd. Current concepts of etiology and treatment of chondromalacia patellae. *Clin Orthop* 1984; 189: 209–228.
8. Bockrath, K, C Wooden, T Worrel, CD Ingersoll, and J Farr. Effects of patella taping on patella position and perceived pain. *Med Sci Sports Exerc* 1993; 25: 989–992.
9. Borg, G, A Holmgren, and I Lindblad. Quantitative evaluation of chest pain. *Acta Med Scand [Suppl]* 1981; 644: 43–45.
10. Bose, K, R Kanagasuntherum, and M Osman. Vastus medialis oblique: An anatomical and physiologic study. *Orthopedics* 1980; 3: 880–883.
11. Boucher, JP, MA King, R Lefebvre, and A Pepin. Quadriceps femoris muscle activity in patellofemoral pain syndrome. *Am J Sports Med* 1992; 20(5): 527–532.
12. Brewerton, DA. The function of the vastus medialis muscle. *Ann Phys Med* 1955; 2: 164–168.
13. Carlsson, AM. Studies on pain assessment and egopsychological analysis of personality in chronic pain patients. Thesis, Karolinska Institute, Stockholm, Sweden 1987.
14. Carlsson, AM, S Werner, C-E Mattlar, G Edman, P Puukka, and E Eriksson. Personality in patients with long-term patellofemoral pain syndrome. *Knee Surg, Sports Traumatol, Arthrosc* 1993; 1: 178–183.
15. Carson, WG. Diagnosis of extensor mechanism disorders. *Clin Sports Med* 1985; 4: 231–246.
16. Caylor, D, R Fites, and TW Worrell. The relationship between quadriceps angle and anterior knee pain syndrome. *JOSPT* 1993; 17(1): 11–16.
17. Cerny, K. Vastus medialis oblique/vastus lateralis muscle activity ratios for selected exercises in persons with and without patellofemoral pain syndrome. *Phys Ther* 1995; 75(8): 672–683.
18. Cesarelli, M, P Bifulco, and M Bracale. Study of the control strategy of the quadriceps muscles in anterior knee pain. *Trans Rehabil Eng* 2000, 8(3): 330–341.
19. Chesworth, BM, EG Culham, GE Tata, and M Peat. Validation of outcome measures in patients with patellofemoral syndrome. *JOSPT* 1989; 10: 302–309.
20. Christou, EA. Patellar taping increases vastus medialis oblique activity in the presence of patellofemoral pain. *J Electromyogr Kinesiol* 2004, 14(4): 495–504.
21. Cowan, SM, KL Bennell, KM Crossley, PW Hodges, and J McConnell. Physical therapy alters recruitment of the vasti in patellofemoral pain syndrome. *Med Sci Sports Exerc* 2002, 34(12): 1879–1885.
22. Cowan, SM, PW Hodges, KL Bennell, and KM Crossley. Altered vastii recruitment when people with patellofemoral pain syndrome complete a postural task. *Arch Phys Med Rehabil* 2002, 83(7): 989–995.
23. Cowan, SM, KL Bennell, PW Hodges. Therapeutic patellar taping changes the timing of the vasti muscle activation in people with patellofemoral pain syndrome. *Clin J Sport Med* 2002, 12(6): 339–347.
24. Cowan, SM, KL Bennell, PW Hodges, KM Crossley, and J McConnell. Simultaneous feedforward recruitment of the vasti in untrained postural tasks can be restored by physical therapy. *J Orthop Res* 2003, 21(3): 553–558.
25. Crossley, KM, KL Bennell, SM Cowan, and S Green. Analysis of outcome measures for persons with patellofemoral pain: Which are reliable and valid? *Arch Phys Med Rehabil* 2004, 85(5): 815–822.
26. D'Amico, JC, and M Rubin. The influence of foot orthoses on the quadrticeps angle. *J Am Podiatry Assoc* 1986; 76: 337–340.
27. DeHaven, KE, WA Dolan, and PJ Mayer. Chondromalacia patellae in athletes. *Am J Sports Med* 1979; 7: 5–11.
28. Doucette, SA, and EM Goble. The effect of exercise on patellar tracking in lateral patellar compression syndrome. *Am J Sports Med* 1992; 20(4): 434–440.
29. Doucette, SA, and DP Child. The effect of open and closed chain exercise and knee joint position on patellar tracking in lateral patellar compression syndrome. *JOSPT* 1996; 23(2): 104–110.
30. Eng, JJ, and MR Pierrynowski. Evaluation of soft foot orthotics in the treatment of patellofemoral pain syndrome. *Phys Ther* 1993; 73(2): 62–70.
31. Engebretsen, L, and E Arendt. Patellofemorale smerter: diagnostikk og behandling. *Tidsskr Nor Laegeforen* 1991; 111: 1949–1952.
32. Fairbank, J, P Pynsent, J van Poortvliet, and H Phillips. Mechanical factors in the incidence of knee pain in adolescents and young adults. *J Bone Joint Surg [Br]* 1984; 66: 685–693.
33. Finestone, A, EL Radin, B Lev, N Shlamkovitch, M Wiener, and C Milgrom. Treatment of overuse patellofemoral pain: Prospective randomized controlled clinical trial in a military setting. *Clin Orthop* 1991; 293: 208–210.
34. Fisher, RL. Conservative treatment of patellofemoral pain. *Orthop Clin North Am* 1986; 17(2): 269–271.
35. Flandry, F, JP Hunt, GC Terry, and JC Hughston. Analysis of subjective knee complaints using visual analog scales. *Am J Sports Med* 1991; 19(2): 112–118.
36. Fox, TA. Dysplasia of the quadriceps mechanism, hypoplasia of the vastus medialis as related to the hypermobile patella syndrome. *Surg Clin North Am* 1975; 55: 199–226.
37. Fritz, GK, EE Bleck, and IS Dahl. Functional versus organic knee pain in adolescents. *Am J Sports Med* 1981; 9: 247–249.
38. Fulkerson, JP. Awareness of the retinaculum in evaluating patellofemoral pain. *Am J Sports Med* 1982; 10: 147.
39. Fulkerson, JP, and DS Hungerford. Biomechanics of the patellofemoral joint. In Fulkerson, JP, and DS Hungerford, eds., *Disorders of the Patellofemoral Joint*, 2nd ed. Baltimore: Williams & Wilkins, 1990, pp. 25–41.

40. Fulkerson, JP, and DS Hungerford. Evaluation and rehabilitation of nonarthritic anterior knee pain. In Fulkerson, JP, and DS Hungerford, eds., *Disorders of the Patellofemoral Joint*, 2nd ed. Baltimore: Williams & Wilkins, 1990, pp. 86–101.

41. Fulkerson, JP, and KP Shea. Current concepts review disorders of patellofemoral alignment. *J Bone Joint Surg [Am]* 1990; 72: 1424–1429.

42. Gajdosik, RL. Effects of static stretching on the maximal length and resistance to passive stretch of short hamstring muscles. *JOSPT* 1991; 14(6): 250–255.

43. Gerrard, B. The patello-femoral pain syndrome: A clinical trial of the McConnell programme. *Austr J Physiother* 1989; 35: 71–80.

44. Gilleard, W, J McConnell, and D Parsons. The effect of patellar taping on the onset of vastus medialis obliquus and vastus lateralis muscle activity in persons with patellofemoral pain. *Phys Ther* 1998; 78(1): 25–32.

45. Goldberg, B. Chronic anterior knee pain in the adolescent. *Pediatric Annals* 1991; 20: 186–193.

46. Goodfellow, J, DS Hungerford, and M Zindel. Patello-femoral joint mechanics and pathology: I. Functional anatomy of the patello-femoral joint. *J Bone Joint Surg [Br]* 1976; 58: 287–290.

47. Grabiner, MD, TJ Koh, and LF Draganich. Neuromechanics of the patellofemoral joint. *Med Sci Sports Exerc* 1994; 26(1): 10–21.

48. Grana, WA, and LA Kriegshauser. Scientific basis of extensor mechanism disorders. *Clin Sports Med* 1985; 4: 247–257.

49. Gruber, MA. The conservative treatment of chondromalacia patellae. *Orthop Clin North Am* 1979; 10: 105–115.

50. Gunther, KP, F Thielemann, and M Bottesi. Anterior knee pain in children and adolescents: Diagnosis and conservative treatment. *Orthopade* 2003, 32(2): 110–118.

51. Hanten. WP, and SS Schulthies. Exercise effect on electromyographic activity of the vastus medialis oblique and vastus lateralis muscles. *Phys Ther* 1990; 70(9): 561–565.

52. Heintjes, E, MY Berger, SM Bierma-Zeinstra, RM Bernsen, JA Verhaar, and BW Koes. Exercise therapy for patellofemoral pain syndrome. *Cochrane Database Syst Rev* 2003; 4: CD003472.

53. Henry, JH, and JW Crosland. Conservative treatment of patellofemoral subluxation. *Am J Sports Med* 1979; 7: 12–14.

54. Hodges, P, and C Richardson. An investigation into the effectiveness of hip adduction in the optimization of the vastus medialis oblique contraction. *Scand J Rehab Med* 1993; 25: 57–62.

55. Hoke, B, D Howell, and M Stack. The relationship between isokinetic testing and dynamic patellofemoral compression. *J Orthop Sports Phys Ther* 1983; 4: 150–153.

56. Hughston, JC, and M Deese. Medial subluxation of the patella as a complication of a lateral retinacular release. *Am J Sports Med* 1988; 16: 383–388.

57. Hungerford, DS, and M Barry. Biomechanics of the patello-femoral joint. *Clin Orthop* 1979; 144: 9–15.

58. Insall, J, V Goldberg, and E Salvati. Recurrent dislocation and high-riding patella. *Clin Orthop* 1972; 88: 67–69.

59. Insall, J. Current concepts review, patellar pain. *J Bone Joint Surg [Am]* 1982; 64: 147–152.

60. Jacobson, KE, and FC Flandry. Diagnosis of anterior knee pain. *Clin Sports Med* 1989; 8: 179–195.

61. Juhn, MS. Patellofemoral pain syndrome: A review and guidelines for treatment. *Am Fam Physician* 1999; 60(7): 2012–2222.

62. Karlsson, J, R Thomeé, and L Swärd. Eleven-year follow-up of patello-femoral pain syndrome. *Clin J Sport Med* 1996; 6: 22–26.

63. Karst, GM, and PD Jewett. Electromyographic analysis of exercises proposed for differential activation of medial and lateral quadriceps femoris muscle components. *Phys Ther* 1993; 73(5): 286–295.

64. Klingman, RE, SM Liaos, and KM Hardin. The effect of subtalar joint position on patellar glide position in subjects with excessive rearfoot pronation. *JOSPT* 1997; 25(3): 185–191.

65. Kowal, MA. Review of physiological effects of cryotherapy. *JOSPT* 1983; 5(2): 66–73.

66. Kowall, MG, G Kolk, GW Nuber, JE Cassisi, and SH Stern. Patellar taping in the treatment of patellofemoral pain: A prospective randomized study. *Am J Sports Med* 1996; 24(1): 61–66.

67. Laprade, J, E Culham, and B Brouwer. Comparison of five isometric exercises in the recruitment of the vastus medialis oblique in persons with and without patellofemoral pain syndrome. *JOSPT* 1998; 27(3): 197–204.

68. Laprade, JA, and EG Culham. A self-administered pain severity scale for patellofemoral pain syndrome. *Clin Rehabil* 2002, 16(7): 780–788.

69. Larsen, B, E Andreasen, A Urfer, MR Mickelson, and KE Newhouse. Patellar taping: A radiographic examination of the medial glide technique. *Am J Sports Med* 1995; 23(4): 465–471.

70. Lieb, F, and J Perry. Quadriceps function. *J Bone Joint Surg [Am]* 1968; 50: 1535–1548.

71. Lin, F, G Wang, JL Koh, RW Hendrix, and LQ Zhang. In vivo and non-invasive three-dimensional patellar tracking induced by individual heads of quadriceps. *Med Sci Sports Exerc* 2004, 36(1): 93–101.

72. Lindh, M. Increase of muscle strength from isometric quadriceps exercise at different angles. *Scand J Rehab Med* 1979; 11: 33–36.

73. Loudon, JK, D Wiesner, HL Goist-Foley, C Asjes, and KL Loudon. Intrarater reliability of functional performance tests for subjects with patellofemoral pain syndrome. *J Athl Train* 2002, 37(3): 256–261.

74. Lysholm, J, M Nordin, J Ekstrand, and J Gillquist. The effect of a patella brace on performance in knee extension strength test in patients with patellar pain. *Am J Sports Med* 1984; 12: 110–112.

75. Mariani, PP, and I Caruso. An electromyographic investigation of subluxation of the patella. *J Bone Joint Surg [Br]* 1989; 61: 169–171.

76. Martin, JA, and BR Londeree. EMG comparison of quadriceps femoris activity during knee extension and straight leg raises. *Am J Phys Med Rehab* 1979; 58: 57–69.

77. McConnell, J. The management of chondromalacia patellae: A long term solution. *Austr J Physiother* 1986; 32(4): 215–223.

78. McConnell, J. Examination of the patellofemoral joint: The physical therapist's perspective. In Grelsamer, RP, and J McConnell, eds., *The Patella: A Team Approach*. Gaithersburg, Maryland: Aspen Publishers, 1998, pp. 109–118.

79. McConnell, J. Conservative management of patellofemoral problems. In Grelsamer, RP, and J McConnell, eds., *The Patella: A Team Approach*. Gaithersburg, Maryland: Aspen Publishers, 1998, pp. 119–136.

80. McKenzie, DK, B Bigeland-Ritchie, RB Gorman, and SC Gandevia. Central and peripheral fatigue of human diaphragm and limb muscles assessed by twitch interpolation. *J Physiol* 1992; 454: 643–656.

81. Michlovitz, SL. Cryotherapy: The use of cold as a therapeutic agent. In Michlovitz, SL, ed., *Thermal Agents in Rehabilitation*, 2nd ed. Philadelphia: FA Davis Company, 1990, pp. 63–86.

82. Milgrom, C, E Kerem, A Finestone, A Eldad, and N Shlamkovitch. Patellofemoral pain caused by overactivity: A prospective study of risk factors in infantry recruits. *J Bone Joint Surg [Am]* 1991; 73: 1041–1043.

83. Miller, JP, D Sedory, and RV Croce. Vastus medialis obliquus and vastus lateralis activity in patients with and without patellofemoral pain syndrome. *J Sport Rehab* 1997; 6: 1–10.

84. Möller, RN, and B Krebs. Dynamic knee brace in the treatment of patellofemoral disorders. *Arch Orthop Trauma Surg* 1986; 104: 377–379.

85. Ninos, JC, JJ Irrgang, R Burdett, and JR Weiss. Electromyographic analysis of the squat performed in self-selected lower extremity neutral rotation and 30° of lower extremity turn-out from the self-selected neutral position. *JOSPT* 1997; 25(5): 307–315.

86. Nisell, R, and J Ekholm. Patellar forces during knee extension. *Scand J Rehab Med* 1985; 17: 63–74.

87. Osborne, AH, and MA Farquharson-Roberts. The aetiology of patello-femoral pain. *J Roy Nav Med Serv* 1983; 69: 97–103.

88. Owings, TM, and MD Grabiner. Motor control of the vastus medialis oblique and vastus lateralis muscles is disrupted during eccentric contractions in subjects with patellofemoral pain. *Am J Sports Med* 2002, 30(4): 483–487.

89. Palmitier, RA, K-N An, SG Scott, and EYS Chao. Kinetic chain exercise in knee rehabilitation. *Sports Med* 1991; 11(6): 404–413.

90. Palumbo, PM. Dynamic patellar brace: patellofemoral disorders: A preliminary report. *Am J Sports Med* 1981; 9: 45–49.

91. Percy, EC, and RT Strother. Patellalgia. *Physician Sports Med* 1985; 13: 43–59.

92. Portney, LG, PE Sullivan, and JL Daniell. EMG activity of vastus medialis obliquus and vastus lateralis in normals and patients with patellofemoral arthralgia. *Phys Ther* 1986; 66: 808.

93. Powers, CM, R Landel, T Sosnick, J Kirby, K Mengel, A Cheney, and J Perry. The effects of patellar taping on stride characteristics and joint motion in subjects with patellofemoral pain. *JOSPT* 1997; 26(6): 286–291.

94. Powers, CM, J Perry J, and HJ Hislop. Are patellofemoral pain and quadriceps femoris muscle torque associated with locomotor function? *Phys Ther* 1997; 77(10): 1063–1075.

95. Price, DD, PA McGrath, A Rafii, and B Buckingham. The validation of visual analog scale measures for chronic and experimental pain. *Pain* 1983; 17: 45–56.

96. Reynolds, L, T Levin, J Medeiros, N Adher, and A Hallum. EMG activity of the vastus medialis oblique and the vastus lateralis in their role in patellar alignment. *Am J Phys Med* 1983; 62: 61–70.

97. Richardson, CA, and MI Bullock. Changes in muscle activity during fast alternating flexion and extension movements of the knee. *Scand J Rehab Med* 1986; 18: 51–58.

98. Sczepanski, TL, MT Gross, PW Duncan, and JM Chandler. Effect of contraction type, angular velocity, and arc of motion on VMO:VL EMG ratio. *JOSPT* 1991; 14(6): 256–262.

99. Sega, L, M Galante, A Fortina, G Squazzini Viscontini, G Bertolotti, and MG Benedetti. Association of dynamic bandage with kinesitherapy in the treatment of patellar instability. *Ital J Sports Traum* 1988; 10: 89–94.

100. Signorile, JF, D Kacsik, A Perry, B Robertson, R Williams, I Lowensteyn, S Digel, J Caruso, and WG LeBlanc. The effect of knee and foot position on the electromyographical activity of the superficial quadriceps. *JOSPT* 1995; 22(1): 2–9.

101. Skalley, TC, GC Terry, and RA Teitge. The quantitative measurement of normal passive medial and lateral patellar motion. *Am J Sports Med* 1993; 21(5): 728–732.

102. Smith, AD, L Stroud, and C McQueen. Flexibility and anterior knee pain in adolescent elite figure skaters. *J Pediatr Orthop* 1991; 11: 77–82.

103. Souza, DR, and MT Gross. Comparison of vastus medialis obliquus:vastus lateralis muscle integrated electromyographic ratios between healthy subjects and patients with patellofemoral pain. *Phys Ther* 1991; 71: 310– 320.

104. Steadman, JR. Nonoperative measures for patellofemoral problems. *Am J Sports Med* 1979; 7: 374–375.

105. Steinkamp, LA, MF Dillingham, MD Markel, JA Hill, and KR Kaufman. Biomechanical considerations in patellofemoral joint rehabilitation. *Am J Sports Med* 1993; 21(3): 438–444.

106. Stiene, HA, T Brosky, MF Reinking, J Nyland, and MB Mason. A comparison of closed kinetic chain and isokinetic joint isolation exercise in patients with patellofemoral dysfunction. *JOSPT* 1996; 24(3): 136–141.

107. Teitge, RA. Iatrogenic medial dislocation of the patella. *Orthop Trans* 1991; 15: 747.

108. Thein Brody, L, JM Thein. Nonoperative treatment for patellofemoral pain. *JOSPT* 1998; 28(5): 336–344.

109. Thistle, HG, HJ Hislop, M Moffroid, and EW Lowman. Isokinetic contraction: A new concept of resistive exercise. *Arch Phys Med Rehab* 1967; 48: 279–282.

110. Thomeé, R. Patellofemoral pain syndrome in young women: Studies on alignment, pain assessment and muscle function, with a model for treatment. Thesis, Göteborg, Sweden, 1995.

111. Thomeé, P, R Thomeé, and J Karlsson. patellofemoral pain syndrome: Pain, coping strategies and degree of well-being. *Scand J Med Sci Sports* 2002, 12(5): 276–281.

112. Tiberio, D. The effect of excessive subtalar joint pronation on patellofemoral mechanics: A theoretical model. *JOSPT* 1987; 9: 160–165.

113. van Kampen, A. The three-dimensional tracking pattern of the patella: In vitro analysis. Thesis, Nijmegen, Holland, 1987.

114. Voight, ML, and DL Wieder. Comparative reflex response times of vastus medialis obliquus and vastus lateralis in normal subjects and subjects with extensor mechanism dysfunction: An electromyographic study. *Am J Sports Med* 1991; 19: 131–137.

115. Werner, S. Patello-Femoral Pain Syndrome: An experimental clinical investigation. Thesis, Karolinska Institutet, Stockholm, Sweden, 1993.

116. Werner, S, H Arvidsson, I Arvidsson, and E Eriksson. Electrical stimulation of vastus medialis and stretching of lateral thigh muscles in patients

with patello-femoral symptoms. *Knee Surg, Sports Traumatol, Arthrosc* 1993; 1: 85–92.

117. Werner, S, and E Eriksson. Isokinetic quadriceps training in patients with patellofemoral pain syndrome. *Knee Surg, Sports Traumatol, Arthrosc* 1993; 1: 162–168.

118. Werner, S, E Knutsson, and E Eriksson. Effect of taping the patella on concentric and eccentric torque and EMG of the knee extensor and flexor muscles in patients with patellofemoral pain syndrome. *Knee Surg, Sports Traumatol, Arthrosc* 1993; 1: 169–177.

119. Werner, S. An evaluation of knee extensor and knee flexor torques and EMGs in patients with patellofemoral pain syndrome in comparison with matched controls. *Knee Surg, Sports Traumatol, Arthrosc* 1995; 3: 89–94.

120. Westfall, DC, and TW Worrell. Anterior knee pain syndrome: role of vastus medialis oblique. *J Sport Rehab* 1992; 1: 317–325.

121. Whittingham, M, S Palmer, and F Macmillan. Effects of taping on pain and function in patellofemoral pain syndrome: A randomized controlled trial. *JOSPT* 2004, 34(9): 504–510.

122. Wild, JJ, TD Franklin, and GW Woods. Patellar pain and quadriceps rehabilitation: An EMG study. *Am J Sports Med* 1982; 10: 12–15.

123. Wilk, KE, GJ Davies, RE Mangine, and TR Malone. Patellofemoral disorders: A classification system and clinical guidelines for nonoperative rehabilitation. *JOSPT* 1998; 28(5): 307–321.

124. Willett, GM, and GM Karst. Patellofemoral disorders: Is timing or magnitude of vastus medialis obliquus and vastus lateralis muscle activity affected by conservative treatment? (Abstract). *JOSPT* 1995; 21(1): 61.

125. Witvrouw, E, C Sneyers, R Lysens, J Victor, and J Bellemans. Reflex response times of vastus medialis oblique and vastus lateralis in normal subjects and in subjects with patellofemoral pain syndrome. *JOSPT* 1996; 24(3) 160–165.

126. Witvrouw, E, R Lysens, J Bellemans, D Cambier, and G Vanderstraeten. Intrinsic risk factors for the development of anterior knee pain in an athletic population: A two year prospective study. *Am J Sports Med* 2000; 28(4): 480–489.

127. Witvrouw, E, L Danneels, D Van Tiggelen, TM Willems, and D Cambier. Open versus closed kinetic chain exercises in patellofemoral pain: A 5-year prospective randomized study. *Am J Sports Med* 2004, 32(5): 1122–1130.

128. Witvrouw, E, S Werner, C Mikkelsen, D Van Tiggelen, L Vanden Berghe, and G Cerulli. Clinical classification of patellofemoral pain syndrome: Guidelines for nonoperative treatment. *Knee Surg, Sports Traumatol, Arthrosc* 2005.

129. Yates, C, and WA Grana. Patellofemoral pain: A prospective study. *Orthopedics* 1986; 9: 663–667.

130. Åstrand, PO, and K Rodahl. *Textbook of Work Physiology*. New York: McGraw-Hill, 1977.

10

Conservative Management of Anterior Knee Pain: The McConnell Program

Jenny McConnell and Kim Bennell

Introduction

Traditionally, conservative management of patellofemoral pain syndrome (PFPS) involved pain-relieving techniques and standard quadriceps strengthening in non-weight-bearing positions. In 1986, an Australian physiotherapist, Jenny McConnell, proposed an innovative management program based on the premise that abnormal patellar tracking plays a key role in the etiology of PFPS.[56] Passive, active, and neural factors predisposing to abnormal patellar tracking were to be identified via a thorough assessment of the patient. Based on the assessment findings, the treatment program aimed first to unload abnormally stressed soft tissue around the patellofemoral joint by optimizing the patellar position, and second to improve the lower limb mechanics. The program included vastus medialis obliquus (VMO) retraining in functional weight-bearing positions combined with patellar taping, patellar mobilization, correction of foot mechanics, and stretching to reduce pain and enhance VMO activation. The McConnell program is now used routinely in Australia and increasingly around the world. There has been much research on the effects of patellar taping but less investigating the efficacy of the overall program. Case series and a recent randomized controlled trial indicate that the program is effective in treating PFPS. This chapter will focus on the McConnell program for conservatively managing PFPS. It will describe factors predisposing to PFPS as a theoretical

rationale for the program and include details of assessment and treatment.

Factors Predisposing to Patellofemoral Pain

Individuals with patellofemoral pain tend to demonstrate a failure of the intricate balance of the soft tissue structures around the joint. This may alter the pressure distribution from the patella to the femur. However, the mechanism of pain production in patellofemoral pain is not fully understood. Patellofemoral pain is most likely due to either tension or compression of the soft tissue structures. Patellofemoral pain may therefore be classified by area of pain as this usually indicates the compromised structure and the possible mechanism for the compromise. For example, lateral pain may be indicative of adaptive shortening of the lateral retinaculum. Those with lateral pain will have chronically tilted patellae (excessive lateral pressure syndrome) and there is often evidence of small nerve injury in the lateral retinaculum when the retinaculum is sectioned histologically.[29] Inferior patellar pain is likely to implicate the infrapatellar fat pad, one of the most pain-sensitive structures in the knee.[2,23] A patient with a recurrently subluxing patella often presents with medial patellofemoral pain because the medial retinaculum is chronically overstretched. It is unusual for this type of patient to have tight lateral structures as the patella is generally mobile in all directions and the VMO is poorly developed.

It is postulated that in individuals who complain of a deep ache in the knee, the articular cartilage has failed such that the load is now borne on the richly innervated underlying subchondral bone.[29] These patients often have the classic chondromalacia patellae where softening and fissuring is present on the undersurface of the patella.

Biomechanical Faults

Although a direct blow or a traumatic dislocation of the patella may precipitate patellofemoral pain, suboptimal mechanics of the patella from biomechanical faults is thought to be the major contributory factor.[29,43,52,68,81] The biomechanical faults may be divided into structural and nonstructural. Structural causes of malalignment may be divided into intrinsic and extrinsic causes and may be quite subtle. The extrinsic factors are more common and magnify the effect of the nonstructural faults.

Intrinsic structural factors relate to dysplasia of the patella or femoral trochlea and the position of the patella relative to the trochlea. Although uncommon, developmental abnormalities such as patella or trochlea dysplasia will create patellofemoral incongruence with resultant instability of the patella.[68,81] Extrinsic structural faults are reported to cause a lateral tracking of the patella.[43,49,52] The extrinsic factors include increased Q angle and tightness of the hamstrings and gastrocnemius muscles.

The Q angle has been used to estimate the angle of pull of the quadriceps muscle group.[52] It forms a valgus vector particularly in extension. The outer limit of Q angle for females is 15°, for males 12°.[49,52] The Q angle varies dynamically, decreasing with knee flexion and increasing with knee extension due to the external rotation of the tibia which occurs during the screw home mechanism to allow full extension to occur.[29,49] Increased femoral anteversion, external tibial torsion, or a lateral displacement of the tibial tubercle can cause an increase in Q angle.[54] Often individuals with an increased Q angle have "squinting" patellae. These individuals usually present with an anteversion of the femur.[54]

Soft Tissue Tightness

Soft tissue tightness is particularly prevalent during the adolescent growth spurt where the long bones are growing faster than the surrounding soft tissues.[60] This leads not only to problems with lack of flexibility and alteration of stress through joints but also to muscle control problems where the motor program is no longer able to appropriately control the limb. A decrease in extensibility of the lateral retinaculum, a reduction in the flexibility of the tensor fasciae latae, hamstrings, gastrocnemius, or rectus femoris will adversely affect patellar tracking.

When the knee flexes, a shortened lateral retinaculum will come under excessive stress as the patella is drawn into the trochlea and the iliotibial band pulls posteriorly on the already shortened lateral retinaculum.[28,29] This will cause a lateral tracking and tilting of the patella and often a weakness of the medial retinaculum.[29] Additionally, a tight TFL, through its attachment into the iliotibial band, will cause a lateral tracking of the patella, particularly at 20° of knee flexion when the band is at its shortest.

Hamstrings and gastrocnemius tightness also cause a lateral tracking of the patella, by increasing the dynamic Q angle.[5,70,77] During running, tight hamstrings will lead to increased knee flexion when the foot lands. Because the knee cannot straighten, an increased amount of dorsiflexion is required to position the body over the planted foot. If the range of full dorsiflexion has already occurred at the talocrural joint, further range is achieved by pronating the foot, particularly at the subtalar joint. This causes an increase in the valgus vector force and hence increases the dynamic Q angle.[77]

Muscle Imbalance

While it would seem that the control and timing of the lower limb muscles, in particular VMO and vastus lateralis (VL), are critical to the smooth functioning of the patellofemoral joint, this is still a controversial area. Voight and Weider[82] found that the reflex response time of the VMO was earlier than the VL in an asymptomatic group, but in a symptomatic patellofemoral group there was a reversal of the pattern. These findings were recently confirmed by Witvrouw and colleagues,[83] but curiously these investigators found that there was a shorter reflex response time in the PF group relative to the control group.[83] Dynamically this issue has been supported by the work of Koh et al.,[48] who examined isokinetic knee extension at 250°s⁻¹, following hamstrings preactivation, finding that the VMO activated 5.6 ms earlier than VL. Even though this finding was statistically significant, these authors questioned the functional relevance. Our research group has shown that the EMG onset of VMO is delayed relative to VL during both stair stepping[9] and postural perturbation tasks[11] in patients with patellofemoral pain compared with asymptomatic controls. However, in the asymptomatic group, VMO onset occurred at the same time as VL and not before. Others have found that the VMO did not fire earlier than the VL in the asymptomatic group and that the VMO was not delayed in the symptomatic group.[30,45,64,65]

There is also contention about whether there is a difference in the ratio of VMO and VL activity.[55,64] Part of the conflict might relate to the problem of normalization of EMG data. Normalization involves obtaining a ratio of the recorded muscle activity and muscle activity from the maximal voluntary contraction (MVC), which then enables comparison of the ratio of one muscle relative to its maximal with another muscle relative to its maximal. There has been some discussion that normalization is affected by the presence of pain that will mask differences as there may be error in the MVC that may appear in the error of the recorded EMG.[74] Furthermore, there is debate about the reliability of the maximal contraction, throwing some concern on the normalization process.[42,85] Where does this leave the clinician and what is the best method of facilitating recovery in a patient with patellofemoral pain? This issue will be addressed in the section concerned with muscle training.

Altered Foot Biomechanics

Altered foot biomechanics such as excessive, prolonged, or late pronation will alter the tibial rotation at varying times through range, thus having an effect on patellofemoral joint mechanics.[70,77] It is essential for the therapist to realize that the foot may be mobile or stiff and that if a foot problem is discovered, orthotics may not necessarily be the only course of action – joint mobilization and muscle training can be extremely effective, particularly if the foot is stiff.

Clinical Examination

In the history, the clinician needs to elicit the location of the pain, the aggravating activities, the history of the pain, its behavior, and any other associated symptoms such as giving way or swelling. Simple outcome measures that are valid and reliable should also be obtained from the patient so that the effectiveness of treatment can be evaluated. These measures include a visual analogue scale for overall usual or worst pain in the past week or the anterior knee pain scale.[16] A change of more than 2 cm out of 10 on the visual analogue scale is needed to represent a clinically important change.

The clinical examination is important to establish the diagnosis and to determine the underlying causative factors of the patient's symptoms so the appropriate treatment can be implemented. The patient is initially examined in standing for assessment of lower extremity alignment. Biomechanical faults are noted so that the clinician has a reasonable indication of how the patient will move. Of particular interest is femoral position, which is easier to see when the patient has the feet together. Internal femoral rotation is a common finding in patients with patellofemoral pain (Figure 10.1). The term internal femoral rotation is preferred to femoral anteversion, because the term rotation implies not only the bony position, but also the soft tissue adaptation that occurs as a result of the femoral anteversion. The soft tissue changes are quite amenable to change by conservative management.

The internal femoral rotation often causes a squinting of the patellae but if the lateral structures of the patellofemoral joint are tight, the patella may appear straight. The clinician is interested in the presence of an enlarged fat pad, which indicates that the patient is standing in hyperextension or a "locked back" knee position. The muscle bulk of the VMO is observed and compared with the other side. The VL and ITB are palpated to determine the resting tension. Presence of varus/valgus and/or torsion of the tibia is noted. The talus is palpated on the medial and lateral sides to check for symmetry of position. In relaxed standing, the patient should be in midstance position, so ideally, the subtalar joint should be in mid-position.[51,70] If the talus is more prominent medially, then the patient's subtalar joint is pronated. The shape of medial and lateral longitudinal arches is noted. If, for example, the medial longitudinal arch is flattened, then the patient will exhibit a prolonged amount of pronation during walking. The great toe and first metatarsal are examined for callus formation as well as position. If the patient has callus on the medial aspect of the first metatarsal or the great toe, or has a hallux valgus, then the therapist should expect the patient to have an unstable push-off in gait. When examined prone this patient will have a forefoot deformity.

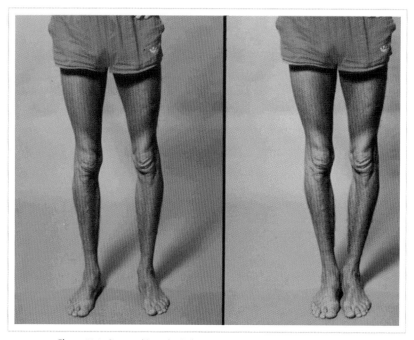

Figure 10.1. Common biomechanical presentation: internal rotation of the femurs.

From the side, the clinician can check pelvic position, to determine whether there is an anterior tilt, posterior tilt, or a sway back posture.[47] Position of hyperextension or lock back knees can be verified looking from the side. From behind, the level of the PSIS is checked, gluteal bulk is assessed, and the position of the calcaneum is observed. If the therapist finds that the calcaneum is in a relatively neutral or inverted position and the talus is more prominent on the medial side, then the therapist could probably expect that the patient would have a stiff subtalar joint. Thus, from a person's static alignment, the clinician can have a reasonable idea of the dynamic picture. Any deviations from the anticipated gives a great deal of information about the muscle control of the activity.

Dynamic Examination

The aim of the dynamic examination is not only to evaluate the effect of muscle action on the static mechanics, but also to reproduce the patient's symptoms so the clinician has an objective reassessment activity to evaluate the effectiveness of the treatment. The least stressful activity of walking is examined first. For example, individuals with patellofemoral pain who stand in hyperextension will not exhibit the nec-essary shock absorption at the knee, at heel strike. Consequently, the femur will internally rotate and the quadriceps will not function well in inner range due to lack of practice. If the patient's symptoms are not provoked in walking, then evaluation of more stressful activities, such as stair climbing, is performed. If symptoms are still not provoked then squat and one-leg squat may be examined and used as a reassessment activity. For the athlete, the clinician will, in many cases, be evaluating the control of the one-leg squat as symptom production in the clinic may be difficult.

Supine Lying Examination

With the patient in supine lying, the clinician gains an appreciation of the soft tissue structures and begins to confirm the diagnosis. Gentle, but careful palpation should be performed on the soft tissue structures around the patella. First, the joint lines are palpated to exclude obvious intrarticular pathology. Second, palpation of the retinacular tissues determine which parts of the retinaculum are under chronic recurrent stress. If pain is elicited in the infrapatellar region on palpation, the clinician should shorten the fat pad by lifting it toward the patella. If on further palpation, the pain is gone, then the clinician can be relatively certain that the patient has a fat pad irritation. If the pain remains, then patellar tendonosis is the most likely diagnosis. The knee is passively flexed and extended with overpressure applied so the clinician has an appreciation of the quality of the end feel. If any of these maneuvers reproduce pain, they can be used as a reassessment sign;[53] for example, the symptoms of fat pad irritation can often be produced with an extension overpressure maneuver.

The hamstrings, iliopsoas, rectus femoris, tensor fascia latae, gastrocnemius, and soleus muscles are tested for length. Tightness of any of these muscles has an adverse effect on patellofemoral joint mechanics and will have to be addressed in treatment. The iliopsoas, rectus femoris, and tensor fascia latae may be tested using the Thomas test.[41,46] Hamstrings flexibility may be examined by a passive straight leg raise, once the lumbar spine is flattened on the plinth and the pelvis is stable.[46] Normal-length hamstrings should allow 80–85° of hip flexion when the knee is extended and the lumbar spine is flattened.[46]

An essential part of patellofemoral evaluation in supine is assessment of the orientation of the patella relative to the femur. In order to maximize the area of contact of the patella with the femur, the patellar position should be optimal before the patella enters the trochlea. The clinician needs to consider the patellar position not with respect to the normal, but with respect to the optimal, because articular cartilage is nourished and maintained by evenly distributed, intermittent compression.[4,37,61]

An optimal patellar position is one where the patella is parallel to the femur in the frontal and the sagittal planes, and the patella is midway between the two condyles when the knee is flexed to 20°.[56,57] The position of the patella is determined by examining four discrete components; glide, lateral tilt, anteroposterior tilt, and rotation, in a static and dynamic manner. Determination of the glide component involves measuring the distance from the midpole of the patella to the medial and lateral femoral epicondyles (Figure 10.2). The patella should be sitting equidistant (+/–5 mm) from each epicondyle when the knee is flexed 20°. A 5 mm lateral displacement of the patella causes a 50% decrease in VMO tension.[1] In some instances, the patella may sit equidistant to the condyles, but moves lateral, out of the line of the femur,

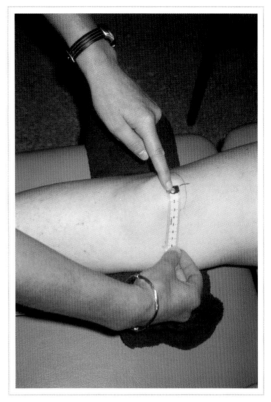

Figure 10.2. Assessment of patellar glide.

when the quadriceps contracts, indicating a dynamic problem. The dynamic glide examines both the effect of the quadriceps contraction on patellar position as well as the timing of the activity of the different heads of quadriceps. If the passive lateral structures are too tight, then the patella will tilt so that the medial border of the patella will be higher than the lateral border and the posterior edge of the lateral border will be difficult to palpate. This is a lateral tilt and, if severe, can lead to excessive lateral pressure syndrome.[29] When the patella is moved in a medial direction, it should initially remain parallel to the femur. If the medial border rides anteriorly, the patella has a dynamic tilt problem that indicates that the deep lateral retinacular fibers are too tight, affecting the seating of the patella in the trochlea.

An optimal position also involves the patella being parallel to the femur in the sagittal plane. A most common finding is a posterior displacement of the inferior pole of the patella (Figure 10.3). This will result in fat pad irritation and often manifests itself as inferior patella pain that

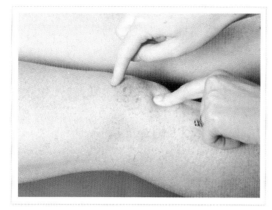

Figure 10.3. Assessment of posterior tilt of the inferior pole of the patella.

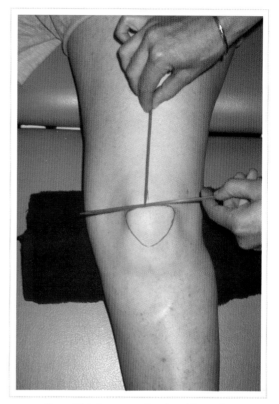

Figure 10.4. Assessment of rotation of the patella.

is exacerbated by extension maneuvers of the knee.[58] A dynamic posterior tilt problem can be determined during an active contraction of the quadriceps muscle as the inferior pole is pulled posteriorly, particularly in patients who hyperextend.

To complete the ideal position, the long axis of the patella should be parallel to the long axis of the femur. In other words, if a line was drawn between the most medial and most lateral aspects of the patella, it should be perpendicular to the long axis of the femur (Figure 10.4). If the inferior pole is sitting lateral to the long axis of the femur, the patient has an externally rotated patella. If the inferior pole is sitting medial to the long axis of the femur, then the patient has an internally rotated patella. The presence of a rotation component indicates that a particular part of the retinaculum is tight. Tightness in the retinacular tissue compromises the tissue and can be a potent source of the symptoms.[29]

Side Lying

The retinacular tissue can be specifically tested for tightness with the patient in side lying and the knee flexed to 20°. The therapist moves the patella in a medial direction, so the lateral femoral condyle is readily exposed. If the lateral femoral condyle is not readily exposed, the superficial retinacular fibers are tight. To test the deep fibers, the therapist places his or her hand on the middle of the patella, takes up the slack of the glide, and applies an anterior-posterior pressure on the medial border of the patella. The lateral should move freely away from the femur, and on palpation the tension in the retinacular fibers should be similar along the length of the patella. This test procedure can also be used as a treatment technique. Iliotibial band tightness may be confirmed further by Ober's test.[41]

Prone

In prone, the clinician may examine the foot to determine whether the patient has a primary foot deformity that is contributing to the patient's patellofemoral symptoms. The deformity will need to be addressed with orthotics or specific muscle training. In the prone position, the clinician is also able to evaluate the flexibility of the anterior hip structures, by examining the patient in a figure of four position, with the underneath foot at the level of the tibial tubercle (Figure 10.5). This position tests the available extension and external rotation at the hip, which is often limited because of chronic adaptive shortening of the anterior structures as a result of the underlying femoral anteversion. The distance of the ASIS from the plinth is measured, so the clinician has an objective measure of change.

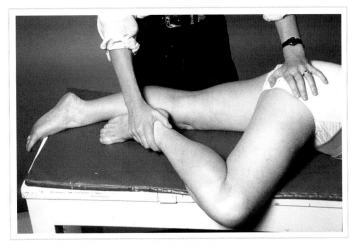

Figure 10.5. Assessment of the flexibility of the anterior hip structures.

A modification of the test position can also be used as a treatment technique. A lumbar spine palpation can be performed at this stage of the examination, if the clinician feels that the knee symptoms have been referred from a primary pathology in the lumbar spine. A summary of the examination process is listed in Table 10.1. Once the patellofemoral joint has been thoroughly examined, and the primary problems have been identified, appropriate treatment can be instigated.

Treatment
Conservative

Most patellofemoral conditions may be successfully managed with physical therapy. Treatment aims to optimize the patellar position and improve lower limb mechanics and thus decrease the patient's symptoms.

Stretching the tight lateral structures and changing the activation pattern of the VMO may decrease the tendency for the patella to track laterally and should enhance the position of the patella. Stretching the tight lateral structures can be facilitated passively by the therapist mobilizing and massaging the lateral retinaculum and the iliotibial band, as well as the patient performing a self-stretch on the retinacular tissue. However, the most effective stretch to the adaptively shortened retinacular tissue may be obtained by a sustained low load, using tape, to facilitate a permanent elongation of the tissues. This utilizes the creep phenomenon, which occurs in viscoelastic material when a constant low load is applied. It has been widely documented that the length of soft tissues can be increased with sustained stretching.[27,38,40,59,80] The magnitude of the increase in displacement is dependent on the duration of the applied stretch.[59,80] If the tape can be maintained for a prolonged period of time, then this, plus training of the VMO to actively change the patellar position, should have a significant effect on patellofemoral mechanics. However, there is some debate as to whether tape actually changes the position of the patella. Some investigators have found that tape changes PF angle and lateral patellar displacement, but congruence angle is not changed.[69] Others have concurred, finding no change in congruence angle when the patella is taped, but congruence angle is measured at 45° knee flexion, so subtle changes in patellar position may have occurred before this.[8] A study of asymptomatic subjects found that medial glide tape was effective in moving the patella medially but ineffective in maintaining the position after vigorous exercise. However, tape seems to prevent the lateral shift of the patella that occurred with exercise.[3] The issue for a therapist, however, is not whether the tape changes the patellar position on x-ray, but whether the therapist can decrease the patient's symptoms by at least 50%, so the patient can exercise and train in a pain-free manner.

Table 10.1. Examination checklist

PATIENT STANDING: Examine for biomechanical abnormalities
Observe alignment from:
1. In front
   - Normal standing
     - position of the feet with respect to the legs
     - Q angle
     - tibial valgum/varum
     - tibial torsion
     - talar dome position
     - navicular position
     - Morton's toe
     - hallux valgus
   - Feet together
     - squinting patellae
     - VMO bulk
     - VL tension
2. Side
   - pelvic position: tilt
   - hyperextension of the knees
3. Behind
   - PSIS position
   - gluteal bulk
   - calf bulk
   - calcaneal position

DYNAMIC EVALUATION: Evaluate the effect of the bony alignment and soft tissue on dynamic activities
1. Walking, if no pain
2. Steps, if no pain
3. Squat, if no pain
4. One leg squat

ASSESSMENT IN SUPINE LYING: Determine the causative factors of the symptoms and formulate a diagnosis
1. Palpation of the tibiofemoral joint line and soft tissue structures of the patellofemoral joint
2. Tibiofemoral tests
3. Meniscal tests
4. Ligament tests
5. Thomas's test: psoas, rectus femoris, tensor fascia lata
6. Tests for hamstrings, gastrocs
7. Slump test for dural length, particularly indicated if the patient complains of lateral knee pain when sitting with the legs out straight.
8. Hip tests (if applicable)
9. Orientation of the patella
   - glide, dynamic glide
   - lateral tilt
   - anteroposterior tilt
   - rotation

ASSESSMENT IN SIDELYING POSITION: Tests for tightness of the lateral structures
1. Medial glide: tests superficial lateral structures
2. Medial tilt: tests deep lateral structures
3. Ober's test for iliotibial band tightness

ASSESSMENT IN THE PRONE POSITION:
1. Lumbar spine palpation (only if applicable, i.e., if dural test positive)
2. Foot assessment
3. Hip rotation
4. Femoral nerve mobility

Patellar Taping

Patellar taping is based on the assessment of the patellar position. The component(s) corrected, the order of correction, and the tension of the tape is tailored for each individual (Figures 10.6 and 10.7). After each piece of tape is applied, the symptom producing activity should be reassessed. The tape should always immediately improve a patient's symptoms by at least 50%. If it does not, then the order in which the tape has been applied or the components corrected should be reexamined. In most cases, hypoallergenic tape is placed underneath the rigid sports tape to provide a protective layer for the skin and if there seems to be additional skin problems a plastic coating, either a spray or a roll-on, may be applied to the skin prior to the tape application. The patient must be taught how to position the tape on him- or herself. The patient should be in long sitting with the leg out straight and the quadriceps relaxed.

If a posterior tilt problem has been ascertained on assessment, it must be corrected first, as taping over the inferior pole of the patella will aggravate the fat pad and exacerbate the patient's pain. The posterior component is corrected together with a glide or a lateral tilt with the nonstretch tape being placed on the superior aspect of the patella, either on the lateral border to correct lateral glide or in the middle of the patella to correct lateral tilt. This positioning of the tape will lift the inferior pole out of the fat pad and prevent irritation of the fat pad.

If there is no posterior tilt problem, the glide may be corrected by placing tape from the lateral patellar border to the medial femoral condyle. At the same time the soft tissue on the medial aspect of the knee is lifted toward the patella to create a tuck or fold in the skin. The skin lift helps anchor the tape more effectively and minimizes the friction rub (friction between the tape and the skin), which can occur when a patient has extremely tight lateral structures.

The mediolateral tilt component is corrected by placing a piece of tape firmly from the middle of the patella to the medial femoral condyle. The object is to shift the lateral border away from the femur so that the patella becomes parallel with the femur in the frontal plane. Again, the soft tissue on the medial aspect of the knee is lifted toward the patella.

External rotation is the most common rotation problem and to correct this the tape is positioned at the inferior pole and pulled upward

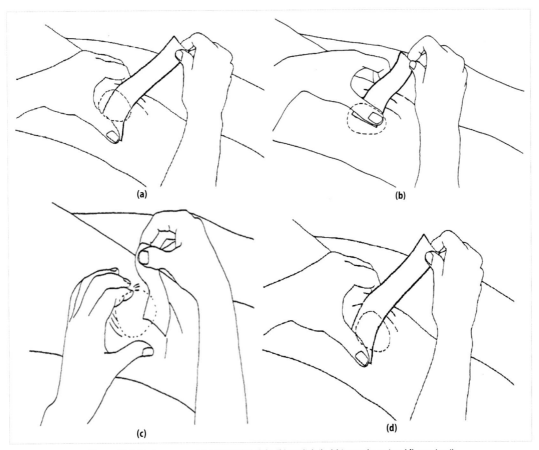

Figure 10.6. Taping components: **(a)** medial glide, **(b)** medial tilt, **(c)** internal rotation, **(d)** anterior tilt.

and medially toward the opposite shoulder while the superior pole is rotated laterally. Care must be taken so that the inferior pole is not displaced into the fat pad. Internal rotation, on the other hand, is corrected by taping from the superior pole downward and medially.

Unloading

The principle of unloading is based on the premise that inflamed soft tissue does not respond well to stretch. For example, if a patient presents with a sprained medial collateral ligament, applying a valgus stress to the knee will aggravate the condition, whereas a varus stress will decrease the symptoms. The same principle applies for patients with an inflamed fat pad, an irritated iliotibial band or a pes anserinus bursitis. The inflamed tissue needs to be shortened or unloaded. To unload an inflamed fat pad, for example a "V" tape is placed below

the fat pad, with the point of the V at the tibial tubercle coming wide to the medial and lateral joint lines (Figures 10.7D and 10.7E). As the tape is being pulled toward the joint line, the skin is lifted toward the patella, thus shortening the fat pad.

Principles of Using Tape to Correct the Patella

The tape is kept on all day, every day, until the patient has learned how to activate his or her VMO at the right time; that is, the tape is like trainer wheels on a bicycle and can be discontinued once the skill is established. The tape is removed with care in the evening allowing the skin time to recover. The tape can cause a breakdown in the skin either through a friction rub or as a consequence of an allergic reaction. Preparation of the skin and skin care advice is essential.

The patient should never train with or through pain or effusion as it has been shown quite conclusively in the literature that pain and effusion have an inhibitory effect on muscle activity.[19,63,75,76] If the patient experiences a return of the pain, the tape should be readjusted. If the activity is still painful, the patient must cease the activity immediately. The tape will loosen quickly if the lateral structures are extremely tight or the patient's job or sport requires extreme amounts of knee flexion.

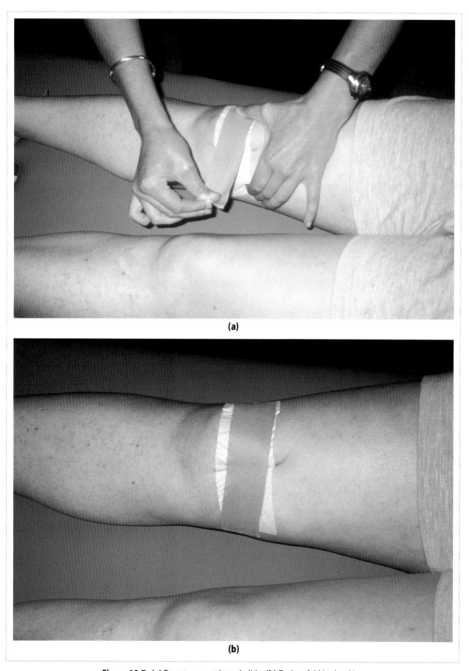

Figure 10.7. (a) Tape to correct lateral glide. **(b)** Tuck or fold in the skin.

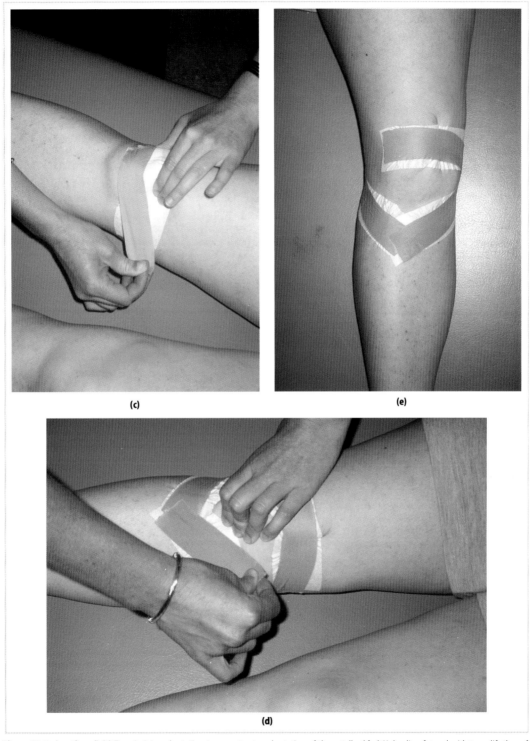

Figure 10.7. (*continued*) **(c)** Tape in internal rotation to correct external rotation of the patella. **(d,e)** Unloading fat pad with tape, lift the soft tissue toward the patella.

Studies Investigating the Effects of Tape

It has been fairly well established that taping the patella relieves pain,[8,34,39] but the mechanism of the effect is still being debated in the literature. This topic has been well reviewed by Crossley et al.[14] As mentioned previously, there is some evidence to show that taping can improve the radiographic position of the patella.[50,69,73] Others have assessed the effect of tape on quadriceps function.[8,34,72] Using isokinetic dynamometry, two studies found that tape significantly increased the quadriceps torque.[8,34] However, the increase in muscle torque with tape did not necessarily correlate with pain reduction. Ernst et al.[26] showed greater knee extensor moments and power during a vertical jump and lateral step-up in a taped condition compared with placebo and no tape conditions in PFPS subjects. It has also been found that during gait, individuals with PFPS decrease the amount of knee flexion in early stance to reduce the patellofemoral joint reaction force.[17,20,32,67] Patellar taping results in small but significant increases in loading response knee flexion in a variety of gait conditions indicating a greater ability to load the knee joint with confidence.[66]

It has been suggested that patellar tape could influence the magnitude of VMO and VL activation, although most studies do not necessarily support this contention.[6,18,39,62,72] Similarly there is conflict with regard to the effect of tape on onset timing of VMO and VL with some showing earlier timing of VMO. Taping the patella of symptomatic individuals such that the pain was decreased by 50% resulted in an earlier activation of the VMO relative to the VL on both step up and step down. Stepping down in particular caused an 8.3° differential between the knee angle at onset of VMO and VL as not only was the VMO activating earlier than the pre-taped condition, but the VL was significantly delayed in the taped condition.[30] Our research group has also found that tape leads to a change in the onset timing of VMO relative to VL compared with placebo tape and no tape.[12]

Muscle Training

There is currently debate about the best type of quadriceps strengthening for rehabilitating the PF joint. Powers concludes that because there is no difference in the activation pattern of the VMO and VL in symptomatic individuals and the ratio of the two muscles is the same, generalized quadriceps strengthening is all that is required.[65] However, this is at odds with our recent research, which demonstrated that a McConnell-based

physiotherapy treatment regime (taping, functional training with biofeedback on VMO and VL) for PFPS alters the motor control of VMO relative to VL in both a functional task[11] and a postural perturbation task.[13]

What types of exercises are most appropriate in training? From the current evidence available, it seems that closed chain exercise (when the foot is on the ground) is the preferred method of training, not only because closed kinetic training has been shown to improve patellar congruence, but muscle training has been found to be specific to limb position.[21] In a group of patients with lateral patellar compression syndrome, it was found that open chain exercise with isometric quadriceps sets at 10° intervals with 3 kg weight resulted in more lateral patellar tilt and glide from 0–20° on CT scan. Closed chain exercise by pushing a foot-plate with resistance cords attached to provide 18 kg resistance led to improved congruence from 0–20°.[21] Another study showed that in closed chain exercises, there is more selective VMO activation than in open chain exercises.[79] However, there is still debate in the literature. Recently a 5-year follow-up of patients in a clinical trial found good maintenance of subjective and functional outcomes in both the open and closed kinetic chain exercise groups.[84]

Specificity of Training

Before examining the issue of exercise prescription for the patellofemoral patient, some discussion on the different philosophies of strength training is required. The traditional strengthening view holds that strength gained in nonspecific muscle training can be harnessed for use in performance, that is, the engine (muscles) is built in the strength training room; learning how to turn the engine on (neural control) is acquired on the field.[71] Strength is therefore increased by utilizing the overload principle, meaning exercising at least 60% of maximal.[31] However, the muscles around the PF joint are stabilizing muscles and need to be endurance trained, so working at 20–30% of maximal is more appropriate. A more recent interpretation of how to facilitate strength is based on the premise that the engine (muscles) and how it is turned on (neural control) should both be built in the strength training room.[71] Training should therefore simulate movement in terms of anatomical movement pattern, velocity, type and force of contraction. Thus, with training the neuromuscular system will tend to become better at generating tension for actions that resemble the muscle actions employed in training, but not necessarily for actions that are dissimilar to those used in training. If the desired outcome of treatment is for the patient to be pain-free on weight-bearing activities, then the therapist must give the patient appropriate weight-bearing training. At no stage should the patient's recovery be compromised by training into pain.

A useful starting exercise is small-range knee flexion and extension movements (the first 30°) with the patient in stance position, where the feet are facing forward and positioned at the width of the pelvis. It is preferable that the patient has a dual channel biofeedback with electrodes on the VMO and the VL so the patient can monitor the timing of the contraction and the amount of activity. This is particularly important for those patients who have trouble activating the VMO. The patient is instructed to squeeze the gluteals and slowly flex the knees to 30° and slowly return to full extension without locking the knees back. The patient is aiming for the VMO to be activated before the VL and remain more than the VL during the activity. This clinical interpretation of the use of EMG biofeedback is at odds with the research application, insofar as the activity of the VMO and the VL has not been normalized. Furthermore, the limited research to date does not necessarily show additional benefit from the incorporation of biofeedback.[22]

Progression of training involves simulation of the knee during the stance phase of walking, so the patient is in a walk-stance position. In this position VMO recruitment is usually poor and the seating of the patella in the trochlea is critical. Again, small-amplitude movements need to be practiced. Again, emphasis should be given to the timing and intensity of the VMO contraction relative to the VL. For a patient who is having difficulty contracting the VMO, muscle stimulation may be used to facilitate the contraction. Further progression of treatment can be implemented by introducing step training. The patients need to practise stepping down from a small height initially. This should be performed slowly, in front of a mirror, so that changes in limb alignment can be observed and deviations can be corrected (Figure 10.8). Specific work on the hip musculature may be necessary to improve

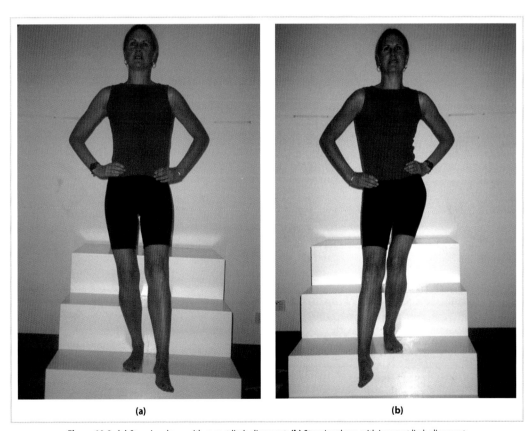

(a)   (b)

Figure 10.8. (a) Stepping down with correct limb alignment. **(b)** Stepping down with incorrect limb alignment.

the limb alignment. Some patients may only be able to do one repetition before the leg deviates. This is sufficient for them to start with, as inappropriate practice can be detrimental to learning. The number of repetitions should be increased as the skill level improves. It is therefore preferable for the therapist to emphasize quality, not quantity. Initially small numbers of exercises should be performed frequently throughout the day. The aim is to achieve a carryover from functional exercises to functional activities. Later, the patient can move to a larger step, initially decreasing the number of contractions and slowly increasing them again. As the control improves, the patient can alter the speed of the stepping activity and vary the place on descent where the stepping action is stopped. Weights may be introduced in the hands or in a backpack. Again, the number of repetitions and the speed of the movement should be decreased initially and built back up again.

Training should be applicable to the patient's activities/sport, so a jumping athlete, for example, should have jumping incorporated in his program. Figure-eight running, bounding jumping off boxes, jumping and turning, and other plyometric routines are particularly appropriate for the high-performance athlete. However, the patient's VMO needs to be monitored at all times for timing and level of contraction relative to the VL. The number of repetitions performed by the patient at a training session will depend on the onset of muscle fatigue. The aim would be to increase the number of repetitions before the onset of fatigue. Patients should be taught to recognize muscle fatigue or quivering, so that they do not train through the fatigue and risk exacerbating their symptoms.

Improving Lower Limb Mechanics

A stable pelvis will minimize unnecessary stress on the knee. Training of the gluteus medius (posterior fibers) to decrease hip internal rotation and the consequent valgus vector force that occurs at the knee is necessary to improve pelvic stability. Weakness of the hip abductors and external rotators has been documented in women with patellofemoral pain compared with pain-free controls.[44] The posterior gluteus medius may be trained in weight bearing with the patient standing side-on to a wall. The leg closest to the wall is flexed at the knee so the foot is off the ground. The hip is in line with the standing hip. The patient should have all the

weight back through the heel of the standing leg, which is slightly flexed. The patient externally rotates the standing leg without turning the foot, the pelvis, or the shoulders. The patient should sustain the contraction for 20 seconds, so a burning can be felt in the gluteus medius region. If this exercise is difficult for a patient to coordinate, then rubber tubing may be used around the ankles to provide resistance as the patient stands on the affected leg while pushing the other leg back diagonally at 45°.

The training may be progressed to standing on one leg where the pelvis is kept level and the lower abdominals and the glutei are worked together while the other leg is swinging back and forward, simulating the activity of the stance phase of gait.

If the patient has marked internal femoral rotation stretching of the anterior hip structures, to increase the available external rotation may be required. The patient lies prone with the hip to be stretched in an abducted, externally rotated and extended position. The other leg is extended and lies on top of the bent leg. The malleolus of the underneath leg is at the level of the tibial tubercle. The patient attempts to flatten the abducted and rotated hip by pushing along the length of the thigh and holding the stretch for 5 seconds. This action activates gluteals in inner range. Although it is not functional, it may facilitate gluteus medius activity in someone who is finding it difficult to activate the muscle in weight bearing.

Muscle Stretching

Appropriate flexibility exercises must be included in the treatment regime. The involved muscles may include hamstrings, gastrocnemius, rectus femoris, and TFL/ITB. A tight gastrocnemius will increase the amount of subtalar joint pronation exhibited in mid-stance phase of gait, so after the stretching, appropriate foot muscle training will be required.

Consideration of Foot Problems

The supinators of the foot, specifically tibialis posterior, should be trained if the patient demonstrates prolonged pronation during the mid-stance in gait. With the foot supinated, the base of the first metatarsal is higher than the cuboid, which will allow the peroneus longus to work more efficiently to increase the stability of the first metatarsal complex for push-off. The therapist can train this action to improve the efficiency of push-off. The position of training is in mid-stance, the patient is instructed to lift the arch while keeping the first metatarsal head on the floor, and then pushing the first metatarsal and great toe into the floor. If the patient is unable to keep the first metatarso-phalangeal joint on the ground when the arch is lifted, then the foot deformity is too large to correct with training alone and orthotics will be necessary to control the excessive pronation. The addition of orthotics to a physiotherapy program in a group of PFPS patients with documented rearfoot varus has been studied. The results showed less knee pain during aggravating activities after 8 weeks when compared with patients issued with a placebo foot insole.[25] Another study showed that patellofemoral pain patients who responded best to off-the-shelf orthotics were those with forefoot valgus of 2°, passive great toe extension of 78°, or navicular drop of 3 mm.[78] Gross and Foxworth[33] provide a review of the role of foot orthoses as an intervention in this condition.

Evaluation of the McConnell Program

Few clinical trials have evaluated the effectiveness of a McConnell-type program for PFPS.[7,24,35] These and other physical interventions for PFPS have been reviewed by Crossley et al.[14] and Heintjes et al.[36] Harrison et al.[35] performed a randomized, blinded, controlled trial investigating three physiotherapy treatment options, one of which best reflects the protocol designed by McConnell.[56] At the end of the one-month intervention period, the subjects in the McConnell-based program showed significant improvements in pain and function compared with a group who had supervised exercises, but did not differ from the group given a home exercises program only. However, the sample size was only sufficient to detect a large effect between the groups. The large dropout rate (up to 48%) at 12 months may have affected the results at this time point, especially since a significantly greater number of subjects in the intervention group who showed substantial improvement were lost to follow-up. The authors concluded that any of the treatments could provide long-term improvements in pain and function.

Clark et al.[7] found that proprioceptive muscle stretching and strengthening aspects of physiotherapy have a beneficial effect at three months sufficient to permit discharge from physiotherapy. These benefits were maintained at three months. While they noted that taping did not influence the outcome, the numbers in each group may not have been large enough to detect independent effects of taping.

We conducted a randomized, double-blind, placebo-controlled trial of the McConnell program in 71 PFPS patients.[10,15] Standardized treatment consisted of 6 treatment sessions, once weekly for both the physiotherapy and placebo groups. Sixty-seven (33 physiotherapy; 34 placebo) subjects completed the trial. The physiotherapy group demonstrated significantly better response to treatment and greater improvements in pain and functional activities than the placebo group. The physiotherapy treatment also changed the onset timing of VMO relative to VL measured using surface electromyography during stair stepping and postural perturbation tasks. At baseline in both groups, VMO came on significantly later than VL. Following treatment, there was no change in muscle onset timing of the placebo group. However, in the physiotherapy group, the onset of VMO and VL occurred simultaneously (concentric) or VMO actually preceded VL (eccentric).[10,13] This study demonstrates that a McConnell-based physiotherapy program significantly improves pain and function and can alter EMG onset of VMO relative to VL compared with placebo treatment.

Conclusion

Management of patellofemoral pain is no longer a conundrum if the therapist can determine the underlying causative factors and address those factors in treatment. It is imperative that the patient's symptoms are significantly reduced. This is often achieved by taping the patella, which not only decreases the pain, but also promotes an earlier activation of the VMO and increases quadriceps torque. Management will need to include specific VMO training, gluteal control work, stretching tight lateral structures, and appropriate advice regarding the foot, be it orthotics, training, or taping.

References

1. Ahmed, A, S Shi, A Hyder et al. The effect of quadriceps tension characteristics on the patellar tracking pattern. *Transactions of the 34th Orthopaedic Research Society,* Atlanta, 1988; 280.
2. Bennell, K, P Hodges, R Mellor, C Bexander, and T Souvlis. The nature of anterior knee pain following injection of hypertonic saline into the infrapatellar fat pad. *J Orthopaed Res 2004;* 22: 116–121.
3. Bockrath, K, C Wooden, T Worrell et al. Effects of patella taping on patella position and perceived pain. *Med Sci Sports Exer* 1993; 25(9): 989–992.

4. Brandt, K. Pathogenesis of osteoarthritis. In Kelley, Harris, Ruddy, Sledge, eds., *Textbook of Rheumatology*. Philadelphia: W.B. Saunders, 1981, Chap. 88.

5. Buchbinder, R, N Naparo, and E Bizzo. The relationship of abnormal pronation to chondromalacia patellae in distance runners. *J Am Pod Assoc* 1979; 69(2): 159–161.

6. Cerny, K. Vastus medialis oblique/vastus lateralis muscle activity ratios for selected exercises in persons with and without patellofemoral pain syndrome. *Phys Ther* 1995; 75(8): 672–682.

7. Clark, DI, N Downing, J Mitchell et al. Physiotherapy for anterior knee pain: A randomised controlled trial. *Ann Rheum Disease* 2000; 59: 700–704.

8. Conway, A, T Malone, and P Conway. Patellar alignment/ tracking Alteration: Effect on force output and perceived pain. *Isokin Exer Sci* 1992; 2(1): 9–17.

9. Cowan, SM, KL Bennell, PW Hodges, KM Crossley, and J McConnell. Delayed electromyographic onset of vastus medialis obliquus and vastus lateralis in subjects with patellofemoral pain syndrome. *Arch Phys Med Rehabil* 2001; 82: 183–189.

10. Cowan, S, K Bennell, K Crossley, P Hodges, and J McConnell. Physical therapy treatment changes electromyographic onset timing of vastus medialis obliquus relative to vastus lateralis in subjects with patellofemoral pain syndrome. *Med Sci Sport Exer* 2002; 34: 1879–1885.

11. Cowan, SM, PW Hodges, KL Bennell, and KM Crossley. Altered vastii recruitment when people with patellofemoral pain syndrome complete a postural task. *Arch Phys Med Rehabil* 2002; 83: 989–995.

12. Cowan, S, K Bennell, and P Hodges. Therapeutic patellar taping changes the timing of vastii muscle activation in people with patellofemoral pain syndrome. *Clin J Sport Med* 2002; 12: 339–347.

13. Cowan, SM, PW Hodges, KL Bennell, KM Crossley, and J McConnell. Simultaneous feedforward recruitment of the vastii in untrained postural tasks can be restored by specific training. *J Orthopaed Res* 2003; 21: 553–558.

14. Crossley, K, S Cowan, J McConnell et al. Patellar taping: Is clinical success supported by scientific evidence? *Manual Ther* 2000; 5: 142–150.

15. Crossley, K, K Bennell, S Green, S Cowan, and J McConnell. Conservative management of patellofemoral pain: A randomised, double-blind controlled trial. *Am J Sport Med* 2002; 30: 857–865.

16. Crossley, K, K Bennell, S Green, and S Cowan. Analysis of outcome measures for persons with patellofemoral pain: Which outcome measures for individuals with patellofemoral pain are reliable and valid? *Arch Phys Med Rehabil* 2004; 85: 815–822.

17. Crossley, KM, SM Cowan, KL Bennell, and J McConnell. Knee flexion during stair ambulation is altered in individuals with patellofemoral pain. *J Orthopaed Res* 2004; 22: 267–274.

18. Christou, EA. Patellar taping increases vastus medialis oblique activing in the presence of patellofemoral pain. *J Electromyogr Kinesiol* 2004; 14: 495–504.

19. de Andrade, J, C Grant, and A Dixon. Joint distension and reflex muscle inhibition in the knee. *J Bone Jt Surg* 1965; 47A: 313.

20. Dillon, P, W Updyke and W Allen. Gait analysis with reference to chondromalacia patellae. *J Orthop Sports Phys Ther* 1983; 5(3): 127–131.

21. Doucette, S, and D Child. The effect of open and closed chain exercise and knee joint position on patellar tracking in lateral patellar compression syndrome. *J Orthop Sports Phys Ther* 1996; 23(2): 104–110.

22. Dursun, N, E Dursun, and Z Kilic. Electromyographic biofeedback-controlled exercise versus conservative care for patellofemoral pain syndrome. *Arch Phys Med Rehab* 2001; 82: 1692–1695.

23. Dye, S. The knee as a biologic transmission with an envelope of function. *Clin Orthop Rel Res* 1996; 325: 10–18.

24. Eburne, J, and G Bannister. The McConnell regimen versus isometric quadriceps exercises in the management of anterior knee pain: A randomised prospective controlled trial. *Knee* 1996; 3: 151–153.

25. Eng, J, and M Pierrynowski. Evaluation of soft foot orthotics in the treatment of patellofemoral pain syndrome. *Phys Ther* 1993; 73(2): 62–70.

26. Ernst, GP, J Kawaguchi, and E Saliba. Effect of patellar taping on knee kinetics of patients with patellofemoral pain syndrome. *J Orthop Sports Phys Ther* 1999; 29(11): 661–667.

27. Frankel, VH, and M Nordin. *Basic Biomechanics of the Skeletal System*. Philadelphia: Lea and Febiger, 1980.

28. Fulkerson, JP. Awareness of the retinaculum in evaluating patellofemoral pain. *Am J Sports Med* 1982; 10(3): 147–149.

29. Fulkerson, J, and D Hungerford. *Disorders of the Patellofemoral Joint*, 2nd ed. Baltimore: Williams & Wilkins, 1990.

30. Gilleard, W, J McConnell, and D Parsons. The effect of patellar taping on the onset of vastus medialis obliquus and vastus lateralis muscle activity in persons with patellofemoral pain. *Phys Ther* 1998; 78(1): 25–32.

31. Grabiner, MD, TJ Koh, and LF Draganich. Neuromechanics of the patellofemoral joint. *Med Sci Sports Exer* 1994; 26(1): 10–21.

32. Greenwald, AE, AM Bagley, FP France et al. A biomechanical and clinical evaluation of a patellofemoral knee brace. *Clin Orthop Rel Res* 1996; 324: 187–195.

33. Gross, MT, and JL Foxworth. The role of foot orthoses as an intervention for patellofemoral pain. *J Orthopaed Sports Phys Ther* 2003; 33: 661–670.

34. Handfield, T, and J Kramer. Effect of McConnell taping on perceived pain and knee extensor torques during isokinetic exercise performed by patients with patellofemoral pain. *Physioth Can Winter* 2000; 39–44.

35. Harrison, EL, MS Sheppard, and AM McQuarrie. A randomized controlled trial of physical therapy treatment programs in patellofemoral pain syndrome. *Physioth Can Spring* 1999; 93–106.

36. Heintjes, E, MY Berger, SM Bierma-Zeinstra, RM Bernsen, JA Verhaar, and BW Koes. Exercise therapy for patellofemoral pain syndrome. *Cochrane Database of Systematic Reviews* 2003; CD003472.

37. Helminen, H, I Kiviranta, M Tammi et al. *Joint Loading*. London: Butterworths, 1987.

38. Herbert, R. Preventing and treating stiff joints. In Crosbie, J, and J McConnell, eds., *Key Issues in Musculoskeletal Physiotherapy*. Oxford: Butterworth-Heinemann, 1993.

39. Herrington, L, and CJ Payton. Effects of corrective taping of the patella on patients with patellofemoral pain. *Physioth* 1997; 83(11): 566–572.

40. Hooley, C, N McCrum, and R Cohen. The visco-elastic deformation of the tendon. *J Biomech* 1980; 13: 521.

41. Hoppenfeld, S. *Physical Examination of the Spine and Extremities.* New York: Appleton-Century-Crofts, 1976.
42. Howard, J, and R Enoka. Maximum bilateral contractions are modified by neurally mediated interlimb effects. *J Appl Physiol* 1991; 70: 306–316.
43. Insall, J. Chondromalacia patellae: Patellar malalignment syndrome. *Orthopaed Clin North Am* 1979; 10: 117–125.
44. Ireland, ML, JD Willson, BT Ballantyne, and IM Davis. Hip strength in females with and without patellofemoral pain. *J Orthopaed Sports Phys Ther* 2003; 33: 671–676.
45. Karst, GM, and GM Willett. Onset timing of electromyographic activity in the vastus medialis oblique and vastus lateralis muscles in subjects with and without patellofemoral pain syndrome. *Phys Ther* 1995; 75(9): 813–823.
46. Kendall, F, and L McCreary. *Muscle Testing and Function.* Baltimore: Williams and Wilkins, 1983.
47. Kendall, HD, FP Kendall, and DA Boynton. *Posture and Pain.* Baltimore: Williams and Wilkinson, 1952.
48. Koh, T, M Grabiner, and R DeSwart. In vivo tracking of the human patella. *J Biomech* 1992; 25(6): 637–643.
49. Kramer, PG. Patella malalignment syndrome: Rationale to reduce excessive lateral pressure. *J Orthop Sports Phys Ther* 1986; 8(6): 301–308.
50. Larsen, BE, A Adreasen, MR Urfer et al. Patellar taping: A radiographic examination of the medial glide technique. *Am J Sports Med* 1995; 23(4): 465–471.
51. Lutter, L. The knee and running. *Clin Sports Med* 1985; 4(4): 685–698.
52. Lyon, L, L Benzl, K Johnson et al. Q angle – A factor: Peak torque occurrence in isokinetic knee extension. *J Orthop Sports Phys Ther* 1988; 9(7): 250–253.
53. Maitland, GD. *Vertebral Manipulation.* London: Butterworths, 1986.
54. Malek, M, and R Mangine. Patellofemoral pain syndromes: A comprehensive and conservative approach. *J Orthop Sports Phys Ther* 1981; 2(3): 108–116.
55. Mariani, P, and I Caruso. An electromyographic investigation of subluxation of the patella. *J Bone Jt Surg* 1979; 61, 169–171.
56. McConnell, J. The management of chondromalacia patellae: A long-term solution. *Aust J Physioth* 1986; 32(4), 215–223.
57. McConnell, J. Training the vastus medialis oblique in the management of patellofemoral pain. *Proceedings Tenth Congress of the World Confederation for Physical Therapy,* Sydney, May 1987.
58. McConnell, J. Fat pad irritation: A mistaken patellar tendonitis. *Sport Health* 1991; 9(4): 7–9.
59. McKay-Lyons, M. Low-load, prolonged stretch in treatment of elbow flexion contractures secondary to head trauma: a case report. *Phys Ther* 1989; 69: 292.
60. Micheli, L, J Slater, E Woods et al. Patella alta and the adolescent growth spurt. *Clin Orthop Rel Res* 1986; 213: 159–162.
61. Mow, V, J Eisenfeld, and I Redler. Some surface characteristics of articular cartilage: II. On the stability of articular surface and a possible biomechanical factor in aetiology of chondrodegeneration. *J Biomech* 1974; 7: 457–467.
62. Ng, GY, and JM Cheng. The effects of patellar taping on pain and neuromuscular performance in subjects with patellofemoral pain. *Clin Rehab* 2002; 16: 821–827.
63. On, AY, B Uludag, E Taskirran, and C Eertekin. Differential corticomotor control of a muscle adjacent to a painful joint. *Neurorehab & Neural Rep* 2004; 18: 127–133.

64. Owings, TM, and MD Grabiner. Motor control of the vastus medialis oblique and vastus laterales is disrupted during eccentric contractions in subjects with patellofemoral pain. *Am J Sports Med* 2002; 30: 483–487.
65. Powers, CM, RF Landel, and J Perry. Timing and intensity of vastus muscle activity during functional activities in subjects with and without patellofemoral pain. *Phys Ther* 1996; 76: 946–955.
66. Powers, CM, R Landel, T Sosnick et al. The effects of patellar taping on stride characteristics and joint motion in subjects with patellofemoral pain. *J Orthop Sports Phys Ther* 1997; 26(6): 286–291.
67. Powers, CM, S Mortenson, D Nishimoto et al. Criterion-related validity of a clinical measurement to determine the medial/lateral component of patellar orientation. *J Orthop Sports Phys Ther* 1999; 29(7): 372–377.
68. Radin, E. A rational approach to treatment of patellofemoral pain. *Clin Orthop Rel Res* 1979; Oct., 144: 107–109.
69. Roberts, JM. The effect of taping on patellofemoral alignment: A radiological pilot study. *Proceedings Sixth Biennial Conference of the Manipulative Therapists Association of Australia,* 1989, pp. 146–151.
70. Root, M, W Orien, and J Weed. *Clinical Biomechanics,* Vol. II. Los Angeles: Clinical Biomechanics Corp., 1977.
71. Sale, D, and D MacDougall. Specificity of strength training: A review for coach and athlete. *Can J Appl Sports Sci* 1981; 6(2): 87–92.
72. Salsich, GB, JH Brechter, D Farwell, and CM Powers. The effects of patellar taping on knee kinetics, kinematics, and vastus laterales muscle activity during stair ambulation in individuals with patellofemoral pain. *J Orthopaed & Sports Phys Ther* 2002; 32: 3–10.
73. Somes, S, TW Worrell, B Corey et al. Effects of patellar taping on patellar position in the open and closed kinetic chain: A preliminary study. *J Sports Rehab* 1997; 6: 299–308.
74. Souza, D, and M Gross. Comparison of vastus medialis obliquus: Vastus lateralis muscle integrated electromyographic ratios between healthy subjects and patients with patellofemoral pain. *Phys Ther* 1991; 71: 310–320.
75. Spencer, J, K Hayes, and I Alexander. Knee joint effusion and quadriceps reflex inhibition in man. *Arch Phys Med* 1984; 65: 171–177.
76. Stokes, M, and A Young. Investigations of quadriceps inhibition: Implications for clinical practice. *Physioth* 1984; 70(11): 425–428.
77. Subotnik, S. The foot and sports medicine. *J Orthop Sports Phys Ther* 1980; 2(2): 53–54.
78. Sutlive, TG, SD Mitchell, SN Maxfield, CL McLean, JC Neumann, CR Swiecki, RC Hall, AC Bare, and TW Flynn. Identification of individuals with patellofemoral pain whose symptoms improved after a combined program of foot orthosis use and modified activity: a preliminary investigation. *Phys Ther* 2004; 84: 49–61.
79. Tang, SF, CK Chen, R Hsu, SW Chou, WH Hong, and HL Lew. Vastus medialis obliquus and vastus lateralis activity in open and closed kinetic chain exercises in patients with patellofemoral pain syndrome: An electromyographic study. *Arch Phys Med Rehab* 2001; 82: 1441–1445.
80. Taylor, D, J Dalton, and A Seaber. Visco-elastic properties of muscle-tendon units. The biomechanical effect of stretching. *Am J Sports Med* 1990; 18: 300.

81. Townsend, PR, and RM Rose. The biomechanics of the human patella and its implications for chondromalacia. *J Biomech* 1977; 10: 403–407.

82. Voight, M, and D Weider. Comparative reflex response times of the vastus medialis and the vastus lateralis in normal subjects and subjects with extensor mechanism dysfunction. *Am J Sports Med* 1991; 10: 131–137.

83. Witvrouw, E, C Sneyers, R Lysens et al. Comparative reflex response times of vastus medialis obliquus and vastus lateralis in normal subjects and subjects with patellofemoral pain syndrome, *J Orthop Sports Phys Ther* 1996; 24(3): 160–166.

84. Witvrouw, E, L Danneels, D Van Tiggelen, TM Willems, and D Cambier. Open versus closed kinetic chain exercises in patellofemoral pain: A 5-year prospective randomized study. *Am J Sports Med* 2004; 32: 1122–1130.

85. Yang, J, and D Winter. Electromyography reliability in maximal contractions and submaximal isometric contractions. *Arch Phys Med Rehab* 1983; 64: 417–420.

11

Skeletal Malalignment and Anterior Knee Pain: Rationale, Diagnosis, and Management

Robert A. Teitge and Roger Torga-Spak

Introduction

Any variation from optimal skeletal alignment may increase the vector forces acting on the patellofemoral joint causing either ligament failure with subsequent subluxation or cartilage failure as in chondromalacia or arthrosis or both ligament and cartilage failure (Figure 11.1). Anterior knee pain may result from these abnormal forces or their consequences.

The mechanical disadvantage provided by a skeleton with a geometrical or architectural flaw distributes abnormal stresses to both the ligaments and the joints of the misaligned limb. Ligament overload and subsequently failure (insufficiency) may occur with a single traumatic episode as well as repetitive episodes of minor trauma or chronic overload. Skeletal malalignment may cause chondromalacia patella and subsequently osteoarthritis by creating an increased mechanical leverage on the patellofemoral joint that can exceed the load capacity of the articular cartilage. A reduction in contact surface area such as a small patella or a high patella or a subluxed patella may also increase the unit area loading beyond the load capacity of the articular cartilage, leading to cartilage failure (osteoarthritis).

Anterior knee pain in association with bony malalignment may be the result of the abnormal tension or compression placed on the capsule, ligaments, synovium, or subchondral bone.

Association of Skeletal Malalignment and Patellofemoral Joint Pathology

Abnormal skeletal alignment of the lower extremity has been associated with various patellofemoral syndromes and biomechanical abnormalities. Our understanding of these associations continues to develop as many references consider only one aspect of the analysis.

In the frontal plane, malalignment has been shown to influence the progression of patellofemoral joint arthritis.[4,12] Varus alignment increases the likelihood of medial patellofemoral osteoarthrosis progression while valgus alignment increases the likelihood of lateral patellofemoral osteoarthrosis progression. Fujikawa[13] in a cadaveric study found a marked alteration of patellar and femoral contact areas with the introduction of increased varus alignment produced by a varus osteotomy.

Lerat et al.[30] noted a statistically significant correlation between increased femoral internal torsion and both patellar chondropathy and instability. Janssen[23] also found patellar dislocation was most commonly combined with increased medial torsion of the femur and speculated that this medial torsion was responsible for the development of dysplasia of the trochlea and of the patella. Takai et al.[41] measured femoral and tibial torsion in patients with

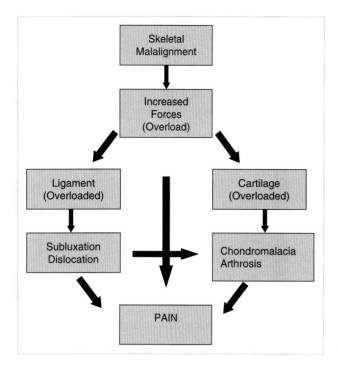

Figure 11.1. Pathogenesis of anterior knee pain.

patellofemoral medial and lateral unicompartmental osteoarthrosis and noted that the correlation of patellofemoral osteoarthritis with increased femoral torsion (23° vs. 9° in controls) was statistically their most significant observation and suggested that excessive femoral torsion is one of the contributory causes of patellofemoral wear.

Turner[43] studied the association of tibial torsion and knee joint pathology and observed that patients with patellofemoral instability had greater than normal external tibial torsion (25° vs. 19°). Eckhoff et al.[11] found the tibia in the extended knee to be 6° more externally rotated than normal controls in a group of patients with anterior knee pain. This was termed knee version. Whether this represents an abnormal skeletal torsion or an abnormal rotation of the tibia on the femur due to knee joint soft tissue laxity or abnormal muscle pull is unknown.

These studies and many others clearly show the importance of abnormal skeletal alignment of the lower extremity in the pathogenesis of various disorders of the patellofemoral joint.

Q-Angle and Skeletal Malalignment

The Q-angle has been implicated as a major source of patellofemoral pathology, but it must be emphasized that the Q-angle is a normal and necessary anatomic fact responsible for balancing the tibiofemoral force transmission. Hvid et al.[19] demonstrated a significant relation between the Q-angle measurement and increased hip internal rotation, thus supporting the existence of a torsional malalignment syndrome of the patellofemoral joint. Insall[20] called an increased Q-angle "patellar malalignment" and noted that it was usually associated with increased femoral anteversion and external tibial torsion so that the motion of the knee occurred about an axis that is rotated medially compared with the axes of the hip and ankle joints, producing "squinting" patella. This type of knee he stated is prone to chondromalacia (clinically "a diffuse aching pain on the anteromedial aspect of the knee"). It should be noted, however, that an increased Q-angle was present in only 40 of 83 (48%) knees in which surgical realignment for chondromalacia was performed. Thus, the problem is not the value of the Q-angle; the problem is that the Q-angle rotates around the coronal plane of the lower extremity.

Finally, it should be perhaps mentioned that Greene et al.[15] showed the reliability of the Q-angle measurement to be poor.

Definitions: Patellofemoral Alignment

There are two common uses for the term *alignment*: (1) malposition of the patella on the femur, and (2) malposition of the knee joint between the body and the foot with the subsequent effect on the patellofemoral mechanics. While it is more common to consider the position of the patella in the trochlea (i.e., subluxation), this view inhibits the more important consideration of what the position of the knee in space relative to the center of gravity of the body has in developing the force that the patellofemoral joint will experience. Tracking is the change in position of patella relative to the femur during knee flexion and extension, and while it is obviously important no clinically useful tracking measurement systems exist and the loading characteristics of the patellofemoral joint are largely unrelated to tracking.

The relationship of the patella to the femur (patellar malalignment) must be viewed in all three planes (Table 11.1). In the coronal plane, one can measure Q-angle and patellar spin. In the sagittal plane one can measure patellar flexion and height; in the horizontal plane one can measure patellar tilt or shift. Lauren[26] noted that shift and mini-tilt may both be manifestations of decreased lateral facet cartilage.

It is a common mistake to consider alignment as referring only to the position of the patella on the femoral trochlea. Alignment refers to the changing relationship of all the bones of the lower extremity and might best be considered as the relationship of the patellofemoral joint to the body. Mechanical alignment is the sum total of the bony architecture of the entire lower extremity from sacrum (center of gravity) to the foot (ground). The position and orientation of patellofemoral joint to the weight-bearing line determines the direction and magnitude of forces that will cross the patellofemoral joint. The relationship of the patellofemoral joint to the body must be defined in all three planes

(Table 11.2). In the frontal plane one can measure varus or valgus and patellar height. In the sagittal plane one can measure the patellar height, distance from the knee joint axis to the patella, depth of the trochlea, and height of the tibial tubercle. In the horizontal plane one can measure the torsion of the acetabulum, femur, tibia and foot, the version of the knee, the position of the tibial tubercle relative to the trochlear groove, and the depth of the groove as well as the "patellofemoral alignment."

Diagnosis of Skeletal Alignment

Malalignment refers to a variation from the normal anatomy; normal is that which is biomechanically optimal. In order to detect and understand deformities of the lower extremity, it is important to establish the limits and parameters of normal alignment based on average values for the general population.

Frontal Plane Alignment

Frontal plane alignment is best determined using longstanding AP radiographs including hip, knee, and ankle joint. To determine the mechanical axis a line is drawn from the center of the femoral head to the center of the ankle joint (Figure 11.2). Typically, normal alignment is defined as the mechanical axis passing just medial to the center of the knee.[34] Valgus alignment refers to the mechanical axis passing lateral to the center of the knee while varus refers to the mechanical axis passing medial to the center of the knee.

Two commonly measured angles are the mechanical tibiofemoral angle (center of femoral head to center of knee to center of talus) and the anatomical tibiofemoral angle (line down center of femoral shaft and line down center of tibial shaft). The mechanical tibiofemoral angle is the angle between the mechanical axis of the femur and the tibia. An angle of $1.2° \pm 2°$ is considered normal (i.e., the limb mechanical axis falls just medial to the center of the knee joint).[6,7,18,34] The anatomical tibiofemoral angle

Table 11.1. Classification of patellar malalignment					
Frontal plane		Sagittal plane		Horizontal Plane	
Internal rotation (spun)	External rotation (spun)	Flexion	Extension	Medial tilt	Lateral tilt
High Q-angle	Low Q-angle	Alta	Baja	Medial shift (translation)	Lateral shift (translation)

Table 11.2. Classification of skeletal malalignment

Frontal plane	Location	Sagittal plane	Location	Horizontal plane	Location
Varus	Femur Tibia Ligaments	Prominent trochlea	Femur	Inward-pointing knee	Femur (internal torsion) Tibia (external torsion) Subtalar joint complex (hyperpronation)
Valgus	Femur Tibia Ligaments	Shallow trochlea	Femur	Outward-pointing knee	Femur (external torsion) Tibia (internal torsion) Subtalar joint complex
		Aplasic tuberosity	Tibia	Increased TT-TG > 20 mm Decreased TT-TG	Tibia

is the angle between the femur shaft and tibia shaft and is usually $5.5° \pm 2°$. Different investigators found no difference between males and females in these angles.[18,44,46]

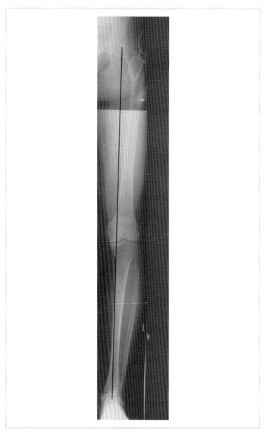

Figure 11.2. Whole limb standing radiograph with mechanical axis added showing varus.

Rotational (Horizontal or Transverse) Plane Alignment

Rotational plane alignment can be determined accurately with the use of axial computed tomography. Common measurements are the torsion of the femur, torsion of the tibia, version or the relationship of the distal femur and proximal tibia, and the relationship between the femur and the tibial tuberosity (TT-TG).

Bone Torsion

Femoral torsion is defined as the angle formed between the axis of the femoral neck and distal femur and is measured in degrees. To assess femoral torsion with CT scan a line from the center point of the femoral head to the center point of the base of the femoral neck is created. This second point is more easily selected by locating the center of the femoral shaft at the level of the base of the neck where the shaft becomes round. Based on the classic tabletop method, the condylar axis is defined as the line between the two most posterior aspects of the femoral condyles. Alternatively a line connecting the epicondyles can be used. Then, the angle formed by the intersection of these two tangents is measured (Figure 11.3).

For assessment of tibial torsion a line is drawn across the center of the tibial plateau. As this line is not easy to locate, some authors use the tangent formed by the posterior cortical margin of the tibial plateau. The femoral epicondylar axis might also be selected as it is easier to locate and would appear to be valid because it is the relationship of the knee joint axis to the ankle joint axis that is of concern. Next a line connecting the center point of the medial malleolus with

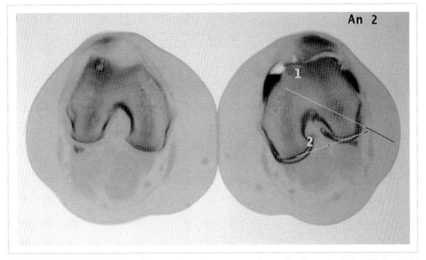

Figure 11.3. CT rotational study shows 43° of femoral anteversion. Line 1 represents the proximal femoral axis; line 2 is the distal femoral axis (tangent to the posterior condyles).

the center point of the lateral malleolus is produced. The angle formed by the intersection of these two lines is measured to determine the tibial torsion (Figure 11.4).

Strecker et al.[39,40] reported the largest series of torsion determinations in normal individuals using CT scan. The authors measured torsion in 505 femurs and 504 tibia and found femoral anteversion of 24.1° ± 17.4° and external tibial torsion of 34.85° ± 17.4°. No correlation to sex could be established. Yoshioka[45] made direct skeletal measurements of femur and tibia and found femoral anteversion to average 13° measuring off the tangent of the distal femoral

condyles and 7° measuring off the epicondylar axis (SD 8°). His values generally agree with those reviewed in the literature that he tabulated. There was no significant difference between males and females. Conversely, lateral tibial torsion averaged 24° with a significant difference between males and females at 21° (SD 5°) versus 27° (SD 11°). Furthermore, even greater differences were noted in the outward foot rotation −5° vs. 11°), which must reflect increases in subtalar position, although this was not mentioned in their paper. These gender differences would explain the higher incidence of patellofemoral disease in females as well as the higher incidence of ACL tears in female athletes. Although this hypothesis is attractive, his findings have not been corroborated by other authors.[35,36]

TT-TG (Tibial Tuberosity–Trochlear Groove)

The relationship of the position of the tibial tuberosity to the trochlear groove will determine the lateralization force acting on the patella through quadriceps contraction. This relationship can be evaluated and quantified by the measurement of the TT-TG. The TT-TG is the distance measured in mm between two perpendiculars to the bicondylar axis.[1] One perpendicular passes through the center of the tibial tuberosity and the other through the center of the trochlear groove. The measurements are taken by superposing two CT scan cuts, one cut

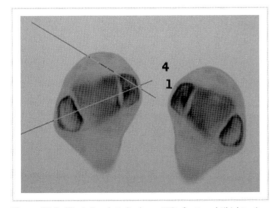

Figure 11.4. CT rotational study shows 55° of external tibial torsion. Line 1 represents the proximal axis (tangent to the posterior femoral condyles); line 4 is the distal axis (line connecting most prominent points of the medial and lateral malleolus).

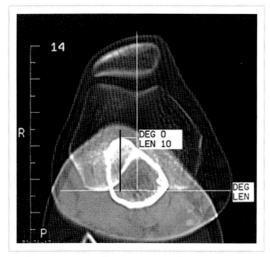

Figure 11.5. CT scan shows measurement of the distance TT-TG.

at the level of the proximal third of the trochlear groove and the other at the superior part of the tibial tuberosity (Figure 11.5). A TT-TG distance of less than 20 mm is considered normal.[14]

Sagittal Plane Alignment

In the sagittal plane the osseous factors to be evaluated include the trochlea, the tibial tuberosity, the patellar height, flexion, and length of the radius of curvature for the trochlea.

Femoral trochlear dysplasia is an abnormality of the shape and depth of the trochlear groove mainly at its cranial part and has been associated with patellar instability and anterior knee pain. Brattström in 1964[2] studied trochlear geometry in recurrent dislocation of the patella and concluded that a shallow femoral groove (i.e., femoral dysplasia) was the most common cause. Trochlear dysplasia can be diagnosed by using a true lateral conventional radiograph of the knee[16,32] (Figure 11.6).

Dejour suggested three criteria to diagnose trochlear dysplasia on the lateral view radiograph: the crossing sign, the trochlear boss or prominence, and the depth of the trochlea. The crossing sign is present when the line representing the floor of the trochlea as it moves proximally crosses the outline of the lateral femoral condyle.[8,9] Dejour's second criterion occurs when the proximal extent of the trochlear floor extends anterior to the anterior femoral cortex. A prominence or boss of greater than 3 mm is considered as a type of trochlear dysplasia.[8,9] This may be a variant of the ridge described by

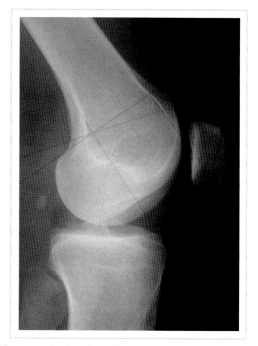

Figure 11.6. True lateral view shows trochlear dysplasia. The trochlear line crosses the contour of the condyles (crossing sign) and a trochlear boss or prominence is present.

Outerbridge. Dejour's third criterion is the actual distance of the floor of the trochlea below the femoral condyles measured at a point in the proximal trochlea. In controls this measured 7.8 mm while in patients with objective patellar instability it measured 2.3 mm.

The shape of the tibial tuberosity is best seen on the lateral radiograph and a hypoplasic tibial tuberosity may be identified. The prominence of the tibial tuberosity will alter the angle of patellar flexion and consequently change compressive forces and contact areas in a manner not yet quantified but speculated as contributing to chondromalacia and pain.

Rotational Malalignment and Contact Pressures in the Patellofemoral Joint

Fixed rotation of either the femur or tibia has been shown to have a significant influence on the patellofemoral joint contact areas and pressures. Lee et al.[27,28,29] investigated the effects of rotational deformities of the lower extremity on patellofemoral contact pressures in a cadaver model. They simulated various types of rotational deformities of the femur by internally and externally rotated the cadaver knees about the axis representing the distal third of the femur. They found that 30 degrees of both internal and external rotation of the femur in their cadaver knee model created a significantly greater peak contact pressure on the contralateral facet of the patella. External rotational deformities of the femur were associated with greater peak contact forces on the medial facet of the patella, while internal rotational deformities were associated with higher peak contact pressures on the lateral facet of the patella.

A study performed in our institution by Kijowski et al.[25] on specimens including the femoral head and foot confirmed Lee's observations (Figure 11.7). When the distal femur was internally rotated about an osteotomy which increased femoral anteversion there was increased contact pressure on the lateral aspect of the patellofemoral joint and decreased contact pressure on the medial aspect of the joint. When femoral torsion was decreased by external rotation osteotomy, there was increased contact pressure on the medial side and decreased contact pressure on the lateral side of the patellofemoral joint.

Rotational Malalignment and Medial Patellofemoral Ligament Strain

Our study also found that internal rotation osteotomy of the femur of 30° results in a significant increase in the strain in all areas of the medial patellofemoral ligament (Figure 11.8).

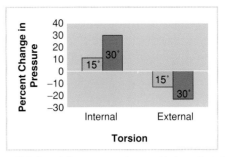

Figure 11.7. Lateral facet pressure change with femoral rotational osteotomy.

The results of this study show that variations in femoral torsion (anteversion-retroversion) caused alterations in the patterns of force transmission across the patellofemoral joint and in the strain present in the medial patellofemoral ligament. The increased strain present in the medial patellofemoral ligament during quadriceps activity in individuals with an internally rotated femur may first result in pain over the medial aspect of the knee joint. The medial patellofemoral ligament may fail as a result of this increase in strain, leading to instability of the patellofemoral joint.

Hefzy et al.[17] used a cadaveric model to study the effects of tibial rotation on the patellofemoral contact pressures and areas. The authors found that internal tibial rotation increases medial patellofemoral contact areas while external tibial rotation increases lateral patellofemoral contact areas at all flexion angles. Lee et al.[28,29] corroborated their findings and they

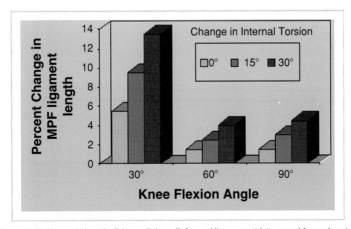

Figure 11.8. Change in length of the medial patellofemoral ligament with increased femoral torsion.

also determined the strain in the peripatellar retinaculum at different tibial rotations. They showed that with increased knee flexion, once the patella is engaged in the trochlea the function of the peripatellar retinaculum is minimal and less affected by tibial rotation.

Effect of Rotational Malalignment on Patellofemoral Joint Position in Space

Maximum gait efficiency with minimal stress is affected by normal limb alignment. Any deviation from normal limb alignment in any plane may also give the same conditions as twisting of the knee. These include femoral anteversion or retroversion, excess internal or external tibial torsion, genu valgum or varus, hyperpronation, Achilles contracture, and so on.

Twisting of the knee away from the limb mechanical axis (inward or outward) will change the direction and magnitude of the patellofemoral compression force and will also add a side-directed vector to the patella. This side-directed vector is resisted by the soft tissue (both the medial and the lateral patellofemoral ligaments) and by the depth and shape of the trochlea. With a more dysplastic trochlea the ligament stress is increased and with a more normal trochlea the trochlear stress is increased.

The foot progression angle (FPA) is generally defined as the angle between the long axis of the foot and the direction of body progression and varies from 10° to 20°.[31] It has been shown that despite congenital or acquired (after fracture) torsional deformities in the lower limb bones, the FPA remains similar.[21,37,42] It is hypothesized that the hip musculature plays a role in accommodating these deformities during gait. For example, in the presence of an internal femoral or external tibial rotational deformity with a normal FPA, the knee joint axis rotates inward and a side force vector is produced, acting on the patella so that both the strain on the medial patellofemoral ligament and the compression on the lateral facet are increased. The opposite situation is present with opposite deformities (see Figures 11.9 to 11.12).

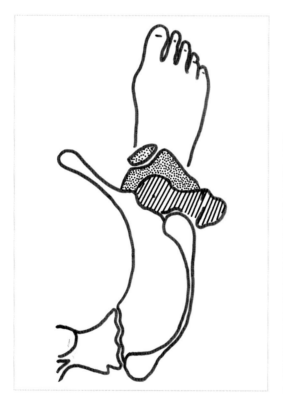

Figure 11.9. Drawing shows 20° excess femoral anteversion. With the foot forward, the knee joint points inward.

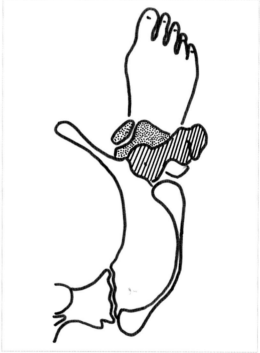

Figure 11.10. Drawing shows 20° excess tibial external torsion. With the foot forward the knee joint points inward, but the hip is also excessively internally rotated.

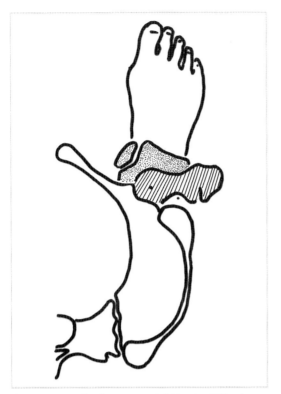

Figure 11.11. Combined excess external tibial torsion (20°) and excess femoral anteversion (20°) with the foot forward. The inward pointing of the knee is the sum of the increase in femoral anteversion plus the excess of external tibial torsion. The hip in this position gains abduction leverage.

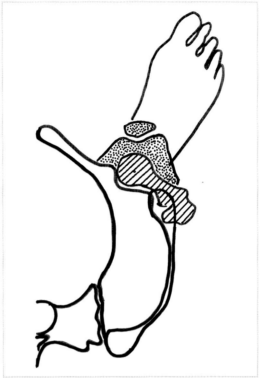

Figure 11.12. Combined 20° excess external tibial torsion and 20° excess femoral anteversion. With the knee joint pointing forward the foot points outward and the hip is in a position of abductor weakness.

Treatment

Treatments are best based on an accurate diagnosis and analysis of the above predisposing factors (Table 11.3). However, we remain limited by the inability to quantify all of the contributing factors. In the history of the treatment of the anterior knee pain, efforts have been made to try to correlate one predisposing factor or one cause as responsible for the pathogenesis of the anterior knee pain. Likewise different authors have proposed different operations to treat patellofemoral pain in a standardized fashion. This approach has led to a high incidence of failure in patellofemoral surgery and a bad reputation.

Abnormal patellofemoral joint mechanics can be the result of many different abnormalities of the alignment. Limb geometry, length, body weight, and muscle forces combine to generate the forces that are to be transmitted through the joint. In the analysis of the pathogenesis it is important to establish a cause and effect. If a primary abnormality is identified, the treatment should be directed to correcting this abnormality. Any soft tissue or intra-articular procedure is destined to failure if this causality has not been determined. In the vast majority of cases a combination of predisposing factors exists. James[22] in 1978 described a "miserable malalignment syndrome," a combination of femoral anteversion, squinting patellae, genu varum, patella alta, increased Q-angle, external tibial rotation, tibia varum, and compensatory feet pronation. A single common surgical procedure such as lateral release or tibial tubercle transfer is not likely to cure anterior knee pain in this setting. It is essential to try and detect all of the bony and soft tissue factors that exist, but when multiple contributors are present the relative contribution of each is not yet quantifiable. In a case with only one variable believed to be responsible for the pathogenesis, that

Table 11.3. Correction of skeletal malalignment associated with patellofemoral pathology

Deformity	Procedure
	Frontal Plane
Genu valgum	Femoral osteotomy (supracondylar)
Genu varum	Tibial osteotomy (infratuberosity)
	Sagittal Plane
Prominent trochlea	Trochleoplasty
Shallow trochlea	Lateral condyle osteotomy
Patella alta	Distal tubercle transfer
Aplasic tuberosity	Maquet osteotomy (maintain normal Q-angle)
	Horizontal Plane
Increased femoral anteversion (>25°)	Proximal femoral external rotation osteotomy (intertrochanteric)
Tibial external torsion (>40°)	Proximal tibial internal rotation (infratuberosity)
Increased AG-TG(>20 mm)	Tibial tubercle medialization
Decreased TT-TG	Lateral tibial tubercle transfer
	Combined Deformities
Valgus + femoral anteversion	Distal femoral varus external rotation osteotomy
Varus + femoral anteversion	Distal femoral valgus external rotation osteotomy
Tibial torsion + increased TT-TG	Proximal tibial osteotomy (supratuberosity)
Femoral anteversion + tibial torsion ("miserable malalignment")	Proximal femoral external rotation osteotomy + proximal tibial internal rotation osteotomy

variable when possible is corrected. For the cases with multiple abnormalities (i.e., femoral anteversion, tibial torsion, genu valgum, and patellar subluxation), our approach is either to correct the deformity that is most abnormal or to correct the factor that we believe contributes most to the symptoms. Multiplane osteotomy is useful when bone geometry is abnormal.

It is important to recognize that with a mechanical overload the most prudent treatment should be a reduction of loading conditions by activity restriction or modification, weight loss, and flexibility and strength training. It might seem too aggressive in some cases to perform a femoral or tibial osteotomy to treat anterior knee pain; however, it has to be understood that the patellofemoral pain is often the expression of a complex problem of skeletal geometry. We have seen patients that experienced not only an improvement of the pain after a corrective femoral osteotomy, but also improvement in the gait pattern, disappearance of compensatory foot pronation and bunions, disappearance of muscle tightness in the thigh and calf, and even improvement in the posture and lumbar pain (Figure 11.13).

It has not been uncommon that the asymptomatic knee becomes symptomatic by comparison to the improved side after correction of deformity. Some patients come to us after five or six unsuccessful procedures around the patella;

these patients presenting with severe instability and chondropathy often have an underlying skeletal malalignment that has gone unrecognized. In such cases it is clear to us that a successful corrective osteotomy performed earlier in the evolution of the disease would not have been too aggressive. In some cases with deformities in two bones, we opt to operate on the more altered bone first and wait for the evolution instead of correcting both bones in the same procedure. It is not unusual that the patient experiences some improvement after recovering from the first operation and asks for the second bone to be corrected or alternatively considers the improvement sufficient to defer other procedures. As Brattström[2] stated in 1964, "Osteotomy is a big operation."

Level of the Osteotomy

With excessive external torsion of the tibia and the foot moving in the line of a normal foot progression angle, the patella is pulled laterally in the trochlear groove, thus increasing the displacement or subluxation force and the lateral articular compression force, while internal torsion of the tibia moves the patella medially within the femoral sulcus. If the TT-TG angle is normal the derotational osteotomy should be performed below the tibial tubercle (Figure 11.14).

An osteotomy above the tibial tubercle will change this normal relationship, leading to a

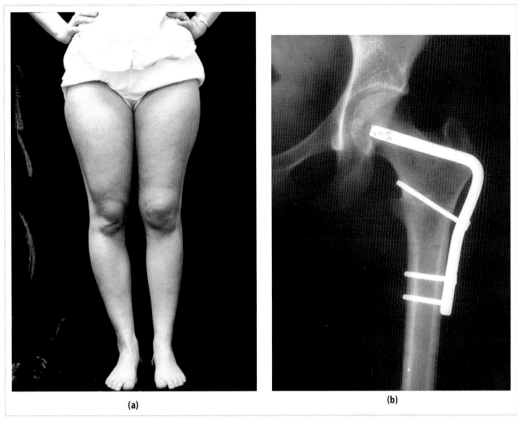

Figure 11.13. (a) Picture shows a patient with excess femoral anteversion. On the left side a proximal intertrochanteric femoral derotational osteotomy was performed; the right lower extremity had no surgery. Observe the difference between right and left in the alignment of the extremity. On the right the patella points inward, the calf muscles are more prominent given a pseudovarus appearance, and the foot is more pronated. **(b)** Postoperative x-rays after proximal femur derotational osteotomy.

reduction in the normal lateral vector with subsequent overload of the medial compartment and the addition of an external rotation vector to the tibial femoral joint. Kelman[24] found that a medial transfer of the tibial tubercle in a knee with normal TT-TG did not pull the patella medially as much as it may pull the tibia into external rotation.

On the femoral side the goal is to create a normal skeletal geometry. With an excessive increase in femoral anteversion we prefer to perform rotational osteotomy at the intertrochanteric femur to reduce the sudden change in direction the quadriceps muscle must make when the osteotomy is located supratrochlear. If two planes need to be corrected, the restoration of a normal tibiofemoral angle usually requires that osteotomy be performed at the distal femur (Figures 11.15). We have noted any difference in patients undergoing rotation osteotomy at the proximal, mid-, or distal femur.

Clinical Experience

Cooke et al.[5] operated on 9 knees in seven patients with inwardly pointing knees and patellofemoral complaints. The authors found this group of patients to have a combined abnormal varus and external torsion of the tibia. The operation performed was derotation valgus Maquet osteotomy with associated lateral release. After a three-year follow-up period the outcome assessments were excellent for all the cases.

Meister and James[33] reported on 8 knees in 7 patients with severe rotational malalignment of the lower extremities associated with debilitating anterior knee pain. The rotational deformity consisted of mild femoral anteversion, severe external tibial torsion, and mild tibia vara and pes planovalgus. Internal rotation tibial osteotomy was performed proximal to the tibial tubercle with an average correction of 19.7°. At 10 years average follow-up all but one patient obtained a

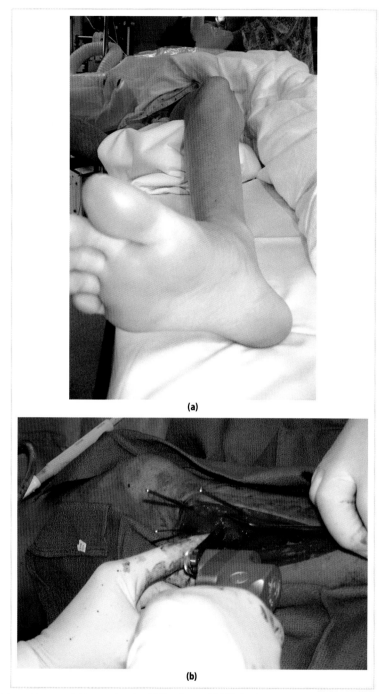

Figure 11.14. (a) Patient with excess tibial external torsion (55°) and normal TT-TG; the foot points outward and the patella points to the front. **(b)** A proximal tibial internal rotation osteotomy is performed below the tibial tubercle.

subjective good or excellent result while functionally all of them had a good or excellent result.

Server et al.[38] performed 35 tibial rotational osteotomies in 25 patients with patellofemoral subluxation secondary to lateral tibial torsion. At 4.3 years follow-up the results were good or excellent in 88.5% of the patients and all the patients but two were satisfied with the procedure.

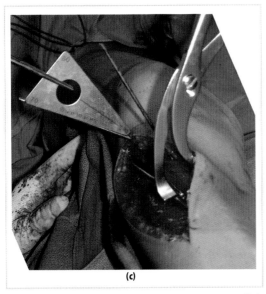

(c)

Figure 11.14. (continued) (c) K-wires show a 30° correction. A blade plate is used for fixation.

Delgado et al.[10] treated operatively 9 patients with 13 affected extremities with patellofemoral pathology related to torsional malalignment. The procedures performed were femoral external rotation osteotomy, tibial internal rotation osteotomy, or both. No additional soft tissue procedure that would alter patellar tracking was carried out. At 2.6 years average follow-up all the patients had an improvement in gait pattern and extremity appearance, and a marked decrease in knee pain.

In a recent publication Bruce and Stevens[3] reviewed the results of correction of miserable malalignment syndrome in 14 patients with 27 limbs. The patients presented significant patellofemoral pain in association with increased femoral anteversion and tibia external rotation. Ipsilateral femoral external rotational osteotomy and tibia internal rotation osteotomy were performed in all the cases. At an average 5.2 years

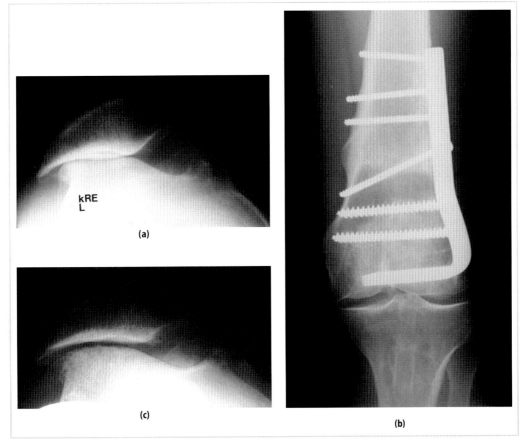

(a)

(c)

(b)

Figure 11.15. (a) Preoperative axial view of a 28-year-old female with history of pain and instability shows collapse of the lateral patellofemoral joint. The patient had valgus and increased femoral anteversion (43°) **(b)** AP postoperative x-rays after distal femoral varus and external rotation osteotomy. **(c)** Axial view taken 5 years postoperative shows widening of the lateral patellofemoral space.

follow-up, all of the patients reported full satisfaction with their surgery and outcomes.

Our Experience

We have recently evaluated the clinical results of 54 intertrochanteric femoral derotational osteotomies in 41 patients performed in our institution from 1998 to 2001. The average time of onset of patellofemoral symptoms was 6.2 years. All the patients were females with an average age of 28 years (14–54). Osteotomies were indicated to correct increased femoral anteversion that was identified as the primary anatomic abnormality. CT rotational studies were available for all the patients and the average preoperative anteversion was 34.9° (18–54°). Patients were evaluated by means of Lysholm scale and Tegner activity level, and were asked if they would have the procedure again. At 7.8 years (3–16) follow-up, 87% of the patients obtained a good or excellent result. All the patients but two would have surgery again.

Conclusions

- Bony architecture dictates where the force vectors acting on the patella will be directed.
- Abnormal skeletal alignment may increase the displacement forces acting on both the ligaments and articular surface of the patella, causing either ligament failure with subsequent instability or cartilage overload with subsequent arthrosis.
- Treatment depends on what is the primary pathology; with large displacement force the best treatment might be osteotomy of long bones.
- Procedures intended to repair soft tissues often fail if the forces directed by the skeletal malalignment are unrecognized or not addressed.
- Osteotomy for patellofemoral arthrosis may be as logical as HTO for varus gonarthrosis.

References

1. Bernageau, J, and D Goutallier. La mesure de la distance TA-GT. In Le scanner ostéo-articulation. *Le genou.* Paris: Vigot, 1991, pp. 132–144.
2. Brattström, H. Shape of the intercondylar groove normally and in recurrent dislocation of patella: A clinical and x-ray anatomical investigation. *Acta Orthop Scan Supplementum* 1964; 68.
3. Bruce, WD, and PM Stevens. Surgical correction of miserable malalignment syndrome. *J Pediatr Orthop* 2004; 24: 392–396.
4. Cahue, S, D Dunlop, K Hayes, J Song, L Torres, and L Sharma. Varus-valgus alignment in the progression of patellofemoral osteoarthritis. *Arthritis Rheum* 2004; 50: 2184–2190.
5. Cooke, TD, N Price, B Fisher, and D Hedden. The inwardly pointing knee: An unrecognized problem of external rotational malalignment. *Clin Orthop* 1990; 260: 56–60.
6. Cooke, TD, J Li, and RA Scudamore. Radiographic assessment of bony contributions to knee deformity. *Ortho Clin. North Am* 1994; 25: 387–393.
7. Chao, EY, EV Neluheni, RW Hsu, and D Paley. Biomechanics of malalignment. *Ortho Clin North Am* 1994; 25: 379–386.
8. Dejour, H, G Walch, P Neyret, and P Adeleine. La dysplasie de la trochlee femorale. *Rev Chir Orthop Reparatrice Appar Mot* 1990; 76: 45–54.
9. Dejour, H, G Walch, L Nove-Josserand, and C Guier. Factors of patellar instability: An anatomic radiographic study. *Knee Surg Sports Traumatol Arthrosc* 1994; 2:19–26.
10. Delgado, ED, PL Schoenecker, MM Rich, and AM Capelli. Treatment of severe torsional malalignment syndrome. *J Pediatr Orthop* 1996; 16: 484–488.
11. Eckhoff, DG, AW Brown, RF Kilcoyne, and ER Stamm. Knee version associated with anterior knee pain. *Clin Orthop* 1997; 339: 152–155.
12. Elahi, S, S Cahue, DT Felson, L Engelman, and L Sharma. The association between varus-valgus alignment and patellofemoral osteoarthritis. *Arthritis Rheum* 2000; 43: 1874–1880.
13. Fujikawa, K, BB Seedhom, and V Wright. Biomechanics of the patello-femoral joint: Part II. A study of the effect of simulated femoro-tibial varus deformity on the congruity of the patello-femoral compartment and movement of the patella. *Engineering in Medicine* 1983; 12: 13–21.
14. Goutallier, D, J Bernageau, and B Lecudonnec. Mesure de l'écart tubérosité tibiale antérieure-gorge de la trochlée (TA-GT). *Rev Chir Orthop*, 1978; 64: 423–428.
15. Greene, CG, TB Edwards, MR Wade, and EW Carson. Reliability of the quadriceps angle measurement. *Am J Knee Surg* 2001; 14: 97–103.
16. Grelsamer, RP, and JL Tedder. The lateral trochlear sign: Femoral trochlear dysplasia as seen on a lateral view roentgenograph. *Clin Orthop* 1992; 281: 159–162.
17. Hefzy, MS, WT Jackson, SR Saddemi, and YF Hsieh. Effects of tibial rotations on patellar tracking and patellofemoral contact areas. *J Biomed Eng* 1992; 14: 329–343.
18. Hsu, RW, S Himeno, MB Coventry, and EY Chao. Normal axial alignment of the lower extremity and load-bearing distribution at the knee. *Clin Ortho* 1990; 255: 215–227.
19. Hvid, I, LI Andersen, and H Schmidt. Chondromalacia patellae: The relation to abnormal patellofemoral joint mechanics. *Acta Orthop Scand* 1981; 52: 661–666.
20. Insall, J, KA Falvo, and DW Wise. Chondromalacia patellae: A prospective study. *J Bone Joint Surg Am* 1976; 58-A: 1–8.
21. Jaarsma, RL, BF Ongkiehong, C Gruneberg, N Verdonschot, J Duysens, and A van Kampen. Compensation for rotational malalignment after intramedullary nailing for femoral shaft fractures: An analysis by plantar pressure measurements during gait. *Injury* 2004; 35: 1270–1278.
22. James, S, BT Bates, and LR Ostering. Injuries to runners. *Am J Sports Med* 1978; 6: 40–50.

23. Janssen, G. Increased medial torsion of the knee joint producing chondromalacia patella. In Trickey, E, and P Hertel, eds., *Surgery and Arthroscopy of the Knee*, 2nd Congress. Berlin: Springer-Verlag, 1986, pp. 263–267.

24. Kelman, GJ, L Focht, JD Krakauer et al. A cadaveric study of patellofemoral kinematics using a biomechanical testing ring and gait laboratory motion analysis. *Orthop Trans* 1989; 13: 248–249.

25. Kijowski, R, D Plagens, SJ Shaeh, and RT Teitge. The effects of rotational deformities of the femur on contact pressure and contact area in the patellofemoral joint and on strain in the medial patellofemoral ligament. Presented at the annual meeting International Patellofemoral Study Group, Napa Valley, San Francisco, September 1999.

26. Lauren, CA, R Dussault, and HP Levesque. The tangential x-ray investigation of the patellofemoral joint: X-ray technique, diagnostic criteria and their interpretation. *Clin Orthop* 1979; 144: 16–26.

27. Lee, TQ, SH Anzel, KA Bennett, D Pang, and WC Kim. The influence of fixed rotational deformities of the femur on the patellofemoral contact pressures in human cadaver knees. *Clin Orthop* 1994; 302: 69–74.

28. Lee, TQ, BY Yang, MD Sandusky, and PJ McMahon. The effects of tibial rotation on the patellofemoral joint: Assessment of the changes in in-situ strain in the peripatellar retinaculum and the patellofemoral contact pressures and areas. *J Rehabil Res Dev* 2001; 38: 463–469.

29. Lee, TQ, G Morris, and RP Csintalan. The influence of tibial and femoral rotation on patellofemoral contact area and pressure. *J Orthop Sports Phys Ther* 2003; 33: 686–693.

30. Lerat, JL, B Moyen et al. Morphological types of the lower limbs in femoro-patellar disequilibrium: Analysis in 3 planes. *Acta Orthop Belg* 1989; 55: 347–355.

31. Lösel, S, MJ Burgess-Milliron, LJ Micheli, and CJ Edington. A simplified technique for determining foot progression angle in children 4 to 16 years of age. *J Pediatr Orthop* 1996; 16: 570–574.

32. Malghem, J, and B Maldague. Depth insufficiency of the proximal trochlear groove on lateral radiographs of the knee: Relation to patellar dislocation. *Radiology* 1989; 170: 507–510.

33. Meister, K, and SL James. Proximal tibial derotation osteotomy for anterior knee pain in the miserably malaligned extremity. *Am J Orthop* 1995; 24: 149–155.

34. Moreland, JR, LW Bassett, and GJ Hanker. Radiographic analysis of the axial alignment of the lower extremity. *J Bone Joint Surg* 1987; 69-A: 745–749.

35. Reikeras, O, and A Hoiseth. Torsion of the leg determined by computed tomography. *Acta Orthop Scand* 1989; June, 60(3): 330–333.

36. Sayli, U, S Bolukbasi, OS Atik, and S Gundogdu. Determination of tibial torsion by computed tomography. *J Foot Ankle Surg* 1994; Mar.–Apr., 33(2): 144–147.

37. Seber, S, B Hazer, N Kose, E Gokturk, I Gunal, and A Turgut. Rotational profile of the lower extremity and foot progression angle: Computerized tomographic examination of 50 male adults. *Arch Orthop Trauma Surg* 2000; 120: 255–258.

38. Server, F, RC Miralles, E Garcia, and JM Soler. Medial rotational tibial osteotomy for patellar instability secondary to lateral tibial torsion. *Int Orthop* 1996; 20: 153–158.

39. Strecker, W, M Franzreb, T Pfeiffer, S Pokar, M Wikstrom, and L Kinzl. Computerized tomography measurement of torsion angle of the lower extremities. *Unfallchirug* 1994; 97: 609.

40. Strecker, W, P Keppler, F Gebhard, and L Kinzl. Length and torsion of the lower limb. *J Bone Joint Surg* 1997; 79-B: 1019–1023.

41. Takai, S, K Sakakida, F Yamashita, F Suzu, and F Izuta. Rotational alignment of the lower limb in osteoarthritis of the knee. *Int Orthop* 1985; 9: 209–215.

42. Tornetta, P, G Ritz, and A Kantor. Femoral torsion after interlocked nailing of unstable femoral fractures. *J Trauma* 1995; 38: 213–219.

43. Turner, MS. The association between tibial torsion and knee joint pathology. *Clin Orthop* 1994; 302: 47–51.

44. Yoshioka, Y, D Siu, and TDV Cooke. The anatomy and functional axes of the femur. *J Bone Joint Surg* 1987; 69-A: 873–880.

45. Yoshioka, Y, and TDV Cooke. Femoral anteversion: Assessment based on function axes. *J Orthop Res* 1987; 5: 86–91.

46. Yoshioka, Y, DW Siu, RA Scudamore, and TDV Cooke. Tibial anatomy and functional axes. *J Ortho Res* 1989; 7: 132–137.

12

Treatment of Symptomatic Deep Cartilage Defects of the Patella and Trochlea with and without Patellofemoral Malalignment: Basic Science and Treatment

László Hangody and Ivan Udvarhelyi

Abstract

Efficacious treatment of chondral and osteo-chondral defects of the patellofemoral surfaces represents an ongoing challenge for the orthopedic surgeon. Treatment options for such full-thickness cartilage defects are discussed in this chapter. Combination of different cartilage repair techniques and appropriate treatment of the underlying biomechanical factors should represent the adequate treatment strategy for these problematic lesions. "Traditional" resurfacing techniques have not stood well to time, based in large part on the poor biomechanical characteristics of the fibrocartilage reparative tissue. During the last decade, efforts have focused on ways to furnish a hyaline or hyaline-like gliding surface for full-thickness lesions. These burgeoning new methodologies embrace several surgical procedures: autologous osteochondral transplantation methods (including osteochondral mosaicplasty); chondrocyte implantation; periosteal and perichondrial resurfacement; allograft transplantation; and also tissue engineering. Experimental background, operative techniques, and clinical results of these new procedures are detailed in this overview.

The early and medium-term experiences with these techniques have provoked a cautious optimism among basic researchers and clinicians alike. Autologous osteochondral mosaicplasty can be an alternative in the treatment of small and medium-sized full-thickness lesions, not only the femorotibial surfaces but also in the patellofemoral junction. The major attractions of the mosaicplasty are the ease of the one-step procedure, relatively brief rehabilitation period, excellent clinical outcome, and low cost. Autologous chondrocyte transplantation represents a promising option in the treatment of larger full-thickness defects. It does require a relatively expensive two-step procedure and longer rehabilitation period, but it seems to be an appropriate treatment of larger defects as well. Similar to other techniques, patellotrochlear use of the chondrocyte transplantation results in less favorable clinical outcome compared with femoral condylar application.

Present recommendations for the transplantation of mushroom-shaped osteochondral allografts are elected cases of advanced degenerative lesions of the patellar surface. The possible indications for perichondrial flapping, biomaterials, and transplantation of engineered tissues have to be cleared.

Full-thickness cartilage damage of the patellotrochlear junction can involve associated problems, not infrequently traumatic or biomechanical in origin. Congenital shape anomalies of the patellotrochlear surfaces, traction malalignment problems, patellofemoral hyperpression, as well as posttraumatic disorders represent the most common background of symptomatic deep cartilage lesions of the patellofemoral junction. Recognition and treatment of these abnormalities are essential to ensure a favorable and enduring outcome. Effective treatment of full-thickness defects on the patellotrochlear surfaces requires careful patient selection, a comprehensive operative plan, and a well-organized treatment course.

Introduction

As regards cartilage lesions, the patellotrochlear junction represents one of the main problematic areas of the knee joint. This articulation serves often as a beginning point of further degenerative processes. Mild or medium-grade damage of the patellar or trochlear chondral surfaces can be initiative factors in early osteoarthritis. Effective treatment of deep cartilage damage of this compartment has an essential role in the prevention of a certain part of osteoarthritic problems.

More effective treatment of full-thickness cartilage defects of the weight-bearing surfaces became one of the most important questions of the orthopedic research in the last two decades. Considerable advances of the basic science as well as the increasing amount of clinical experiences have already made it clear that cartilage damage of the patellofemoral articulation has less favorable chances for promising clinical outcome than other joint surfaces. Presence of these disadvantageous aspects of the patellotrochlear junction requires a sensitive diagnostical approach, very well-planned treatment strategy, and a demanding rehabilitation.

Anatomy and Pathophysiology of the Articular Cartilage

Articular cartilage represents a well-organized complex structure that provides an excellent conduit for pain-free motion in the joint and tolerance of a wide range of cyclical stresses on its gliding surfaces.[124,128] The articular hyaline cartilage with its remarkable ultrastructure and durability is the only tissue that can serve these high requirements. Living cells of this tissue are embedded within a highly organized extracellular matrix composed of macromolecules. This complex arrangement contains mainly different types of proteoglycans, collagens and other proteins in combination with water and electrolytes.[24,124,127,132] Cells and matrix together bind about 60–80% water. This relatively high amount of water contributes to nutrition of the chondrocytes and also participates in joint lubrication. The dynamic alliance of cells, matrix, and water plays a major role in the unique mechanical properties of the hyaline cartilage.[25,124,128,132]

The solid phase of the cartilage constitutes a three-dimensional framework of collagen network noncovalently bound with the negatively charged aggrecans through which water and electrolytes flow at controlled rates. Proteoglycan monomers and aggregates consisting of a central protein core and several bounded sulfated glycoseaminoglycans are electronically active chains. Their negative charges bind cations and water, and on the other hand the glycoseaminoglycan side chains repel each other. This interactive feature keeps the molecules in a distended state. Proteoglycans tend to absorb a very high amount of water. In the normal articular hyaline cartilage they are only partially hydrated because of the "compressive effect" of the collagen framework.[25,124,128,132] Any damage on the collagen structure can cause swelling of the matrix as the proteoglycans absorb more water, resulting in an expansion of the matrix. Consequent to this process, the cartilage will loose its elasticity and became softer.[25,124,128,132]

As mentioned, collagen structure contributes a "compressive effect" on the partially hydrated glycoseaminoglycan chains. The three-dimensional structure of collagen network in the hyaline cartilage consists of 90–95% type II collagen.[25,127,132] Other collagen types – mainly I, IX, and X – are frequent in other connective or supportive tissues, such as meniscus, annulus fibrosus, tendon, and bone, but high content of type II collagen is unique to hyaline cartilage. This highly organized collagen network confers high biomechanical value for the hyaline cartilage particularly during compressive and shear stress. Loading forces on the gliding surfaces result in a relatively quick outflow from the compressed area, but when the load is removed the elastic structure will regain its original shape and interstitial fluid can flow back to its original place. This process is limited by the low permeability of the hyaline cartilage and therefore the solid phase – in case of "normal loading" – is protected from permanent deformation. Not only does this biphasic nature promote tolerance of intensive cyclic stresses, but it ensures constant movement of the fluid for the nutrition of cartilage and metabolic activities of the chondrocytes.[25,124,128,132]

Chondrocytes are the cellular elements of this highly organized tissue. They produce the extracellular matrix and later maintain the homeostasis of the entire structure. Their synthetic function is altered by chemical and mechanical changes of the matrix. Prior to skeletal maturation, chondrocytes show high activity – they proliferate and actively synthesize extracellular matrix. Upon completion of growth, cellular activity becomes lower and dividing ability and matrix-producing capability will lessen.[24,29,103]

Articular cartilage serves our joints well and can remain virtually intact over the span of human life. Columnar organization of this wonderful structure can tolerate various types of mechanical loading including shear forces. Yet when it deteriorates or is injured, which unfortunately occurs with significant regularity, great challenges unfold for its substitution. From our present understanding the only reliable treatment options are to imitate the structure or produce the same tissue.

While hyaline cartilage has a wide tolerance among physiological circumstances, it has only moderate capability for healing.[76,91,104,105,161] As is clear from anatomical and physiological aspects, chondrocytes are key elements in the responses of the cartilage tissue. These cells control the components of the matrix and are responsible for the homeostasis and turnover of the whole tissue. It is well known that in adults, chondrocytes have a limited capacity to reproduce themselves and this feature seems to be essential in their behavior in repairing actual damage or injury of the gliding surfaces. Another disadvantage in cartilage healing is the location of the chondrocytes. In mature tissues chondrocytes are embedded in their matrix and this situation provides only limited and paced contact with the circulatory system.[25,88,105,132]

Important components for a good healing response would be the availability of a full array of circulatory resources, multipotential cells, important cellular factors (cytotactic, chemotactic, and mitogenic factors; growth factors), and other bioactive molecules. These components are necessary for an effective repair process. As hyaline cartilage itself is a bradytroph structure, such vascular components can originate only from a neighboring tissue, in this case from the underlying bone.[103,132,161]

Further disadvantages of cartilage's response in healing are the matrix inhibitory factors. Articular cartilage matrix contains inhibitor factors that can decrease invasion of cellular elements and clot formation. Experimental studies

eliminating the effect of such inhibitors demonstrated a better repair capability of superficial cartilage injuries.[124,132,162]

In another regard, several authors have noted that partial-thickness injuries have poor healing capability. Chondrocytes next to the injury demonstrate only a very brief mitotic and matrix synthetic activity without effective repair ability. This limited proliferation is represented as some cluster formation at the margin of the injured area, but no real repair mechanism can develop. In spite of their poor healing activity, according to clinical experiences, these superficial injuries have only a low tendency to progress.[1,25,26,40,50,55]

A few experimental studies have reported complete healing of small-sized deep cartilage defects. Cartilage flow observed in these trials can fill only very small defects. Lesions larger than 2 to 3 mm in diameter will not heal in such a manner, suggesting that they must heal by different mechanisms.[35,55,124]

Numerous authors described the repair response of the articular cartilage in the case of a full-thickness defect.[24,25,28,35,51,89,106,115] The first period involves bleeding due to the injury, which penetrates through the subchondral plate or – in degenerative cases – from small, superficial fissures of the same cortical layer. This bleeding results in clot formation from which bioactive molecules (cytokines, chemotactic factors, etc.) induce further vascular invasion and migration of pluripotential mesenchymal stem cells. These cells have the capability to reproduce themselves and can differentiate in various directions.[25,28,90,132]

In the second phase, inflammatory reactions are predominant. Exudative and transudative products result in a formation of a fibrinous network, which will serve as a base for the next remodeling period. Vascular granulating tissue will develop from the former fibrinous network. Deeper layers of this cellular mass are involved in bone formation to reconstruct the subchondral bony plate, while superficial parts of the same tissue will produce cartilage.[24,25,51,91,132] It is worth mentioning that other studies investigating the behavior of the multipotential cambium cells of perichondrial and periosteal flaps have demonstrated very similar processes. High oxygen tension promotes bone formation while poor oxygenation favors cartilage production.[38,82,93,148]

Through metaplasia of the repair tissue, hyaline-like tissue can be produced. Notwithstanding this replication, several features of the newly formed tissue are different from the articular cartilage. In addition to a certain amount of type II collagen, a relatively high content of type I can be found. Furthermore, proteoglycan content is not as high when compared to healthy hyaline cartilage, and decreases with time. One of the most important differences is the poorly organized collagen structure. Missing superficial collagen layer and low proteoglycan content seem to be the main causes of the limited biomechanical value of the repair tissue. The important differences appear to be inferior organization of the collagen network, absent superficial collagen layer, and time-dependent low concentrations of proteoglycans.[24,28,35,51,91,105,115,116]

Notably, integration of the repair tissue with the surrounding host cartilage is fragile. Often, microscopic or macroscopic gaps are visible between the two types of cartilage. Occasionally, suggestions of deep matrix integration can be observed but these junctions cannot tolerate the physiological shear forces of normal daily activity. According to Shapiro et al.,[154] Mow et al.,[127] and other authors, in a relatively short period (6 months) the new tissue becomes more typical of fibrocartilage, and early degenerative changes can be observed. Beyond six months, these changes become more pronounced, leading to signs of osteoarthritis.[51,116,127,132,151,154,161]

The tissue produced by such a mechanism has quantitative as well as qualitative inferiority to the preexisting cartilage. In degenerative full-thickness lesions, repetitive microtraumas to the underlying bone result in a sequester layer.[89,90] Spreading of the repair tissue is not possible because this dead bony layer prevents fixation of the repair tissue to the bony base. Thus, instead of contiguous gliding surface, only fibrocartilage islands develop, which do not spread to adjacent defective areas. Mechanical elimination of this layer may promote the healing response.[12,89]

Therapeutical Options for Cartilage Lesions of the Patellofemoral Joint

"From Hippocrates to the present age, it is universally allowed that ulcerated cartilage is a troublesome thing and that once destroyed it is not repaired." Since this declaration of Sir William Hunter (1743), the peculiar response of cartilage to insult has continued to draw the attention of medical researchers and clinicians alike.[76] Intense and productive basic research as

to the nature of cartilage, coupled with clinical application of new surgical techniques over the past decade, suggests that we are at the threshold of a complete understanding of this tissue's pathways to degeneration and repair. Beside bony and soft tissue techniques to reconstruct the correct alignment and congruency, different ways of cartilage repair may promote an effective treatment of patellofemoral cartilage defects. At present, attention is being focused on hyaline or hyaline-like substitution resurfacement for such defective articular surfaces.[124,132]

Combination of an effective treatment of the underlying causes and improved results of different cartilage repair techniques may present a step forward in delaying or preventing the cascading osteoarthritic processes.

Conservative Treatment

Introduction of conservative treatment options (rest, restriction of activity, quadriceps training, NSAIDs, McConnell's rehabilitation program, cryotherapy, chondroprotective drugs, etc.) isn't a goal of this chapter. In spite of recent advances of modern diagnostic techniques (new MRI sequences, ultrasound, CT-arthrography, etc.), exact diagnosis of full-thickness cartilage damage and osteochondral lesions of the patellofemoral joint are usually verified at an actual arthroscopy. Before this diagnosis certain forms and amounts of conservative treatment have already been introduced for a patient suffering with patellofemoral complaints. Perhaps one of the most effective tools to improve mild retropatellar pain is a well-performed physiotherapy educating the patient to better muscle balance. Strengthening of the vastus medialis has a crucial role in this process. Isokinetic exercises can also provide certain improvement. Certain types of physical therapies (cool therapy, electrotherapy, ultrasound, etc.) may provide some improvement in anterior knee pain. Chondroprotective drugs and nonsteroid anti-inflammatory medications and relaxants have less efficacy in this stage.[81,111]

Treatment of the Underlying Causes

Deep cartilage damage of the patellar or trochlear surfaces is usually based on some kind of biomechanical disturbance of the affected junction. Alignment problems of the quadriceps traction, patellofemoral hyperpression, and congruency anomalies of the patellar and trochlear surfaces are the most common problems resulting in chondral or osteochondral damage.[81] Correction of such biomechanical conditions represents one of the tasks to improve the clinical symptoms and support the prognosis of the actual cartilage repair.

Lessening of the Patellofemoral Hyperpression

Too-tight contact between patellar and trochlear surfaces (lateral patellar compression syndrome) is a common factor of mild or severe chondral damage in the patellofemoral joint. Documented patellar tilt is a usual indication for lateral retinacular release. In spite of the fact that an objective measurement of this increased pressure is usually not possible, open or arthroscopic release of the lateral retinaculum is a technique often used to lessen the excessive patellofemoral pressure. As the physiological or increased femorotibial valgus position represents a predisposing factor of this problem, longitudinal incision of the tight lateral retinaculum may promote the lessening of the patellofemoral hyperpression. Incision by normal or diathermic blades also represents a potential, partial denervation of the patella, which can have an advantageous influence on the retropatellar pain.[113,118]

Clinical results of open versus arthroscopic lateral retinacular release are controversial in the literature. There are advantages and disadvantages to both of these techniques. Excessive postoperative bleeding is a potential complication of the lateral release, therefore meticulous hemostasis and intra-articular drainage is recommended. From the first postoperative days the patient is instructed to start range-of-motion exercises actively and passively (the use of CPM may be beneficial), and weight bearing as tolerated. Exercises to restore the quadriceps strength – especially the vastus medialis – have an essential role in the rehabilitation.[109,113,118]

Elevation of the tibial tubercle has been recommended by Maquet and Bandi to reduce patellofemoral contact pressures.[6,107,108] According to the biomechanical rationale of this technique, ventral advancement of the tibial tuberosity would yield a reduction of the patellofemoral compressive forces. Besides good results reported by Bandi and later Maquet, a significant number of complications were also reported by different authors. Heatly et al. and Engebretsen et al. reported less advantageous clinical outcome and, according to their reports,

results deteriorated with increasing follow-up.[42,69] In 1983, Fulkerson also published a technique to correct the patellofemoral conditions by anteromedialization of the tibial tuberosity.[49] In his procedure an oblique osteotomy in a posterior and lateral direction results in a medial and anterior displacement of the tibial tubercle. Morshuis et al. evaluated the Fulkerson technique in an independent center.[126] Repeated follow-up at 12 and 30 months in a series of 25 knees gave decreasing success rate both in the objective and subjective results.

Summarizing, it seems that, in spite of promising early results, elevation of the tibial tuberosity has less successful long-term outcomes and should be used only in carefully selected cases. Lateral retinacular release has fewer complications and can provide some improvement.

Correction of the Malalignment

Patellar subluxation or dislocation as well as malalignment of the quadriceps traction often cause patellotrochlear cartilage damage. As lateral retinacular release is insufficient to treat such problems, more extended soft tissue techniques are usually used to create better traction conditions. Insall's proximal realignment is one of the most popular soft tissue procedures to alter the line of pull of the quadriceps muscle. During this procedure traction realignment is effected by advancing the medial flap containing the vastus medialis laterally and distally. There are also other soft tissue techniques, but distal and combined realignment techniques are more frequently used to correct the traction line. Procedures in which the tibial attachment of the patellar ligament is detached and transferred medially and distally to reduce the Q-angle and correct the height of the patella represent distal or combined realignment techniques. While in the Hughston procedure the tibial tubercle is transplanted medially and distally as a free flap, the Elmslie-Trillat technique preserves a distal osteoperiosteal bridge to promote and earlier bony healing of the tibial tubercle in its new place. Both of these techniques involve a lateral retinacular release and may be combined by tightening of the medial retinacular structures.[75,81,164]

Improvement of the Congruency

From a therapeutic point of view, shape anomalies of the patellar or trochlear surfaces represent one of the most difficult problems of the patellotrochlear junction. Wiberg analyzed the horizontal section of the patella and determined three main types according to morphological appearance.[165] Baumgartl gave a fourth type ("Jaegerhut" shape) to this classification to describe the most frequent shape anomalies.[8] Grelsamer et al. created a different classification, determining three types according to the radiological appearance in the sagittal plane.[58] The morphological analyzation of the femoral trochlea didn't result in similar widely accepted classifications, but a flat or severely asymmetric trochlear groove can also be a pathogenetic factor of cartilage damage.

Osteotomies on the patella and especially on the femoral trochlea are rare and less popular techniques to have a positive influence on the congruency conditions. In a few selected cases we have performed such osteotomies to improve the congruency of the patellar and trochlear surfaces. In spite of the good and satisfactory results, such an aggressive approach should be used only in exceptional cases (Figure 12.1).

Additional Techniques

Spongialization recommended by Ficat represents nowadays only a historical option to treat effectively patellar cartilage damage.[46] Prosthetic

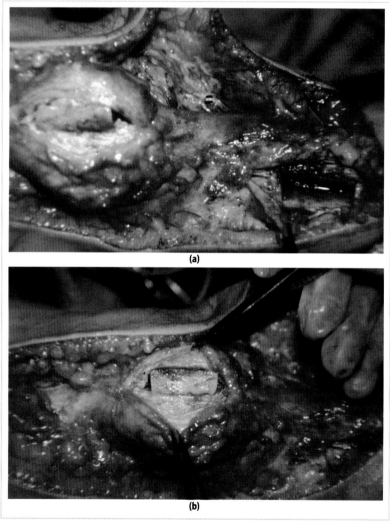

(a)

(b)

Figure 12.1. Sagittal patellar opening wedge osteotomy. **(a)** Graft harvest of a cortical-cancellous bone graft from the upper-medial tibia. **(b)** The graft opens the osteotomy.

resurfacement of the patellofemoral joint described by McKeever and different types of patellectomies also have some clinical experience, but these operations cannot be recommended to treat cartilage damage of the patellotrochlear surfaces.[16,20,114]

Cartilage Repair

Surgical management of full-thickness, focal chondral, or osteochondral defects represents a special problem. In such cases, most of the gliding surfaces are covered by healthy hyaline cartilage and only a limited area has been destroyed. Although some studies have observed that such defects may have limited correlation with clinical symptoms,[1,117,151] most of the publications report further degenerative processes following an initial focal derangement.[24,76,105,157] According to the majority, small-sized cartilage defects can lead to early

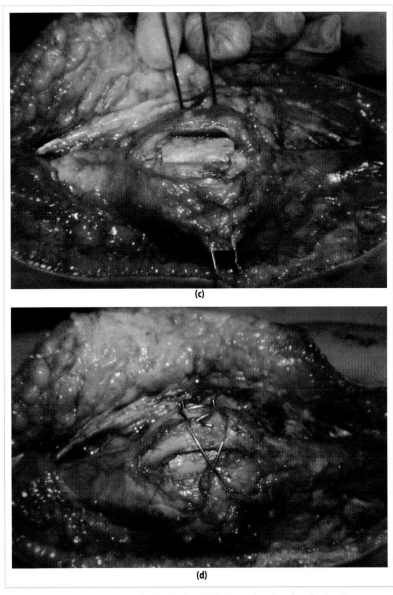

(c)

(d)

Figure 12.1. (c) Situation fixed by K-wires. **(d)** K-wires and cerclage fixes the situation.

(*continued*)

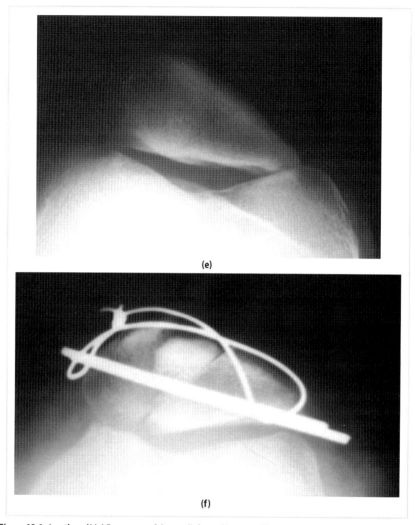

Figure 12.1. *(continued)* **(e)** Preop x-ray of the patellofemoral junction. **(f)** Postop x-ray of the patellofemoral junction.

osteoarthritis. Deterioration of surrounding cartilage surfaces is quicker on the weight-bearing areas; thus chondral resurfacement of these defects in the initial phase of the degenerative process may prevent the extension of the cartilage damage.

There are several treatment options in the surgical armamentarium that aim to serve as long-lasting and successful chondral resurfacement. These operative treatment options can be classified into two main groups: "traditional" and "modern" cartilage repair procedures.

Traditional resurfacing techniques rely on the natural regenerative potential of certain elements of the subchondral bone marrow. Multipotential mesenchymal stem cells can be mobilized from the subcortical cancellous bone cavities toward the articular surface where they can produce repair tissue. This connective tissue can undergo a fibrous metaplasia to cover the defect by fibrous cartilage. Traditional cartilage repair techniques require a sufficient direct connection between the bone marrow cavity of the spongiosa and the articular surface. Because of the limited mechanical characteristics of the reparative fibrous tissue, these techniques have only a limited value. In response to these limitations, several researchers have carried out extended experimental and clinical studies presenting a new trend of resurfacing strategies.

Modern resurfacing techniques try to produce a hyaline or hyaline-like surface in the region of a localized, full-thickness cartilage defect. The main goal is to create a gliding surface appropriate for demands of weight-bearing areas. Such procedures may shield the joint from further degeneration.

Traditional Techniques

The main goal of these techniques is to promote the natural healing process. As this repair results in only fibrocartilage, these treatment options have only a limited value because of the poor biomechanical features of the fibrous tissue.

Debridement

A primary goal in any treatment of cartilage continues to be the prevention of further degenerative processes and abatement of further deleterious effects initiated by the very disruption of the articular surface. Debridement addresses these issues, and may alleviate symptoms even when damage is extensive.[7,12,13,83,100,120,147]

Biochemical changes due to degenerative processes of the gliding surfaces result in an altered biochemical environment, which among other alternations, stimulates inflammatory responses. Mere shaving of the damaged surface does not appear to achieve a positive restorative effect,[91,121] but removal of fragmented cartilage may lessen the reactive synovitis, thus expressing a positive influence on the intra-articular milieu. When originally proposed, surgical cleaning of the joint had been recommended to treat severe osteoarthritic problems.[100] Over time and with accumulated clinical experience, the trend has been shifted to early stage treatment by minimally invasive techniques incorporating lavage as a major component. At the very least, the partial success of arthroscopic debridement and lavage has fostered a renaissance in the effects of minimal intra-articular surgical approaches.[7,13,83,90,147] The procedure, when used in conjunction with correction of underlying biomechanical alterations and attentive physical therapy, represents a viable option when endoprosthetic replacement is contradicted. Patellotrochlear cartilage damage is often the subject of such arthroscopic shaving techniques. Overall objective evaluation of the end results of the procedure remains elusive in large part due to the

variable combination with the aforementioned attendant treatments.[12,26,83,90,120]

Some reports have expressed a limited effect of debridement alone.[90,120,132] On the other hand, relatively good results of debridement have been reported by other authors. Jackson[84] found 68% improved in 1988, Bert[13] 66% in 1989, Baumgartner[7] 52% in 1990, and Rand[147] 67% in 1991. However, in the case of full-thickness focal cartilage defects, most authors believe that we cannot only expect fair results from debridement in the long term. Formal open debridement arthrotomy is now, by and large, reserved for selected rheumatoid cases.

Pridie Drilling

Debridement alone cannot promote a spontaneous fibrocartilage repair in the region of a full-thickness cartilage defect.[88,89,90,120] During the natural healing, small fissures on the bony base of the defect provide a conduit for marrow blood vessels and multipotential cellular elements to engage in the repair process. Theoretically, surgical perforation of the subchondral cortical bony layer should enhance the benefit of debridement by expanding what occurs in the unaided healing response. Penetration of the subchondral cortical plate creates more uniform communication between the subchondral cancellous bone and the joint space, and in this way, increases the potential to mobilize more mesenchymal stem cells from the bone marrow to the joint surface.[31,79,122,146]

One and a half to five mm drill holes are the widely used diameters to provide these direct contacts to promote bloodborne healing. Experimental studies of Mitchell and Shephard[122] demonstrated that initially hyaline-like cartilage is produced, but soon it degrades, and fibrous elements become dominant in the newly formed tissue. Interestingly, in addition to numerous clinicians such as Pridie,[146] Insall,[79] and Johnson,[90] we[60] have observed immediate pain relief after the Pridie decompression. This effect may be the result of the decompression of the subchondral cancellous bone structure and thus decreasing the elevated intraosseous pressure under the defect. Unfortunately, this effect is transient, explainable by the rapid capping of the perforations by scar tissue. Pridie drilling of the trochlear surfaces in certain cases can be performed arthroscopically but patellar drilling usually requires an open approach. Predictable deterioration with time has been the rule as a

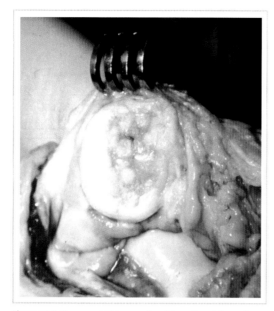

Figure 12.2. Five-year-old intraoperative picture of a patellar surface treated by Pridie drilling.

suitable weight-bearing surface cannot be produced (Figure 12.2). Another disadvantage of the procedure is that the thick and deep holes can weaken the subchondral layer to such an extent that the bone can collapse, producing areas of articular incongruity.[79,120,132,146]

Abrasion Arthroplasty

Maintenance of the original curvature of the gliding surfaces is better assured if the resurfacing technique is less aggressive than the drilling. Johnson[88,89,90] has recommended removing this sequester layer and the creation of small cavities to connect the marrow cavities and joint space. He has developed an arthroscopic burr that can abrade the sequestrated barrier and make small punctual bleeding craters in the subchondral cortical plate. According to him, removal of the superficial sequester layer of the subchondral cortical plate is critical to the success of the resurfacement, as this layer prevents the spreading of the regenerative tissue.

By his account, this technique can produce a hyaline-like cartilage or, at least, a contiguous fibrocartilage layer. In 1986, Johnson[89] reported 77% good results. Unfortunately, others have not substantiated the long-lasting value of the procedure. Friedman[48] reported good results in 60% of the cases in 1984, Bert[13] 51% in 1989, and Rand[147] 50% in 1991. In light of these results,

application of Johnson's abrasion arthroplasty has declined in popularity.

Microfracture

Upon analysis of abrasion arthroplasty, the use of small surface cavities for punctuate bleeding could be improved upon for the deliverance of marrow healing elements to the surface. This consideration led to the development of the microfracture technique.

Steadman et al.[159,160] have developed small surgical awls, curved in different angles, to reach all parts of the articular surface during an arthroscopic procedure. In the course of the treatment, the superficial bone layer must be penetrated and the whole base of the defect carefully fractured. The surgical awls are tapped into the subchondral cortical bone to a 3–4 mm depth at 3–5 mm intervals. In the postoperative course the beneficial effect of the use of CPM has been reported.[149] According to Steadman et al.,[160] this technique can result in cartilage of hyaline-like quality. In the opinion of several authors, however, the microfracture technique, like its predecessors, cannot produce more than fibrocartilage in the long term. Nonetheless, this procedure is a step forward since the regenerated tissue is more extensive and contiguous than that produced by earlier traditional cartilage producing techniques. Presently it represents the most widely accepted and used operation among the traditional cartilage surface producing techniques.[120,149,159,160] Unfortunately, reports of long-term evaluation of the microfracture technique – especially in the patellofemoral junction – are still missing.

Modern Resurfacing Techniques

Over the past two decades, considerable effort has been made in developing new options for the production of a long-lasting hyaline-like gliding surface. Areas of research and application have been in the directions of hyaline cartilage regeneration and hyaline cartilage transplantation.

Considerable basic science supports the development of these new techniques but controversy abounds. Most of the procedures have been preceded by animal trials, some have promising early results in the human practice, but few have even medium-term clinical evaluation.

Correct and critical evaluation of the new resurfacing techniques is difficult. These surgical procedures are, indeed, quite different, making an objective evaluation difficult. An objective comparison would require standard evaluation forms. Such detailed and critical evaluations, by standardized format, are under development by a number of scientific societies. New diagnostic possibilities promote the pre-operative and postoperative conditions, but unfortunately their use is sometimes restricted because of their invasiveness. It is suggested that, in addition to these initial controls, support of modern imaging techniques, critical histological assessments, and independent, multicenter, prospective, randomized comparative studies are required to determine the final efficacy of these techniques.

Periosteal Flapping

Transplantation of periosteum and osteoperiosteal grafts is one of the new techniques having the longest history among these procedures.[43,44,71,86,134,138,150] Animal trials were already carried out with this approach in 1940. In 1982 Rubak[150] produced neochondrogenesis in osteochondral defect with periosteum transplantation. Details of operative technique and rehabilitation protocol have undergone a great deal of change. Theoretically, multipotential cells of the cambium layer of the periosteum are used to produce hyaline-type regenerative tissues. The postoperative status seems to have a determining role in whether neochondrogenesis or bone formation will be the actual response of the transplanted tissue. Poor oxygenization of the transplanted tissue and continuous passive motion promote cartilage formation; whereas better circulation to the recipient site and immobilization of the joint result in mineralization of the graft.[38,87,129,137,148]

From experimental models, some unsolved questions regarding the role of the cambium layer in the neochondrogenesis have arisen. In a few trials the periosteum has been implanted in the opposite position, namely, the cambium layer facing to the joint space. According to the experiments of Jaroma and Ritsila,[86] there has been no difference in the results of the two types of implantation techniques.

Kreder et al.[94] investigated the efficacy of allogeneic periosteum flaps in the resurfacement in a rabbit model. They concluded that grafts harvested from mature animals gave superior results compared with immature donors.

There have been limited clinical experiences with the periosteum transplantation. O'Driscoll[139] reported good results but mentioned relatively high frequency of periosteum calcification or other failure. A well-developed rehabilitation algorithm seems to be essential in an advantageous clinical outcome. Experimental works of Salter et al.[152] and clinical investigations of Alfredson and Lorentzon,[2] O'Driscoll,[139] and Moran et al.[125] emphasized the important role of CPM in rehabilitation. Recently O'Driscoll also remarked on the importance of proper graft harvesting in the success of the transplantation. Regarding the implantation, several authors recommended drilled tunnels on the bony base of the defect as fixation points for the free periosteal flap.[2,99,137]

Alfredson and Lorentzon,[2] Hoikka et al.,[71] Niedermann et al.,[134] Sandelin et al.,[153] and O'Driscoll[139] published promising patellofemoral applications. Jensen and Bach[87] also reported successful clinical outcome. The most recent study of Lorentzon[99] reported excellent patellofemoral results.

Other authors, including Brittberg et al.,[14] used the periosteum as a free flap to secure the autologous chondrocyte transplantation. These applications are detailed later (autologous chondrocyte implantation).

We had only moderate results with periosteal flapping of the femoral condyles, but achieved slightly better clinical outcome on the patellar surface. According to our experiences, transplantation of free periosteal flaps can be an alternative in the treatment of severe, extended patellar lesions. Acceptable clinical outcome can be achieved only by combination of periosteal flapping and correction of the underlying biomechanical problems (Figure 12.3).

An increasing number of reports on application of free periosteal flaps demonstrate improving results.[71,87,99,139,148,153] According to these papers the periosteum is taken from the proximal part of the tibia, in the region of the pes anserinus insertion. It can form, through an incompletely understood mechanism, a new sliding articular surface. According to O'Driscoll[139] this surface material resembles hyaline cartilage biochemically, but has significant structural differences. Summarizing these controversial data, it seems that transplantation of free periosteal flaps can provide an alternative in the treatment of full-thickness patellar defects. Further documentation of the sequence of metaplasia and durability of the resultant tissue and clinical experience will be needed prior to broader application of the technique.

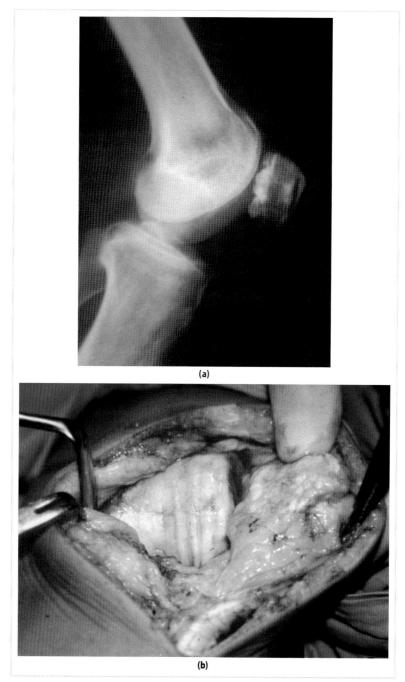

Figure 12.3. Case report of a periosteal transplantation of a 29-year-old woman having patellofemoral rest pain and having received mushroom-shaped frozen allograft implantation two years before. **(a)** Preop lateral x-rays. **(b)** Intraoperative picture of the severely damaged patellotrochlear surfaces.

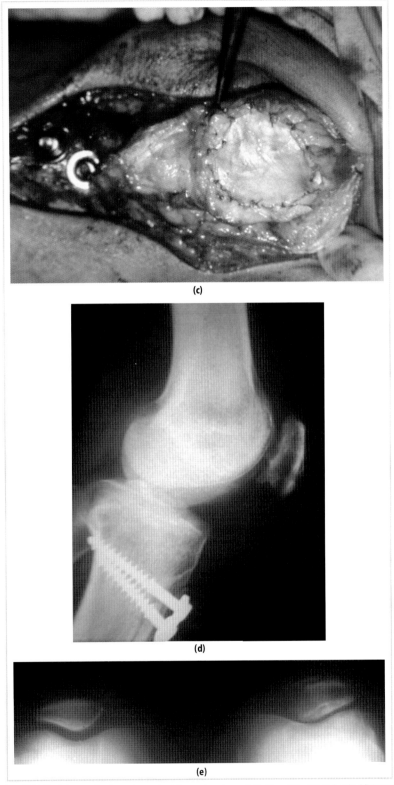

Figure 12.3. *(continued)* **(c)** Final picture of periosteal transplantation and ventromedialization of the tibial tubercle. **(d)** Lateral x-rays half-year-old postop. **(e)** Axial x-rays one-year-old postop.

(continued)

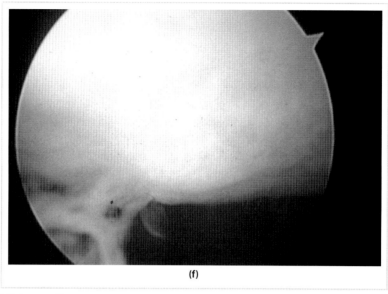

Figure 12.3. *(continued)* **(f)** One-year-old control arthroscopy of the resurfaced patella: good fibrocartilage coverage with slight fibrillation. The patient is free of pain.

Perichondrium Transplantation

In contrast to periosteal transplantation, there is less experience with the use of perichondrium. The first most important reports in this field originated from Skoog et al.[155] in 1972, Engkvist[44] in 1979, and Hvid and Andersen[77] in 1981. Experimental transplantations of autogenous free perichondrial flaps on dogs by Engkvist[44]; on rabbits by Coutts et al.,[37] Ohlsen,[141] and Homminga et al.[73]; and on sheep by Bruns et al.[22] provided basic scientific support for further research.

While Coutts et al.[37] achieved hyaline-like resurfacement in 60% Bruns[22,23] obtained successful transplantation in a higher percent. Bruns's experimental study had been performed on 36 sheep. He divided the animals in three groups: In Group A the sheep received rib perichondrial grafts secured by collagen sponges, in Group B the same grafts were fixed by fibrin glue, and Group C served as the control in which the created defects were left bare.

After 4, 8, 12, and 16 weeks histological evaluations revealed that non-weight-bearing resurfacements had given superior results to weight-bearing repairs and control specimens. A parallel study carried out in vitro investigated the behavior of the same tissue on three different matrices: collagen sponges, fibrin glue, and cellulose acetate filter. Clear differentiation of perichondrial cells toward a chondrocyte-like cell shape was noticed in all matrices.

Allogenous perichondrocyte and perichondrium transfer have also been investigated by Chu et al.[34] and Homminga et al.[72] Homminga's group implanted rabbit rib perichondrium flaps into full-thickness defects of sheep knees. A gliding surface containing 74% type II collagen was achieved.

In 1980 Engkvist and Johansson[43] published the results of 26 cases; in 1990 Homminga et al.[74] reported 30 autologous perichondrium transplantations on 25 patients. Each group fixed the free perichondrial flap to the debrided bone by fibrin glue. The cambium layer of the transplant has been positioned facing to the joint. It is worth referring to Kulick et al.,[95] who demonstrated that there has been no significant difference between positioning this layer toward or away from the articular surface. Second looks between 3 and 12 months demonstrated cartilage-covered defects in 90%. Histological evaluations did not show degenerative changes in the cartilage tissue, but according to the radiological data calcification signs occurred.

Later Bruns – based upon his advantageous experimental findings – began the clinical use of free autogenous rib perichondrial grafts.[21]

Full-thickness cartilage defects in the knee (most of the defects located on the femoral condyles), ankle, and hip joint in 27 selected patients were treated. After the transplantation of the free perichondrial flaps the operated extremities were immobilized for one week. The first week was followed by a CPM period up to 12 weeks. Non-weight-bearing was ordered for 8–12 weeks. Indomethacin was administered to avoid calcification of the grafts. No complications (infections, transplant loosening, limitation of range of motion) were reported. Only 14 patients were followed up at least one year postoperatively. All of them have demonstrated significant improvement. Average HSS score from 78.5 to 95.9 and Lysholm score from 60.9 to 92.5 improved. Bruns states that the transplantation of free perichondrial flaps can be an alternative for deep cartilage defects. Long-term follow-up of these resurfacements result will be of interest.

Comparing this technique to periosteal transplantation, the disadvantages may be the demanding operative technique, and the requirement of two incisions. Ritsilä et al.[148] in 1994 published a paper comparing the periosteum and perichondrium transplantations.

Autologous Chondrocyte Implantation

In the last few years considerable interest and discussion has been focused on autologous chondrocyte transplantation. In 1965, Smith,[156] and in 1968, Chesterman and Smith[30] had already reported isolation of chondrocytes. They had implanted these cells into articular defects in rabbit humeri and into the iliac crest. Later Bentley and Greer,[10] Aston and Bentley,[4] Green,[57] and Grande et al.[56] published results of rabbit studies in which transplantation of isolated chondrocytes had been performed. In the last report, Grande et al.[56] observed 82% neocartilage formation on the patellar implantations at one year. Autologous chondrocyte transplantations gave superior results compared with allogeneic transfer of the same cells.

Brittberg et al. tested the chondrocyte transplantation in rabbits in four different groups.[19] Chondrocyte cultures had been implanted under free periosteal flaps with or without carbon scaffolds. Both of these implantations had a control group (no chondrocytes used). The best hyaline-like tissue formation came from the chondrocyte-periosteum group, but some cluster formation of chondrocytes had also been observed in the newly formed cartilage. In 1994 Brittberg et al. published the first clinical results of autologous chondrocyte implantation in the *New England Journal of Medicine*.[18]

These authors worked out an animal trial model using autologous chondrocyte transplantation and managed to achieve, in two-thirds of the cases, hyaline-like cartilage regeneration. In 1987 the concept obtained approval from the medical faculty of the University of Göteborg to use the technique in clinical practice. Lars Peterson, Mats Brittberg, and their associates[18,19] developed the operative technique of the reimplantation of cultured autologous chondrocytes during a two-step operative procedure.

The first operation involves an arthroscopic examination to establish the presence of a localized full-thickness cartilage defect, simultaneously providing the opportunity to obtain a biopsy from the healthy cartilage of the medial periphery of the medial femoral condyle at the level of the patellofemoral joint. These samples are sent to the laboratory, where the cartilage is minced and enzymatically digested to separate the cells from their matrix. The cells are then cultured in a medium, which is composed of 10% of the patient's own serum. The activated and expanded population of chondrocytes is then reimplanted by arthrotomy exposure.

During the second operation the devitalized tissue of the defect is excised, the base debrided, and a periosteum flap is harvested from the medial side of the medial upper part of the tibia from the region of the pes anserinus. The defect is covered with this periosteum flap with the cambium layer facing down to the bone. The periosteal flap, approximately the same size as the defect, is then sutured to the edges of the defect with resorbable 6 × 0 sutures and sealed with fibrin glue to achieve a waterproof coverage over the defect. The last step is the introduction of the chondrocytes under the periosteum flap to repopulate the defect and effect production of new cartilage. Postoperatively the patients are kept on non-weight-bearing for 12 weeks. Monitored rehabilitation generally requires 6 to 9 months.

The article published in the *NEJM* in 1994 reported the results of 23 patients: 14 out of 16 femoral implantations had very good or good results, 2 out of 7 patellar implantations had good results.[18] Hyaline-like quality cartilage was achieved in 11 out of 15 femoral implantations and in 1 out of 7 patellar resurfacements. The disappointing patellar results were explained by the insufficient correction of the biomechanical factors. Mandelbaum et al.[102] referred to an international cartilage repair data collection, which has been developed with support from the Genzyme Tissue Repair Corporation to evaluate the Carticel method. The Cartilage Repair Registry gave an account of the actual results of follow-up every six months. Clinical outcome was controlled by several scoring systems (modified Cincinnati, Lysholm, Knee Society Score, WOMAC score, etc.) and compared to a baseline. Complications and adverse effects were also registered. These results are much better, especially for the patella, than the earlier ones in 1994.

In addition to these promising attributes, the procedure has certain disadvantages. This technique requires two operations. The second one must be a relatively extended arthrotomy and the rehabilitation period lasts a minimal of 6 to 8 months, but usually is longer. Furthermore, the technique is expensive: The cost of the laboratory process alone is US$10,000. These features of the operation could be improved.

Some scientific data have also been published that have not supported the efficacy of this technique. In 1997 a canine study was reported, revealing comparative data of the autologous chondrocyte transplantation.[17] In this animal model 44 operations on 14 dogs were performed in three groups: In the first group, the control group, the defect of the weight-bearing area was left untreated; in the second group, the defect was covered with a periosteal flap; and in the third group, an autologous chondrocyte suspension was injected under the periosteal flap. The procedure in the second group was analogous with that of the chondrocyte transplantation. By macroscopic and histological analysis a majority of the results were not satisfactory and, significantly, no differences were found in the three groups. In the two groups in which periosteum was sutured to the surrounding articular cartilage, degenerative changes had been observed that appeared to be suture related. Other complications of the human practice have also been reported.[131]

Autologous chondrocyte transplantation technique appears to be a promising method now supported by several research studies. Concerns based upon the distinct disadvantages of the procedure are being concurrently debated. Final evaluation can only be given by independent, multicenter long-term follow-up studies.

Biomaterials, Tissue Engineering, and Cartilage Repair Stimulating Factors

Synthetic materials are also under investigation as possible options in cartilage repair. After successful applications of so-called "designer tissues" (such as liver, skin, intestinal lumen, and blood vessel), tissue engineering expresses efforts to provide biodegradable materials to promote cartilage repair or scaffolds for mesenchymal stem cells or cultured chondrocytes. Tissue engineers are vigorously searching for biodegradable materials to promote cartilage repair or scaffolds for mesenchymal stem cells or cultured chondrocytes Fibrinogen-based materials, Teflon and Dacron substances, polylactic and polyglycolic acids, carbon fiber rods and pads, and collagen gels and plugs are notable materials being tested in animal and limited human trials to serve as a framework for a better cartilage repair.[11,98,133,136]

Bioactive molecules are also under investigation as to their specific influence on cartilage repair. Different types of bone morphogenetic protein (BMP) and growth factors, chondroprotective agents, and polymerized fibrin-IGF composites are the most widely scrutinized substances. These options may support the natural healing processes and the cartilage repair techniques as well.[70,123,135]

Osteochondral Allograft Transplantation

The first publication on this topic appeared in 1908 by Lexer.[96] In his work the whole or half of the joint was replaced with fresh allografts for severe osteochondral destruction. These implantations were performed without tissue typing or detailed microbiological examination, with very poor results by today's standards.

Over the past 25 years there has been a great deal of experience with allografts. Reports on different sizes and types of transplanted osteochondral allografts have been published. Mankin et al.,[103] McDermott et al.,[112] and Mahomed et al.[101] published their long-term follow-up results. In their opinion, the implantation of fresh or tissue bank osteochondral allografts showed good results. It must be emphasized that these patients often had very severe joint instability and deformity with extensive osteochondral destruction. The success was gauged by the degree of functional improvement over the pretransplantation status, a reasonable standard of measurement in these cases.

Several authors have reported their experience with transplantation of fresh osteochondral allografts.[9,36,53,59,96,101,119,140] In contrast to the transplantation of bone where transfer of living cells isn't necessary, a successful substitution of cartilage requires viable chondrocytes. Therefore, transplantation of fresh osteochondral allografts seems to be a reasonable solution, as they contain living chondrocytes in a higher percentage than preserved or frozen transplants. As indicated in these reports, the long-term viability of these cells in transplanted fresh grafts certainly supports this contention.

Hyaline cartilage has several advantages for transplantation from an immunological perspective. Avascularity provides a shield against the immunological system; and chondrocytes deeply embedded in the matrix do not send rejection antigens to the surface. However, beneath and intimately connected is the subchondral bone, which has many immunogenic cells ready to provoke immune responses.[39,47]

The use of fresh osteochondral allotransplants always brings the risk of disease transmission. Present laboratory techniques and monitoring can reduce the chance of such misfortune, but cannot eliminate it.[3,59] Frozen grafts gain an advantage by decreasing the immunogenicity of the bony part, and inhibiting viral transmission, but at the expense of killing all but the hardiest of the chondrocytes. In this regard, even with the most careful and slow freezing techniques (from 0 to $-40°C$) and use of cryoprotective agents, the number of viable chondrocytes is drastically reduced. As such, in spite of difficulties in proper preparation and availability, fresh osteochondral grafts remain popular due to their viability potential.[47,59,132] Mahomed et al.[101] report good results of 92 implantations in 91 patients with smaller, fresh allografts instead of massive ones: 70% good results at 5 years, 64% at 10 years, and 63% good results at 14 years. The operations were performed because of posttraumatic osteoarticular defects. Unipolar transplantations faired slightly better than bipolar implantations. Gross[59] has one of the longest follow-ups and highest success rates of fresh allografts. He emphasized the importance of the correct alignment, good matching to protect the graft from excessive loading and appropriate fixation. According

to Gross there is about 1:500,000 risk ratio of viral transmission. Tomford et al.[163] reemphasized the value of fresh allografts because of a higher percent of viable chondrocytes in fresh allografts.

Other authors prefer to use frozen allografts. Ottolenghi,[142] Parrish,[145] and Mankin et al.[103] reported on massive frozen allografts. While Ottolenghi[142] and Parrish[145] used a store temperature between $-15°C$ and $-25°C$, Mankin et al.[103] used cryoprotective materials and lower temperature. Bakay and Csönge[5] achieved good results with cryopreserved osteochondral allografts in Hungary. They have also developed a special design (mushroom-shaped osteochondral allograft) for patellar resurfacing. Frozen allografts have the special indication for replacing massive cartilage and bone loss in tumor cases.

Some researchers in this field report long-term survival of the transplanted hyaline cartilage, while others believe the transplanted hyaline cartilage will transform into fibrocartilage, and therefore, long-lasting hyaline-quality sliding surface cannot be expected from this method. Presently the general opinion grants that allograft transplantation may be the best, if imperfect, option in the treatment of severe and extensive osteochondral destruction. Large osteochondral defects combined with instability and/or malalignment appear appropriate complex problems for these procedures.[59,103,142,145,163]

Osteochondral Autograft Transplantation

According to several authors, autologous hyaline cartilage survives the process of transplantation allowing a hyaline cartilage surface to be produced at the site of the defect.[27,45,97,143,166] The major overall advantages of this technique are (1) the hyaline cartilage is transplanted as a unit with its subchondral bone base, thus preserving the very important hyaline cartilage-bone interface; (2) the graft is, by its very nature, protected from immunological reaction; and (3) it does not carry the risk of viral transmission.

Single Block Transplantation. Campanacci et al.,[27] Fabricciani et al.,[45] Outerbridge et al.,[143] and Yamashita et al.[166] have had good medium- and long-term experiences by transplantation of single block osteochondral autografts. Their publications reported long-term survival of transplanted hyaline cartilage. Lindholm et al.[97] emphasized the importance of graft congruity, since in its absence the grafts will degenerate. Graft procurement represents a problematic point of this technique. It is difficult to find suitable donor sites for defects larger than 10 mm in diameter without violating the weight-bearing articular surfaces.

Mosaicplasty. To eliminate the donor site and congruency problems, transplantation of multiple small-sized grafts could provide advantages compared with single block transfer. The first successful transplantation of multiple cylindrical osteochondral grafts was reported by Matsusue in 1993.[110] His case report was of an autogenous osteochondral transplantation of 3 cylinders 9 mm long and 5 mm in diameter into a defect on the medial femoral condyle associated with an ACL deficient knee. His 37-year-old male patient had no complaint at 3-year follow-up examination. Slight subchondral sclerosis at the recipient site on the x-rays was reported.

The autologous osteochondral mosaicplasty was developed in Hungary in 1991. Conceptually, the technique specifically addressed problems of congruency at the recipient site by the implantation of small-sized grafts sequentially arrayed in a mosaic-like pattern.[65] Inherent to the technique design has been the procurement of these small grafts from less weight-bearing surfaces, thus reducing the potential of donor site morbidity.[61–66,92] Following several series of animal trials, cadaver research, and the development of special instrumentation, this technique was introduced into clinical practice in 1992.

During the procedure, edges of the defect are excised back to healthy hyaline cartilage. Then the base of the lesion is abraded to viable subchondral cortical bone to refreshen the bony base and to remove the sequester layer. The number and size of the grafts for the ideal covering of the defect are determined by special instrumentation (Mosaicplasty™ Complete System, Smith and Nephew Endoscopy Inc., Andover, MA). The next step is taking small-sized osteochondral cylinders from the edges of the medial or lateral femoral condyles. These grafts are harvested from the less weight-bearing supracondylar ridge of the patellofemoral joint by compressive tubular chisels. The last step is a mosaic-like implantation of the osteochondral transplants by press fit technique into drilled holes of recipient area (Figures 12.4 to 12.7). Specially designed instrumentation serves the same operative technique for open procedures and arthroscopic implantations.

During rehabilitation, a full range of motion and non-weight-bearing period for 2 to 3 weeks and partial loading (30–40 kg) for 2 weeks are advised in accordance with site and extent of the defect. Full weight bearing after 4 or 5 weeks and normal daily activity from 6 to 8 weeks is allowed, but sport activity is not recommended during the first postoperative 4 to 6 months. The use of CPM (6 hours per day) in the first 7 to 10 days can promote the rehabilitation.

The aim of this procedure is to create a composite cartilage surface at the site of the defect.

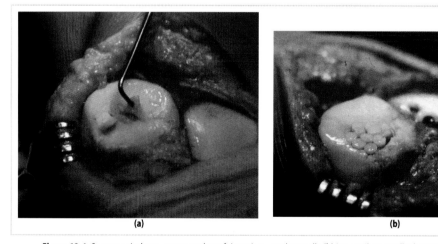

Figure 12.4. Open mosaicplasty – anterograde graft insertion – on the patella (**b**) in a cartilage patellar lesion grade III-IV (**a**).

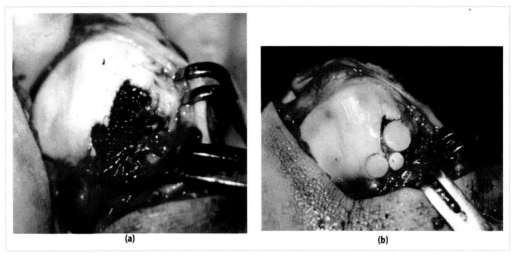

Figure 12.5. (a) Fresh osteochondral fracture of the patella. **(b)** Resurfacement by 3 plugs: 8.5, 6.5, and 4.5 mm diameters.

This composite cartilage layer consists, on an average, of 70–80% transplanted hyaline cartilage, and 20–30% integrated fibrocartilage. Mathematically, the use of same-sized contacting rings results in a theoretical 78.5% filling. But, filling the dead spaces with smaller sizes can improve the coverage of the defect. The special design of the instrumentation can accommodate a 100% filling rate but, naturally, such transplantation requires more graft harvesting. Long-term experience has taught that an 80% filling rate correlates with good a clinical outcome.

Fibrocartilage results from the natural healing process of the refreshened bony base of the defect. According to experimental data, this fibrocartilage fills the space between the transplanted grafts and also eliminates the minimal

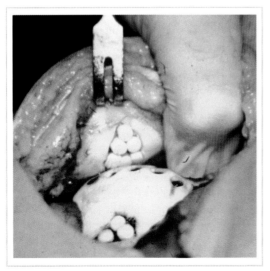

Figure 12.6. Patellar and trochlear mosaicplasties: Kissing lesions are exceptional indications.

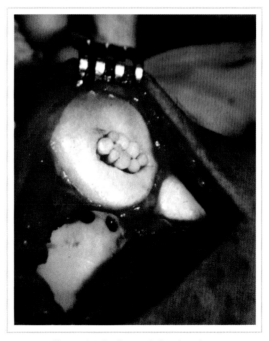

Figure 12.7. Patellar mosaicplasty by 8 plugs.

incongruities of the surface.[63] Shapiro et al.[154] and Desjardins et al.,[41] in separate experimental studies, have reported that newly formed or transplanted hyaline cartilage are not well integrated with the surrounding host cartilage. In contrast, Hangody et al. in German Shepherd dog and Bodó et al. in horse mosaicplasty trials have demonstrated that deep matrix integration is possible between transplanted and surrounding hyaline cartilage, as well as hyaline cartilage and reparative fibrocartilage.[15,63] Histological evaluations of these interfaces of animal and human biopsies showed that such integration was the rule, but in some sections gaps remained between the two types of tissues.[15,63,79,80,92] Further studies have been planned to investigate bioactive materials and factors, which may trigger a better integration process.

The donor site behavior is similar to that prevailing after Pridie drilling. The holes fill by cancellous bone during the first 4 postoperative weeks. Its surface will be covered by early regenerative tissue at 6 weeks and final coverage will be finished by a central fibrocartilage cap and peripheral hyaline cartilage at the eighth to tenth weeks. This partially nonhyaline coverage of the donor holes separated by host articular cartilage appears to be adequate surface for the biomechanical requirements of the less weight-bearing area.[63,66,92] Donor site selection still represents a subject of debate among autologous osteochondral investigators. Hangody et al. prefer the less weight-bearing peripheries of the medial and lateral femoral condyles at the level of the patellofemoral joint.[61,65] Bobic[14] also harvested grafts from the notch area, while Johnson et al. (88) reported graft harvest from the proximal tibiofibular joint. Several studies have been published to investigate possible donor site morbidity.[33,66,158] According to Stäubli et al.,[158] dynamic analyses of opposing articular cartilage contact zones of the patellofemoral joint autografts harvesting from the superolateral aspect of the lateral part of the femoral trochlea should be avoided.

Follow-up examinations and control arthroscopies over the last eight years have demonstrated good preliminary clinical results confirming the data from preclinical animal trials. The latest summary of the clinical results involves 612 cases. Femoral and tibial condylar implantation demonstrated 92% good and excellent results using modified HSS and modified Cincinnati activity scores, while patellofemoral implantation gave only 84%

good to excellent outcome.[66,92] Refinement of the technique by miniarthrotomy and arthroscopic application combined with reproducibility has resulted in a worldwide popularity of the mosaicplasty as an effective, inexpensive, one-step resurfacing technique.[61,62,92] Possible donor site morbidity, as controlled by the Bandi score, has been less than 3%. This morbidity has been uniform: patellofemoral complaints with strenuous physical activity. Other failures have been 4 deep septic complications and 45 painful postoperative hemarthroses. Most of these bleeds have been treated by needle arthrocentesis, while the remaining cases, and the septic failures, needed open or arthroscopic debridement.[66,92] Separate evaluations in different subgroups (such as osteochondral resurfacements[65]; 3 to 7 years follow-up[66]; mosaicplasties among athletes[92]) also gave near to 90% success rate.

Besides femoral and patellar use, tibial (Hangody et al.[67]); talar (Jakob et al.,[85] Imhoff et al.,[78] Hangody et al.[64]); capitulum humeri (Hangody et al.[67,68]); and femoral head transplants (Jakob et al.,[85] Gautier et al.[54]) have been published as further successful applications. Talar implantations have medium-term results. Two to six years follow-up of 31 mosaicplasties for osteochondral lesions gave 95% good and excellent results according to the Hannover scoring system.[67,68] Five cases have had minor donor site complaints up to the end of the first postop year. The second-look arthroscopies demonstrated talar recipient site surfaces that appeared and palpated as normal as well as being congruent with their environs. The biopsy specimens were analyzed histologically using various stains (HE, picrosirius red, toluidin blue, orcein, etc.) and polarization, collagen typing, and enzymhistochemistry. These slides show staining specific for type II collagen and articular proteoglycans, lending histological evidence to our other observations that the hyaline cartilage survives intact and bonds to the talus.

MRI controls have documented good integration of the implanted grafts to the surrounding tissue. Seventy-three control arthroscopies, recipient and donor site biopsies, and, in some cases, indentometric measurements have connoted the hyaline-like character of the replaced area and the fibrocartilage covering of the donor area.[60-68] Cartilage stiffness measurements (by indentometry) at the recipient site have produced matching values for graft and surrounding healthy hyaline cartilage. Several independent, multicentric studies have also supported the results of Hangody, Kárpáti, Kish et al.[33,52] Christel et al.[33] in a French multicenter study have found a similar success rate as Hangody et al.

Beside the mosaicplasty technique, similar multiple cylindrical grafting options have also been developed. Bobic,[14] Jakob,[85] Chow and Barber,[32] and others[52,78] have produced similar promising results. Increasing numbers of successful transplantations by these techniques support the theoretical considerations of multiple autologous osteochondral transfer. Disadvantages, both projected and practical, such as early and long-term donor site morbidity,[66,81,92] incomplete healing of transplanted tissue to the host cartilage,[144] and technical difficulties[92,130] compromise the procedure. Addressing these issues must be the subject of further investigation to reduce the morbidity rate and validate the long-term results.

As at any other type of cartilage repair, mosaicplasties of the patellofemoral joint have less advantageous clinical outcome than femoral or talar applications. Causative factors of these moderate results are well known: Biomechanical problems of the patellotrochlear joint have less effective treatment options than femoral or tibial cartilage damage. In spite of these disadvantageous experiences a well-considered therapeutical strategy can promote an acceptable clinical outcome.

According to the follow-up results, autologous osteochondral mosaicplasty seems to be an efficacious alternative in the treatment of the focal chondral and osteochondral defects. Naturally, as with every other modern resurfacing technique, long-term results and prospective, multicentric, comparative studies are required to determine the final role of this technique in prevention of osteoarthritis.

Considerations for Treatment Strategy

Over the past decade, progress in the pursuit of solutions for lasting and functional repair of articular cartilage loss has accelerated. Hunter's tissue, after centuries, has become less enigmatic. Innovative procedures such as autogenous chondrocyte transplantation and autogenous osteochondral grafting have met mid-term success in providing durable hyaline-like and hyaline resurfacements to focal chondral defects. These successes are also their limitations: Indications

are for focal defects in the younger population, and long-term critical analysis has yet to occur. Perhaps their enduring contributions, from their concepts, will have been as broad links across the disciplines of basic science and surgical application to create a unified understanding of cartilage. In dealing with the arthritic and articular cartilage deficient patients, the orthopedic surgeon should understand the indications for all the available cartilage procedures and the specifics of their techniques, and above all, use restraint in their application. Patellofemoral applications of the new cartilage repair techniques require a more cautious approach than femoral condylar use as biomechanics of this junction are less clear than the femorotibial contact. Meticulous diagnostics, careful patient selection, well-developed therapeutical algorithm, and appropriate postoperative rehabilitation are the key elements for a better clinical outcome in this problematic joint.

References

1. Abernethy, PJ, PR Townsend, RM Rose, and EL Radin. Is chondromalacia patellae a separate clinical entity? *J Bone Joint Surg* 1978; 60-B: 205–211.
2. Alfredson, H, and R Lorentzon. Superior results with continuous passive motion compared to active motion after periosteal transplantation: A retrospective study of human patella cartilage defect treatment. *Knee Surg Sports Traumatol Arthrosc* 1999; 7: 137–143.
3. Asselmeier, MA, RB Caspari, and S Bottenfield. A review of allograft processing and sterilization techniques and their role in transmission of the human immunodeficiency virus. *Am J Sports Med* 1993; 21: 170–175.
4. Aston, JE, and G Bentley. Culture of articular cartilage as a method of storage: Assessment of maintenance of phenotype. *J Bone Joint Surg* 1982; 64B: 384–388.
5. Bakay, A, L Csönge, and L Fekete. A mushroom-shaped osteochondral patellar allograft. *Int Orthop* 11996; 20:370–375.
6. Bandi, W. Chondromalacia patellae and femoropatellare arthrose. *Chir Acta Suppl* 1972; 1:3.
7. Baumgaertner, MR, WD Cannon, Jr., JM Vittori et al. Arthroscopic debridement of the arthritic knee. *Clin Orthop* 1990; 253: 197–202.
8. Baumgartl, F. *Das Kniegelenk*. Berlin: Springer Verlag, 1944.
9. Beaver, RJ, M Mahomed, D Backstein et al. Fresh osteochondral allografts for post-traumatic defects in the knee: A survivorship analysis. *J Bone Joint Surg* 1992; 74-B:105–110.
10. Bentley, G and RB Greer, III. Homotransplantation of isolated epiphyseal and articular cartilage chondrocytes into joint surfaces of rabbits. *Nature* 1971; 230: 385–388.
11. Bentley, G, D Norman, and FS Haddad. An 8-year experience of cartilage repair by the matrix support prosthesis. *Proceedings 2nd Symposium of International Cartilage Repair Society*, Boston, MA, November 16–18, 1998.

12. Bert, JM. Role of abrasion arthroplasty and debridement in the management of osteoarthritis of the knee. *Rheum Dis Clin North Am* 1993; 19: 725–739.

13. Bert, JM, and K Maschka. The arthroscopic treatment of unicompartmental gonarthrosis: A five-year follow up study of abrasion arthroplasty plus arthroscopic debridement and arthroscopic debridement alone. *J Arthrosc* 1989; 5: 25–32.

14. Bobic, V. Arthroscopic osteochondral autograft transplantation in anterior cruciate ligament reconstruction: A preliminary clinical study. *Knee Surg Sports Traumatol Arthrosc* 1996; 3: 262–264.

15. Bodó, G, L Hangody, Zs Szabó, D Girtler, V Peham, and M Schinzel. Arthroscopic autologous osteochondral mosaicplasty for the treatment of subchondral cystic lesion in the medial femoral condyle in a horse. *Acta Vet Hung* 48(3): 343–354.

16. Boyd, HB, and BL Hawkins. Patellectomy: A simplified technique. *Surg Gynecol Obstet* 1948; 86:357.

17. Breinan, HA, T Minas, HP Hsu et al. Effect of cultured chondrocytes on repair of chondral defects in a canine model. *J Bone Joint Surg* 1997; 79-A: 1439–1451.

18. Brittberg, M, A Lindahl, A Nilsson et al. Treatment of deep cartilage defects in the knee with autologous chondrocyte transplantation. *NE J Med* 1994; 331: 889–895.

19. Brittberg, M, A Nilsson, A Lindahl et al. Rabbit articular cartilage defects treated with autogenous cultured chondrocytes. *Clin Orthop* 1996; 326: 270–283.

20. Brooke, R. The treatment of fractured patella by excision: A study of morphology and function. *Br J Surg* 1937; 24:733.

21. Bruns, J, P Behrens, and J Steinhagen. Autogenous rib perichondrial grafts for the treatment of osteochondral defects. *Proceedings 2nd Symposium of International Cartilage Repair Society*, Boston, November 16–18, 1998.

22. Bruns, J, P Kersten, A Weiss, and M Silbermann. Morphological results after grafting of autologous rib perichondrium in experimentally induced ostechondral lesions in the sheep-knee joint and tissue culture on three different culture soils. *Proceedings 2nd Symposium of International Cartilage Repair Society*, Boston, November 16–18, 1998.

23. Bruns, J, P Kersten, W Lierse, M Silbermann. Autologous rib perichondrial grafts in experimentally induced osteochondral lesions in the sheep-knee joint: morphological results. *Virchows Arch A Pathol Anat Histopathol* 1992; 421:1–12.

24. Buckwalter, JA, E Hunziker, L Rosenberg et al. Articular cartilage: Composition and structure. In Woo, SL-Y, and JA Buckwalter, eds., *Injury and Repair of the Musculoskeletal Soft Tissues*. Park Ridge, IL: AAOS, 1988, pp. 405–425.

25. Buckwalter, JA, and HJ Mankin. Articular cartilage. Part II: Degeneration and osteoarthritis, repair, regeneration and transplantation. *J Bone Joint Surg* 1997; 79A: 612–632.

26. Buckwalter, JA, LC Rosenberg, and EB Hunziker. Articular cartilage: Composition, structure, response to injury and methods of facilitating repair. In Ewing, JW, ed., *Articular Cartilage and Knee Joint Function: Basic Science and Arthroscopy*. New York: Raven Press, 1990, pp. 19–56.

27. Campanacci, M, C Cervellati, and U Dontiti. Autogenous patella as replacement for a resected femoral or tibial condyle: A report of 19 cases. *J Bone Joint Surg* 1985; 67B: 557–563.

28. Campbell, CJ. The healing of cartilage defects. *Clin Orthop* 1969; 64: 45–63.

29. Caplan, AI. Mesenchymal stem cells. *J Orthop Res* 1991; 9: 641–650.

30. Chesterman, PJ, and AU Smith. Homotransplantation of articular cartilage and isolated chondrocytes: An experimental study in rabbits. *J Bone Joint Surg* 1968; 50B: 184–197.

31. Childers, JC Jr., and SC Ellwood. Partial chondrectomy and subchondral bone drilling for chondromalacia. *Clin Orthop* 1979; 144: 114–120.

32. Chow, JC. Autologous osteochondral transplantation by the COR system. *Seventeenth Annual Cherry Blossom Seminar, Book of Abstracts,* Washington, DC, April 16–18, 1998.

33. Christel, P, G Versier, Ph Landreau, and P Djian. Les greffes osteo-chondrales selon la technique de la mosaicplasty. *Maitrise Orthopédique* 1998; 76, 1–13.

34. Chu, CR, RD Coutts, M Yoshioka et al. Articular cartilage repair using allogeneic perichondrocyte-seeded biodegradable porous polylactic acid (PLA): A tissue engineering study. *J Biomed Mater Res* 1995; 29: 1147–1154.

35. Convery, FR, WH Akeson, and GH Keown. The repair of large osteochondral defects: An experimental study in horses. *Clin Orthop* 1972; 82: 253–262.

36. Convery, FR, WH Akeson, and MH Meyers. The operative technique of fresh osteochondral allografting of the knee. *Operative Tech Orthop* 1997; 7: 340–344.

37. Coutts, RD, SL Woo, D Amiel et al. Rib perichondrial autografts in full-thickness articular cartilage defects in rabbits. *Clin Orthop* 1992; 275: 263–267.

38. Curtin, WA, WJ Reville and MP Brady. Quantitative and morphological observations on the ultrastructure of articular of articular tissue generated from free periosteal grafts. *J Electron Microsc (Tokyo)* 1992; 41: 82–90.

39. Czitrom, AA, T Axelrod, and B Fernandes. Antigen presenting cells and bone allotransplantation. *Clin Orthop* 1985; 197: 27–31.

40. DePalma, AF, CD McKeever, and DK Subin. Process of repair of articular cartilage demonstrated by histology and autoradiography with tritiated thymidine. *Clin Orthop* 1966; 48: 229–242.

41. Desjardins, MR, MB Hurtig, and NC Palmer. Heterotopic transfer of fresh and cryopreserved autogenous articular cartilage in the horse. *Vet Surg* 1991; 20: 434–445.

42. Engebretsen, L, S Svenningsen, and P Benum. Advancement of the tibial tuberosity for patellar pain: A 5-year follow-up. *Acta Orthop Scand* 1989; 60: 20.

43. Engkvist, O, and SH Johansson. Perichondrial arthroplasty: A clinical study in twenty-six patients. *Scand J Plast Reconstr Surg* 1980; 14: 71–87.

44. Engkvist, O. Reconstruction of patellar articular cartilage with free autologous perichondrial grafts: An experimental study in dogs. *Scand J Plast Reconstr Surg* 1979; 13: 361–369.

45. Fabbricciani, C, A Schiavone Panni, A Delcogliano et al. Osteochondral autograft in the treatment of osteochondritis dissecans of the knee. *AOSSM Annual Meeting,* Orlando, FL, 1991.

46. Ficat, RP, C Ficat, P Gedeon et al. Spongialization: A new treatment for diseased patellae. *Clin Orthop* 1979; 144: 74–83.

47. Friedlaender, GE, and MC Horowitz. Immune responses to osteochondral allografts: Nature and significance. *Orthopedics* 1992; 15: 1171–1177.
48. Friedman, MJ, DO Berasi, JM Fox, WD Pizzo, SJ Snyder, and RD Ferkel. Preliminary results with abrasion arthroplasty in the osteoarthritic knee. *Clin Orthop* 1984; 182: 200–205.
49. Fulkerson, JP. The etiology of patellofemoral pain in young active patients: A prospective study. *Clin Orthop* 1983; 179:129.
50. Fuller, JA, and FN Ghadially. Ultrastructural observations on surgically produced partial-thickness defects in articular cartilage. *Clin Orthop* 1972; 86: 193–205.
51. Furukawa, T, DR Eyre, S Koide et al. Biochemical studies on repair cartilage resurfacing experimental defects in the rabbit knee. *J Bone Joint Surg* 1980; 62A: 79–89.
52. Gambardella, RA. Osteochondral grafting: A multicenter review of clinical results. *Proceedings 2nd Symposium of International Cartilage Repair Society*, Boston, November 16–18, 1998.
53. Garrett, JC. Treatment of osteochondritis dissecans of the distal femur with fresh osteochondral allografts. *Arthroscopy* 1986; 2: 222–226.
54. Gautier, E, K Ganz, N Krügel, and R Ganz. Osteochondral autografts in the hip joint: Anatomic considerations and surgical approaches. *Proceedings 2nd Symposium of International Cartilage Repair Society*, Boston, November 16–18, 1998.
55. Ghadially, JA, and FN Ghadially. Evidence of cartilage flow in deep defects in articular cartilage. *Virchows Arch B Cell Path* 1975; 18: 193–204.
56. Grande, DA, MI Pitman, L Peterson et al. The repair of experimentally produced defects in rabbit articular cartilage by autologous chondrocyte transplantation. *J Orthop Res* 1989; 7: 208–218.
57. Green, WT Jr. Articular cartilage repair: Behavior of rabbit chondrocytes during tissue culture a subsequent allografting. *Clin Orthop* 1977; 124: 237–250.
58. Grelsamer, RP, CS Proctor, and AM Bazos. Evaluation of patellar shape in the sagittal plane: A clinical analysis. *Am J Sports Med* 1994; 22: 61.
59. Gross, A. Fresh osteochondral allografts for posttraumatic knee defects: Surgical technique. *Oper Tech Orthop* 1997; 7: 334–339.
60. Hangody, L, G Kish, Z Kárpáti, and R Eberehardt. Osteochondral plugs: Autogenous osteochondral mosaicplasty for the treatment of focal chondral and osteochondral articular defects. *Oper Tech Orthop* 1997; 7: 312–322.
61. Hangody, L, and Z Kárpáti. A new surgical treatment of localized cartilaginous defects of the knee. *Hung J Orthop Traumat* 1994; 37: 237–243.
62. Hangody, L, G Kish, Z Kárpáti et al. Arthroscopic autogenous osteochondral mosaicplasty for the treatment of femoral condylar articular defects. *Knee Surg Sports Traumatol Arthrosc* 1997; 5: 262–270.
63. Hangody, L, G Kish, Z Kárpáti et al. Autogenous osteochondral graft technique for replacing knee cartilage defects in dogs. *Orthop Int Ed* 1997; 5: 175–181.
64. Hangody, L, G Kish, Z Kárpáti et al. Treatment of osteochondritis dissecans of the talus: The use of the mosaicplasty technique – preliminary report. *Foot and Ankle Int* 1997; 18: 628–634.
65. Hangody, L, G Kish, and Z Kárpáti. Osteochondral plugs: Autogenous osteochondral mosaicplasty for the treatment of focal chondral and osteochondral articular defects. *Oper Tech Orthops* 1997; 7: 312–322.
66. Hangody, L. The biology of cartilage repair. In *European Instructional Course Lectures* 1999; 4: 112-118. British Editorial Society of Bone and Joint Surgery.
67. Hangody, L. *Mosaicplasty*. In Insall, J, and N Scott, *Surgery of the Knee*. Churchill Livingstone, 2000, pp. 357–361.
68. Hangody, L. Autologous osteochondral mosaicplasty in the treatment of focal chondral and osteochondral defects of the weight-bearing articular surfaces. *Osteologie*, 2000; 9: 63–69.
69. Heatly, JH, PR Allen, and JH Patrick. Tibial tubercle advancement for anterior knee pain: A temporary or permanent solution. *Clin Orthop* 1986; 208: 215.
70. Hills, R, L Belanger, and E Morris. The effects of BMPs 2, 9, and 13 on the metabolism of bovine chondrocytes grown in explant culture. *Proceedings 2nd Symposium of International Cartilage Repair Society*, Boston, November 16–18, 1998.
71. Hoikka, VE, HJ Jaroma, and VA Ritsilä. Reconstruction of the patellar articulation with periosteal grafts: four year follow-up of 13 cases. *Acta Orthop Scand* 1990; 61: 36–39.
72. Homminga, GN, SK Bulstra, R Kuijer et al. Repair of sheep articular cartilage defects with rabbit costal perichondrial graft. *Acta Orthop Scand* 1991; 62: 415–418.
73. Homminga, GN, TJ van der Linden, EAW Terwindt-Rouwenhorst et al. Repair of articular defects by perichondrial grafts: Experiments in the rabbit. *Acta Orthop Scand* 1989; 60: 326–329.
74. Homminga, GN, SK Bulstra, PSM Bouwmeester, and AL Van der Linden. Perichondrial grafting for cartilage lesions of the knee. *J Bone Joint Surg* 1990; 72-B: 1003–1007.
75. Hughston, JC, and WM Walsh. Proximal and distal reconstruction of the extensor mechanism for patellar subluxation. *Clin Orthop* 1979; 144: 36.
76. Hunter, W. On the structure and diseases of articulating cartilages. *Philos Trans R Soc Lond* 1743; 42B: 514–521.
77. Hvid, J, and LL Andersen. Perichondrial autograft in traumatic chondromalacia patellae: Report of a case. *Acta Orthop Scand* 1981; 52: 91–98.
78. Imhoff, AB, GM Oettl, A Burkart, and S Traub. Extended indication for osteochondral autografts in different joints. *Proceedings 2nd Symposium of International Cartilage Repair Society*, Boston, November 16–18, 1998.
79. Insall, JN. The Pridie debridement operation for osteoarthritis of the knee. *Clin Orthop* 1974; 101: 61–67.
80. Insall, JN, AJ Tria, and P Aglietti. Resurfacing of the patella. *J Bone Joint Surg Am* 1980; 62: 933.
81. Insall, JN, and WN Scott. *Surgery of the Knee I-II*. Churchill Livingstone, 2000.
82. Itay, S, A Abramovici, and Z Nevo. Use of cultured embryonal chick epiphyseal chondrocytes as grafts for defects in chick articular cartilage. *Clin Orthop* 1987; 220: 284–303.
83. Jackson, RW, R Silver, and R Marans. Arthroscopic treatment of degenerative joint disease. *Arthroscopy* 1986; 2: 114.
84. Jackson, RW, HJ Marans, and RS Silver. Arthroscopic treatment of degenerative arthritis of the knee. *J Bone Joint Surg* 1988; 70-B: 332–341.
85. Jakob, RP, P Mainil-Varlet, C Saager, and E Gautier. Mosaicplasty in cartilaginous lesions over 4 square cm

and indications outside the knee. *Cartilage Repair, 2nd Fribourg International Symposium, Book of Abstracts,* 1997.

86. Jaroma, HJ, and V Ritsilä. Reconstruction of patellar cartilage defects with free periosteal grafts: An experimental study. *Scand J Plast Reconstr Surg* 1987; 21: 175–181.

87. Jensen, LJ, and KL Bach. Periosteal transplantation in the treatment of osteochondritis dissecans. *Scand J Med Sci Sports* 1992; 2: 32–36.

88. Johnson, LL, SD Martin, DB Golden et al. Autogenous osteochondral grafts from the proximal tibiofibular joint: A novel donor site. *Proceedings 2nd Symposium of International Cartilage Repair Society,* Boston, November 16–18, 1998.

89. Johnson, LL. Arthroscopic abrasion arthroplasty: Historical and pathological perspective: Present status. *Arthroscopy* 1986; 2: 54-69.

90. Johnson, LL. Surgical Arthroscopy: Principles and Practice. St. Louis: CV Mosby, 1986.

91. Kim, HKW, ME Moran, and RB Salter. The potential for regeneration of articular cartilage in defects created by chondral shaving and subchondral abrasion: An experimental investigation in rabbits. *J Bone Joint Surg* 1991; 73A: 1301–1315.

92. Kish, G, L Módis, and L Hangody. Osteochondral mosaicplasty for the treatment of focal chondral and osteochondral lesions of the knee and talus in the athlete. *Clin Sports Med* 1999; 18: 45–66.

93. Korkala, O, and H Koukkannen. Autogenous osteoperiosteal grafts in the reconstruction of full thickness joint surface defects. *Int Orthop* 1991; 15: 233–237.

94. Kreder, HJ, M Moran, FW Keeley et al. Biologic resurfacing of a major joint defect with cryopreserved allogeneic periosteum under the influence of continuous passive motion in a rabbit model. *Clin Orthop* 1994; 300: 288–296.

95. Kulick, MI, B Brent, and J Ross. Free perichondrial graft from the ear to the knee rabbits. *J Hand Surg* 1984; 9A: 213–215.

96. Lexer, E. Substitution of whole or half joints from freshly amputated extremities by freeplastic operation. *Surg Gynecol Obstet* 1908; 6: 601–607.

97. Lindholm, TS, K Osterman, P Kinnunen, TC Lindholm, and HK Osterman. Reconstruction of the joint surface using osteochondral fragments. *Scand J Rheumatol (Suppl)* 1982; 44: 5–12.

98. Lohmann, CH, Z Schwartz, GG Niederauer et al. Ability of chondrocytes to form neocartilage on porous PLG-scaffolds varies with donor site. *Proceedings 2nd Symposium of International Cartilage Repair Society,* Boston, November 16–18, 1998.

99. Lorentzon, R, H Alfredson, and CH Hildingsson. Treatment of deep cartilage defects of the patella with periosteal transplantation. *Knee Surg Sports Traumatol Arthrosc* 1998; 6: 202–208.

100. Magnuson, PB. Technique of debridement of the knee joint for arthritis. *Surg Clin North Am* 1946; 26:249–258.

101. Mahomed, MN, RJ Beaver, and AE Gross. The long-term success of fresh, small fragment osteochondral allografts used for intra-articular post-traumatic defects in the knee joint. *Orthopedics* 1992; 15:1191–1199.

102. Mandelbaum, BR, JE Browne, F Fu et al. Articular cartilage lesions of the knee. *Am J Sportsmed* 1998; 26: 853–861.

103. Mankin, HJ, SH Doppelt, and WW Tomford. Clinical experience with allograft implantation: The first 10 years. *Clin Orthop* 1093; 174: 69–83.

104. Mankin, HJ. Chondrocyte transplantation – one answer to an old question. *NE J Med* 1994; 331: 940–941.

105. Mankin, HJ. The reaction of articular cartilage to injury and osteoarthritis I-II. *NE J Med* 1974; 291: 1285–1292; 1335–1340.

106. Mankin, HJ. The response of articular cartilage to mechanical injury. *J Bone Joint Surg* 1982; 64A: 460–466.

107. Maquet, P. Advancement of the tibial tuberosity. *Clin Orthop* 1976; 115: 225.

108. Maquet, P. Mechanics and osteoarthritis of the patellofemoral joint. *Clin Orthop* 1979; 144: 70.

109. Marumoto, JM, C Jordan, and RA Atkins. A biomechanical comparison of lateral retinacular releases. *Am J Sports Med* 1995; 23: 151.

110. Matsusue, Y, T Yamamuro, and M Hama. Arthroscopic multiple osteochondral transplantation to the chondral defect in the knee associated with anterior cruciate ligament disruption: Case report. *Arthroscopy* 1993; 9: 318–321.

111. McConnell, J. The management of chondromalacia patellae: A long-term solution. *Aust J Physiother* 1986; 32: 215.

112. McDermott, AGP, F Langer, KPH Pritzker et al. Fresh small-fragment osteochondral allografts: Long-term follow-up study on first 100 cases. *Clin Orthop* 1985; 197: 96–102.

113. McGinty, JB, and JC McCarthy. Endoscopic lateral retinacular release: A preliminary report. *Clin Orthop* 1981; 158: 120.

114. McKeever, DC. Patellar prosthesis. *J Bone Joint Surg Am* 1955; 37: 1074.

115. Meachim, G, and C Roberts. Repair of the joint surface from subarticular tissue in the rabbit knee. *J Anat* 1971; 109: 317–327.

116. Messner, K, and C Wei. Healing chondral injuries. *Sports Med Arthrosc Rev* 1998; 6: 13–24.

117. Messner, K, and W Maletius. The long-term prognosis for severe damage to weight-bearing cartilage in the knee: A 14-year clinical and radiographic follow-up in 28 young athletes. *Acta Orthop Scand* 1996; 67: 165–168.

118. Metcalf, RW. An arthroscopic method for lateral release of subluxating or dislocating patella. *Clin Orthop* 1982; 167: 9.

119. Meyers, MN, W Akeson, and R Convery. Resurfacing of the knee with fresh osteochondral allografts. *J Bone Joint Surg* 1989; 71-A: 704–714.

120. Minas, T. Treatment of chondral defects in the knee. *Orthop Spec Ed* 1997; Summer, 69–74.

121. Mitchell, N, and N Shepard. Effect of patellar shaving in the rabbit. *J Orthop Res* 1987; 5: 388–392.

122. Mitchell, N, and N Shepard. The resurfacing of adult rabbit articular cartilage by multiple perforations through the subchondral bone. *J Bone Joint Surg* 1976; 58A: 230–233.

123. Miura, Y, CN Commisso, JS Fizsimmons, and SW O'Driscoll. Brief (30 minutes) exposure to high dose TGF-β1 enhances periosteal chondrogenesis in vitro. *Proceedings 2nd Symposium of International Cartilage Repair Society,* Boston, November 16–18, 1998.

124. Módis, L. *Organization of the Extracellular Matrix: A Polarization Microscopic Approach.* Boca Raton, FL: CRC, 1991, pp. 75–97.

125. Moran, ME, HK Kim, and RB Salter. Biological resurfacing of full thickness defects in patellar articular cartilage of the rabbit: Investigation of autogenous periosteal grafts subjected to continuous passive motion. *J Bone Joint Surg* 1992; 74B: 659–667.
126. Morshuis, WJ, PW Pavlov, and KP DeRooy. Anteromedialization of the tibial tuberosity in the treatment of patellofemoral pain and malalignment. *Clin Orthop* 1990; 255: 242.
127. Mow, VC, GA Ateshian, and A Ratcliffe. Anatomic form and biomechanical properties of articular cartilage of the knee joint. In Fineman, GAM, and FR Noyes, eds., *Biology and Biomechanics of the Traumatized Synovial Joint: The Knee as a Model.* Rosemont, IL: AAOS, 1992, pp. 55–81.
128. Mow, VC, MH Holmes, WM Lai et al. Fluid transport and mechanical properties of articular cartilage: A review. *J Biomech* 1984; 17: 377–394.
129. Nakahara, H, VM Goldberg, and AI Caplan. Culture-expanded human periosteal-derived cells exhibit osteochondral potential in vivo. *J Orthop Res* 1991; 9: 465–476.
130. Navarro, RA. Intraoperative complications with O.A.T. *Proceedings 2nd Symposium of International Cartilage Repair Society,* Boston, November 16–18, 1998.
131. Nehrer, S, M Spector, and T Minas. Complications after autologous chondrocyte implantation: A histological analysis of retrieved tissue. *Proceedings 2nd Symposium of International Cartilage Repair Society,* Boston, November 16–18, 1998.
132. Newman, AP. Articular cartilage repair. *Am J Sport Med* 1998; 26: 309-324.
133. Niederauer, GG, MA Slivka, NC Leatherbury et al. Polymeric implants for osteochondral cartilage repair. *Proceedings 2nd Symposium of International Cartilage Repair Society,* Boston, November 16–18, 1998.
134. Niedermann, B, S Boe, J Lauritzen, and JM Rubak. Glued periosteal grafts in the knee. *Acta Orthop Scand* 1985; 56: 457–460.
135. Nixon, AJ, LA Fortier, and G Lust. Insulin-like growth factor-I facilitates chondrocyte-based articular cartilage resurfacing in vivo. *Proceedings 2nd Symposium of International Cartilage Repair Society,* Boston, November 16–18, 1998.
136. Nixon, AJ, LA Fortier, J Williams, and HO Mohammed. Polymerized fibrin-IGF-I composites for repair of full-thickness articular defects. *Proceedings 2nd Symposium of International Cartilage Repair Society,* Boston, November 16–18, 1998.
137. O'Driscoll, SW, AD Recklies, and AR Poole. Chondrogenesis in periosteal transplants. *J Bone Joint Surg Am* 1994; 76: 1042–1051.
138. O'Driscoll, SW, and RB Salter. The repair of major osteochondral defects in joint surfaces by neochondrogenesis with autogenous osteoperiosteal grafts stimulated by continuous passive motion: An experimental investigation in the rabbit. *Clin Orthop* 1986; 208: 131–140.
139. O'Driscoll, SW. Cartilage regeneration through periosteal transplantation: Basic scientific and clinic studies. Presented at the 64th Annual Meeting of the AAOS in San Francisco, California, February 13–17, 1997.
140. Oakeshott, RD, J Farine, KPH Pritzker et al. A clinical and histological analysis of failed fresh osteochondral allografts. *Clin Orthop* 1988; 233: 283–294.
141. Ohlsen, L. Cartilage formation from free perichondral grafts: An experimental study in rabbits. *Br J Plast Surg* 1976; 29: 262–267.
142. Ottolenghi, CE. Massive osteo- and osteo-articular bone grafts: Technique and results of 62 cases. *Clin Orthop* 1972; 87: 156–164.
143. Outerbridge, HK, AR Outerbridge, and RE Outerbridge. The use of a lateral patellar autogenous graft for the repair of a large osteochondral defect in the knee. *J Bone Joint Surg* 1995; 77-A: 65–72.
144. Paletta, GA Jr., J Hannafin, C Ibarra et al. Histologic, biomechanical and MR image evaluation of autogenous osteochondral plug transplantation in a dog model. *Proceedings 2nd Symposium of International Cartilage Repair Society,* Boston, November 16–18, 1998.
145. Parrish, FF. Allograft replacement of all or part of the end of a long bone following excision of a tumor. *J Bone Joint Surg* 1973; 55A: 1–22.
146. Pridie, KH. A method of resurfacing osteoarthritic knee joint. *J Bone Joint Surg* 1959; 41-B: 618–619.
147. Rand, JA. Role of arthroscopy in osteoarthritis of the knee. *Arthroscopy* 1991; 7: 358–363.
148. Ritsilä, VA, S Santavirts, S Alhopuro et al. Periosteal and perichondrial grafting in reconstructive surgery. *Clin Orthop* 1994; 302: 259–265.
149. Rodrigo, JJ, JR Steadman, JF Silliman et al. Improvement of full-thickness chondral defects healing in the human knee after debridement and microfracture using continuous passive motion. *Am J Knee Surg* 1994; 7: 109–116.
150. Rubak, JM, M Poussa, and V Ritsilä. Chondrogenesis in repair of articular cartilage defects by free periosteal grafts in rabbits. *Acta Orthop* 1982; 53:187–191.
151. Sahlström, A, O Johnell, and I Redlund-Johnell. The natural course of arthrosis of the knee. *Acta Orthop Scand Suppl* 1993; 63 (248): 57–64.
152. Salter, RB, DF Simmonds, BW Malcolm, EJ Rumble, D MacMichael, and ND Clements. The biological effect of continuous passive motion on the healing of full thickness defects in articular cartilage: An experimental investigation in the rabbit. *J Bone Joint Surg Am* 1980; 62: 1232–1251.
153. Sandelin, HVJ, AK Harilainen, and VA Ritsilä. Reconstruction of patellar articular defects with periosteal grafts: A 13-year follow-up. *Proceedings 2nd Symposium of International Cartilage Repair Society,* Boston, November 16–18, 1998.
154. Shapiro, F, S Koide, and MJ Glimcher. Cell origin and differentiation in the repair of full-thickness defects of articular cartilage. *J Bone Joint Surg* 1993; 75A: 532–553.
155. Skoog, T, L Ohlsen, and SA Sohn. Perichondrial potential for cartilaginous regeneration. *Scand J Plast Reconstr Surg* 1972; 6: 123–125.
156. Smith, AU. Survival of frozen chondrocytes isolated from cartilage of adults mammals. *Nature* 1965; 205: 782–784.
157. Spector, TD, JE Dacre, PA Harris, and EC Huskisson. Radiological progression of osteoarthritis: An 11-year follow-up study of the knee. *Ann Rheum Dis* 1992; 51: 1107–1110.
158. Stäubli, HU, U Dürrenmatt, B Porcellini, and W Rauschning. Patellofemoral articular cartilage contact zones and potential trochlear cartilage harvesting sites. *Proceedings 2nd Symposium of International Cartilage Repair Society,* Boston, November 16–18, 1998.

159. Steadman, JR, WG Rodkey, SB Singleton, and KK Briggs. Microfracture technique for full thickness chondral defects: Technique and clinical results. *Oper Tech Orthop* 1997; 7: 300–304.

160. Steadman, JR, and WI Stereet. The surgical treatment of knee injuries in skiers. *Med Sci Sports Exerc* 1995; 27(3): 328–337.

161. Suh, JK, A Aroen, TS Muzzonigro et al. Injury and repair of articular cartilage: Related scientific issues. *Oper Tech Orthop* 1997; 7: 270–278.

162. Thompson, RC. An experimental study of surface injury to articular cartilage and enzyme responses within the joint. *Clin Orthop* 1975; 107: 239–248.

163. Tomford, WW, DS Springfield, and HJ Mankin. Fresh and frozen articular cartilage allografts. *Orthopedics* 1992; 15: 1183–1192.

164. Trillat, A, H DeJour, and A Couette. Diagnostic et traitement des subluxations recidivantes de la rotule. *Rev Chir Orthop* 1964; 50: 813.

165. Wiberg, G. Roentgenographic and anatomic studies on the patellofemoral joint: With special reference to chondromalacia patellae. *Acta Orthop Scand* 1941; 12: 319.

166. Yamashita, F, K Sakakida, F Suzu, and S Takai. The transplantation of an autogenic osteochondral fragment for osteochondritis dissecans of the knee. *Clin Orthop* 1985; 210: 43–50.

13

Autologous Periosteum Transplantation to Treat Full-Thickness Patellar Cartilage Defects Associated with Severe Anterior Knee Pain

Håkan Alfredson and Ronny Lorentzon

Introduction

Articular cartilage injuries have an extremely limited potential for repair or regeneration,[4,17] and full-thickness defects of the patellar articular cartilage are often, but not always, associated with disabling anterior knee-pain and inability to take part in knee-loading daily activities. However, it is important to know that the natural course of cartilage injuries is unknown,[4] and not all cartilage injuries progress and are associated with pain.[30,33] For patients with severe and disabling anterior knee-pain from a full-thickness patellar cartilage defect (Figure 13.1), there is an urgent need to find a treatment that can accomplish regeneration of hyaline (Figure 13.2) (or hyaline-like) cartilage and pain-freeness, or at least a diminished level of anterior knee-pain, during daily living activities. From experimental studies it is well known that the cells in the cambium layer of the periosteum are pluripotent and can differentiate into hyaline (or hyaline-like) cartilage. In a few clinical studies, using different surgical techniques and postoperative rehabilitation models, autologous periosteum transplants alone have been used in the treatment of full-thickness patellar cartilage defects in the knee joint.[1,10,15,16] The results from these studies are varying. A method where chondrocyte transplantation is combined with autologous periosteum transplantation (sutured as a roof on the defect) has shown poor results on patellar cartilage defects.[3]

At our clinic, we treat patients with chronic full-thickness patellar cartilage defects and severe anterior knee pain with autologous periosteum transplantation, followed by continuous passive motion and a carefully controlled rehabilitation program. We started to use this treatment method in 1991, and have treated altogether 85 patients with isolated patellar cartilage defects.

In this chapter we discuss the background of why autologous periosteum can be used with the purpose to form hyaline or hyaline-like cartilage. Experimental and clinical studies are being reviewed. We also introduce our indications for treatment, the surgical technique we use, our type of postoperative rehabilitation model, and the clinical results achieved at our clinic.

Background

The periosteum (Figure 13.3) contains two main layers, the outer fibrous layer and the inner cambium layer. The bone-forming capacity of the cells in the periosteum was demonstrated already 1867 by Ollier.[24] However, the relatively undifferentiated mesenchymal cells in the cambium layer (bottom or inner layer) of the periosteum are also capable of producing cartilage.[7] A cartilaginous callus is produced by the periosteum at a fracture site that is subjected to movement,[13] and periosteal grafts exposed to motion in a synovial joint have demonstrated a chondrogenic potential.[29]

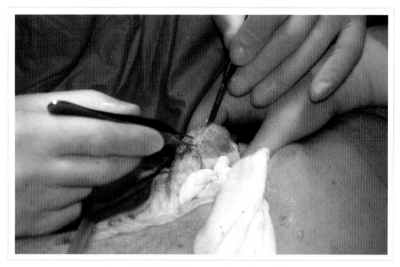

Figure 13.1. A full-thickness patellar cartilage defect.

There are several experimental studies, with different designs, that have investigated the chondrogenic potential of the periosteum. Free periosteal grafts have been demonstrated to mainly differentiate through the enchondral ossification phase.[25] However, the graft environment seems to be of great importance, and in a chondrotrophic environment the differentiation of the periosteum seems to favor cartilage formation.[26] Furthermore, different chondrotrophic environments seem to have different chondrogenic potential. In growing rabbits, the behavior of the cells in free periosteal grafts was studied in three different chondrotrophic environments (costal cartilage, ear cartilage, and synovial fluid of the knee joint).[26] The results showed that the periosteal grafts first formed cartilage, which was transformed rather rapidly

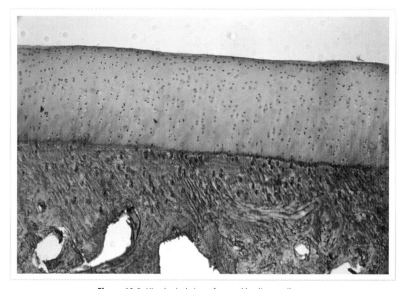

Figure 13.2. Histological view of normal hyaline cartilage.

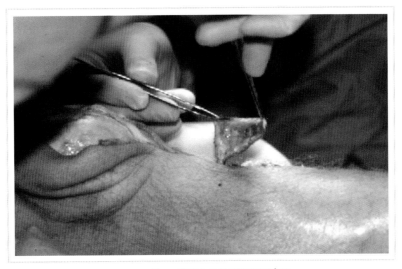

Figure 13.3. A periosteum transplant.

into bone in the costal cartilage, but more slowly in the ear cartilage. However, in the knee-joint no bone formation was found.

Free periosteal grafts transplanted into created deep cartilage defects (sutured with its cambium layer facing the spongious bone) in rabbit knee joints, followed by free mobility immediately after the operation, have been demonstrated to differentiate into hyaline-like cartilage tissue resembling the surrounding original cartilage histologically.[12,27,28] The chondrous tissue formation was strongest at six weeks after implantation, and after 20 weeks the tissue was thick and resembled hyaline cartilage. In control defects where no periosteum was transplanted into the defect, no real cartilage, but a mixture of fibrous tissue and fibrocartilage was found. Using the design with a periosteal graft that is transplanted into a created full-thickness cartilage defect, there is a possibility that the cartilage tissue originates from either the periosteum or the subchondral bone. Therefore, with the use of an isolating filter hindering the penetration of cells, it was demonstrated that the cartilage tissue that proliferated into the defect originated from the periosteum graft and not from the subchondral bone.[28] Studies on horses have confirmed the chondrogenic potential of periosteal grafts in the repair of full-thickness cartilage defects.[34]

The importance of the postoperative treatment regimen for the growth of the healing tissue

has been evaluated especially using a rabbit model. Salter and colleagues have demonstrated that continuous passive motion improves the healing and regeneration of cartilage tissue in full-thickness articular cartilage defects in rabbits.[31,32] The effect of continuous passive motion was compared with the effects of immobilization and that of intermittent active motion. The metaplasia of the healing tissue within the defects, from undifferentiated mesenchymal tissue to hyaline articular cartilage, was shown to be much more rapid and much more complete with continuous passive motion than with immobilization or intermittent active motion. Also, free intra-articular periosteum autografts placed under the influence of continuous passive motion was shown to give superior healing tissue compared to autografts placed in immobilized knee joints of adolescent rabbits.[20] The results showed that the grafts in the immobilized joints were soft and small, whereas the grafts in the joints that had been treated with continuous passive motion had the gross appearance of articular cartilage and had grown larger. Histologically, cartilage was the dominant tissue in 59% of the grafts in the limbs exposed to continuous passive motion, compared to 8% of the grafts in the immobilized limbs.[20] A graft of tibial periosteum transplanted to a full-thickness cartilage defect in the patellar groove in adolescent and adult rabbits (sutured with its cambium layer facing the joint), and under the influence of continuous passive motion for four weeks, can repair the defect by producing a tissue that resembles articular cartilage grossly, histologically, and biochemically, and that contains predominantly type II collagen.[21] The durability of the cartilage-like tissue in rabbit knees has been demonstrated to be good at a one-year follow-up.[22] There were no signs of deterioration with time or degenerative changes in the adjacent cartilage. The positioning of the periosteal graft with the cambium layer facing the cancellous bone or with the cambium layer facing the joint have been shown to give similar results in terms of cartilage-like tissue.[12]

Some criticism, or questions, can be raised when discussing the experimental studies. In most of the experimental studies by Salter and O'Driscoll and others, the periosteum transplant has been anchored in the defects by being sutured toward the surrounding cartilage. However, the cartilage in the rabbit knee is very thin and it is in fact questionable if it is possible at all, or at least if it is possible to achieve a safe anchoring of the transplant, by using this technique. It is our experience that it is impossible to get a safe anchoring of the periosteum transplant that can withstand shearing forces in the rabbit knee with the use of the technique described above.

O'Driscoll and colleagues have investigated the effects of different culture conditions and of adding transforming growth factor-β1 in rabbit periosteal explants cultured in vitro, in order to improve the effectiveness of periosteal chondrogenesis in vivo.[23] The optimum conditions for enhancement of chondrogenesis in vitro was found to be when the explant had been cultured in an agarose gel combined with transforming growth factor-β1. Isolated chondrocytes can retain or regain their cartilaginous phenotype in agarose,[2] but the mechanism behind this effect on the cells is not known. Also, in vitro, higher doses of transforming growth factor-β1 have been shown to be more effective than lower concentrations for the stimulation of chondrogenesis.[18]

In vitro studies have shown that basic fibroblast growth factor can stimulate proliferation of the undifferentiated mesenchymal stem cells in the periosteum, but inhibit osteochondrogenic proliferation.[11] The interaction and combined effect of transforming growth factor-β1 and basic fibroblast growth factor on the undifferentiated mesenchymal cells in the periosteum is, to our knowledge, not known.

To study the relationship of donor site to chondrogenic potential of the periosteum, periosteal explants from different bones (skull, ilium, scapula, medial proximal tibia, posterior tibia, and distal tibia) in rabbits were cultured in vitro.[6] The iliac periosteum was shown to exhibit the best overall chondrogenic potential, but periosteum from the traditionally used medial proximal tibia was also excellent. There was a positive association between the total cell count of the cambium layer and the chondrogenic potential.[8]

Mesenchymal stem cells from periosteum and also from bone marrow have been demonstrated to be able to be cultured in vitro without loosing their ability to form cartilage.[9,19] These cultured cells were then embedded in a type-I collagen gel, and transplanted into full-thickness defects in the weight-bearing articular surface of the knee in rabbits.[35] The rabbits returned to nonrestricted activity immediately after the operation. The results showed that the mesenchymal cells had differentiated into chondrocytes throughout the defects two weeks after transplantation, and the subchondral bone was completely repaired by means of endochondral replacement of the basal cartilage after 24 weeks. There was no apparent difference between the results obtained with the cells from the periosteum and those from the bone marrow. Rabbit marrow stromal cells embedded in alginate has shown the best chondrogenic potential in vivo, compared to stromal cells embedded in agarose or type I collagen gels.[5]

Clinical Studies

There are relatively few clinical studies on the treatment of patellar cartilage defects with autologous periosteum transplants, and in these studies the surgical technique and postoperative rehabilitation is varying.[1,10,15,16] Unfortunately, the surgical technique, and especially the postoperative treatment regimen, is often poorly described. Therefore, comparisons and discussions of the results achieved in the different reports are difficult to make. O'Driscoll and his research group have performed a majority of the experimental studies dealing with periosteum transplants, but strangely enough, they have not presented any clinical reports.

Hoikka and colleagues reported the results of reconstruction of the patellar articulation with free periosteal grafts in 13 patients with chronic knee-pain caused by lesions of the articular surface.[10] The etiology to the lesions was direct trauma in 8 patients, dislocation of the patella in 2 patients, and chondromalacia in 3 patients. Debridement of the damaged articular surface was made, osteophytes were excised, and multiple drillholes down in the cancellous bone were done. A periosteal graft that was scraped loose from the underlying anterior surface of the tibia was in 7 patients sutured (resorbable sutures) to the surrounding cartilage with its cambium layer facing the subchondral bone, and in 6 patients also glued to the articular surface. In 2 patients, both the patellar and also "kissing lesions" at the femoral surfaces were covered with periosteum. In 3 patients, an anterior tibial tubercle elevation was also done. Postoperatively 10 patients were immobilized in a cast for 1 to 6 weeks, and 3 patients were allowed immediate mobilization. The results showed that 8 patients were graded as good (had no restrictions of daily activities and no or only slight pain), 4 were graded as fair (considerable alleviation of pain and able to work), and 1 was graded as poor (persistent intense pain). The patient that was graded poor was 55 years old. Radiographic examination showed congruent patellar position in 8 patients and a slight subluxation of the patella in 5 patients. The slight subluxation of the patella was not associated with a less favorable result compared to a congruent patellar position. No biopsies were taken. In a follow-up, signs of a poor outcome in most of these patients have been reported (personal communication with Dr. Jerker Sandelin, Finland).

In 1995 Korkala and Kuokkanen presented the results of 7 consecutive patients with full-thickness articular cartilage defects at the patella treated with free autogenous osteoperiosteal grafts.[15] Three patients had acute traumatic patellar cartilage defects, three patients had chondromalacia (grade-4), and one patient had a fresh multifragmented osteochondral fracture of the patella. The loose chondral fragments were removed followed by fixation (sutured to the surrounding cartilage with absorbable sutures) of the osteoperiosteal graft into the defect (with its bony surface and cambium layer facing the cancellous bone). In 4 patients fibrin glue was added, injected under the transplant (between the raw surfaces of the bone and graft). Postoperatively, 2 patients were immobilized in a cast initially, while for the other patients continuous passive motion in

a CPM machine and active exercises in a brace with restricted motion (0–30°) was instituted. The patients were allowed full weight-bearing immediately, and sports were permitted 2 months after the operation. At follow-up (1.5–6.5 years after operation) 5 knees were graded as excellent or good, and 2 were graded as fair. Of the 4 fresh cases, 3 ended up as excellent. There was no radiographic follow-up, and no biopsies were taken.

At our clinic, we started to treat patients with localized full-thickness patellar cartilage defects and severe anterior knee-pain with autologous periosteum transplantation in 1991. The following text includes our indications for treatment with this method, the surgical technique and type of postoperative rehabilitation we use, our methods for evaluation of the results, and the clinical results we have achieved.

Indications for Treatment

At our clinic, we carefully evaluate the patients before surgical treatment. To be able to draw any conclusions of the results, we believe that the treatment group needs to be well defined. Several factors needs to be taken into account: the type (traumatic or nontraumatic) and localization of injury, grading of the lesion (full-thickness defect), duration and severity of symptoms, other injuries or diseases affecting the knee joint, previous treatment, and possibility (mental and physical capability) to manage the postoperative rehabilitation.

Our indications for treatment are:

- A long duration (> 1 year) of pain symptoms from a full-thickness patellar cartilage defect.
- No other full-thickness cartilage defects in the knee.
- Pain when walking on flat ground.
- Traditional conservative treatment, including eccentric quadriceps training, without effect.
- Traditional surgical treatment (arthroscopic lavage, debridement/shaving) without effect.
- Physical and mental capability to manage the postoperative rehabilitation.
- No joint disease (rheumatoid arthritis, Mb Bechterew, collagen diseases etc.).
- Age between 16 and 55 years.
- Traumatic etiology of injury (fracture, dislocation, contusion).*

*(New indication [1999]: Before, patients with the diagnosis chondromalacia NUD [no known trauma] were also included.)

Preoperative Evaluation

Preoperatively, all patients are examined with a clinical examination, regular x-ray, and arthroscopy. The patients are carefully informed that this type of operation is a new method that still is under development and nothing can be said about the prognosis of this treatment. They are also informed that the goal with the operation and rehabilitation is to regain the ability to walk without pain and a return to a not-too-heavy knee-loading work.

The ethical committee of the Faculty of Medicine at the University of Umeå have given their approval for performing this operation and using this type of postoperative rehabilitation.

Surgical Technique

The findings during arthroscopy (a full-thickness cartilage defect) are verified through a medial mini-arthrotomy. Thereafter the medial incision is lengthened proximally and distally, the quadriceps tendon is incised, and the patella is partially or totally everted depending on the size and localization of the cartilage defect.

The surgical procedure for the periosteum transplantation is visualized in Figures 13.4 and 13.5. The chondral lesion is excised, sclerotic subchondral bone is removed, and multiple drilling through the remaining subchondral bone into the cancellous bone is done. Drillholes through the patella are placed in the corners and at the sides of the defect, close to the borders of the surrounding cartilage. The periosteum is taken from the proximal tibia with the use of a sharp dissector in order to preserve the cambium layer of the periosteum, and is anchored to the underlying bed with the cambium layer (inner layer) turned inward (i.e., facing the bone). The anchoring procedure is performed with resorbable throughout sutures, Polyglactin 910 resorbable sutures (Vicryl® 2/0), with knots at the ventral side of the patella. Before the last suture is knotted, fibrin glue (Tisseel®) is injected under the transplant. The operation is performed in a bloodless field, and after the fixation of the transplant is done, compression onto the transplant is applied and the bloodless field is released. Compression is held for 3 to 4 minutes and is followed by inspection of the fixation of the transplant to the underlying bed. No blood accumulation beneath the periosteum is allowed.

Postoperative Treatment Regimen

The patients are treated with morphine pump or continuous epidural anesthesia the first 3 to 5 days postoperatively, which is necessary for the

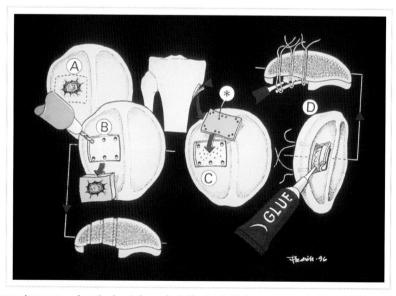

Figure 13.4. Autologous periosteum transplantation (surgical procedure). The chondral lesion is excised and sclerotic subchondral bone is removed (**a**). Through drilling close to the borders of the defect, and multiple drilling into the cancellous bone (**b**). The periosteum is taken from the proximal medial tibia and fitted into the defect with the cambium layer (inner layer) facing the cancellous bone (**c**). A fibrin sealant is injected under the transplant and the sutures are knotted on the dorsal side of the patella (**d**). (Reproduced with permission from reference 16.)

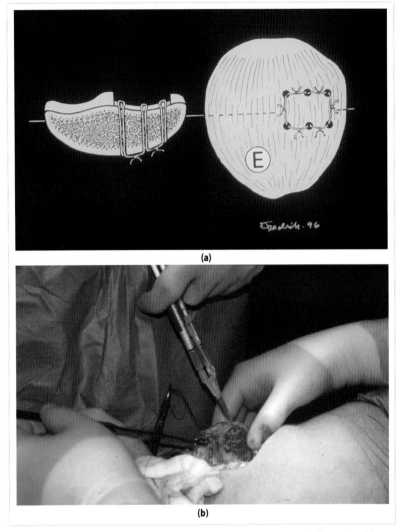

Figure 13.5. The periosteal transplant is fixed to the bottom of the defect with through sutures **(a)** and a fibrin sealant **(b)**. (Part A reproduced with permission from reference 16.)

ability to start treatment with continuous passive motion (CPM) (Figure 13.6). CPM treatment (0–70° flexion in the knee joint) is started the day after operation, and is done one hour every three hours six times a day for four to five days. At day 5–6 postoperatively, the CPM regimen is extended to 0–90°. Active flexion (0–90°) plus isometric quadriceps training is added, and partial weight bearing with crutches is introduced. At day 6–7 the patient leaves the hospital with a home training program containing isometric quadriceps training and active flexibility

training to a full range of motion. No weight-bearing loading of the femoropatellar joint is allowed during the first 12 weeks. Thereafter, slowly progressing strength training and weight-bearing activities are introduced. The patient is followed regularly by the operating doctor and physiotherapist. Pain and effusion in the knee joint are defined as signs of overloading, and lead to a lowered (less loading and less repetitions) rehabilitation level. The patients are informed that the duration of the postoperative rehabilitation period is at least one year.

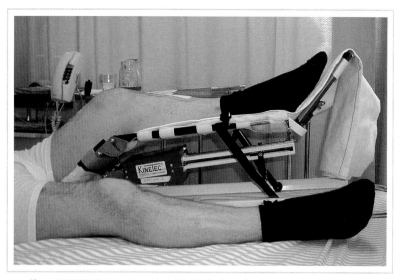

Figure 13.6. CPM (continuous passive motion) in the immediate postoperative period.

Evaluation

Our goal with the treatment is no knee-pain during rest and when walking, and a return to a not-too-heavy knee-loading work. Strenuous knee-loading activities are not encouraged. Therefore, on this group of patients, there is no appropriate score to use for the postoperative evaluation. However, in an often-cited article, presenting a method for treatment of deep cartilage defects in the knee with autologous chondrocyte transplantation plus autologous periosteum transplants,[3] a symptom score is used for the evaluation of results (see below). Therefore, we have decided to use that score in the clinical evaluation of our group of patients.

Brittberg Score for Clinical Grading

Excellent: No pain, swelling, or locking with strenuous heavy knee-loading activity (soccer, icehockey, floor ball, downhill skiing, rugby etc.)

Good: Mild aching with strenuous activity, walking (on flat ground) without pain, no swelling or locking

Fair: Moderate pain with strenuous activity, occasional swelling but no locking

Poor: Pain at rest, swelling, and locking

To try to minimize the risks of bias, we also use a questionnaire assessing patient satisfaction with the treatment. This questionnaire is filled in by the patients at home, and is not under any influence of the investigators.

When we started to use this method (autologous periosteum transplanation) we decided to use clinical examination, patient satisfaction outcome (questionnaire), MRI, biopsy from the transplanted area, and x-ray as tools for the evaluation.

MRI (T1 and T2 weighted examination) was done in 15 patients, and we took biopsies from the transplanted area in five randomly selected patients, all more than one year postoperatively. However, we have now stopped using MRI and biopsies for the postoperative evaluation. This is because the only information we get from MRI (with the methods in use at our hospital) is whether the defect is filled with tissue. In our patients, repeated MRI examinations showed progressive and finally complete filling of the articular defects. Nothing could be said about the type or quality of the tissue that was filling the defect. For biopsies, all our five biopsies showed hyaline-like cartilage, but the only information we get is about the tissue at that exact spot were the biopsy is taken. We know nothing at all about the rest of the transplanted area. It is our experience that the quality of the tissue is varying between different parts of transplanted area, making it questionable to draw any conclusions from the result of one or two minor biopsies. It is demonstrated that in two cases the biopsy showed hyaline-like cartilage but the clinical results were poor and fair, and in one case where the biopsy showed no signs of hyaline-like cartilage the clinical result was good. Another experience is that quite often it is difficult to see the borders between the transplanted area and surrounding cartilage, making it difficult to be really sure that your biopsy is taken from the correct area.

Radiographic examination (x-ray-frontal and lateral view in a standing position, patellofemoral view bilaterally) was done in 18 patients. There were no large differences between the findings at x-ray examinations preoperatively and postoperatively. An irregular bone-surface of the patella was often seen (10 patients), but the irregular surface was also seen preoperatively (9 patients). Minor degenerative changes at the edges of the patella (6 patients), minor loose bodies (3 patients), minor reduction of femoropatellar joint space (3 patients), minor calcification (3 patients), and fragment (1 patient), were other findings. The x-ray findings seemed to have no association with the clinical outcome and activity level postoperatively.

Therefore, we are no longer using these tools (MRI, biopsy, x-ray) for evaluation of our group of patients. Instead, we have to trust the results of the clinical grading and the patient satisfaction outcome (questionnaire). We are waiting for a method where the transplanted area can be evaluated in terms of type and quality of the tissue. Hopefully, new MRI programs can solve this problem in the future.

Results

The cartilage defects ranged in size from 0.75 to 20.0 cm^2 and were all full-thickness defects (grade 4). Varying amounts of sclerotic bone were seen in the defect. In all patients, the subchondral bone plate was macroscopically abnormal.

Postoperatively, there were few complications. One patient had a temporary peroneal nerve paresis, and two patients had an intra-articular postoperative hematoma that was evacuated.

Clinically, most patients (n = 75) had a normal range of motion by three months postoperatively, and all patients (n = 77) had a normal range of motion by six months postoperatively. However, quadriceps atrophy was more prolonged.

A follow-up of 77 patients, all more than 2 years postoperatively (range 24–152 months), showed that 20 patients were graded as excellent, 34 patients were graded as good, 12 patients were graded as fair, and 11 patients were graded as poor according to the Brittberg symptom score. Eleven of the fair and poor cases had nontraumatic (chondromalacia NUD) patellar cartilage defects.

Sixteen patients resumed sports or recreational activities at their desired level (ranging from recreational jogging to the highest national level of rugby). The size of the cartilage defect seemed to have no influence on the possibility to return to previous sports activity.

Follow-up arthroscopy was performed in 26 patients (range 8–36 months postoperatively). In 21 cases, the transplanted area was totally or partially covered with a thin fibrous layer that had the appearance of periosteum. The surface under the periosteum macroscopically had a varying degree of cartilage-like appearance. In some cases the surface was smooth and it was difficult to see the borders between the transplanted area and the surrounding cartilage. In other cases, the transplanted area was irregular and parts of the borders to the surrounding cartilage could be identified. When probed, some cases had similar stiffness as the surrounding cartilage, while in other cases the transplanted area was slightly harder than the surrounding cartilage. The macroscopic findings at arthroscopy did not always correlate with the clinical outcome. The three cases that had sustained a trauma postoperatively, and two other cases, all had full-thickness defects in the transplanted area, and were clinically graded as fair and poor.

Comments

We believe that with our surgical technique and model for postoperative rehabilitation the results of treatment with autologous periosteum transplantation in patients with traumatic full-thickness patellar cartilage defects are good. However, until randomized studies comparing different methods and results of long-term follow-ups of large groups of patients have been performed, it is our opinion that this method is going to be used only for carefully selected patients with severe anterior knee pain and traumatic full-thickness patellar cartilage defects.

Our group of patients all had severe pain when walking and had undergone several other operations previously. Therefore, the periosteum transplantation was a kind of salvage operation, and the main goal was the ability to walk freely without any anterior knee pain. Even though we do not encourage our patients to return to knee-loading sports, some of the patients returned to very strenuous knee-loading sports like rugby, soccer, and downhill skiing without having any knee pain. Therefore, it seems that there is definitely a possibility for regeneration of a cartilage-like tissue that can withstand high loadings.

It should be heavily stressed that our major end point was in this study simply the clinical outcome. Quite another kind of question is whether the periosteum transplantation resulted in regeneration of hyaline cartilage. We have seen postoperative MRI examinations (n = 15) that show filling of the defect with a tissue that resembles the surrounding cartilage, and also biopsies that show hyaline-like cartilage, but it has to be remembered that these examinations do not tell anything at all about the quality of the new-grown tissue. Arthroscopic probing of the transplanted area has also been done, but this is a very subjective method and cannot be used in the evaluation. Therefore, the patient's answers on the questions considering pain at rest, the ability to walk or take part in more strenuous knee-loading activities, swelling and locking, seem thus far to be the best predictors of the quality of the tissue.

In this up-dating follow-up, the clinical results presented are not as good as those presented about three years ago. We believe that this most likely could be explained by increasing patient age, and consequently higher risks for cartilage degenerative disorders. Eleven patients in our material are more than 50 years of age today, and 7 of them now have signs of general arthrosis in the knee joint.

It also needs to be mentioned that the reason why our material has not been increased by more than 15 patients during the last 3 years is because of hospital economical reasons. To try to save money, the hospital did not allow us to operate on full capacity during this period.

There are few previous clinical studies using periosteum transplants on cartilage defects at the patella. Their results are not as encouraging as ours, but it is difficult to compare these studies with ours because the surgical technique and postoperative rehabilitation was different. We believe that the anchoring technique of the transplant is very important to prevent loosening of the transplant during the rehabilitation period. The articular surfaces sustain high loads and theoretically wearing effects of the trans-

plant may occur during rehabilitation. In the study by Hoikka and colleagues[10] the transplant was sutured to the surrounding cartilage in seven patients and in six patients also anchored with the use of fibrin glue, while Korkala and Koukkanen[15] sutured the transplant to the surrounding cartilage. With our method, the periosteum transplant is anchored to the bottom of the cartilage defect with the use of throughout sutures tied on the ventral side of the patella and with fibrin glue (Tisseel®) injected under the transplant, to minimize the risk of loosening during rehabilitation training. The postoperative rehabilitation completely differs between the other studies and ours. While most of the patients in the studies by Hoikka and colleagues and Korkala and Koukkanen were immobilized in a cast postoperatively, our patients were treated by CPM followed by active motion (flexion/extension) in the early postoperative period. We believe that the type of postoperative rehabilitation may be of significant importance, and that rigorous immediate postoperative motion plays a central role in the differentiation of the mesenchymal cells in the periostal cambium layer into chondrocytes and finally hyaline-like cartilage. We have demonstrated that CPM in the immediate postoperative period was associated with better clinical results than active motion.[1]

Another factor that may be of importance for the possibilities of regeneration of articular cartilage is the time for introduction of weight-bearing loading on the transplanted area postoperatively. Hypothetically, overloading of the transplanted area could be harmful to the newly built tissue. We do not allow weight-bearing loading on the transplanted area for 3 months postoperatively. After that period, weight-bearing loading is gradually instituted, but if there is pain and/or effusion, the weight-bearing loading is again diminished. In our model of postoperative rehabilitation, we regard pain and effusion as signs of overloading.

We do not know whether it is the mesenchymal cells in the periosteum or the mesenchymal cells in the subchondral bone, or a combination of these cells and other factors such as growth factors, that is responsible for the cartilage-like tissue that is formed after autologous periosteum transplantation. In our surgical method, the sclerotic part of the subchondral bone is always removed, and the bone-plate is perforated. Thereby, theoretically, there are possibilities for mesenchymal stem cells, growth factors, and other factors from the subchondral spongious bone to be involved in the remodeling process beneath the periosteum.

Summary

Full-thickness patellar cartilage defects are troublesome injuries often associated with disabling anterior knee-pain and inability to take part in regular daily activities. Today, there are many methods in use with the purpose of treating cartilage defects; however, despite many years of research there is no method that scientifically has been proven to be superior to others. Consequently, there is no treatment of choice for this condition.

We have used autologous periosteum transplantation since 1991. It is well known that the cells in the cambium layer of the periosteum are pluripotent and can differentiate into hyaline (or hyaline-like) cartilage, especially in a joint environment and under the influence of continuous passive motion. At our clinic, autologous periosteum transplantation alone, followed by continuous passive motion (CPM) in the immediate postoperative period and non-weight-bearing loading for 3 months, has shown promising clinical results. The best clinical results have been achieved on traumatic (fracture, contusion, dislocation) cartilage defects, where 54 out of 77 patients (70%) have been clinically graded as excellent or good at follow-up (>2 years postoperatively). For nontraumatic patellar cartilage defects (chondromalacia NUD) the results are poor, with only 35% of patients being graded as excellent or good. Therefore, we believe that nontraumatic patellar cartilage defects (chondromalacia NUD) are less suitable for treatment with autologous periosteum transplants, and are at our clinic no longer included for this type of treatment.

References

1. Alfredson, H, and R Lorentzon. Superior results with continuous passive motion than active motion after periosteum transplantation: A retrospective study of human patella cartilage defect treatment. *Knee Surg, Sports Traumatol Arthrosc* 1999; 7: 232–238.
2. Benya, PD, and JD Shaffer. Dedifferentiated chondrocytes reexpress the differentiated collagen phenotype when cultured in agarose gels. *Cell* 1982; 30: 215–224.
3. Brittberg, M, A Lindahl, A Nilsson et al. Treatment of deep cartilage defects in the knee with autologous chondrocyte transplantation. *NE J Med* 1994; 331: 889–895.
4. Buchwalter, JA, LC Rosenberg, and EB Hunziker. Articular cartilage: Composition, structure, response to injury and methods of facilitating repair. In Ewing, JW, ed., *Articular Cartilage and Knee Joint Function: Basic Science and Arthroscopy*. New York: Raven Press, 1990, pp. 19–56.
5. Diduch, DR, LCM Jordan, CM Mierish et al. Marrow stromal cells embedded in alginate for repair of osteochondral defects. *Arthroscopy* 2000; 16: 571–577.
6. Fang, HC, YK Yuan, and LJ Miltner. Osteogenic power of tibial periosteum. *Proc Soc Exp Biol Med* 1934; 31: 1239–1240.
7. Fell, HB. The osteogenic capacity in vitro of periosteum and endosteum isolated from the limb skeleton of fowl embryos and young chicks. *J Anat* 1932; 66: 157–180.
8. Gallay, SH, Y Miura, CN Commisso et al. Relationship of donor site to chondrogenic potential of periosteum in vitro. *J Orthop Res* 1994; 12: 515–525.
9. Goshima, J, VM Goldberg, and AI Caplan. The osteogenic potential of culture-expanded rat marrow mesenchymal cells assayed in vivo in calcium phospate ceramic blocks. *Clin Orthop* 1991; 262: 298–311.
10. Hoikka, VEJ, H Jaroma, and V Ritsilä. Reconstruction of the patellar articulation with periosteal grafts. *Acta Orthop Scand* 1990; 61: 36–39.
11. Iwasaki, M, H Nakahara, K Nakata et al. Regulation of proliferation and osteochondrogenic differentiation of periosteum-derived cells by transforming growth factor-β1 and basic fibroblast growth factor. *J Bone Joint Surg* 1995; 77-A: 543–554.
12. Jaroma, H, and V Ritsilä. Reconstruction of patellar cartilage defects with free periosteal grafts. *Scand J Plast Reconstr Surg* 1987; 21: 175–181.
13. Kernek, CB, and JB Wray. Cellular proliferation in the formation of fracture callus in the rat tibia. *Clin Orthop* 1973; 91: 197–209.
14. Korkala, O, and H Kuokkanen. Autogenous osteoperiosteal grafts in the reconstruction of full-thickness joint surface defects. *Int Orthop* 1991; 15: 233–237.
15. Korkala, O, H Kuokkanen. Autoarthroplasty of knee cartilage defects by osteoperiosteal grafts. *Arch Orthop Trauma Surg* 1995; 114:253–256.
16. Lorentzon, R, H Alfredson, and C Hildingsson. Treatment of deep cartilage defects of the patella with periosteal transplantation. *Knee Surg, Sports Traumatol Arthrosc* 1998; 6: 202–208.
17. Mankin, HJ. Current concepts review: The response of articular cartilage to mechanical injury. *J Bone Joint Surg* 1982; 64-A: 460–466.
18. Miura, Y, JS Fitzsimmons, CN Commisso et al. Enhancement of periosteal chondrogenesis in vitro: Dose-response for transforming growth factor-β1. *Clin Orthop* 1994; 301: 271–280.
19. Nakahara, H, VM Goldberg, and AI Caplan. Culture-expanded periosteal-derived cells exhibit osteochondrogenic potential in porous calcium phosphate ceramics in vivo. *Clin Orthop* 1992; 276: 291–298.
20. O'Driscoll, SW, and RB Salter. The induction of neochondrogenesis in free intra-articular periosteal autografts under the influence of continuous passive motion. *J Bone Joint Surg* 1984; 66-A: 1248–1257.
21. O'Driscoll, SW, FW Keeley, and RB Salter. The chondrogenic potential of free autogenous periosteal grafts for biological resurfacing of major full-thickness defects in joint surfaces under the influence of continuous passive motion. *J Bone Joint Surg* 1986; 68-A: 1017–1035.

22. O'Driscoll, SW, FW Keeley, and RB Salter. Durability of regenerated articular cartilage produced by free autogenous periosteal grafts in major full-thickness defects in joint surfaces under the influence of continuous passive motion. *J Bone Joint Surg* 1988; 70-A: 595–606.

23. O'Driscoll, SW, AD Recklies, and AR Poole. Chondrogenesis in periosteal explants. *J Bone Joint Surg* 1994; 76-A: 1042–1050.

24. Ollier, L. *Traité Experimental et Clinique de la Regeneration des Os et de la Production Artificielle du Tissue Osseaux.* Vol 1. Paris: Victor Masson et Fils, 1867.

25. Poussa, M, and V Ritsilä. The osteogenic capacity of free periosteal and osteoperiosteal grafts. *Acta Orthop Scand* 1979; 50: 491–499.

26. Poussa, M, J Rubak, and V Ritsilä. Differentiation of the osteochondrogenic cells of the periosteum in chondrotrophic environment. *Acta Orthop Scand* 1981; 52: 235–239.

27. Rubak, JM. Reconstruction of articular cartilage defects with free periosteal grafts: An experimental study. *Acta Orthop Scand* 1982; 53: 175–180.

28. Rubak, JM, M Poussa, and V Ritsilä. Chondrogenesis in repair of articular cartilage defects by free periosteal grafts in rabbits. *Acta Orthop Scand* 1982; 53: 181–186.

29. Rubak, JM, M Poussa, and V Ritsilä. Effects of joint motion on the repair of articular cartilage with free periostal grafts. *Acta Orthop Scand* 1982; 53: 187–191.

30. Sahlström, A, O Johnell, and I Redlund-Johnell. The natural course of arthrosis of the knee. *Acta Orthop Scand (Suppl 248)* 1993; 63: 57.

31. Salter, RB, DF Simmonds, BW Malcolm et al. The biological effect of continuous passive motion on the healing of full-thickness defects in articular cartilage: An experimental investigation in the rabbit. *J Bone Joint Surg* 1980; 62-A: 1232–1251.

32. Salter, RB, RR Minister, N Clements et al. Continuous passive motion and the repair of full-thickness articular cartilage defects: A one-year follow-up. *Orthop Trans* 1982; 6: 266–267.

33. Spector, TD, JE Dacre, PA Harris et al. Radiological progression of osteoarthritis: An 11-year follow-up study of the knee. *Ann Rheum Dis* 1992; 51: 1107–1110.

34. Vachon, AM, CW McIlwraith, and FW Keeley. Biochemical study of repair of induced osteochondral defects of the distal portion of the radial carpal bone in horses by use of periosteal autografts. *Am J Veter Res* 1991; 52: 328–332.

35. Wakitani, S, T Goto, SJ Pineda et al. Mesenchymal cell-based repair of large, full-thickness defects of articular cartilage. *J Bone Joint Surg* 1994; 76-A: 579–592.

14

Patella Plica Syndrome

Sung-Jae Kim

Introduction

The anatomy of the synovial folds, or plicae, in the knee joint was first described through cadaver dissection by Mayeda[1] in 1918, followed by Hohlbaum,[2] Pipkin,[3,4] Hughston,[5] and Harty and Joyce.[6] Embryologically, although there is no consensus about the development of the joint cavity, it has been widely believed that the knee joint is originally composed of three compartments: medial and lateral synovial compartments and suprapatellar bursa.[7,8] These compartments are partitioned by synovial septums. At about 3 months of fetal age, these synovial septa begin to disappear little by little, and then they vanish completely or remain in part. The folds were not delineated fully in the past, but with the advancement of arthroscopy, their classification and incidences are reported in recent papers.[9,10-12] The plicae are classified according to their corresponding anatomic sites of the knee, as suprapatellar, mediopatellar, infrapatellar, and lateral patellar plicae. Although the three-cavitation theory for development of the knee joint may explain the formation of the suprapatellar and infrapatellar plicae, that of the mediopatellar plica and the lateral patellar plica remains uncertain. Moreover, the theory cannot explain the variety of shapes of the plica. Thus, the variety of patterns of the plica can be chosen as evidence supporting the multiple cavitations theory for development of the knee joint proposed by Gray and Gardner[7] and Ogata[8] and backed up by Kim.[12] There was no consensus concerning the incidence of synovial plicae. In literature review, the reported incidence of each plicae is controversial.[2,3,6,10,11,13-16] In our study including 400 knees in 363 patients,[12] incidence of the synovial plica at the knees were: suprapatellar plica, 87.0%; mediopatellar plica, 72.0%; infrapatellar plica, 86.0%; and lateral patellar plica, 1.3%. These plicae were at first considered abnormal when seen at arthroscopy and then excised. However, the plicae are now recognized as normal structures that represent remnants of synovial membranes in embryonic development of the knee. When chronic inflammation is developed by trauma or the presence of other pathological knee conditions, the pliability of synovial folds might be affected. When a plica of the synovial membrane loses its normal elasticity and becomes fibrotic, it might cause dynamic derangement of the knee called "pathologic plica syndrome."

Suprapatella Plica
Anatomy

The suprapatella plica is a persistent remnant of the embryonic synovial membrane that lies between the suprapatella pouch and the knee joint proper. The suprapatella plica is attached on the superomedial and superolateral wall of the knee joint and also on the undersurface of the quadriceps tendon region in axial plane. When the knee is flexed beyond 90°, the suprapatella plica folds longitudinally rather than in a transverse fold. The incidence rate of suprapatella plica has been widely reported to be from 20% to 87%.[4,10,12,17] The suprapatella plica has a variety of shapes and sizes. Zidorn[11] presented a classification of the suprapatella plica, which classified it into four groups: complete septum type, perforated septum type, residual septum type, and extinct septum type. We also classified each plica as one of the following patterns: absent, vestigial, medial, lateral, arch, hole, or complete septum type, of which the arch type is most frequent (Figures 14.1 and 14.2).[12] Although suprapatella plica is found frequently in the knee joint in variable shapes and sizes, the pathologic suprapatella plica is rarely reported. There have been some reports of symptomatic suprapatella plica, or combination of the suprapatella and medial patella plica.[18,19] Dupont[20] reported 3 symptomatic suprapatella plicae in 12,000 arthroscopies. We reported a case of arch type pathologic suprapatella plica that was excised using an arthroscopic technique (Figure 14.3).[21] The pathophysiology of symptomatic plica has not

been clearly defined. Complete or near-complete type suprapatella plica has been reported to cause intermittent painful swelling of the knee because of its one-way valvular mechanism.[4,22] Some investigators have suggested that synovial changes result from a variety of causes. Blunt trauma, localized hemorrhage, and joint laxity can create symptomatic synovial plica.[23,24] Whatever the reason, as a result, the synovium loses its elasticity, thickens, and becomes inflammatory. This inflammatory process eventually causes fibrosis of the synovial plica followed by serious intra-articular disturbances. The thickened and inflexible structural degeneration of the plica interferes with the patellofemoral gliding mechanism and may

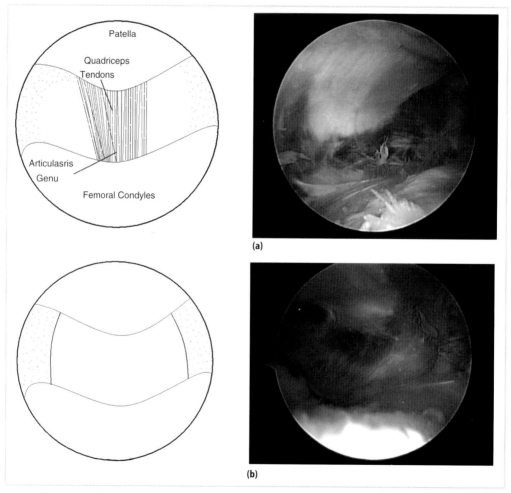

Figure 14.1. Illustrations and arthroscopic findings for patterns of suprapatella plica in the right knee. **(a)** Absent type: No sharp-edged fold of synovium between the suprapatella pouch and the knee joint cavity. **(b)** Vestigial type: A plica with a less than 1 mm protrusion of the synovium.

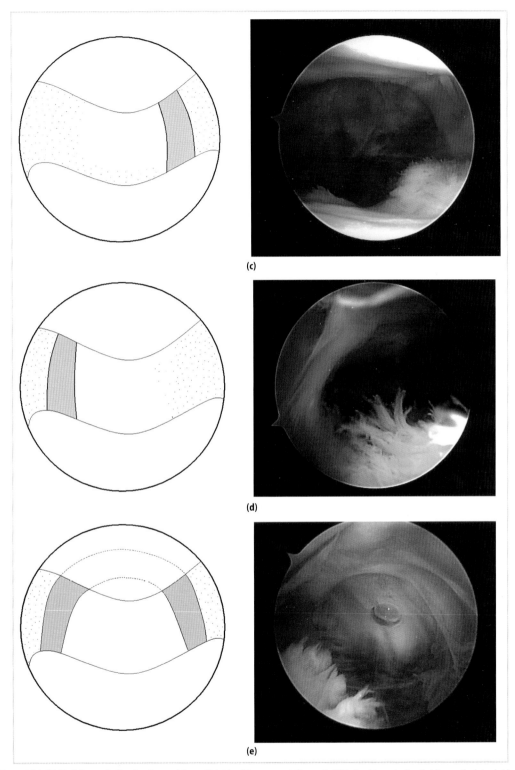

Figure 14.1. (c) Medial type: A plica that lies on th0e medial side of the suprapatella pouch. **(d)** Lateral type: A plica that lies on the lateral side of the suprapatella pouch. **(e)** Arch type: A plica that is present on the medial, lateral, and anterior aspects of the suprapatella pouch but not over the anterior surface of the femur.

(*continued*)

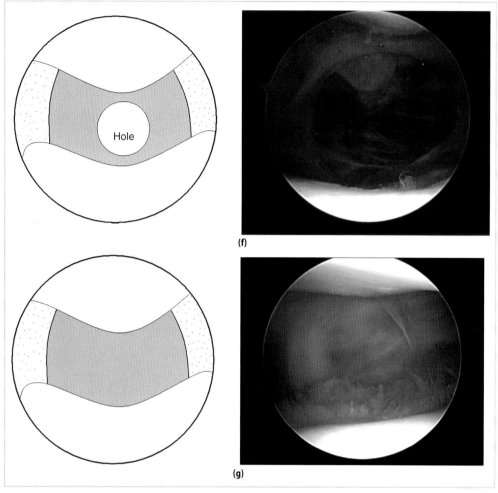

Figure 14.1. *(continued)* **(f)** Hole type: A plica extending completely across the suprapatella pouch but with a central defect. **(g)** Complete septum type: A plica dividing the suprapatella pouch into two separate compartments. Each pattern may have lateral cave, or nothing.

cause changes in the articular surfaces of the patella and femoral condyle. This may be the mechanism of compression of the femoral condyle.[24,25]

Clinical Significance

The clinical characteristics of the pathologic suprapatella plica included chronic intermittent pain of the superior aspect of the knee joint and exercise-related swelling. A palpable bandlike mass on the suprapatella pouch with local tenderness and swelling may be present. The pain was aggravated during stair climbing and while sitting for a long time while the knee was flexed from 45° to 90°. Strover et al.[26] and Kim[21] confirmed that suprapatella plica

impinges between the femoral condyle and quadriceps mechanism when the knee is flexed 70° to 100°. Sometimes, a high-pitched snap can be heard during knee motion. The high-pitched sound characterizes the plica syndrome and differentiates this snap from sounds associated with meniscal derangements and loose bodies, which are lower in pitch.[17,27] The suprapatella plica can provide a good hiding place for loose bodies, especially in complete septum type of plica, in which we cannot identify the insertion of the articularis genu. Diagnosis of the suprapatella plica syndrome is made by recognizing characteristic symptoms and by physical examination. Plain radiography is of little help in establishing a diagnosis.

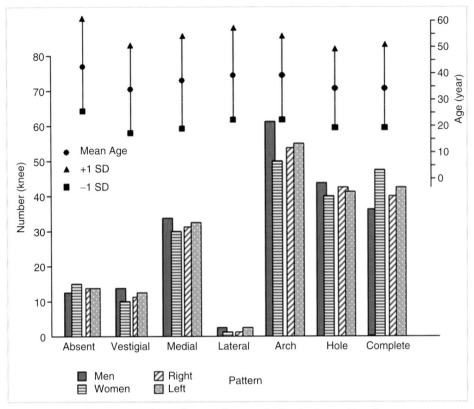

Figure 14.2. Distribution of patterns of suprapatella plica related to sex, side, and age.

Arthrography and magnetic resonance imaging can be of some assistance, but arthroscopy is the gold standard for diagnosing plica syndrome. Plicae that are soft, wavy, vascularized, and synovial-covered are normal findings. However, thick, rounded, or shredded fibrotic plicae with white inner borders should be suspected for pathological changes. Only those plicae that have been confirmed as pathological should be excised meticulously.

Medial Patellar Plica Anatomy

The medial patellar plica is a synovial fold that originates on the medial wall of the knee joint, runs obliquely down in coronal plane, and inserts into the medial synovial lining of the infrapatellar fat pad. Synovial plicae are thin, pink, and flexible. It may be connected with the suprapatellar plica, but is usually separated. The incidence of medial patellar plicae reported in the literature has ranged from 18.5% to 72.0%.[9,12,28-30] The

appearance of each plica was classified in one of the following patterns according in its shape: absent, vestigial, shelf, reduplicated, fenestra, or high riding (Figures 14.4 and 14.5).

Sometimes the wide shelf type obstructed arthroscopic examination of the medial compartment. The incidence of medial patella plica reported has ranged from 18.5% to 72% of the knees. The most common pattern is the shelf.[12]

Medial Patellar Plica (MPP) Syndrome

The normal synovial folds in the knee are asymptomatic. The pathogenic processes of a medial patellar plica are initiated by various etiologic factors, from direct trauma such as direct blow or strain during athletic activity to the intrinsic conditions that develop into synovitis. The incidence rate of pathologic MPP has been reported as from 3.25% to 11% of cases.[18,31-36]

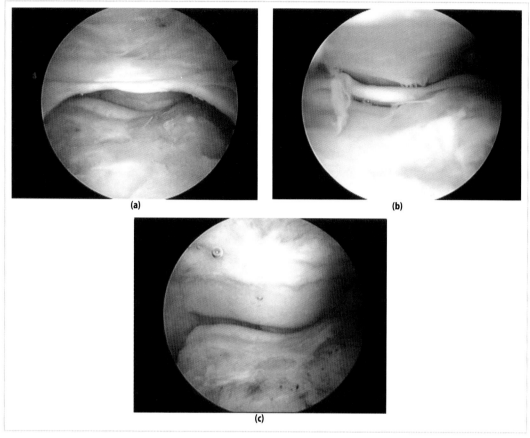

Figure 14.3. The pathologic suprapatella plica seen from the superomedial portal. **(a)** Full extension. **(b)** 100° flexion. Impingement of plica between the femoral condyle and quadriceps femoris tendon. **(c)** View following excision of pathologic suprapatella plica.

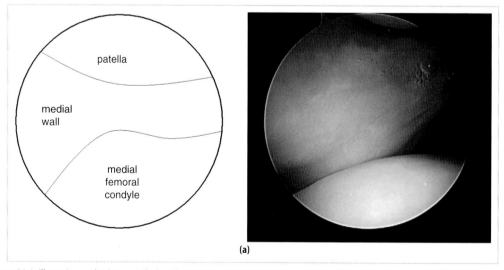

Figure 14.4. Illustrations and arthroscopic findings for patterns of medial patella plica. **(a)** Absent type: The pattern was considered to be absent if the synovial shelf did not exist on the medial wall.

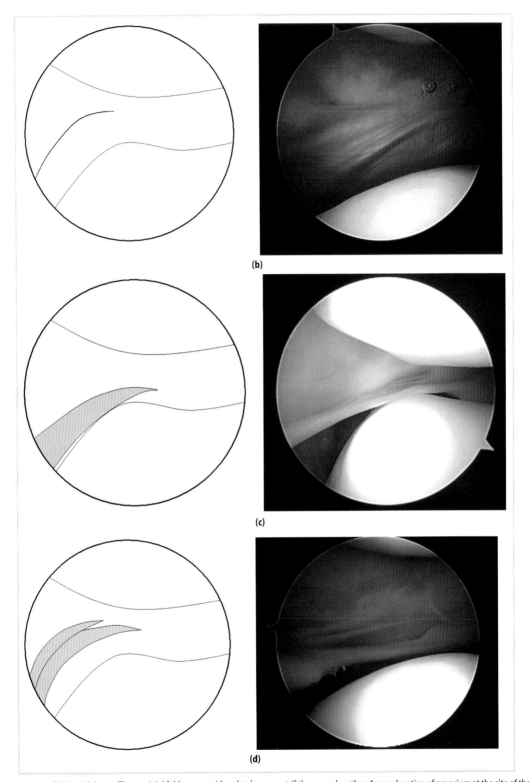

Figure 14.4. (b) Vestigial type: The vestigial fold was considered to be present if there was less than 1 mm elevation of synovium at the site of the shelf. It may disappear under outside digital compression. **(c)** Shelf: The synovium that formed a complete fold with a sharp free margin was classified as shelf. **(d)** Reduplicated: Two or more shelves ran parallel on the medial wall of the knee. The shelves all varied in size.

(continued)

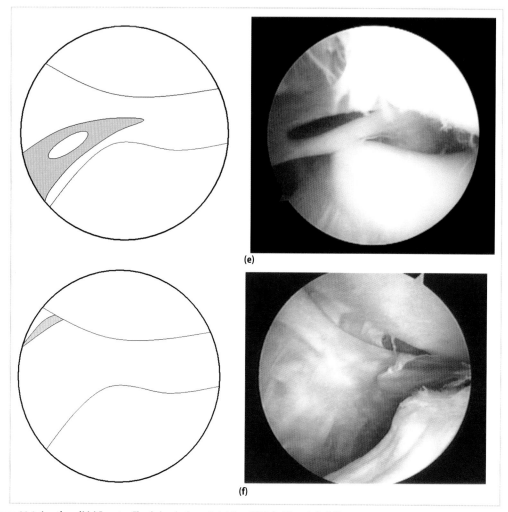

Figure 14.4. *(continued)* **(e)** Fenestra: The shelves had a central defect. **(f)** High-riding: A shelf-like structure was sometimes seen anterior to the posterior aspect of the patella, in a position where it could not touch the femur.

Then inflammatory reaction eventually causes fibrosis of the synovial plica, which loses its elasticity and becomes a thick and inflexible structure. As a result, hardened, bow-stringing plica over the medial femoral condyle impinges the condyle and is entrapped between the patella and the femoral condyle (Figure 14.6). Chondromalacia on one side or both sides of the patellofemoral joint is observed in over half the cases (93 knees [65%] among the 142 symptomatic MPP in our series).

The principal symptom of the pathologic MPP is intermittent anterior knee pain, which is exacerbated by activity such as descending with or without ascending stairs and associated with painful clicking, giving way, and the feeling of catching in the knee.[19] Tender bend may be palpable approximately on fingerbreadth medial from the patella and rolling over the medial femoral condyle may be palpable with the knee motion (rolling over sign).

MPP syndrome may be difficult to differentiate from chondromalacia patella,[37-39] patellofemoral subluxation,[40,41] patellar compression syndrome,[42] and meniscal tears[43] due to similar symptom complex.

Tests

Although diagnostic accuracy is improving with the use of magnetic resonance imaging, diagnosis of pathologic MPP has been troublesome to orthopedic surgeons. A carefully documented

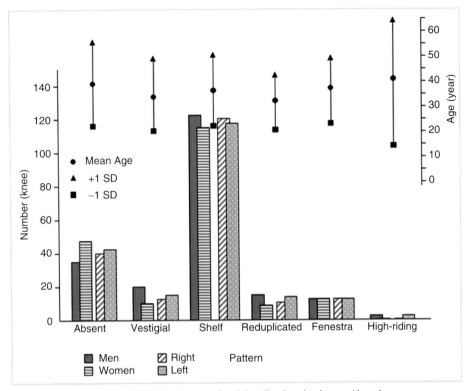

Figure 14.5. Distribution of patterns of medial patellar plica related to sex, side, and age.

history and physical examination remain the most important for the diagnosis of MPP syndrome. Some clinical tests have been introduced to improve the diagnostic accuracy, such as MPP test,[44] knee extension test,[4] flexion test,[45] rotation valgus test, and holding test.[46]

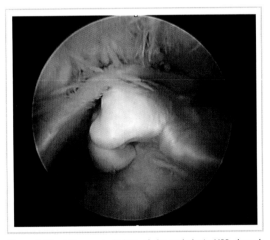

Figure 14.6. Arthroscopic finding of the pathologic MPP through superolateral view.

- *MPP test.* The MPP test was conducted with the patient supine and the knee extended. Using the thumb, manual force was applied to press the inferomedial portion of the patellofemoral joint, so as to insert the medial plica between the medial femoral condyle and the patella causing tenderness (Figures 14.7 and 14.8).

  While maintaining this force, the knee was flexed at 90°. The MPP test was defined to be positive when the patient experienced pain with the knee in extension and eliminated or markedly diminished pain with the knee in 90° of flexion (Figure 14.9). The symptomatic knee was compared with the knee on the opposite side.

- *Knee extension test.* The knee extension test is performed by extending the knee from 90 degrees of flexion, while internally rotating the leg and pushing the patella medially. The knee typically pops as a consequence of the presence of a pathologic plica between 60 degrees and 45 degrees of flexion. However, the popping disappears during the day because of formation of effusion in the knee.

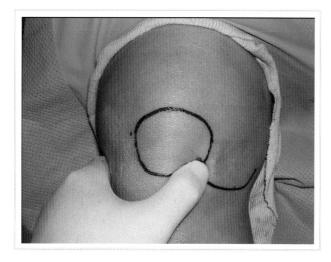

Figure 14.7. Using the thumb, manual force was applied to press the inferomedial portion of the patellofemoral joint.

- *Flexion test.* While gentle pressure is maintained over the plica, the knee is passively flexed no more than 6 times. The test is positive when the patient experiences pain or discomfort that corresponds to their presenting symptoms.
- *Rotation valgus test.* The examiner flexes the patient's knee and forces it into a valgus position, with the patella pushed medially and the lower leg internally or externally rotated. Knee pain with or without a palpable click of the shelf is a positive sign.

- *Holding test.* The knee is held in the fully extended position. The examiner flexes the knee against patient's extension with the patella pushed medially. Knee pain with or without a palpable click of the shelf is a positive sign.

Management

Suspected diagnosis of MPP syndrome should be managed conservatively. Conservative therapy is especially effective in younger patients with short duration symptoms. Nonoperative modalities

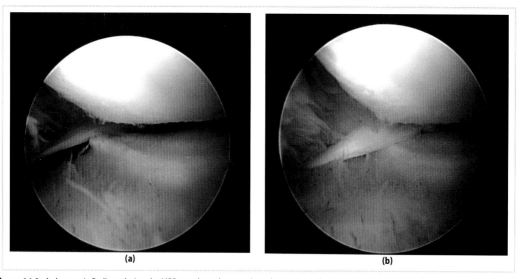

Figure 14.8. Arthroscopic findings during the MPP test through superolateral view. **(a)** Before MPP test. **(b)** With thumb pressure on the inferomedial portion of the patellofemoral joint, the medial plica is entrapped between the medial femoral condyle and the patella causing tenderness.

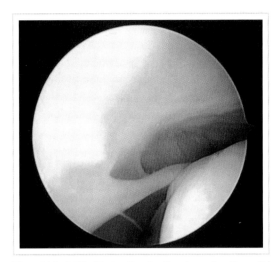

Figure 14.9. At 90° of flexion, the plica slipped away from the medial femoral condyle.

include rest, nonsteroidal anti-inflammatory agents, hamstring stretches, and quadriceps-strengthening exercise. If the clinical syndrome fails to subside after 3 to 6 months of nonoperative management, then arthroscopic excision of pathologic MPP should be considered rather than division or release to avoid recurrence.

Arthroscopic Technique

Two portals are used: high anterolateral portal and superolateral portal. For the diagnosis of associated intra-articular pathological conditions and pathologic MPP, the arthroscope is positioned through a high anterolateral portal. Then the arthroscope is moved into superolateral portal, allowing the plica to be viewed from above. While viewing through the superolateral portal, the MPP test was done without overdistension of the knee joint. After pathologic MPP was confirmed, total arthroscopic excision was performed using basket forceps and motorized shaver.

Infrapatellar Plica

The infrapatellar plica is the vestigial remnant of the embryological vertical septum. It is commonly called as the ligamentum mucosum. It is a synovial fold that originates from the intercondylar notch, runs parallel to and above the anterior cruciate ligament, and attaches to the infrapatellar fat pad. Posteriorly, the plica is separated from the anterior cruciate ligament, but it may be attached to the anterior cruciate ligament either completely or partially.[47] The appearance of the plica was classified as one of the following patterns according to its shape: absent, separate, split, vertical septum, or fenestra. (Figures 14.10 and 14.11).[12]

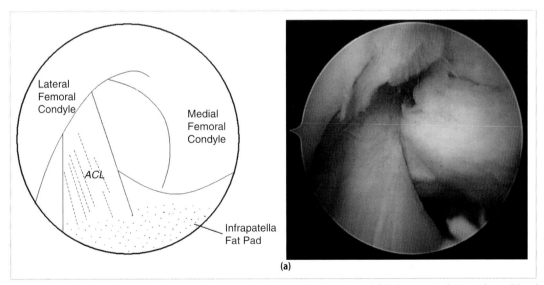

(a)

Figure 14.10. Illustrations for patterns of infrapatellar plica in the right knee. **(a)** Absent: Synovial fold does not exist between the condyles of the femur.

(continued)

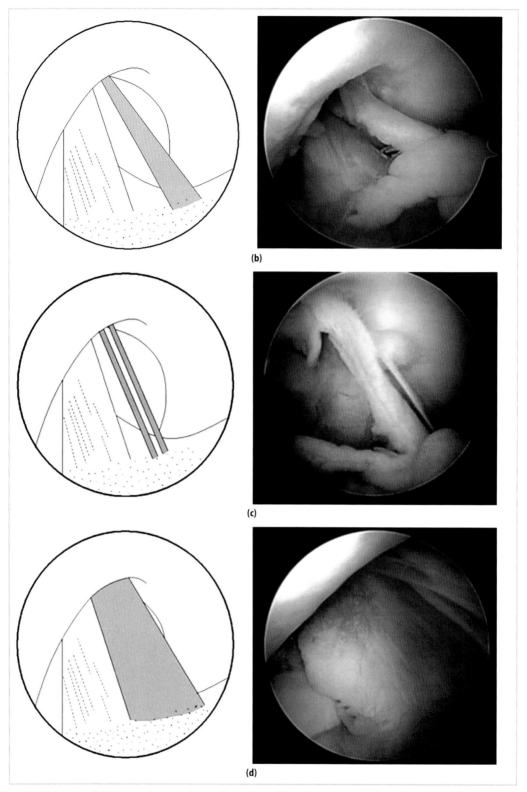

Figure 14.10. *(continued)* **(b)** Separate: Synovial fold is completely separated from the anterior cruciate ligament. It comes in various thicknesses: slender or thick. **(c)** Split: Synovial fold is not only separated from the anterior cruciate ligament but also divided into two or more bands. **(d)** Vertical septum: Synovial fold is a complete vertical synovial septum, in continuity with the anterior cruciate ligament. The plica divides the anterior joint cavity into the medial and lateral compartments.

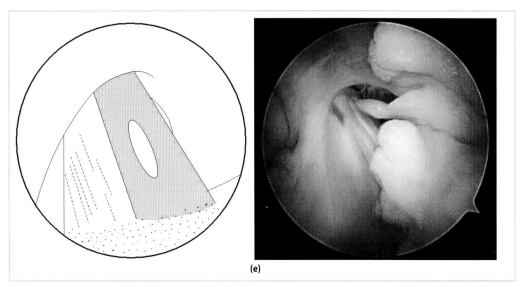

(e)

Figure 14.10. *(continued)* **(e)** Fenestra: If the vertical septum has a hole, the plica is classified as fenestra pattern.

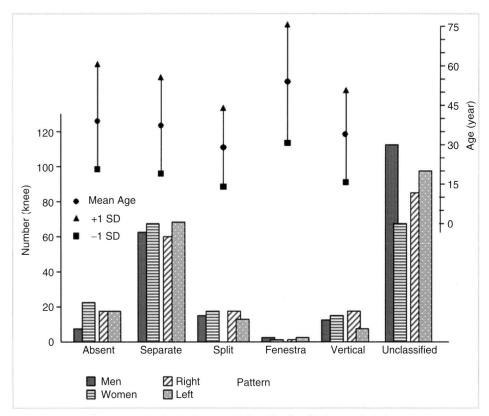

Figure 14.11. Distribution of patterns of infrapatellar plica related to sex, side, and age.

On occasion, a plica may become symptomatic. It is then responsible for the so-called plica syndrome.[17] Chronic inflammation initiated by trauma or other pathological knee conditions affects the pliability of the synovial folds. When a plica of the synovial membrane loses its normal elasticity and becomes fibrotic, it can be a cause of dynamic derangement of the knee.[48,49] Mediopatellar plica and suprapatellar plica cause symptoms occasionally.[24,50] Although it is generally agreed that the infrapatellar plica does not cause symptoms,[17,24,50] we have experiences with pathologic infrapatellar plica with limitation in knee extension in three cases.[51,52] On the physical examinations, these patients revealed flexion contractures of 20 to 25 degrees and atrophy of the thigh musculature. Two patients' cases were vertical septum patterns (Figure 14.12), and the other case exhibited fenestra pattern (Figure 14.13) on the arthroscopic examination. After arthroscopic excision and immediate postoperative exercise, full active range of motion of the knee was gained in all these patients.

The thick type of separate pattern or the vertical septum pattern frequently accompanies the hypertrophy of the infrapatellar fat pad; thus it may obstruct the arthroscopic view.

Lateral Patellar Plica

Lateral plica is rare. It originates in the lateral wall above the popliteus hiatus of the lateral gutter and attaches to the infrapatellar fat pad in axial plane. It prevents viewing of the popli-

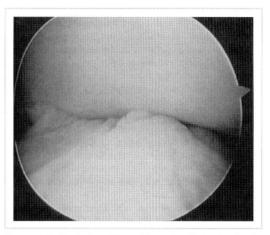

Figure 14.12. The thickened fibrotic infrapatellar plica impinged to the intercondylar trochlea, resulting in limitation of extension of the knee.

teus hiatus or manipulation of the arthroscope from the anterolateral portal into the lateral gutter. The pattern of each plica is classified as absent, shelf, or fenestra (Figures 14.14 and 14.15).[12]

Unusually, lateral plica may produce symptoms. In the literature review, pathologic lateral plica syndrome is reported.[53-56] Patients complain of chronic pain and frequent painful snapping at the lateral side of patella. On examination, a cordlike painful thickening may be palpable. Pain is alleviated and the snapping disappears after the arthroscopic excision of lateral plica.

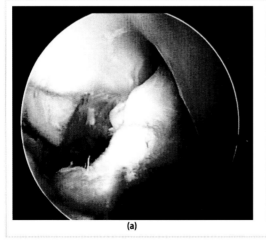
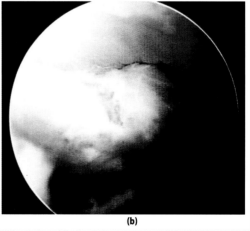

(a)   (b)

Figure 14.13. The fenestra type of infrapatellar plica was thickened and fibrotic and had lost its elasticity. **(a)** In flexion. **(b)** In extension.

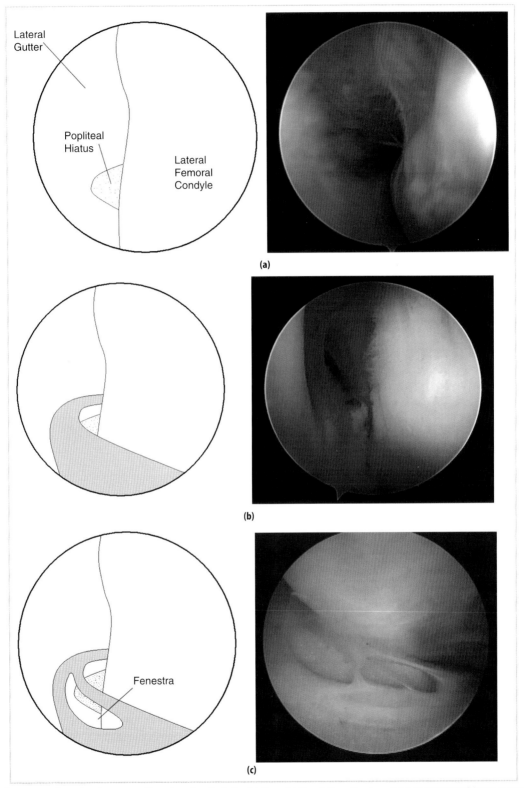

(a)

(b)

(c)

Figure 14.14. Illustrations for patterns of lateral patellar plica in the right knee. **(a)** Absent: The pattern is considered to be absent if the synovium at the site of the shelf was completely smooth. **(b)** Shelf: The synovium forms a complete shelf with a sharp free margin. Thus, it looks like a shelf under arthroscopy. **(c)** Fenestra: If the shelves have a central defect, the plica is described as fenestra.

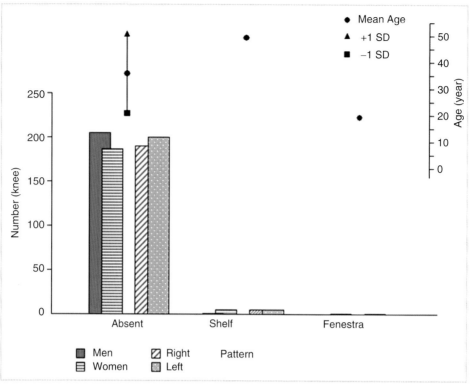

Figure 14.15. Distribution of patterns of lateral patellar plica related to sex, side, and age.

References

1. Mayeda, T. Uber das Strangartige Gebilde in der Knigelenkhle (Chorda cavi articularis Genu). *Mitt Med Fak Kaiserl Univ Tokyo* 1918; 21: 507–553.
2. Hohlbaum, J. Die bursa suprapatellaris und ihre Beziehungenzum Kniegelenke: Ein Beitrag zur Endwicklung der angeborenen Schleimbeutel. *Beitr Z Klin Chir* 1923; 128: 481–498.
3. Pipkin, G. Lesions of the suprapatellar plica. *J Bone Joint Surg Am* 1950; 32: 363–369.
4. Pipkin, G. Knee injuries: The role of suprapatella plica and suprapatella bursa in simulating internal derangement. *Clin Orthop* 1971; 74: 161–176.
5. Hughston, JC, GS Whatley, RA Dodelin, and MM Stone. The role of the suprapatellar plica in internal derangement of the knee. *Am J Orthop* 1963; 5: 25–27.
6. Harty, M, and JJ Joyce III. Synovial folds in the knee joint. *Orthop Rev* 1977; 6: 91–92.
7. Gary, DJ, and E Gardner. Prenatal development of the human knee and superior tibiofibular joints. *Am J Anat* 1950; 86: 235–287.
8. Ogata, S, and HK Uhthoff. The development of synovial plicae in human knee joints: an embryologic study. *Arthroscopy* 1990; 6: 315–321.
9. Sakakibara, J. Arthroscopic study on Iino's band (plica synovialis mediopatellaris). *J Jpn Orthop Assoc* 1976;50: 513–522.
10. Dandy, DJ. Anatomy of the medial suprapatellar plica and medial synovial shelf. *Arthroscopy* 1990; 6: 79–85.
11. Zidorn, T. Classification of the suprapatellar septum considering ontogenetic development. *Arthroscopy* 1991; 8: 459–464.
12. Kim, SJ, and WS Choe. Arthroscopic findings of the synovial plicae of the knee. *Arthroscopy.* 1997; Feb., 13: 33–41.
13. Patel, D. Arthroscopy of the plicae synovial folds and their significance. *Am J Sports Med* 1978; 6: 217–225.
14. Kenji, Y. über dei Schleimbeutel und Nebenhohlen des Kniegelenkes bei den Japanern. *Folia Anat Jpn* 1928; 6: 191–240.
15. Schafer, H. Die Synovialhhle des Kniegelenkes und ihre grossen kommunizierenden Bursen. *Fortschr Rontgenstr* 1989; 150: 32–38.
16. Watanabe, M, S Takeda, H Ikeuchi, and J Sakakibara. On the chorda cavi articularis genu (Mayeda) from the viewpoint of arthroscopy. *Clin Orthop Surg(Japanese)* 1972; 7: 986–991.
17. Hardaker, WT Jr, TL Whipple, and FH Bassett III. Diagnosis and treatment of the plica syndrome of the knee. *J Bone Joint Surg Am* 1980; 62: 221–225.
18. Dorchak, JD, RL Barrack, JS Kneisl, and AH Alexander. Arthroscopic treatment of symptomatic synovial plica of the knee: Long-term follow-up. *Am J Sports Med* 1991; 19: 503–507.
19. Johnson, DP, DM Eastwood, and PJ Witherbow. Symptomatic synovial plica of the knee. *J Bone Joint Surg Am* 1993; 75: 1485–1496.

20. Dupont, JY. Les replies synoviaux du genou: Aspects anatomiques, physiopathologiques et cliniques. *J Traumatol Sport* 1990; 7: 25–38.

21. Kim, SJ, SJ Shin, and TY Koo. Arch type pathologic suprapatella plica. *Arthroscopy* 2001; 17: 536–538.

22. Ross, KR, and MMS Glasscow. The suprapatella plica. *J Bone Joint Surg Br* 1984; 66: 280.

23. Patel, D. Plica as a cause of anterior knee pain. *Orthop Clin North Am* 1986; 17: 273–277.

24. Tindel, NL, and B Nisonson. The plica syndrome. *Orthop Clin North Am* 1992; 23: 613–618.

25. Amatuzzi, M, A Fazzi, and MH Varella. Pathologic synovial plica of the knee. Results of conservative treatment. *Am J Sports Med* 1990; 18: 466–469.

26. Strover, AE, E Rouholamin, N Guirguis, and H Behdad. An arthroscopic technique of demonstrating the pathomechanics of the suprapatella plica. *Arthroscopy* 1991; 7: 308–310.

27. Bae, DK, GU Nam, SD Sun, and YH Kim. The clinical significance of the complete type of suprapatella membrane. *Arthroscopy* 1998; 14: 830–835.

28. Lino, S. Normal arthroscopic findings in the knee joint in adult cadavers. *J Jpn Orthop Assoc* 1939; 14: 467–523.

29. Aoki, T. The "ledge" lesion in the knee. *Proceedings 12th Congress of the International Society of Orthopaedic Surgery and Traumatology. Excerpta Medica International Congress Series,* No. 291, Amsterdam, Excerpta Medica, 1973, p. 462.

30. Jackson, RW, DJ Marshall, and Y Fujisawa. The pathologic medical shelf. *Orthop Clin North Am* 1982; Apr., 13(2): 307–312.

31. Munzinger, U, J Ruckstuhl, H Scherrer, and N Gschwend. Internal derangement of the knee joint due to pathologic synovial folds: The mediopatellar plica syndrome. *Clin Orthop.* 1981; Mar.–Apr., 155: 59–64.

32. Nottage, WM, NF Sprague III, BJ Auerbach, and H Shahriaree. The medial patellar plica syndrome. *Am J Sports Med* 1983; July–Aug., 11(4): 211–214.

33. Broom, MJ, and JP Fulkerson. The plica syndrome: a new perspective. *Orthop Clin North Am* 1986; Apr., 17(2): 279–281.

34. Brabants, K, S Geens, and L Blondeel. Plica synovialis mediopatellaris. *Acta Orthop Belg* 1988; 54(4): 474–476.

35. Richmond, JC, and JB McGinty. Segmental arthroscopic resection of the hypertrophic mediopatellar plica. *Clin Orthop* 1983; Sep., 178: 185–189.

36. Glasgow, M, DJ McClelland, J Campbell, and RW Jackson. The synovial plica and its pathological significance in the knee. *J Bone Joint Surg Br* 1981; 63: 630.

37. Aleman, O. Chondromalacia post traumatic patellae. *Acta Chir Scandinavica* 1928; 63: 149–189.

38. Dehaven, KE, WA Dolan, and PJ Mayer. Chondromalacia patellae in athletes: Clinical presentation and conservative management. *Am J Sports Med* 1979; Jan.–Feb., 7(1): 5–11.

39. Ficat, RP, J Philippe, and DS Hungerford. Chondromalacia patellae: A system of classification. *Clin Orthop* 1979; Oct., 144: 55–62.

40. Broom, HJ, and JP Holkerson. The plica syndrome: A new perspective. *Orthop Clin North America* 1986; 17: 297–281.

41. Sherman, RMP, and RW Jackson. The pathologic medial plica: Criteria for diagnosis and prognosis. *J Bone and Joint Surg* 1989; 71-B(2): 351.

42. Larson, RL, HE Cabaud, DB Slocun, SL Hanes, T Keenan, and T Hutchison. The patellar compression syndrome: surgical treatment by lateral retinacular release. *Clin. Orthop* 1978; 134: 158–167.

43. Dandy, DJ, and RW Jackson. The diagnosis of problems after meniscectomy. *J Bone and Joint Surg* 1975; 57-B(3): 349–352.

44. Kim, SJ, JH Jeong, YM Cheon, SW Ryu. MPP test in the diagnosis of medial patellar plica syndrome. *Arthroscopy* 2004; Dec., 20(10): 1101–1103.

45. Flanagan, JP, S Trakru, M Meyer, AB Mullaji, and F Krappel. Arthroscopic excision of symptomatic medial plica. *Acta Orthop Scand* 1994; 65: 408–411

46. Koshino T, and R Okamoto. Resection of painful shelf (Plic synovialis mediopatellaris) under arthroscopy. *Arthroscopy* 1985; 1: 136–141.

47. Kim, S-J, B-H Min, and H-K Kim. Arthroscopic anatomy of the infrapatellar plica. *Arthroscopy* 1996;12: 561–564.

48. Patel, D. Synovial lesions: Plicae. In McGinty, JB, ed., *Operative Arthroscopy.* New York: *Raven,* 1996, pp. 447–458.

49. Mital, M, and J Hayden. Pain in the knee in children: The medial plical shelf syndrome. *Orthop Clin North Am* 1979; 10: 713–722.

50. Subotnick, SI, and P Sisney. The plica syndrome: A cause of knee pain in the athlete. *J Am Pediatric Med Assoc* 1986; 76: 292–293.

51. Kim, S-J, and W-S Choe. Pathologic infrapatellar plica: A report of two cases and literature review. *Arthroscopy* 1996; 12: 236–239.

52. Kim, S-J, J-Y Kim, and J-W Lee. Pathologic infrapatellar plica. *Arthroscopy* 2002; 18(5): E25.

53. Bough, BW, and BF Regan. Medial and Lateral synovial plicae of the knee: Pathological significance, diagnosis and treatment by arthroscopic surgery. *Irish Med J* 1985; 78: 279–282.

54. Fujisawa, Y, N Matsumoto, S Shiomi et al. Problems caused by the medial and lateral synovial folds of the patella (in Japanese). *Kansetsukyo* 1976; 1: 40–44.

55. Kurosawa, S, S Koide, T Yaota et al. Disorders of the knee caused by synovial plicae: So-called plica syndrome. *Clin Orthop Surg* 1979; 11: 231–237.

56. Kurosaka, M, S Yoshiya, M Yamada, and K Hirohata. Lateral synovial plica syndrome. A case report. *Am J Sports Med* 1992; 20(1): 92–94.

15

Patellar Tendinopathy:
Where Does the Pain Come From?

Karim M. Khan and Jill L. Cook

Introduction

The aim of this chapter is to address the question: Where is the pain coming from in patellar tendinopathy? Although a traditional answer would be "inflammatory cells," this is unlikely to be correct. In this chapter we first summarize the evidence that overuse patellar tendon injury (henceforth called patellar tendinopathy) is not primarily an inflammatory condition.[1] We then outline some noninflammatory mechanisms that may produce patellar tendon pain. This topic is clinically relevant because patient management will be greatly simplified when we eventually understand what causes the pain of patellar tendinopathy.

Overuse Tendinosis – Not Tendinitis

It has been widely assumed that patellar tendon overuse caused inflammation, and therefore, pain. Despite the pervasiveness of this dogma, a large body of evidence contradicts this assumption.[2-4] It has become clear that the true cause of pain lies elsewhere: It may be mechanical discontinuity of collagen fibers, biochemical irritation that results from damaged tendon tissue activating nociceptors[5,6] or neovascularization.[7] Alternatively, unique anatomical features may produce pain at the patellar tendon, such as impingement[8] or stress shielding.[9]

For many years, it was widely believed[10] that patellar tendinopathy had an inflammatory basis (Figure 15.1). Pain and inflammation have been linked since Celsus (AD 14–37) reported the association of "rubor et tumor cum calor et dolor."[11,12] The clinical label "patellar ten-

donitis" implies that inflammation is present. Furthermore, nonsteroidal and corticosteroidal anti-inflammatory agents are popular treatment modalities. Ultrasound[13] and magnetic resonance imaging[14] papers have reported the presence of "inflammatory fluid" around symptomatic patellar tendons and thus reinforced this model.

As long ago as 1976, Giancarlo Puddu of Rome documented that the pathology in what was clinically known as "Achilles tendonitis" was separation and fragmentation of collagen, which he labeled "tendinosis."[15] Since then, numerous authors have shown that tendinosis is the predominant pathology in patellar tendinopathy[4] and these findings are briefly reviewed here and discussed in detail in the next chapter.

Macroscopically, the patellar tendon of patients with patellar tendinopathy contains soft, yellow-brown and disorganized tissue in the deep posterior portion of the patellar tendon adjacent to the lower pole of the patella.[16-18] This macroscopic appearance is often described as "mucoid" degeneration.[19,20] Under the light microscope, there is a loss of the normal tightly bundled parallel collagen fiber appearance; instead fibers are in disarray and separated by increased ground substance. Collagen degeneration with variable fibrosis and neovascularization was a consistent feature across studies.[21]

When imaging studies in athletes with patellar tendinopathy were correlated with histopathology, areas of hypoechogenicity on ultrasonography[3] and increased signal on MR imaging[2,3] corresponded with collagen and mucoid degeneration.

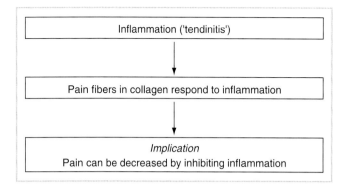

Figure 15.1. The classical "inflammatory" model of tendon pain.

Does a Short-term Inflammatory "Patellar Tendinitis" Precede the Noninflammatory Tendinosis?

Some consider that tendinosis is the end-stage of a continuum that begins with normal tendon and passes through a period of painful "tendinitis" (Figure 15.2). Although this is plausible, there is no evidence for a significant interim phase of "tendinitis" in overuse tendinopathy. Data to explore this question comes from biopsy samples in athletes with patellar tendinopathy, biopsies taken in cases of patellar tendon rupture, and animal models of tendinopathy.

In our histopathological study of athletes who underwent surgery for jumper's knee,[3] several subjects were operated on after only 4 months of pain, and even in these cases inflammatory cells were absent. Patellar tendinopathy is thought to progress distally from the proximal pole with time, as the hypoechoic region enlarges.[22] Thus, we identified the proximal patellar attachment of the specimens obtained at surgery with a suture, and the histopathologist was able to carefully scrutinize the transition from abnormal to normal[3] (Figure 15.3). If tendinitis were to always precede tendinosis, then this region

should contain evidence of tendinitis. However, there were no inflammatory cells at this transition area, suggesting that if there is such a phase of tendinitis, it is rather brief.

Further human evidence for tendinosis arising without a period of painful tendinitis comes from studies of tendon ruptures. Pekka Kannus and Laszlo Józsa examined tendon tissue in cases of spontaneous patellar tendon rupture and found preexisting degenerative tendon pathology (tendinosis) at sites near, but distinct from, the rupture even in patients who had never had any tendon symptoms.[23] By deduction, painful tendinitis is not a prerequisite for tendinosis.

There are no animal models of patellar tendinopathy but experiments causing overuse tendinopathy of the plantaris tendon and Achilles tendon provide important histopathological specimens of tendon tissue soon after injury. This provides insight as to the length of any inflammatory tendinitis that precedes collagen degeneration.

In a rat plantaris tendinopathy model[24] tendons were examined at 1 and 2 weeks. At both these times there was no evidence of inflamma-

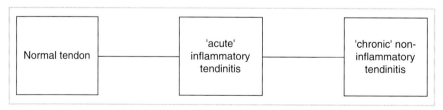

Figure 15.2. Proposed transition from normal tendon, through "tendinitis," to tendinosis.

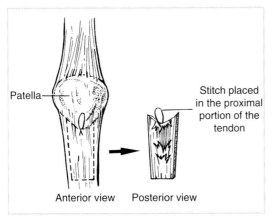

Figure 15.3. A method to examine histopathology of tendon tissue that may only recently have become abnormal. In patients who underwent patellar tendon surgery for chronic jumper's knee, the abnormal tissue was excised completely as shown (dotted line) and a stitch of 4/0 silk was placed in the proximal portion so that the histopathologist could orient the specimen. It would be expected that the distal tendon tissue had become abnormal more recently than the proximal tendon as patellar tendinopathy normally extends distally from the proximal pole with time. Tendinosis diminished in severity with distance from the patella but there was no evidence of a transition zone of "tendinitis" at the border between normal and abnormal tissue.[3]

tion but there was strong evidence of tendon repair, as quiescent fibroblasts had transformed into rounded, active cells. These cells were identical to those found in human overuse tendinopathy.

Backman and colleagues developed a rabbit model to study overuse Achilles tendinopathy using transcutaneous stimulation of the calf muscle.[25] They reported degenerative collagen changes ("fibrillation") and neovascularization, together with some inflammatory cells in the adipose tissue close to the paratenon. They considered this histopathology to be "identical to those reported in biopsy material from professional runners and joggers with sustained Achilles tendon complaints admitted for surgery after months or years of non-beneficial conservative management."[25]

Chukuka Enwemeka from Kansas examined the issue of duration of tendon inflammation in a surgical tenotomy model.[26] This surgical model is known to generate much more inflammation than an overuse model. In this experiment, rats had the Achilles tendon severed transversely and then reapproximated and sutured with three loops of 3/0 surgical silk. The skin was closed and the limb immobilized. This intervention produced a prominent inflam-

matory response that peaked at 5 days and disappeared by day 18. Thus, even in a model predicted to stimulate considerably more inflammation than an overuse injury model, inflammatory cells disappeared within 3 weeks of surgical insult. Although healing of rat tendons does not necessarily translate directly into healing in humans, these data suggest that inflammation is not a lengthy process in tendon repair, even after surgical tenotomy.

Thus, human and animal data downplay the role of inflammation in the pain of chronic patellar tendinopathy. Although there may be a period of inflammation for a few days after certain tendon injuries, symptoms that are present for more than one week must arise from a noninflammatory mechanism. Noninflammatory mechanisms that may explain pain include mechanical models (collagen separation, tissue impingement), neurovascular models (neovascularization), and biochemical models. These models are the focus of the rest of this chapter.

Can Noninflammatory Mechanisms of Tendon Pain Explain the Pain-relieving effect of Corticosteroid Injections?

We cannot exhort the reader to abandon the inflammatory model of chronic tendinopathy without discussing the effect of corticosteroid injections. One of the most frequent questions we are asked when presenting these histopathological findings in tendinopathy is "Why do corticosteroids work?" Whether or not corticosteroids benefit patients with tendinopathy is an issue that is the focus of other articles.[27-32] Nevertheless, both clinical experience and randomized studies[33,34] have shown these medications provide at least short-term pain relief. Also, the protease inhibitor aprotinin has been shown to relieve tendon pain.[35]

It has been postulated that any chemical agent (e.g., corticosteroids) may bathe the region of tendinosis and alter the chemical composition of the matrix (e.g., pH level).[21] Fenestration of an area of tendinosis with needling may promote beneficial bleeding into new channels created through degenerated mucoid tissue. This mechanical disruption may transform a failed intrinsic healing response into a therapeutic extrinsic one. At present, the mechanism of pain relief from these agents remains unknown – and this will likely remain the case until the mechanism of pain in tendinosis itself is understood.

Mechanical Models of Pain in Tendinopathy

Mechanical models of patellar tendon pain include those that attribute pain to damage to collagen fibers and those associated with tissue catching between the patella and the proximal tibia. We begin with theories of pain arising from collagen damage.

Collagen Fiber Disruption and Patellar Tendon Pain

This model is based on the premise that collagen fibers are pain free when intact and painful when disrupted (Figure 15.4). This is analogous to the mechanism of acute ligament sprain. While nobody would deny that acute tearing of collagen causes pain (e.g., acute partial tendon tears), we have observed numerous situations where tendons are not completely intact, yet remain pain free. These observations are listed to highlight that tendon pain may not be due to a straightforward relationship between mechanical collagen separation and pain.

Observations about Tendon Pain and Surgical Findings

Two types of surgery performed on the patellar tendon – ACL autograft reconstruction and tenotomy for painful jumper's knee – illuminate the relationship between collagen and tendon pain. Consider first the middle third patellar tendon autograft ACL reconstruction. Individuals who undergo this operation have minimal donor site knee pain, yet collagen has been excised (Figure 15.5). Even at 2 years postoperatively, the donor site may have significant histological abnormality, yet remain pain free.[36,37]

Some would argue that completely excised collagen contains no intact fibers to produce pain, just as a complete ligament rupture is less painful than a substantial partial rupture. Nevertheless, in the postoperative period some patients develop pain consistent with patellar tendinopathy, indicating that healing collagen can become painful.[38] When imaged, the painful tendon donor site remains indistinguishable from that in individuals who remain pain free.[38,39] This indicates that the relationship between pain and collagen status is not one that can be detected at the macroscopic level.

Clinical observations in athletes undergoing surgery for jumper's knee also provide thought-provoking data regarding collagen and pain. We monitored athletes recovering from open patellar tenotomy with both ultrasound (3 monthly) and MR imaging (6 monthly) for one year.[40] Tendons remained largely abnormal to imaging, but this correlated poorly with pain. In a retrospective study of a similar postoperative population, ultrasound imaging at a mean of 4 years also did not correlate with pain and function.[41] Both of these studies confirm that even substantial degrees of collagen insult do not automatically produce tendon pain.

Jumper's knee can also be treated by arthroscopic debridement of the posterior border of the patellar tendon,[42] and this provides particularly interesting evidence regarding the role of collagen defects in tendon pain. In this procedure, the surgeon first debrides the adherent fat pad to expose the posterior aspect of the tendon (Figure 15.6) and then removes the cheesy, tendinosic tissue itself. The body of the tendon, however, remains largely untouched and postoperative ultrasonography reveals that the

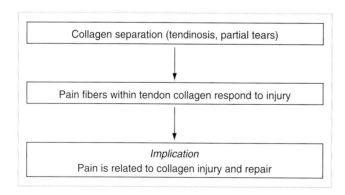

Figure 15.4. The "mechanical" model of collagen separation causing tendon pain.

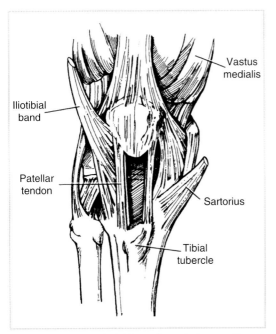

Figure 15.5. The middle third of the patellar tendon is removed in autograft ACL reconstruction. Although a great deal of collagen is removed, the patient is generally pain free soon after the operation. Complete tendon regeneration takes up to two years, but morphology does not correspond with pain of patellar tendinopathy in those patients who develop it.

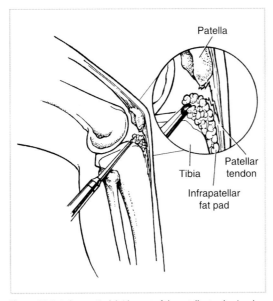

Figure 15.6. Arthroscopic debridement of the patellar tendon involves mainly excision of the fat pad adhering to the posterior aspect of the proximal patellar tendon near its junction with the patella. At surgery, the mucoid degeneration of the posterior portion of the patellar tendon is clearly evident as a cheesy adhesion to the normal tendon. Surgery does little to disturb the tendon itself, yet patients often report that their patellar tendon pain is absent postoperatively.

intratendinous hypoechoic region (so often considered pathognomonic of this condition) is still evident, yet pain is significantly reduced.

This form of treatment could relieve pain by a number of mechanisms, including denervation. However, the proportion of patients who reported skin paresthesia or numbness after patellar tendon surgery was the same after arthroscopic or open patellar tenotomy, suggesting a similar degree of denervation in both anterior and posterior approaches to the patellar tendon.[41]

Longitudinal tenotomy is a well-established treatment for overuse tendinopathy at various body sites including the patellar tendon.[43] This causes new injury to tendon and, although the tenotomy is directed longitudinally so as not to sever the tendon, it is inevitable that collagen is divided because of the normal spiraling of tendon. Nevertheless the procedure is often therapeutic rather than deleterious. This phenomenon cannot be explained by invoking a purely mechanical model of pain in tendinopathy.

Observations about Tendon Pain and Imaging Appearances

A variant of the structural model of pain in tendinopathy outlined above argues that it is not *torn* collagen that hurts per se, but the persisting *intact* collagen that is placed under greater load because adjacent collagen is injured, and thus becomes painful. Pain is presumed to occur when the proportion of collagen injured reaches a critical threshold and persisting collagen is stressed beyond its normal capacity into a painful overload zone. This model predicts that greater degrees of tendinosis should be more painful than lesser degrees, until complete tendon rupture, in which case pain disappears because there is no longer any collagen left under tension. Data from numerous imaging studies argue against this model.

In patients with patellar tendon pain, size of collagen abnormality as measured on ultrasound does not correspond with pain, either in cross-sectional studies[44,45] or in longitudinal observational studies where change in area of abnormal tissue was monitored.[22] Patients with patellar tendinopathy can also have a normal MR scan.[46] This is seen in clinical practice where a patient may have a very small, or no, morphological abnormality, yet have significant symptoms.

In parallel studies conducted in large numbers of asymptomatic athletes, ultrasonographic hypoechoic regions (abnormal collagen) were common, even in subjects with no past history of jumper's knee.[44,45,47] Another study using MR imaging in asymptomatic controls found an abnormal signal consistent with collagen degeneration.[46] These examples demonstrate that there is more to tendon pain than discontinuity of collagen.

Tissue Impingement Causing Patellar Tendon Pain

Both the patellar tendon and the fat pad are in a position where they could be pinched between the patella and the proximal tibia. Could this be the cause of pain in patellar tendinopathy?

Impingement as a Mechanism of Patellar Tendon Pain

Impingement is a form of mechanical load, and adds compressive or shearing load to the tendon's normal tensile load. Johnson and colleagues[8] argued that tension failure of the patellar tendon would affect the superficial fibers more than the deep surface, which is not the case in patellar tendinopathy. Thus, they proposed an alternative mechanism of the pain and the lesion of jumper's knee: impingement of the inferior pole of the patella on the patellar tendon during knee flexion (Figure 15.7).

Three clinical observations are inconsistent with deep knee flexion (and impingement) causing jumper's knee pain. First, pain commences in the early phase of landing from a jump, with quadriceps muscle contraction while the knee is still relatively extended. Second, patients with severe jumper's knee have pain on muscle contraction even when the knee is fully extended and unloaded (e.g., lying in bed), whereas patients with impingement syndromes generally obtain substantial relief when the joint is moved away from the impinging direction. Third, the pain of jumper's knee does not disappear and may actually increase when palpation is performed with the knee in full extension.

A dynamic magnetic resonance study investigated this hypothesis[48] and found there was no difference in patellar movement between symptomatic tendons and those tendons without pain and pathology. The angle of the tendon to the patella either with or without quadriceps contraction was similar in both these groups, suggesting that impingement was not a causative factor.

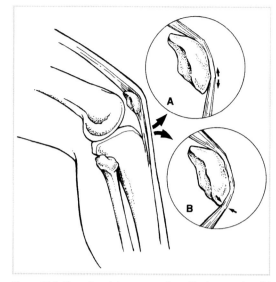

Figure 15.7. Illustration of the argument for an "impingement" model of pain in patellar tendinopathy. Assuming that the insertion of the patellar tendon to the patella was of a uniform strength, tension on the tendon with the knee flexed should generate more force superficially (large arrows) than deeply. Thus, an impingement model was proposed whereby pain, and pathology, was caused by the patellar impinging against the tendon tissue (see text).

Furthermore, Johnson's argument that tension failure of the patellar tendon would affect the superficial fibers more than the deep surface is only valid if the superficial and deep fiber attachments are equally strong. Biomechanical studies, however, found the superficial attachment to be far stronger than the deep.[49,50] Thus, tension failure can influence the deep fibers preferentially. In combination, clinical and research findings suggest that impingement from the patella may not be a factor in patellar tendinopathy.

Another theory more recently proposed by Louis Almekinders from North Carolina is the "stress-shielding" theory.[51,52] The stress-shielding theory considers tendinopathy to be a combined overuse-underuse injury, where the superficial portion of the tendon bears too much of the tensile load while the deep portion of the tendon bears too little of the same load. Further investigation is required; however, it is clear that critical etiological questions such as the nature of tendon load must be answered quickly, as it is the essence of adequate management.

The Role of the Fat Pad in Patellar Tendon Pain

Duri[53] speculated that the fat pad has "an important role in the production of intense pain in patellar tendonitis" when it adheres to the back of the patellar tendon and causes "synovitis." The infrapatellar fat pad is an extremely sensitive region[54,55] with many nociceptors. However, surgical management of the main body of the patellar tendon in athletes revealed no macroscopic abnormality of the fat pad.[56] Intuitively, one would be loath to attribute tendon symptoms to a structure found only at one or two anatomical sites (i.e., the patellar fat pad, Kager's triangle) when tendinopathy occurs at various sites. On the other hand, the fat pad may be a specific form of the nociceptive peritendinous tissue that is sensitive to biochemical irritants. That is, the fat pad in the patellar tendon may play the same role as the paratenon in Achilles tendinopathy and the subacromial bursa in rotator cuff tendinopathy.

Note that the fat pad undoubtedly plays a role in anterior knee pain independently of any role in patellar tendinopathy. Jenny McConnell, the Australian physiotherapist renowned for her work in patellofemoral pain syndrome,[57] recognized fat pad impingement as a cause of anterior knee pain (not necessarily tendon pain) over 10 years ago. Most clinicians would agree that some patients appear to suffer a chronic version of anterior knee pain aggravated by knee extension, similar to the condition referred to as Hoffa's syndrome, when presenting with acute trauma to the anterior knee.[58]

Biochemical Models of Pain in Tendinopathy

If one discards the inflammatory model of pain production, and has reservations about a purely mechanical model for the reasons listed above, the biochemical irritant model becomes increasingly attractive.[6,21] (Figure 15.8). Bob Nirschl said, "We suspect that the cause of pain in tendinosis is chemical irritation due to regional anoxia and the lack of phagocytic cells to remove noxious products of cellular activity."[21] It may be that the pain of tendon overuse injury is largely due to biochemical factors activating peritendinous nociceptors.

The elusive noxious agent could include matrix substances and minor collagens that are only currently being characterized in normal tissues. For example, chondroitin sulphate exposed through tendon damage may stimulate nociceptors.[6,30,59] In the knee, nociceptors are located in the retinaculum, fat pad, synovium, and periosteum,[60] and all these structures may play a role in the mechanism of pain in patellar tendinopathy. In 39 cadaver dissections of the proximal patellar tendon,[3] we consistently identified a thin layer of fat adherent to the posterior portion of the patellar tendon. In the corresponding tissue specimens from patients operated on for chronic jumper's knee, this fat tissue contained increased Alcian Blue stain (and thus, glycosaminoglycans)

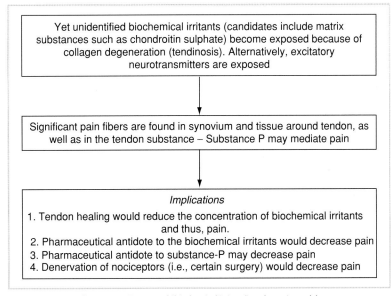

Figure 15.8. A proposed "biochemical irritant" tendon pain model.

that had presumably extravasated from the adjacent region of tendinosis.

Another potential candidate is glutamate, which has been recognized as a mediator of pain[61] and has been demonstrated in several tendons of the body at significantly higher levels in pathological tendons than in normal tendons.[5,62,63] Certain ionotropic glutamate receptors are present in unmyelinated and myelinated sensory axons,[64] and glutamate antagonists reduced the pain that rats felt when given a test dose of formalin. Using in vivo microdialysis, Hakan Alfredson and colleagues[63] found that the neurotransmitter glutamate was present in higher intratendinous concentrations in subjects with patellar tendinopathy than controls. However, their more recent studies have found that the levels of glutamate do not decrease in those tendons that become asymptomatic after eccentric exercise treatment,[65] suggesting that glutamate is not as important as first thought with regard to mediating tendon pain.

Substance-P, and the related neuropeptide, calcitonin gene related peptide (CGRP), has also been found in nerve afferents around the feline knee[66] and are thought to be involved in joint nociception.

A structural relationship has been observed between neuropeptide containing nerve fibers and collagen.[66] However, how tendon injury is transduced into nerve impulses, and perhaps a pain signal, remains unclear. Although there are some data on innervation of tendon,[30,67] and there is ultrastructural evidence of all four categories of nerve endings (Ruffini corpuscles, Vater-Pacini corpuscles, Golgi tendon organs, and free nerve endings or pain receptors) in normal tendons,[30] this field requires a great deal more work before the mechanism of tendon pain is unraveled. If substance-P proved to be a significant agent in tendinopathy, its already developed nonpeptide antagonists could be appropriate for a therapeutic trial.[68]

Can the Biochemical Model Explain the Therapeutic Effect of Eccentric Tendon Strengthening?

The mechanism whereby eccentric strengthening reduces tendon pain remains to be fully elucidated. Al Banes's group at the University of North Carolina have used in vivo animal models, intact tendon specimens and cell cultures to investigate the relationship between mechanical loading and tenocyte response. These authors have provided seminal evidence that tenocytes communicate in response to mechanical load via gap junctions and the cytoskeleton within tenocytes.[69-71] It is therefore possible that eccentric strengthening may stimulate a positive tendon response and therefore also potentially affect tendon pain. Although it is far too early to correlate these findings with the pain-reducing effect of eccentric strength programs, it is apparent that the painful training program that may initially increase, but then decrease, the pain of Achilles and patellar tendinopathy[72-74] may provide the type of mechanical stimulus that Banes has shown promotes DNA and collagen production. Banes's model, and the data that underpin it, is consistent with the clinical evidence that tendon repair can be stimulated by mechanical loading, without a need to invoke any inflammatory pathways. The interested reader is directed to the referenced papers for detailed explanation of the pathway between mechanical stimulus and collagen production in tendon.[75]

Clinical Implications if Pain Were Due to Biochemical Irritants

If the "biochemical irritant" model of tendon pain proves to have some validity, it would mean that clinical management would aim to modify the biochemical milieu. Collagen repair would, of course, contribute to resolving tendinopathy, but researchers would be encouraged to pursue a pharmaceutical approach focused on reducing the irritant (but not necessarily inflammatory) biochemical compounds around the tendon.

Neural and Vascular Models of Pain in Tendinopathy

Normal tendons have a low vascularity, but have sufficient supply for their metabolic needs. In the pathological tendon, increases in vascularity (neovascularization) have been demonstrated histopathologically,[21] with imaging on Doppler ultrasound,[7,76,77] and with laser flowmetry[78,79] (Figure 15.9). Further investigations have demonstrated that neovascularization has been associated with pain and, furthermore, sclerosing or obliterating the neovascularization decreases tendon pain.[80]

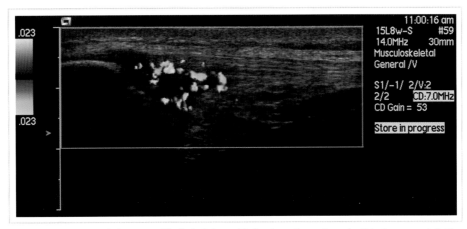

Figure 15.9. Color Doppler ultrasound of a 19-year-old volleyball player with chronic patellar tendinopathy. Note the neovascularization within the hypoechoic region of his patellar tendon.

Neovascularization may be associated with nerve fibers,[63] including those immunoreactive to substance P and CGRP.[81] The association between pain and neovascularization is not absolute, as some studies demonstrate that tendons with neovascularization may not be painful.[82,83] Conversely, pathological tendons without neovascularization may also be painful. However, there is evidence that there is more pain in pathological tendons with neovascularization compared to pathological tendons without neovascularization.[84] Longitudinal studies demonstrate that neovascularization may come and go, and the stimulus for this and the relation to pain is currently undefined 84a.

David Hart and colleagues at the University of Calgary have proposed that the close proximity between neural elements and tissue mast cells in tendon would permit the mast cell–neurite "unit" to stimulate what they termed "neurogenic inflammation."[85] As paratenon is more highly innervated and vascularized than tendon itself, it has been proposed that neurotransmitters such as substance P can influence mast cell degranulation and secretory activity. Neural activity could be amplified, via a feedback mechanism, when mast cells release a panel of biologically active molecules that impact on vascular elements and fibroblasts. Theoretically, the mediators contained in mast cells such as cytokines and growth factors could influence a number of potentially pain-producing factors such as cellular edema and chemotaxis for inflammatory cells. The pro-

ponents of this mechanism argue that the release of low amounts of these mediators could be part of the normal regulatory system, while higher levels may contribute to the adaptive response of tissues.[85]

This type of "neurogenic inflammation" has been seen in various body tissues, although not proven in tendon. The authors refer to this as an "endogenous inflammatory system," in contrast to the "exogenous inflammatory system" composed of bloodborne cells generally associated with inflammation.[85] One criticism of this model as it stands is that mast cells are not prominent in tendon tissue. Nevertheless, the model may apply to paratenonitis, and it may explain the process of neovascularization in tendinosis.

Conclusions

There is little doubt that overuse tendinopathy is noninflammatory. Although collagen fiber injury is almost certainly involved in production of pain in tendinopathies, it may not fully explain the mechanism of tendon pain. Numerous observations illustrate that there is no perfect correlation between collagen injury and pain.

Any model of the pain mechanism in patellar tendinopathy must be consistent with the following observations:

- The pathology underlying tendinopathy is tendinosis.
- Abnormal tendon morphology on imaging confers a risk, but not a guarantee, of symptoms.

- Various surgical treatments including longitudinal tenotomy and arthroscopic tendon debridement can alleviate pain without directly affecting pathological tissue.
- Medical treatment such as corticosteroid injection and aprotinin can relieve the pain quickly, but not necessarily permanently.
- Eccentric strength training is effective in pain relief and can promote tendon healing.

Ideally, the model would apply at numerous sites of the clinically relevant tendinopathies.

Currently, the cause of tendon pathology and pain is unknown. Experimental and clinical research is clarifying aspects of the aetiology of tendon pain and pathology but the relationship between them is still unclear. Until we discover the cause of patellar tendon pain, options for ameliorating tendon pain will remain limited.

References

1. Maffulli, N, KM Khan, and G Puddu, Overuse tendon conditions. Time to change a confusing terminology. *Arthroscopy* 1998; 14: 840–843.
2. Yu, JS et al. Correlation of MR imaging and pathologic findings in athletes undergoing surgery for chronic patellar tendinitis. *Am J Radiology* 1995; 165: 115–118.
3. Khan, KM et al. Patellar tendinosis (jumper's knee): Findings at histopathologic examination, US and MR imaging. *Radiology* 1996; 200: 821–827.
4. Khan, KM et al. Histopathology of common overuse tendon conditions: Update and implications for clinical management. *Sports Med* 1999; 6: 393–408.
5. Alfredson, H, K Thorsen, and R Lorentzon. In situ microdialysis in tendon tissue: high levels of glutamate, but not protoglandin E$_2$ in chronic Achilles tendon pain. *Knee Surg, Sports Traumatol, Arthrosc* 1999; 7: 378–381.
6. Khan, K et al. Where is the pain coming from in tendinopathy? It may be biochemical, not only structural, in origin. *Br J Sports Med* 2000; 34(2): 81–83.
7. Ohberg, L, R Lorentzon, and H Alfredson. Neovascularisation in Achilles tendons with painful tendinosis but not in normal tendons: An ultrasonographic investigation. *Knee Surg Sports Traumatol Arthrosc* 2001; 9: 233–238.
8. Johnson, DP, CJ Wakeley, and I Watt. Magnetic resonance imaging of patellar tendonitis. *J Bone & Joint Surg* 1996; 78-B(3): 452–457.
9. Almekinders, LC, JH Vellema, and PS Weinhold. Strain patterns in the patellar tendon and the implications for patellar tendinopathy. *Knee Surg Sports Traumatol Arthrosc* 2002; 10(1): 2–5.
10. Thurston, AJ. Conservative and surgical treatment of tennis elbow: A study of outcome. *Aust & New Zealand J Surg* 1998; 68(8): 568–72.
11. Scott, A et al. What is inflammation? Are we ready to move beyond Celsus? *Brit J Sports Med* 2004; 38: 248–249.
12. Scott, A et al. What do we mean by the term "inflammation"? A contemporary basic science update for sports medicine. *Brit J Sports Med* 2004; 38: 372–380.
13. Fritschy, D, and RD Gautard. Jumper's knee and ultrasonography. *Amer J Sports Med* 1988; 16: 637–640.
14. McLoughlin, RF et al. Patellar tendinitis: MR features, with suggested pathogenesis and proposed classification. *Radiology*, 1995; 197: 843–848.
15. Puddu, G, E Ippolito, and F Postacchini. A classification of Achilles tendon disease. *Amer J Sports Med* 1976; 4: 145–150.
16. Raatikainen, T et al. Operative treatment of partial rupture of the patellar ligament. *Int J Sports Med* 1994; 15: 46–49.
17. Karlsson, J et al. Partial rupture of the patellar ligament: Results after operative treatment. *Amer J Sports Med* 1991; 19: 403–408.
18. Karlsson, J et al. Partial rupture of the patellar ligament. *Amer J Sports Med* 1992; 20(4): 390–395.
19. Cook, JL et al. A cross-sectional study of 100 cases of jumper's knee managed conservatively and surgically. *Brit J Sports Med* 1997; 31(4): 332–336.
20. Colosimo, AJ, and FH Bassett. Jumper's knee: Diagnosis and treatment. *Orthop Revs* 1990; 29: 139–149.
21. Kraushaar, B, and R Nirschl. Tendinosis of the elbow (tennis elbow): Clinical features and findings of histological, immunohistochemical, and electron microscopy studies. *J Bone & Joint Surg Amer* 1999; 81(2): 259–278.
22. Khan, KM et al. Patellar tendon ultrasonography and jumper's knee in elite female basketball players: A longitudinal study. *Clin J Sports Med* 1997; 7: 199–206.
23. Kannus, P, and L Jozsa. Histopathological changes preceding spontaneous rupture of a tendon. *J Bone & Joint Surg* 1991; 73A: 1507–1525.
24. Zamora, AJ, and JF Marini. Tendon and myotendinous junction in an overloaded skeletal muscle of the rat. *Anat & Embryol* 1988; 179: 89–96.
25. Backman, C et al. Chronic Achilles paratenonitis with tendinosis: An experimental model in the rabbit. *J Orth Res* 1990; 8(4): 541–547.
26. Enwemeka, CS. Inflammation, cellularity, and fibrillogenesis in regenerating tendon: Implications for tendon rehabilitation. *Phys Ther* 1989; 69: 816–825.
27. Fredberg, U. Local corticosteroid injection in sport: Review of literature and guidelines for treatment. *Scand J Med & Sci in Sports* 1997; 7: 131–139.
28. Matheson, GO et al. Scintigraphic uptake of 99mTc at non-painful sites in athletes with stress fractures: The concept of bone strain. *SM* 1987; 4: 65–75.
29. Shrier, I, G Matheson, and G Kohl. Achilles tendinitis: Are corticosteroid injections useful or harmful? *Clin J Sports Med* 1996; 6(4): 245–150.
30. Józsa, L, and P Kannus. *Human Tendons*. Champaign, IL: Human Kinetics, 1997, p. 576.
31. Almekinders, L, and J Temple. Etiology, diagnosis, and treatment of tendonitis: an analysis of the literature. *Med & Sci in Sport and Exercise*, 1998; 30(8): 1183–1190.
32. Smidt, N et al. Corticosteroid injections, physiotherapy, or wait-and-see policy for lateral epicondylitis: A randomised controlled trial. *Lancet* 2002; 359: 657–662.
33. Stahl, S, and T Kaufman The efficacy of an injection of steroids for medial epicondylitis: A prospective study of sixty elbows. *J Bone & Joint Surg Amer* 1948; 79(11): 1648–1652.
34. Hay, EM et al. A pragmatic randomised controlled trial of local corticosteroid injection and physiotherapy for the treatment of new episodes of unilateral shoulder pain in primary care. *Annals Rheum Diseases* 2003; 62(5): 394–399.

35. Capasso, G et al. Aprotinin, corticosteroids and nor-mosaline in the management of patellar tendinopathy in athletes: A prospective randomized study. *Sports Exer & Injury* 1997; 3: 111–115.

36. Kartus, J et al. Evaluation of harvested and normal patellar tendons: A reliability analyses of magnetic resonance imaging and ultrasonography. *Knee Surg Sports Traumatol Arthrosc* 2000; 8: 275–280.

37. Nixon, RG et al. Reconstitution of the patellar tendon donor site after graft harvest. *Clin Orthop* 1995; 317: 162–171.

38. Kiss, ZS et al. Postoperative patellar tendon healing: An ultrasound study. *Australasian Radiol* 1998; 42: 28–32.

39. Adriani, E et al. Healing of the patellar tendon after harvesting of its mid-third for anterior cruciate ligament reconstruction and evolution of the unclosed donor site defect. *Knee Surg Sports Traumatol Arthrosc* 1995; 3: 138–143.

40. Khan, KM et al. Correlation of US and MR imaging with clinical outcome after open patellar tenotomy: prospective and retrospective studies. *Clin J Sports Med* 1999; 9(3): 129–137.

41. Coleman, BD et al. Outcomes of open and arthroscopic patellar tenotomy for chronic patellar tendinopathy: A retrospective study. *Amer J Sports Med* 2000; 28(2): 1–8.

42. Coleman, BD et al. Studies of surgical outcome after patellar tendinopathy: Clinical significance of methodological deficiencies and guidelines for future studies. *Scand J Med & Sci in Sports* 2000; 10(1): 2–11.

43. Testa, V et al. Ultrasound guided percutaneous longitudinal tenotomy for the management of patellar tendinopathy. Med & Sci in Sport & Exercise 1999; 31(11): 1509–1515.

44. Cook, JL et al. Asymptomatic hypoechoic regions on patellar tendon US do not foreshadow symptoms of jumper's knee: A 4 year follow-up of 46 tendons. *Scand J Sci & Med in Sports* 2000; 11(6): 321–327.

45. Lian, O et al. Relationship between symptoms of jumper's knee and the ultrasound characteristics of the patellar tendon among high level male volleyball players. *Scand J Med & Sci in Sports* 1996; 6: 291–296.

46. Shalaby, M, and LC Almekinders. Patellar tendinitis: The significance of magnetic resonance imaging findings. *Amer J Sports Med* 1999; 27(3): 345–349.

47. Cook, JL et al. Patellar tendon ultrasonography in asymptomatic active athletes reveals hypoechoic regions: A study of 320 tendons. *Clin J Sports Med* 1998; 8: 73–77.

48. Schmid, MR et al. Is impingement the cause of jumper's knee? Dynamic and static magnetic resonance imaging of patellar tendinitis in an open-configuration system. *Amer J Sports Med* 2002; 30(3): 388–395.

49. Evans, EJ, M Benjamin, and DJ Pemperton. Fibrocartilage in the attachment zones of the quadriceps tendon. *J Anat (Lond.)* 1990; 171: 155–162.

50. Evans, EJ, M Benjamin, and DJ Pemperton. Variation in the amount of calcified tissue at the attachments of the quadriceps tendon and patellar ligament in man. *J Anat (Lond.)* 1991; 174: 145–151.

51. Almekinders, LC, PS Weinhold, and N Maffulli. Compression etiology in tendinopathy. Clinics in Sports Med 2003; 22(4): 703–710.

52. Almekinders, LC, PS Weinhold, and N Maffulli Compression etiology in tendinopathy. 2003; 703–710.

53. Duri, ZAA, and PM Aichroth. Patellar tendonitis: Clinical and literature review. *Knee Surg Sports Traumatol Arthrosc* 1995; 3: 95–100.

54. Dye, SF, GL Vaupel, and CC Dye. Conscious neurosensory mapping of the internal structures of the human knee without intraarticular anesthesia. *Amer J Sports Med* 1998; 26(6): 773–777.

55. Sanchis-Alfonso, V, and E Rosello-Sastre. Anterior knee pain in the young patient: What causes the pain? "Neural model." *Acta Orthop Scand* 2003; 74(6): 697–703.

56. Maffulli, N et al. Surgical management of tendinopathy of the main body of the patellar tendon in athletes. *Clin J Sport Med* 1999; 9(2): 58–62.

57. McConnell, J. The management of chondromalacia patellae: A long term solution. *Austral J Physiother* 1986; 32(4): 215–223.

58. Brukner, P, and K Khan. *Clinical Sports Medicine,* 2nd ed. Sydney: McGraw-Hill Companies, 2001.

59. Benazzo, F, G Stennardo, and M Valli. Achilles and patellar tendinopathies in athletes: pathogenesis and surgical treatment. *Bull Hosp Joint Disease* 1996; 54: 236–240.

60. Witonski, D, and M Wagrowska-Danielewicz. Distribution of substance-P nerve fibers in the knee joint in patients with anterior knee pain syndrome: A preliminary report. *Knee Surg, Sports Traumatol, Arthrosc* 1999; 7(3): 177–183.

61. Dickenson, AH. NMDA receptor antagonists: interactions with opioids. *Acta Anaesthesiol Scand* 1997; 41(1 Pt 2): 112–115.

62. Alfredson, H et al. In vivo investigation of ECRB tendons with microdialysis technique: No signs of inflammation but high amounts of glutamate in tennis elbow. *Acta Orthop Scand* 2000; 71(5): 475–479.

63. Alfredson, H et al. In vivo microdialysis and immunohistochemical analyses of tendon tissue demonstrated high amounts of free glutamate and glutamate receptors, but no signs of inflammation, in Jumper's knee. *J Orthop Res* 2001; 19: 881–886.

64. Coggeshall, RE, and SM Carlton. Ultrastructural analysis of NMDA, AMPA, and kainate receptors on unmyelinated and myelinated axons in the periphery. *J Comp Neurol* 1998; 391(1): 78–86.

65. Alfredson, H, and R Lorentzon. Intratendinous glutamate levels and eccentric training on chronic Achilles tendinosis: A prospective study using microdialysis technique. *Knee Surg Sports Traumatol Arthrosc* 2003; 11: 196–199.

66. Marshall, KW, E Theriault, and DA Homonko. Distribution of substance P and calcitonin gene related peptide immunoreactivity in the normal feline knee. *J Rheumatol* 1994; 21(5): 883–889.

67. Andres, KH, MV During, and RF Schmidt. Sensory innervation of the Achilles tendon by group III and IV afferent fibres. *Anat & Embryol* 1985; 172: 145–156.

68. Baby, S et al. Substance P antagonists: The next breakthrough in treating depression? *J Clin Pharma & Therapeutics* 1999; 24(6): 461–469.

69. Banes, AJ et al. Tendon cells of the epitenon and internal tendon compartment communicate mechanical signals through gap junctions and respond differentially to mechanical load and growth factors. In Gordon, SL, SJ Blair, and LJ Fine, eds., *Repetitive Motion Disorders of the Upper Extremity*. Park Ridge: American Academy of Orthopaedic Surgeons, 1995, pp. 231–245.

70. Banes, AJ et al. Mechanoreception at the cellular level: the detection, interpretation, and diversity of responses

to mechanical signals. *Biochem & Cell Biol* 1995; 73(7-8): 349–365.

71. Banes, AJ, P Weinhold, and X Yang. Gap junctions regulate responses of tendon cells ex vivo to mechanical loading. *Clin Orthop & Rel Res* 1999; 367S: 357–370.
72. Niesen-Vertommen, SL et al. The effect of eccentric versus concentric exercise in the management of Achilles tendonitis. *Clin J Sports Med* 1992; 2: 109–113.
73. Alfredson, H et al. Heavy-load eccentric calf muscle training for the treatment of chronic Achilles tendinosis. *Amer J Sports Med* 1998; 26(3): 360–366.
74. Young, M et al. Eccentric decline squat protocol offers superior results at 12 months compared to traditional eccentric protocol for patellar tendinopathy in volleyball players. *Brit J Sports Med* 2005; 392: 102–105.
75. Ohberg, L, R Lorentzon, and H Alfredson. Eccentric training in patients with chronic Achilles tendinosis: Normalised tendon structure and decreased thickness at follow up. *Brit J Sports Med* 2004; 38(1): 8–11.
76. Terslev, L et al. Ultrasound and power Doppler findings in jumper's knee: Preliminary findings. *Eur J Ultrasound* 2001; 13: 183–189.
77. Alfredson, H, L Ohberg, and S Forsgren. Is vasculo-neural ingrowth the cause of pain in chronic Achilles tendinosis? An investigation using ultrasonography and colour Doppler, immunohistochemistry, and diagnostic injections. *Knee Surg, Sports Traumatol, Arthrosc* 2003; 11(5): 334–338.
78. Astrom, M, and N Westlin. Blood flow in chronic Achilles tendinopathy. *Clin Orthop* 1994; 308: 166–172.

79. Astrom, M, and N Westlin. Blood flow in the normal Achilles tendon assessed by laser Doppler flowmetry. *J Orthop Res* 1994; 12(2): 246–252.
80. Ohberg, L, and H Alfredson. Ultrasound guided sclerosis of neovessels in painful chronic Achilles tendinosis: Pilot study of a new treatment. *Brit J Sports Med* 2002; 36: 173–177.
81. Ljung, B, S Forsgren, and J Friden. Substance P and calcitonin gene-related peptide expression at the extensor carpi radialis brevis muscle origin: Implications for the etiology of tennis elbow. *J Orthop Res* 1999; 17(4): 554–559.
82. Zanetti, M et al. Achilles tendons: Clinical relevance of neovascularization diagnosed with power Doppler US. *Radiology* 2003; 227: 556–560.
83. Khan, KM et al. Are ultrasound and magnetic resonance imaging of value in assessment of Achilles tendon disorders? A two year prospective study. *Brit J Sports Med* 2003; 37(2): 149–154.
84. Cook, JL et al. Neovascularisation and pain in abnormal patellar tendons of active jumping athletes. *Clin J Sports Med* 2004; 14(5): 296–299.
84a. Cook, JL, Malliaras P, Luca JD, et al. Vascularity and pain in the patellar tendon of adult jumping athletes: a 5 month longitudinal study. *Br J Sports Med* 2005; 39: 458.
85. Hart, DA, CB Frank, and RC Bray. Inflammatory processes in repetitive motion and overuse syndromes: Potential role of neurogenic mechanisms in tendons and ligaments. In Gordon, SL, SJ Blair, and LJ. Fine, eds., *Pathophysiology: Connective Tissue*. Park Ridge, IL: American Academy of Orthopaedic Surgeons, 1995, pp. 247–262.

16

Patellar Tendinopathy:
The Science Behind Treatment

Karim M. Khan, Jill L. Cook, and Mark A. Young

Introduction

Patellar tendon injuries constitute a significant problem in a wide variety of sports.[1] Despite the morbidity associated with patellar tendinopathy, clinical management remains largely anecdotal[2,3] as there have been few well-designed treatment studies. The goal of this chapter is to update the reader on basic science as it relates to the patellar tendon, and then to discuss the evidence supporting current patient management.

Anatomy and Histopathology

When examined under a light microscope, abnormal tendon from patients with chronic patellar tendinopathy differs from normal tendon in several key ways. It has a loss of collagen continuity (Figure 16.1) and an increase in ground substance, vascularity, and cellularity. Special light microscopy staining[4] and electron microscope studies[5] confirm that cellularity results from the presence of fibroblasts and myofibroblasts, not inflammatory cells. As discussed in the previous chapter, inflammatory cells are absent in patients who have chronic overuse tendinopathies.[6]

Clinical Presentation of Patellar Tendinopathy

In the patient with patellar tendinopathy, knee pain may arise insidiously. Patients who can recall when the pain began often recall one heavy training session or, less commonly, a specific jump that initiated the pain. In addition, they often remember a specific activity that seemed to make the pain worse. Pain is usually precisely localized to the inferoanterior patellar region, and many patients notice tenderness at the inferior pole of the patella even before they present for a medical examination.

Early in the clinical course, the patient's knee pain and discomfort may ease completely while exercising. In this case, the player often disregards the injury and does not seek treatment. With time and continued activity, however, pain worsens and limits sporting performance. Eventually, pain can develop during activities of daily living and can even be present at rest.[7]

Examination reveals tenderness at the junction of the patella and the patellar tendon, and this is most evident when the knee is fully extended and the inferior pole of the patella is raised. This clinical scenario has a number of names, including jumper's knee, patellar tendinopathy, patellar tendinosis, and patellar tendinitis. The preferred diagnostic term is patellar tendinopathy,[8,9] with the terms tendonitis and tendinosis best reserved for histopathology findings only.

Palpation of the tendon attachment at the inferior pole of the patella has been the classic physical examination technique for detecting patellar tendinopathy, but mild tenderness at this site is not unusual in a normal tendon.[10] Only moderate and severe tenderness is significantly associated with tendon abnormality as defined by ultrasonography. Thus, mild patellar tendon tenderness should not be overinterpreted, and may be a normal finding in active athletes.

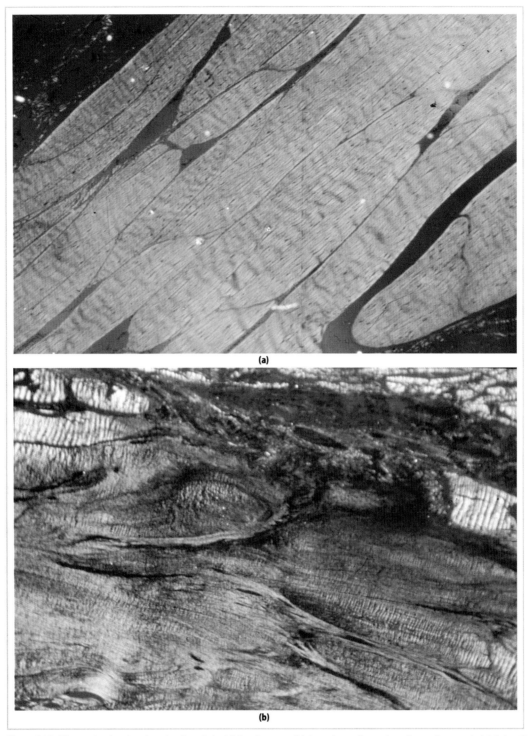

Figure 16.1. Micrographs of tendon viewed under polarized light microscopy. **(a)** A specimen of normal patellar tendon reveals tightly bundled collagen with characteristic golden reflectivity, also referred to as birefringence. **(b)** A specimen of tendon tissue obtained at surgery. The 26-year-old patient had 4 months of patellar tendon pain. Polarized light microscopy reveals separation of collagen fibers and the presence of an amorphous (mucoid) ground substance.

Patients with chronic symptoms may exhibit quadriceps wasting. Thigh circumference may be diminished, and calf muscle atrophy may or may not be apparent. Testing the functional strength of the quadriceps may be done by comparing the ease with which the patient can perform 10 single-leg step-downs. The athlete bends at the knee and then straightens again without letting the other foot touch the floor (Figure 16.2A). Alternatively, a 25-degree decline board (Figure 16.2B) can be utilized to assess squat function. Craig Purdam and his colleagues from the Australian Institute of Sport have developed the decline board to enable greater specificity when loading the patellar tendon.[11] The downward angle decreases calf contribution to the squat, and by keeping the trunk upright this minimizes gluteal function and enables the knee extensors to be loaded maximally. The decline board is also a useful tool in the management of patellar

tendinopathy.[12,13] Work capacity of the calf is assessed by asking the patient to perform single-leg heel raises. Jumping athletes should be able to do at least 30 raises. It is important to monitor both the onset of fatigue and the quality of movement (e.g., control, as measured by wobbling) as either can be affected in the symptomatic limb. Pelvic stability is also assessed, as poor pelvic control is a common feature of the athlete with jumper's knee. Weakness of the gluteal, lower abdominal, quadriceps, and calf muscles can lead to fatigue-induced aberrant movement patterns that may alter forces acting on the knee. It is therefore imperative that proximal and distal muscle groups be assessed in patients with chronic patellar tendinopathy.

In general, the clinical features of patellar tendinopathy make diagnosis relatively straightforward.[14] In some cases, however, patellofemoral pain syndrome (PFPS) or fat pad symptoms

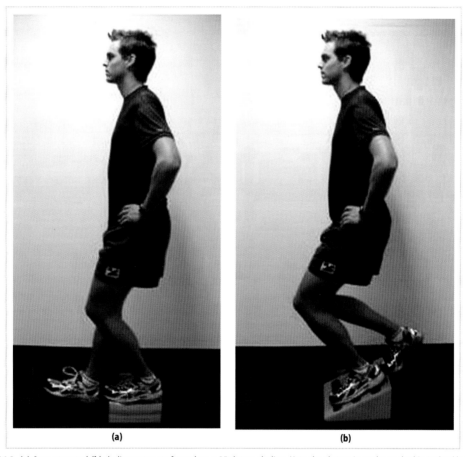

(a) (b)

Figure 16.2. (a) Step squat and **(b)** decline squat, performed on a 25-degree decline. Note the change in angles at the hip and ankle enabling increased load through the knee extensors.

may be difficult to differentiate from patellar tendinopathy, or the conditions may coexist. Typically, pain is localized to the inferior pole of the patella with PT, and tends to warm up with activity as opposed to PFPS, which is poorly localized and becomes worse with activity.

A useful clinical tool for assessing the athlete with jumper's knee is the Victorian Institute of Sport Assessment (VISA) score[7] (Figure 16.3). Ranging from 0 to 100, the VISA score consists of 8 questions assessing symptoms, simple tests of function and ability to play sport. A maximum score of 100 points represents full pain-free function. Competing athletes with patellar tendinopathy commonly record a score between 50 and 80 points. The VISA score enables both the therapist and the patient to objectively measure progress, and allows early detection of any worsening of symptoms.

Imaging Appearances

Magnetic resonance (MR) imaging and ultrasound (US) are the investigations of choice in the jumping athlete with knee pain. Here we summarize the typical findings in a patient with patellar tendinopathy and we discuss the clinical utility of the imaging modalities.

Magnetic Resonance Imaging

The abnormal patellar tendon contains an oval or round area of high signal intensity on T1 and T2 images, or a focal zone of high signal intensity in the deep layers of the tendon insertion[4,15,16] (Figure 16.4). Tendons with patellar tendinopathy have an increased anteroposterior diameter in the affected region.[15] The T2 weighted sequences (particularly the T2 GRE weighted sequences) have better sensitivity than the T1 weighted protocols,[4,17] but even T1 weighted sequences reveal most cases of patellar tendinopathy.

In clinical practice, MR scans can identify the exact location and extent of tendon involvement, and help exclude other clinical conditions such as bursitis and chondromalacia.[16] Surgeons often use MR to assess the extent of the pathology and provide guidance as to how much tendon to excise.

Disadvantages of MR include cost, and the slow, often incomplete, resolution of signal changes after surgical intervention.[18,19] Furthermore, when Shalaby and colleagues investigated the significance of MR findings in patellar tendinopathy, they found that in younger patients with relatively mild symptoms, MR images did not show significant changes. Also, in older, active patients changes may be present in asymptomatic knees[20] (Figure 16.5).

Abnormal signal without change in size must be interpreted with caution, as the normal patellar tendon has a range of appearances due to technical factors and intrinsic fiber differences.[21] In particular, the "magic angle" phenomenon can result in false-positive high signal intensity on T2 GRE weighted images of normal tendon.[22,23]

Ultrasonography

Sonographic studies in athletes with the clinical features of patellar tendinopathy should include both knees using high-resolution linear array 10 or 12 MHz ultrasound transducers. The tendon must be examined with the probe exactly perpendicular to the tendon to avoid a false positive image due to artifactual hypoechogenicity.[24]

Sonographic appearances in jumper's knee reveal a focal hypoechoic area (Figure 16.6) combined with an enlargement of the surrounding tendon. Note that in some cases, the tendon can have an enlarged appearance without any presence of a hypoechoic region.

A proportion of asymptomatic athletes have sonographic hypoechoic regions in their patellar tendons. Among volleyball players, 54% of asymptomatic knees contained patellar tendons with hypoechoic regions on US.[25] Similarly, 15% of basketball players with no past history of knee pain had abnormal tendon morphology on US.[26] Furthermore, longitudinal studies found that hypoechoic US regions did not predict subsequent development of symptoms in sportswomen[27] or sportsmen,[28,29] but conferred relative risk of patellar tendinopathy in 16- to 18-year-old basketball players.[29] These data suggest that ultrasound appearance alone would be a poor guide to prognosis and management. Also, a sonographic hypoechoic region is not of itself an indication for surgery.[29] Surgeons have, however, used US to accurately locate the area of tendinopathy to allow correct placement of the scalpel blade when performing multiple percutaneous longitudinal tenotomies.[30]

Conservative Management of Patellar Tendinopathy

Given the degree of morbidity associated with chronic tendon problems, and the extent of

Name _____   Date _____

The Modified VISA Score

Please mark **R** for **RIGHT knee** and **L** for **LEFT knee** and complete both sides of the form.

The term "pain" refers specifically to pain in the patellar tendon region.

1.   For how many minutes can you sit pain free?

0 mins
0 1 2 3 4 5 6 7 8 9 10
100 mins

2.   Do you have pain walking downstairs normally?

Severe Pain / Unable
0 1 2 3 4 5 6 7 8 9 10
No pain

3.   Whilst sitting down, do you have pain at the front of the knee when straightening your leg?

Severe Pain / Unable
0 1 2 3 4 5 6 7 8 9 10
No pain

4.   How much pain do you have in the front leg when doing a full lunge?

Severe Pain / Unable
0 1 2 3 4 5 6 7 8 9 10
No pain

5.   Do you have pain when squatting?

Severe Pain / Unable
0 1 2 3 4 5 6 7 8 9 10
No pain

6.   Do you have pain during and/or after doing 10 single leg hops? (If you cannot do 10 then your score is 0)

Severe Pain / Unable
0 1 2 3 4 5 6 7 8 9 10
No pain

Figure 16.3. Visa score questionnaire.

(*continued*)

7.   Are you currently undertaking full training?

0 ☐   Not at all

4 ☐   Modified training ± modified competition

7 ☐   Full training ± competition but not at same level as when symptoms began

10 ☐   Competing at the same or higher level as when symptoms began

8.   Please complete EITHER A, B or C in this question.

A. If you have no pain while undertaking activity please complete **Q8a only**.

B. If you have pain while undertaking sport but it does not stop you from completing the activity, please complete **Q8b only**.

C. If you have pain that stops you from completing sporting activities, please complete **Q8c only**.

8a.   If you have no pain while playing sport, for how long can you train?

Nil	0 – 20 mins	20 – 40 mins	40 – 60 mins	> 60 mins
☐	☐	☐	☐	☐
0	7	14	21	30

8b.   If you have some pain while playing sport, but it does not stop you from completing your training, for how long can you train?

Nil	0 – 10 mins	10 – 20 mins	20 – 30 mins	> 30 mins
☐	☐	☐	☐	☐
0	5	10	15	20

8c.   If you have pain that stops you from playing sport, for how long can you train?

Nil	0 – 5 mins	5 – 10 mins	10 – 15 mins	> 15 mins
☐	☐	☐	☐	☐
0	2	5	7	10

TOTAL VISA SCORE _____

Figure 16.3. *(continued)*

knowledge in certain areas of medical treatment, there is a surprising lack of scientific rationale for tendon treatment.[31] Conservative and operative treatments for tendinopathies vary considerably among surgeons and across countries. Unfortunately, there is little scientific evidence for the majority of treatments proposed and used for chronic tendon problems.[19] There is, however, a growing body of evidence for a small number of treatments.

We discuss conservative management of the athlete with patellar tendinopathy under four broad headings: (1) decreasing load on the tendon, (2) eccentric strengthening, (3) electrotherapy and massage, and (4) pharmacological management. Finally, we discuss surgical options.

Decreasing Load on the Tendon

In jumping sports, forces generated in landing are substantially greater than those that produce

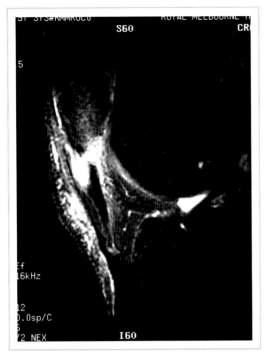

Figure 16.4. A T2 weighted gradient echo MRI of the patellar tendon in an 18-year-old jumping athlete shows an area of markedly increased signal intensity relative to that of the remainder of the tendon. This appearance corresponds with tendinosis (collagen degeneration).

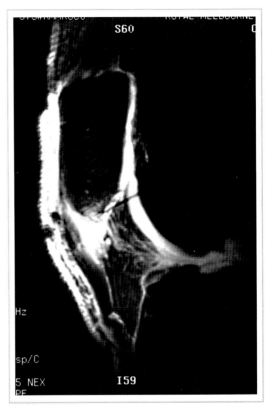

Figure 16.5. A T2 weighted MRI image of the patellar tendon illustrating that symptoms do not necessarily correlate with imaging appearance. An MRI shows the tendon from a 40-year-old man with an excellent clinical outcome but marked increases in signal in the patellar tendon.

the jump.[32] Therefore, correcting biomechanics improves the energy-absorbing capacity of the limb both at the affected musculoskeletal junction and at the hip and ankle. The ankle and calf are critical in absorbing the initial landing load, and any functional compromise of these structures increases the load transmitted to the knee. Animal studies estimate that about 40% of landing energy is transmitted proximally.[33] Thus, the calf complex must absorb a major portion of the load that would otherwise be transmitted proximally to the patellar tendon–quadriceps complex. Jumping and running technique is therefore important. Compared with flat-foot landing, forefoot landing generates lower ground reaction forces; if this technique is combined with a large range of hip or knee flexion, vertical ground reaction forces in landing can be reduced by a further 25%.[34]

The practical implication of these data is that, aside from the standard joint, muscle, and kinetic chain assessments, the practitioner should assess the patient's functional biomechanics. Some static abnormalities, such as pes planus, may be evident during static assessment, but others, such as excessively rapid pronation, may only be evident during dynamic evaluation. Inflexibility of the quadriceps, hamstrings, iliotibial band, or calf have the potential to restrict range of motion at the knee and ankle joints and are thought to increase the load on the patellar tendon. Posterior leg tightness (decreased sit and reach test) is associated with increased prevalence of patellar tendinopathy.[35] Although clinically biomechanical assessment is important, evidence to support its contribution to patellar tendinopathy management is unclear.[36]

Eccentric Exercise Protocols: The Evidence

Eccentric strengthening has long been recognized as the keystone to successful management of tendinopathies.[37] Surprisingly, only a few studies have investigated the benefits of strengthening

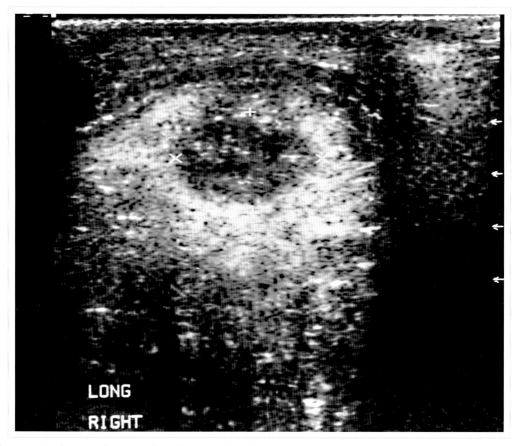

Figure 16.6. An ultrasonographic image in the axial (transverse) plane of the patellar tendon of a 31-year-old man reveals a characteristic hypoechoic region in the patellar tendon. This appearance corresponds with tendinosis (collagen degeneration).

for patellar tendinopathy.[38-40] In contrast, well-designed studies have demonstrated the efficacy of strengthening as a treatment for both Achilles and adductor tendinopathies.[41-43]

Traditionally, when eccentrically loading the patellar tendon,[44] the key exercise is a single-leg squat from standing to about 70–90° of knee flexion. Patients perform 3 sets of 10 repetitions per session (one session daily). This traditional treatment program emphasizes training specificity, maximal loading, and progression.[37,45] Maximal loading occurs when patients feel their tendon pain in the final set of 10 repetitions. Progression is achieved by increasing the speed of movement or by increasing the external resistance, again using pain as a guide. Ice is used to cool the tendon after the eccentric training.

Following the success of a pain-based eccentric exercise program in the treatment of Achilles tendinopathy,[41] we recently investigated the effect of painful eccentric training using decline boards during the rehabilitation of volleyballers with patellar tendinopathy.[12,13] We found that the use of a decline board and training into pain offers greater clinical gains than the traditional squat programs in athletes who continue to train and play with pain. These programs are particularly useful to athletes who have failed a pain-free conservative program during the season. They are best completed during the off-season, when training commitments are greatly reduced.

Prescribing Eccentric Exercise: Clinical Experience

Therapists often have concerns as to when and how they should begin a strengthening program. A rehabilitation program should always begin

Table 16.1. Outline of strengthening program for treatment of patellar tendinopathy

Timing	Type of overload	Activity
0–3 months	Load endurance	Hypertrophy and strengthen the affected muscles; focus attention on the calf as well as the quadriceps and gluteals
3–6 months	Speed endurance	Weight-bearing and speed-specific loads
6+ months	Combinations dependent on sport (e.g., load, speed, jumping)	Sports-specific rehabilitation

with strengthening exercises. Table 16.1 presents a strength program embracing the activities and timelines that our clinical experience has shown to be effective. Even athletes with severe patellar tendinopathy should be able to begin some exercise, at the very least standing calf strength and isometric quadriceps work. On the other hand, the athlete who has not lost appreciable knee strength and bulk can progress quickly to the speed part of the program.

Both pain and the musculotendinous unit's ability to do work should guide the amount of strengthening activity. If pain is a limiting factor, then the program must be modified so that the majority of the work occurs relatively pain free, and does not cause delayed symptoms, commonly pain in the morning after exercise. However, some recent studies challenge this theory,[12,13] and exercising into tendon pain appears a viable option, especially in the chronic athlete who is between seasons.

In most cases, if pain is under control, then the practitioner supervising the program should monitor the control and quality with which the patient performs the exercises. Athletes should only progress to the next level of the program if the previous workload is easily managed, pain is controlled, and function is satisfactory.

Because athletes with patellar tendinopathy tend to "unload" the affected limb to avoid pain, the symptomatic leg is not only weak, but also displays abnormal motor patterns that must be corrected. Strength work must progress to single-leg exercises, as bilateral exercises only offer options to continue to unload the tendon. Some physicians and therapists maintain that quadriceps-only exercises such as leg extensions have a place in the rehabilitation of patellar tendinopathy, specifically to load the quadriceps exclu-

sively, thus not allowing the calf and gluteal muscles to take over the exercise. Similarly, we have found that squats performed on a 25 degree decline board are effective in reducing the influence of the calf group in retarding knee flexion such as occurs in a normal squat done with the heels fixed.[11] The therapist can help the patient progress by adding load and speed to the exercises, and then endurance can be introduced once the patient can do these exercises well. After that, combinations such as load (weight) and speed, or height (e.g., jumping exercises) and load can be added. These end-stage eccentric exercises can provoke tendon pain, and are only recommended after a sufficiently long rehabilitation period and when the sport demands intense loading. In several sports it may not be necessary to add height to the rehabilitation program at all, whereas in some sports (volleyball, for example), it is vital.

Failure in rehabilitation strength programs can stem from many sources. They include too rapid a progression of rehabilitation; inappropriate loads (e.g., not enough strength or speed work, eccentric work too early or aggressively, insufficient single-leg work); too many passive treatments, such as electrotherapeutic modalities; and lack of monitoring patients' symptoms during and after therapy. Rehabilitation and strength training must also continue once returning to sport, rather than ending immediately on return. Finally, plyometric training must be undertaken with care, as it is often performed inappropriately or poorly tolerated.

Electrotherapy and Deep Tissue Massage

To control initial tissue response to tendon injury most clinicians advise rest, cryotherapy, and anti-inflammatory medication.[46] Cryotherapy may limit tissue damage by decreasing blood flow and metabolic rate. Electrical modalities that have been used in patellar tendinopathy include ultrasound, heat, interferential therapy, magnetic fields, pulsed magnetic and electromagnetic fields, TENS, and laser. The true effects of all of these modalities remain unknown, with equivocal results thus far.[40,47]

Remedial massage aims to decrease load on tendons by improving muscle stretch. Deep friction massage may activate mesenchymal stem cells to stimulate a healing response.[48,49] A controlled study failed to find any positive effects of massage treatment in patients with patellar tendinopathy.[50]

Pharmacotherapy

The main pharmaceutical agents used to treat patellar tendinopathy have been nonsteroidal anti-inflammatory drugs (NSAIDs) and corticosteroids. After discussing these, we review the data regarding novel agents for treating tendinopathies.

Although the biological basis for using NSAIDs in tendinopathies is not obvious,[6] these drugs are undoubtedly the most commonly used symptomatic therapy.[51] In a double-blind placebo-controlled study of NSAIDs in tendinopathy, piroxicam did not benefit patients with Achilles tendinopathy.[52] Although the use of "anti-inflammatory" medication seems paradoxical in a degenerative condition, NSAIDs act in ways beyond their well-known anti-inflammatory mode.[53-55] For example, in tendons, some NSAIDs stimulate, and some inhibit, glycosaminoglycan synthesis.[56] This suggests a mechanism whereby NSAIDs could influence the extracellular matrix. Thus, it would appear premature to rule out any potential benefit of this class of medication merely because tendinopathy is not an inflammatory condition.

Injection and infiltration of corticosteroids by means such as iontophoresis has a dramatic effect on symptoms arising from inflamed synovial structures.[57] However, the role of corticosteroids in management of tendinopathy remains controversial.[58,59] Józsa and Kannus's[31] guidelines for appropriate use of corticosteroid injections should be adhered to in the absence of scientific evidence as to when these injections may be most appropriate. Although corticosteroids injected into tendons are catabolic, this type of injection is now rarely performed, and the effect of corticosteroids on the surrounding tendon structures is unknown.

Aprotinin

Aprotinin has been trialled in the management of patellar tendinopathy.[60] Aprotinin is a polyvalent inhibitor of the proteases collagenase, elastase, metalloprotease, kallikrein, plasmin, and cathepsin C. At least in the short term, aprotinin (two to four injections of 62,500 IU with local anesthetic in the paratendinous space) seems to offer a greater chance of pain relief than corticosteroids. However, patients with an insertional tendinopathy fared less well than those with tendinopathy of the main body of the tendon.

Another promising development in pharmacotherapy is the use of nitrous oxide. Topically applied nitric oxide has been shown, in animal models, to be effective for the treatment of fractures and cutaneous wounds through mechanisms that may include stimulation of collagen synthesis in fibroblasts.[61] Recent positive findings in the treatment of extensor and Achilles tendinopathies[61,62] indicate that treatment of patellar tendinopathy may be enhanced by the addition of nitrous oxide.

Surgical Management

Patellar tendon surgery[63-67] is generally performed when the patient has not improved after at least six months of conservative management. A variety of surgical methods for treatment of jumper's knee have been described.[68] These include: drilling of the inferior pole of the patella, resection of the tibial attachment of the patellar tendon with realignment,[69] excision of macroscopic necrotic areas,[70] repair of macroscopic defects,[71] scarification (i.e., longitudinal tenotomy/tenoplasty of the tendon),[72] percutaneous needling,[73] percutaneous longitudinal tenotomy,[30] and arthroscopic debridement.[74] Surgical technique is based on each surgeon's opinion/experience, as the pathophysiology of patellar tendinopathy is not known.

Patellar tendon surgery has a rather unpredictable outcome. A review of 23 papers found that authors reported surgical success rates of between 46% to 100%.[75] In the three studies that had more than 40 patients, authors reported combined excellent and good results of 91%, 82%, and 80% in a series of 78, 80, and 138 subjects respectively. The mean time for return to pre-injury level of sport varied from 4 months to greater than 9 months. A long-term study of outcome in patients who underwent open patellar tenotomy for patellar tendinosis showed that only 54% were able to return to their previous level of sporting activity.[74] In two prospective studies that evaluated time to return to sport, most subjects required more than 6 months, and often 9 months, to return to full sporting competition.[18,30]

Unfortunately, several factors confound analysis of outcome of surgery.[75] Surgeons differ in their diagnostic criteria, selection of cases for surgery, the actual operation performed, and their postoperative protocols. Different types of surgery result in a difference in the amount of bone either excised or drilled, the margin of normal tissue excised around the macroscopically degenerative tissue, the use or avoidance of longitudinal tenotomies, and the type of closure of the tendon after surgery. Intersurgeon technical ability is another major factor whose influence has never been studied.

Recently, we have shown that the scientific methodology behind published articles on the outcome of patellar tendinopathy after surgery is poor, and that the poorer the methodology, the higher the success rate.[75] Obviously, improving study design would provide clinicians with a more rigorous evidence-base for treating patients who have recalcitrant patellar tendinopathy.

Conclusions

Patellar tendinopathy is a degenerative, not inflammatory, condition of the patellar tendon most likely resulting from excessive load bearing. Clinical assessment is the key to diagnosis, although the presence of US or MR abnormalities increases the likelihood that the patient's symptoms arise from the patellar tendon. Imaging appearances should not dictate management, which, for the time being, remains based on clinical experience rather than scientific rationale.

A variety of management modalities exist, including correcting perceived underlying biomechanical problems, local physical modalities such as ice and, when the patient is pain free, a graduated strengthening program emphasizing functional exercises including eccentric training. Eccentric training protocols appear most promising, and training into tendon pain is a viable option to relieve long-standing symptoms. To prescribe exercise effectively requires thorough assessment of the patient's functional capacity and a skillful approach to gradually increasing the demand that the athlete imposes on the tendon. Many athletes tend to cycle between full load and complete rest, while it is far more effective to aim for gradual increases in activity.

Surgery is indicated after a 6- to 9-month trial of appropriate conservative management. Open patellar tenotomy is the conventionally accepted surgical treatment of insertional patellar tendinopathy but often requires 6 to 12 months' rehabilitation. Arthroscopic debridement has been proposed, and, although randomized controlled trials are lacking, this procedure may permit earlier return to sport than traditional open surgery, even though both techniques have an equal success rate at 12 months.[74]

References

1. Ferretti, A. Epidemiology of jumper's knee. *Sports Med* 1986; 3: 289–295.
2. Almekinders, LC. Tendinitis and other chronic tendinopathies. *J Amer Acad Orth Surg* 1998; 6: 157–164.
3. Khan, K, and N Maffuli. Tendinopathy: An Achilles' heel for athletes and clinicians. *Clin J Sports Med* 1998; 8(3): 151–154.
4. Khan, KM et al. Patellar tendinosis (jumper's knee): Findings at histopathologic examination, US and MR imaging. *Radiology* 1996; 200: 821–827.
5. Kraushaar, B, and R Nirschl. Tendinosis of the elbow (tennis elbow): Clinical features and findings of histological, immunohistochemical, and electron microscopy studies. *J Bone & Joint Surg Amer* 1999; 81(2): 259–278.
6. Khan, KM et al. Histopathology of common overuse tendon conditions: Update and implications for clinical management. *Sports Med* 1999; 6: 393–408.
7. Visentini, PJ et al. The VISA score: An index of the severity of jumper's knee (patellar tendinosis). *J Sci & Med in Sport* 1998; 1: 22–28.
8. Maffulli, N, KM Khan, and G Puddu. Overuse tendon conditions: Time to change a confusing terminology. *Arthroscopy* 1998; 14: 840–843.
9. Cook, J et al. Overuse tendinosis, not tendinitis: Applying the new approach to patellar tendinopathy. *Phys & Sports Med* 2000; 28(6): 31–46.
10. Cook, J et al. Reproducibility and clinical utility of tendon palpation to detect patellar tendinopathy in young basketball players. *Brit J Sports Med* 2001; 35: 65–69.
11. Purdam, CR et al. Discriminative ability of functional loading tests for adolescent jumper's knee. *Phys Ther in Sport* 2003; 4(1): 3–9.
12. Purdam, CR et al. A pilot study of the eccentric decline squat in the management of painful chronic patellar tendinopathy. *Brit J Sports Med* 2004; 38(4): 395–397.
13. Young, M et al. Eccentric decline squat protocol offers superior results at 12 months compared with traditional eccentric protocol for patellar tendinopathy in volleyball players. *Brit J Sports Med* 2005; 39: 102–105.
14. Blazina, M et al. Jumper's knee. *Ortho Clin North America* 1973; 4: 665–678.
15. Yu, J et al. MR imaging of injuries of the extensor mechanism of the knee. *Radiographics* 1994; 14(3): 541–551.
16. El-Khoury, GY et al. MR imaging of patellar tendinitis. *Radiology* 1992; 184: 849–854.
17. McLoughlin, RF et al. Patellar tendinitis: MR features, with suggested pathogenesis and proposed classification. *Radiology* 1995; 197: 843–848.
18. Khan, KM et al. Correlation of US and MR imaging with clinical outcome after open patellar tenotomy: Prospective and retrospective studies. *Clin J Sports Med* 1999; 9(3): 129–137.
19. Sandmeier, R, and P Renstrom. Diagnosis and treatment of chronic tendon disorders in sport. *Scand J Med Sci Sports* 1997; 7: 96–106.
20. Shalaby, M, and LC Almekinders. Patellar tendinitis: The significance of magnetic resonance imaging findings. *Amer J Sports Med* 1999; 27(3): 345–349.
21. Pope, CF. Radiologic evaluation of tendon injuries. *Clin Sports Med* 1992; 11: 579–599.
22. Erickson, SJ et al. Effect of tendon orientation on MR imaging signal intensity: A manifestation of the "magic angle" phenomenon. *Radiology* 1991; 181: 389–392.

23. Erickson, SJ, RW Prost, and ME Timins. The "magic angle" effect: Background physics and clinical relevance. *Radiology* 1993; 188: 23–25.

24. Fornage, BD. The hypoechoic normal tendon: A pitfall. *J Ultrasound in Med* 1987; 6: 19–22.

25. Lian, O et al. Relationship between symptoms of jumper's knee and the ultrasound characteristics of the patellar tendon among high level male volleyball players. *Scand J Med & Sci in Sports* 1996; 6: 291–296.

26. Cook, JL et al. Patellar tendon ultrasonography in asymptomatic active athletes reveals hypoechoic regions: A study of 320 tendons. *Clin J Sports Med* 1998; 8: 73–77.

27. Khan, KM et al. Patellar tendon ultrasonography and jumper's knee in elite female basketball players: A longitudinal study. *Clin J Sports Med* 1997; 7: 199–206.

28. Cook, JL et al. Asymptomatic hypoechoic regions on patellar tendon US do not foreshadow symptoms of jumper's knee: A 4 year follow-up of 46 tendons. *Scand J Sci & Med in Sports* 2000; 11(6): 321–327.

29. Cook, JL et al. Prospective imaging study of asymptomatic patellar tendinopathy in elite junior basketball players. *J Ultrasound in Med* 2000; 19: 473–479.

30. Testa, V et al. Ultrasound guided percutaneous longitudinal tenotomy for the management of patellar tendinopathy. *Med & Sci in Sport and Exercise* 1999; 31(11): 1509–1515.

31. Józsa, L, and P Kannus. *Human Tendons.* Champaign, IL: Human Kinetics, 1997, p. 576.

32. Richards, DP et al. Knee joint dynamics predict patellar tendinitis in elite volleyball players. *Amer J Sports Med* 1996; 24(5): 676–683.

33. Prilutsky, BI, W Herzog, and T Leonard. Transfer of mechanical energy between ankle and knee joints by gastrocnemius and plantaris muscles during cat locomotion. *J Biomech* 1996; 391–403.

34. Prapavessis, H, and PJ McNair. Effects of instruction in jumping technique and experience jumping on ground reaction forces. *J Orthrop Sports Phys Ther* 1999; 29: 352–356.

35. Cook, JL et al. Posterior leg tightness and vertical jump are associated with US patellar tendon abnormality in 14-18-year old basketball players: A cross-sectional anthropometric and physical performance study. *Brit J Sports Med* 2004; 38: 206–209.

36. Richards, DP SV Ajemian, SP Wiley, et al. Relation between ankle joint dynamics and patellar tendinopathy in elite volleyball players. 2002; 12: 266–272.

37. Curwin, S, and WD Stanish. *Tendinitis: Its Etiology and Treatment.* Lexington: Collamore Press, 1984.

38. Cannell, LJ et al. A randomised clinical trial of the efficacy of drop squats or leg extension/leg curl exercises to treat clinically diagnosed jumper's knee in athletes: Pilot study. *Brit J Sports Med* 2001; 35: 60–64.

39. Jensen, K, and RP Di Fabio. Evaluation of eccentric exercise in treatment of patellar tendinitis. *Phys Ther* 1989; 69(3): 211–216.

40. Stasinopoulos, D, and I Stasinopoulos. Comparison of effects of exercise programme, pulsed ultrasound and transverse friction in the treatment of patellar tendinopathy. *Clin Rehab* 2004; 18: 347–352.

41. Alfredson, H et al. Heavy-load eccentric calf muscle training for the treatment of chronic Achilles tendinosis. *Amer J Sports Med* 1998; 26(3): 360–366.

42. Holmich, P et al. Effectiveness of active physical training as treatment for long-standing adductor related groin pain in athletes: Randomised trial. *Lancet* 1999; 353: 439–443.

43. Mafi, N, R Lorentzon, and H Alfredson. Superior short-term results with eccentric calf muscle training compared to concentric training in a randomized prospective multi-center study on patients with chronic Achilles tendinosis. *Knee Surg Sports Traumatol Arthrosc* 2001; 9: 42–47.

44. Fyfe, I, and WD Stanish, The use of eccentric training and stretching in the treatment and prevention of tendon injuries. *Clin Sports Med* 1992; 11(3): 601–624.

45. El Hawary, R, WD Stanish, and SL Curwin. Rehabilitation of tendon injuries in sport. *Sports Med* 1997; 24: 347–358.

46. Kannus, P. Tendon pathology: Basic science and clinical applications. *Sports Exer & Inj* 1997; 3: 62–75.

47. Lee, E et al. Pulsed magnetic and electromagnetic fields in experimental Achilles tendonitis in the rat: A prospective randomised study. *Arch Phys Med & Rehab* 1997; 78: 399–404.

48. Davidson, C et al. Rat tendon morphological and functional changes resulting from soft tissue mobilization. *Med & Sci in Sports & Exer* 1997; 29: 313–319.

49. Gehlsen, G, L Ganton, and R Helfst. Fibroblast responses to variation in soft tissue mobilisation pressure. *Med & Sci in Sport & Exer* 1999; 31(4): 531–535.

50. Pellecchia, G, H Hamel, and P Behnke. Treatment of infrapatellar tendinitis: A combination of modalities and transverse friction massage versus iontophoresis. *J Sport Rehab* 1994; 3: 315–345.

51. Rolf, C et al. An open, randomized study of ketoprofen in patients in surgery for achilles or patellar tendinopathy. *J Rheumatol* 1997; 24: 1595–1598.

52. Astrom, M, and N Westlin. No effect of piroxicam on achilles tendinopathy: A randomized study of 70 patients. *Acta Orthop Scand* 1992; 63: 631–634.

53. Weiler, JM. Medical modifiers of sports injury: The use of nonsteroidal anti-inflammatory drugs (NSAIDs) in sports soft tissue injury. *Clin in Sports Med* 1992; 11(3): 625–644.

54. Almekinders, LC. The efficacy of nonsteroidal anti-inflammatory drugs in the treatment of ligament injuries. *Sports Med* 1990; 9: 137–142.

55. Almekinders, L, and J Temple. Etiology, diagnosis, and treatment of tendonitis: An analysis of the literature. *Med & Sci in Sport & Exer* 1998; 30(8): 1183–1190.

56. Riley, GP et al. Inhibition of tendon cell proliferation and matrix glycosaminoglycan synthesis by non-steroidal anti-inflammatory drugs in vitro. *J Hand Surg (Brit & Eur Vol)* 2001; 26B(3): 224–228.

57. Leadbetter, WB. Tendon Overuse Injuries: Diagnosis and Treatment. In Renstrom, PAFH, ed., *Sports Injuries: Basic Principles of Prevention and Care.* London: Oxford, 1993, pp. 449–476.

58. Fredberg, U, and L Bolvig. Jumper's knee. *Scand J Med & Sci in Sports* 1999; 9: 66–73.

59. Shrier, I, G Matheson, and G Kohl. Achilles tendinitis: Are corticosteroid injections useful or harmful? *Clin J Sports Med* 1996; 6(4): 245–150.

60. Capasso, G et al. Aprotinin, corticosteroids and normosaline in the management of patellar tendinopathy in athletes: A prospective randomized study. *Sports Exer & Inj* 1997; 3: 111–115.

61. Paoloni, JA, RC Appleyard, J Nelson et al. Topical nitric oxide application in the treatment of chronic extensor tendinosis at the elbow: A randomized, double-blinded, placebo-controlled clinical trial. *AM J Sports Med* 2003; 915–920.

62. Paoloni, JA Appleyard RC, Nelson J, et al. Topical glyceryl trinitrate treatment of chronic noninsertional achilles

tendinopathy: A randomized, double-blind, placebo-controlled trial. *J Bone Joint Surg AM* 2004; 916–922.

63. Popp, JE, JS Yu, and CC Kaeding. Recalcitrant patellar tendinitis. Magnetic resonance imaging, histologic evaluation and surgical treatment. *Amer J Sports Med* 1997; 25(2): 218–222.

64. Karlsson, J et al. Partial rupture of the patellar ligament: Results after operative treatment. *Amer J Sports Med* 1991; 19: 403–408.

65. King, J et al. Patellar tendinopathy. *Sports Med & Arthrosc Rev* 2000; 8: 86–95.

66. Ferretti, A, E Ippolito, P Mariani, and G Puddu. Jumper's knee. *Amer J Sports Med* 1983; 11: 58–62.

67. Colosimo, AJ, and FH Bassett. Jumper's knee: Diagnosis and treatment. *Orth Rev* 1990; 29: 139–149.

68. Binfield, PM, and N Maffulli. Surgical management of common tendinopathies in the lower limb. *Sports Exer & Inj* 1997; 3: 116–122.

69. Biedert, R, U Vogel, and NF Friedrichs. Chronic patellar tendinitis: A new surgical treatment. *Sports Exer & Inj* 1997; 3: 150–154.

70. Raatikainen, T et al. Operative treatment of partial rupture of the patellar ligament. *Int J Sports Med* 1994; 15: 46–49.

71. Martens, M et al. Patellar tendonitis: Pathology and results of treatment. *Acta Orth Scand* 1982; 53: 445–450.

72. Puddu, G et al. Jumper's knee and other forms of tendinitis about the knee. In *The Hughston Clinic Sports Medicine Book*. Baltimore: Williams and Wilkins, 1995, pp. 429–439.

73. Leadbetter, WB et al. The surgical treatment of tendinitis: Clinical rationale and biologic basis. *Clin in Sports Med* 1992; 11(4): 679–712.

74. Coleman, BD et al. Outcomes of open and arthroscopic patellar tenotomy for chronic patellar tendinopathy: A retrospective study. *Amer J Sports Med* 2000; 28(2): 1–8.

75. Coleman, BD et al. Studies of surgical outcome after patellar tendinopathy: Clinical significance of methodological deficiencies and guidelines for future studies. *Scand J Med & Sci in Sports* 2000; 10(1): 2–11.

17

Prevention of Anterior Knee Pain after Anterior Cruciate Ligament Reconstruction

K. Donald Shelbourne, Scott Lawrance, and Ron Noy

Introduction

Anterior knee pain is a poorly understood entity that has not been well studied in the literature. One reason for this is because "anterior knee pain" is not specific, and the cause for this symptom may encompass many different etiologies. Studies vary with their own particular definitions, and thus comparisons and conclusions are difficult to interpret. It is, therefore, important when one discusses anterior knee pain that a specific definition be initially offered. This chapter will describe anterior knee pain after anterior cruciate ligament reconstructive surgery. After a definition is made, discussions will include incidence and possible etiologies. Prevention of anterior knee pain will be addressed, including preoperative, intraoperative, and postoperative concerns. Finally, treatment options will be offered. It has been the practice in our clinic to evaluate patients carefully with regular follow-up, scrutinizing their results so that we may learn from them and continually improve our techniques and outcomes. Through the course of the chapter, we will interject our findings where appropriate in an effort to shed light on this complicated subject.

Definition

Anterior knee pain after reconstruction of the ACL has been documented as a frequent complaint of patients in many studies in the literature.[2-5,7,14,20] It is important, however, to differentiate pain in the knee into two broad categories. A knee that functions well until a specific injury causes a change can be understood by the patient as being broken, as opposed to when the knee gradually becomes painful or sore from overuse. Patients can easily distinguish between these two entities, and this distinction becomes helpful during history taking for narrowing a differential diagnosis. Both these entities can occur after ACL reconstruction surgery. The former encompasses all the different injuries that can occur in any knee regardless of previous surgery. These injuries must be identified and treated, but are not within the scope of this chapter. Knee soreness after surgery is more commonly the complaint of the patient. This pain is often vague and cannot be specifically localized with one finger. The patient, when asked to point to where it hurts, will often sweep his fingers along both sides of the patellar tendon, from the sides of the patella to the tibia tubercle. Often, the patient will think of this as "kneecap" symptoms.

Etiology

A review of the literature offers many possible factors leading to anterior knee pain in patients who have not had surgery. These include malalignment, muscular imbalance, improper training mechanics and overuse, biochemical substance changes, and psychological issues.[10] The speculation that these factors are involved in the cause of postoperative pain has altered operative and rehabilitative protocols at some institutions.

Alignment of the lower extremity has been implicated in the literature as a possible cause of anterior knee pain.[10] The quadriceps angle (Q-angle) in particular has been thought to be a significant issue. It is defined as the angle created by drawing lines from the anterior superior iliac spine to the middle of the patella to the tibia tubercle. The average Q-angle is 10 to 15 degrees with knee extended. An increased Q-angle theoretically places more stress on the lateral portion of the patella as the knee is flexed as the contact area decreases. This may result in tilting, subluxation, or even frank dislocation. Of these, tilting is most common especially in women and may cause poor patella tracking and excess wear. Some surgeons will perform a lateral retinacular release in conjunction with anterior cruciate ligament reconstruction if tilting of the patella is present. Because patella tilt is usually asymptomatic in these patients before injury, it has been our experience that a lateral release is usually not necessary and we no longer perform it unless properly indicated.

Muscle imbalance has also been proposed as a cause of tilt and subluxation.[10] A relative weakness of the vastus medialis muscle has often been taught to be a key component of muscle imbalance, and physical therapy protocols have been designed to selectively strengthen this muscle. However, it has recently been shown by EMG analysis that it is difficult if not impossible to isolate the vastus medialis using the proposed exercises, and in reality the entire quadriceps is being rehabilitated together.[6,11] After injury to the anterior cruciate ligament, swelling in the knee causes a temporary shutdown of the quadriceps muscles, causing it to be weak. While many preoperative protocols stress regaining quadriceps strength before surgery, we mainly emphasize the return of full range of motion and leg control in the injured knee.[1,12] Since 1998, we have been routinely harvesting the graft from the contralateral extremity, which has allowed us to focus the preoperative and postoperative rehabilitation on regaining range of motion and leg control without an immediate concern for gaining strength.[21] Strengthening exercises for the graft-donor site can begin immediately after surgery without a concern for loss of range of motion or an effusion. Separating the postoperative rehabilitation between knees allows for an earlier return of range of motion in the ACL reconstructed knee and a quicker return of strength in graft-donor knee. Ultimately, patients are able to return to normal activities and sports sooner.

Overuse of any muscle or tendon may cause soreness, and this is no exception after anterior cruciate ligament reconstruction. Although we believe that this is a completely different entity from the anterior knee pain that we are discussing in this chapter, it should be included in the differential diagnosis when an ipsilateral bone-patellar tendon-bone autograft technique is utilized. Some of our patients who have undergone the contralateral graft procedure have complained of soreness in the graft-donor knee after completing a few successive "two-a-day" practices. The soreness in this setting is simply overuse-related patella tendon pain. We reached this conclusion by realizing that the graft-donor knee does not share many of the same concerns as the injured knee, which therefore excludes many possible sources of pain. Assuming the graft-donor leg is normal (no previous injuries or congenital abnormalities), there are no other associated pathologies such as cartilage damage or meniscus tears that could cause anterior knee pain. Harvesting the graft is an extra-articular procedure; therefore, iatrogenic intra-articular damage that may cause pain is excluded. Given that knee range of motion and strength are normal preoperatively, and are easily regained postoperatively, the contributions by these factors to pain are minimized. Furthermore, the athletes do not complain of pain during the first few days of the new practice week, but only after many successive practices, and rest usually alleviates their symptoms. We realized that we were overworking the tendon and not allowing it to recuperate between workouts. For the same reason that weightlifters alternate which body region they concentrate on each day, the patella tendon and quadriceps muscle need a day to rest between heavy strengthening workouts. We have therefore recently changed our contralateral donor-graft leg strengthening workouts to be performed every other day, and this is still under review. What this clearly shows is that the harvesting of the tendon itself is probably not the cause of the anterior knee pain syndrome.

Of much lesser prevalence is a psychosomatic basis for this pain.[23] This should be low on the differential diagnosis list, but should not be dismissed altogether should an organic cause for the pain not be found. Sustaining an anterior cruciate ligament injury, while certainly not as career threatening and ominous as it may have been only a few short years ago, can have a very strong effect on an athlete's mental state. We must remember that we are treating the patient and not just the knee injury.

Although much of the above may have some role in causing anterior knee pain post anterior cruciate ligament reconstructive surgery, other factors have much greater implications. First and foremost, the most important contributor to this syndrome is a lack of regaining full hyperextension as compared with the pre-injured state. Related to this concept are poor tunnel placement and graft-notch mismatch. Also, previous underlying patellofemoral disease has been implicated as a source of anterior knee pain, as is other intra-articular pathology such as meniscus tears and articular surface chondral lesions. Lastly, tibia hardware may also present itself as a cause of pain and needs to be addressed.

By far, the most important issue is the lack of regaining full hyperextension.[14,15,20] After anterior cruciate ligament rupture, an intra-articular hemarthrosis usually occurs acutely. The resulting pain and swelling cause the patient to keep the affected knee bent for comfort. Upon initial evaluation, patients will have a flexion contracture, even if they are seen quickly after injury. Most uninjured knees will hyperextend past zero degrees (Figure 17.1) and it is from this hyperextended position that lack of extension must be measured.[18] Because it is impossible to know what the full hyperextension on the injured knee was before injury, we compare the injured knee to the normal contralateral knee. Caution must be observed if the patient has had any previous injury or condition affecting the other knee

because the injury can lead to an inaccurate assessment of full hyperextension, which in turn can lead to erroneous operative planning. If less than full normal hyperextension, then the graft maybe set tensioned too tightly in an attempt to match the other leg, resulting in less hyperextension. Even a small amount of flexion contracture can greatly impact performance, especially for athletes who require full knee extension to jump and run well, and must not be taken lightly. In the non-athlete, these changes can also have a significant effect on future lifestyle issues. We extensively reviewed 602 patients from 1987 to 1992 regarding anterior knee pain after anterior cruciate ligament reconstruction. These knees were reconstructed using a standard ipsilateral bone-patellar tendon-bone autograft with a mini-arthrotomy technique. We observed an apparent association between knee flexion contracture and anterior knee pain, and this observation was similar to reports published by Sachs and colleagues.[9] We implemented a perioperative rehabilitative protocol that emphasized regaining full hyperextension before surgery was performed and during the first week postoperatively. Physical therapy programs used by others during the same time period had concerns regarding extension of the reconstructed knee beyond 30° of flexion as it was thought that full extension unduly stressed the graft before it healed.[15,17] We have shown in other studies,

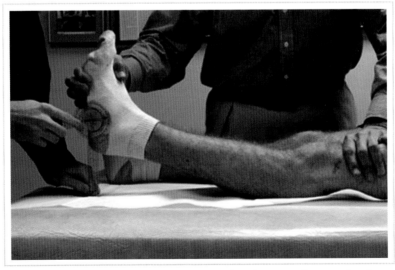

Figure 17.1. Most patients' knees have some degree of hyperextension. To evaluate the amount of hyperextension, place one hand above the knee to hold the thigh and place the other hand on the patient's foot to life the heel off of the examination table.

however, that if the graft is placed properly in its isometric position with the appropriate amount of tension, the graft can withstand the forces applied with an aggressive rehabilitation program.[8] In fact, side-to-side KT-1000 arthrometer testing showed no significant loss of stability in patients who underwent this protocol. These patients all returned an anterior knee pain questionnaire with an average follow-up of 3.6 years. Their results were compared with those of a control group, which consisted of 122 young healthy asymptomatic athletes, averaging 20.3 years old. Full hyperextension was achieved in all patients and the average loss of flexion was five degrees at 2.3 years after initial surgery. It was necessary for 21 of these patients to undergo arthroscopic lysis of adhesions at an average of 6.8 months post-op because of lack of full hyperextension, but all of these patients eventually regained full extension symmetrical to the noninjured knee. Out of a possible 100 points, the ACL-reconstructed patients scored 89.5 points, which was not significantly different from the control group (90.2 points). We concluded from these results that regaining hyperextension was the key to decreasing the incidence of anterior knee pain.[20]

The intraoperative requirement for regaining hyperextension has to do with obtaining the proper fit of the graft within the notch. When proper graft placement, appropriate tensioning, and adequate notchplasty are simultaneously performed, full hyperextension should be achievable if it was obtained preoperatively (Figure 17.2). If full extension is not maintained postoperatively, the graft will hypertrophy and block full knee extension. When the graft fits properly within the notch with the leg in full hyperextension, it will conform to this space during its healing stages and therefore allow normal motion.

Previously existing patellofemoral chondromalacia has been thought by some orthopedic surgeons to be a relative contraindication to harvesting a bone-patellar tendon-bone autograft. The existence of patellofemoral chondromalacia can be diagnosed with history, physical examination, radiographs, and MRI. Some have tried other types of screening studies such as bone scan and thermography.[22] These special tests (other than history and physical) can be costly, invasive, and inaccurate. Furthermore, some surgeons will perform an initial diagnostic arthroscopy to evaluate the patellofemoral joint and then use this information as a basis of choosing a different source of graft, including hamstring or allograft. Both of these grafts are far inferior choices as they do not allow for an accelerated rehabilitative program, which may result in longer return to sport intervals.[8] In our experience, we have not found chondromalacia of the patellofemoral joint to be of any significance in postoperative performance or symptoms other than a mild increased incidence of pain with sports and kneeling. In the previously mentioned

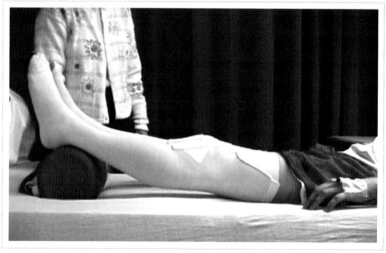

Figure 17.2. Immediately after surgery, patients should be able to obtain full hyperextension in the ACL-reconstructed knee equal to the normal knee. The heel prop exercise shown in this figure is an easy method for achieving full extension.

study, we noticed that of 49 patients that reported anterior knee pain preoperatively on a modified Noyes survey, only 4 of these were found to have grade 3 or 4 disease when inspected intraoperatively. Therefore, even history is inaccurate in assessing the extent of disease in this area.[20] We did not alter our operative technique based on patellofemoral chondromalacia. Postoperatively, patients with patellofemoral disease did not have significantly different anterior knee pain scores from other patients without any patellofemoral disease or from the control group of young athletes without any disease. We believe that choosing a different source for the graft based on patellofemoral chondromalacia is unwarranted. The advantages of the bone-patellar tendon-bone autograft far outweigh the slightly increased risk of symptoms with kneeling and sports.

Associated pathology found during surgery most often includes meniscus damage and chondromalacia of the articular surfaces. It can also include other ligament damage and osteochondral defects, although much less commonly. Meniscus lesions are addressed during surgery either with trephination and left in situ, partial resection, or repair. A meniscus tear is most often in the posterior horn and should not give the type of symptoms seen with anterior knee pain. The pain is usually more localized posteriorly, or is perceived by the patient to be deep in the joint. Physical findings are more specific with joint line tenderness posteriorly and a positive McMurray test. Because meniscus lesions are addressed intraoperatively, it theoretically should not cause any pain postoperatively. However, an iatrogenic source of pain after meniscus repair can occur, especially with placement of devices such as absorbable arrows, which can overpenetrate the capsule and cause sharp pain. However, meniscus arrows do not usually cause vague anterior pain, and the pain can usually be localized.

Proposed treatment of articular cartilage lesions varies greatly in aggressiveness. Debridement using an arthroscopic shaver or a thermal probe (coblation) is very popular. The long-term effects of the latter have yet to be shown, and the viability of cartilage cells has come into question. More invasive treatments including mosaicplasty and cartilage cell transfers have also been suggested, but are still under review. While large loose flaps should be debrided, it has been our experience that the remainder of the lesion does not need to be addressed surgically. Shelbourne and colleagues[13] studied the outcome of untreated articular cartilage defects in conjunction with ACL reconstruction. From 1987 to 1999, 125 patients met the study criteria of having an articular cartilage defect rated as Outerbridge grade 3 or 4 but had both menisci intact. The mean defect size was 1.7 cm^2. The objective and subjective results of the study group were compared with a matched control group of patients who had intact menisci and no articular cartilage damage. At a mean follow-up time of 8.7 years after surgery, the mean subjective score was 92.8 points in the study group versus 95.9 in the control group. This difference was statistically significantly different, but both scores represent a good outcome. The radiographic results were not statistically significantly different between the study group and the control group. The study by Shelbourne and colleagues[13] provides baseline information that can be used to compare the results of procedures designed to treat articular cartilage defects.

Retained tibia hardware can also be a source of anterior knee pain after surgery. Many fixation devices, including screws with washers, interference screws, staples, and buttons, have been used depending on graft technique. Recent design improvements, such as low-profile head-on screws, have been made in an effort to minimize irritation that can become symptomatic. In addition, careful technique in covering the device with soft tissue should be performed when possible because even suture knots may become symptomatic. Despite these advances and precautions, these hardware devices still can be a problem and may necessitate a second operation to remove the device once the graft is fully incorporated and healed. This pain, however, can also be localized over the device by palpation and usually results in a different pain pattern.

Prevention

Prevention of anterior knee pain following anterior cruciate ligament reconstruction is an essential key to success. These measures can be subdivided into preoperative, intraoperative, and postoperative concerns.

Preoperative

Preoperative prevention begins with proper history and physical evaluation. Pre-injury knee pain or dysfunction should be elicited from the patient. If the patient complains of preexisting pain, then the cause of this should be sought and proper planning of surgery can then be performed. The overall alignment of the leg should be checked. Patella tracking through full range of motion can be quickly evaluated, and a "J" sign can be elicited if present. Direct palpation of the articular surface of the patella as well as mobility, tilt, and apprehension are checked. Range of motion of the knee is compared with the contralateral extremity. If the knee is still markedly swollen, cold/compression (Cryo/Cuff, Aircast, Inc. Newark NJ), elevation, and physical therapy have been shown to reduce the swelling effectively in a short period of time. Any lack of hyperextension must be regained before proceeding with surgery. Physical therapy exercises consisting of heel props, towel extension exercises (Figure 17.3), prone leg hangs, and the use of a hyperextension device can also be added to regain full hyperextension (Figure 17.4). In addition to therapeutic exercises, patients must be made conscious of how to maintain full extension throughout the day. Extension habits, including sitting heel prop and standing on the involved extremity with the knee locked out and forced into full hyperextension by an active quadriceps contraction are performed by the patients whenever they are sitting or standing. Once this has been achieved, surgery can then be performed with the best chance for obtaining full hyperextension and preventing anterior knee pain postoperatively.

Intraoperative

Intraoperative concerns are easily dealt with as long as the surgeon is aware of them and proficient in his or her craft. Graft choice is the first consideration. When using hamstring grafts, it has been recommended to avoid full hyperextension in the postoperative period because the stress may stretch the graft. The ability to regain full hyperextension when it is not initially obtained in the early postoperative period can be difficult. Given that the lack of full hyperextension causes anterior knee pain after ACL reconstruction, choosing a bone-patellar tendon-bone graft that allows immediate full hyperextension after surgery should reduce the incidence of anterior knee pain postoperatively.

Placement of incision is a subject that is not often addressed. We use an offset incision medial to the patella tendon as opposed to directly over the tendon. This location not only aids in visualization, but avoids a scar and subcutaneous scar tissue directly where patients kneel. Furthermore, by using a contralateral graft and a mini-arthrotomy approach, extensive subcutaneous dissection anterior to the

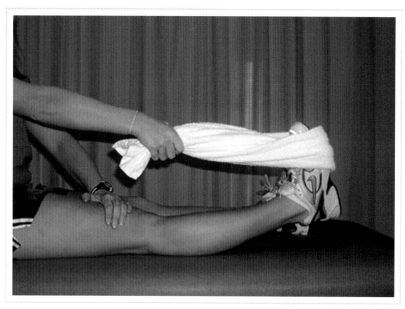

Figure 17.3. Towel stretch exercise: A towel is looped around the arch of the foot and the patient holds onto both ends of the towel with one hand. The other hand pushes down on the top of the thigh while using the towel to pull up on the foot. This maneuver allows the patient to bring the knee into hyperextension passively.

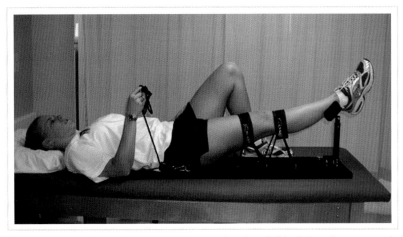

Figure 17.4. Elite seat extension device: The ankle of the affected leg is propped on the end of the device and straps are attached above and below the knee. The device has a pulley system that allows the patient to progressively extend the knee while lying completely supine, which allows the patient's hamstring muscles to relax fully. The hyperextension stretch should be held for approximately 10 minutes at a time.

ipsilateral tendon can be avoided. This again should decrease scar formation in this region, which may allow more motion and less pain.

Proper placement of the tunnels and notchplasty are important. Precise placement of the tibial tunnel will prevent superior roof impingement, thereby alleviating the need for superior notchplasty. As seen on a lateral radiograph taken with the knee in full hyperextension, the anterior portion of the tibial tunnel should be parallel to Blumensaat's line. Preoperative evaluation of x-rays can help the surgeon visualize the proper orientation of the tibial tunnel and to evaluate placement of the guide wire. Proper placement of the tibial tunnel also minimizes the amount of lateral wall resection that is needed to allow for the proper fit of the new 10 mm graft. The amount of lateral notch resection that is necessary is accurately measured with a caliper, and the appropriate amount of bone is removed. Proper placement of the femoral tunnel is equally as important. Placement of the femoral tunnel that is too anterior will result in impingement and a decrease in knee range of motion. The femoral tunnel should leave a one-millimeter posterior cortical rim and slightly overlap the lateral border of the posterior cruciate ligament. Impingement should be checked with the knee in full hyperextension, and any correction should be made before surgery is completed. When the graft fits properly within the notch, it remodels to fit that space as it heals. Improper

placement of either tunnel or an inadequate notchplasty can result in impingement, which blocks extension. If the graft does not sit in the notch correctly, it hypertrophies as it heals, further preventing full hyperextension.[3] The result is a flexion contracture, which can cause anterior knee pain. In addition, pain may also occur due to the actual impingement itself.

The next issue of great importance is that of placing the proper tension of the graft. Many orthopedic surgeons try to put the graft in as tight as possible. Securing the graft too tightly does not allow full hyperextension, which results in a tight knee that can be painful.[8] If the tension in the graft is not set with the knee in full hyperextension, then full hyperextension should be forced after graft fixation to allow the graft tension to adjust and allow full hyperextension. It is more preferable to have a slightly lax knee than an overly tight knee, because a stiff stable knee is painful. Our operative technique incorporates a press fit technique, placing both bone blocks from inside out, securing the graft on both sides with buttons. We are able to make subtle adjustments on the graft tension as we test for full motion and stability. The result is a stable knee with full hyperextension and flexion.

Another issue is repairing the tendon defect and bone plug defects. As previously described, repairing the tendon together with the paratendon should eliminate the patellar tendon defect as a source of pain. It decreases the amount of fibrous scar tissue filling the defect as well as the surrounding subcutaneous tissue. Leaving the defect unrepaired allows excessive scar formation that can persist up to the patella and displace it, as shown on postoperative CT scans.[7] Bone grafting the defects resulting from harvesting the bone plugs allows quicker and more uniform healing of these areas. While not proven, leaving defects in the patella and tibia may act as stress risers, as can the defect in the patellar tendon. While bone grafting the plug sites may decrease the incidence of patella and tibia fractures, it has been shown to have no effect on the incidence of anterior knee pain.[2]

Postoperative

Postoperatively, the most important issue clearly is retaining full hyperextension. While regaining full flexion also needs to be addressed, obtaining full hyperextension immediately after surgery will prevent anterior knee pain and afford the patient the best opportunity to return to his or her pre-injury level of play. A postoperative program can be set up to attain this goal. The first step is to discuss with the patient and family members step by step what is to occur after surgery on a daily basis, and what is expected of them and why. Immediately after surgery, a Cryo/Cuff is applied to the knee and the leg is placed in a continuous-passive-motion machine. Patients remain in the hospital overnight for administration of intravenous ketorolac,[16] patient education, and supervision of the postoperative exercises. Range-of-motion exercises are done once every two hours for a total of 6 times daily. Extension exercises are performed as described previously, including towel stretches, heel props with the addition of prone hangs, or use of an extension device as needed depending on the patient's extension. Flexion exercises include maximal CPM machine flexion to 125° and held for 3 minutes. Next a heel slide is performed to maximal flexion and measured using a yardstick. The yardstick is set with the knee fully extended so that the end of the yardstick is lined up with the heel. A measurement is taken when maximal flexion is reached by recording the number of centimeters the heel has traveled. If the patient demonstrates any restriction in full extension range of motion, all flexion exercises should be held until full extension returns and efforts focused on regaining full passive extension. These exercises are done in conjunction with using the

Cryo/Cuff to dramatically reduce swelling, which would otherwise restrict motion, and cause pain and poor wound healing. During the first postoperative week, the patient is made to remain lying down with the leg elevated in a CPM so that the knee remains above the level of the heart as much as possible to keep the swelling to a minimum. Patients may place full weight on both legs while ambulating with crutches, but this should be restricted to ambulating to the bathroom only for the first week remaining supine with their leg elevated. Cryotherapy, continuous passive movement, and hyperextension/flexion exercises are continued at home. The patients are given the goals for their one-week follow-up appointment of full terminal hyperextension, flexion greater than or equal to 110°, normal gait pattern, minimal swelling, and good leg control. During the second week of rehabilitation, towel extensions and heel props are continued and prone leg hangs and/or an extension devise may be added to the regimen if necessary. Extension habits are again reviewed and reinforced for use when both sitting and standing. Once full range of motion and normal gait are achieved, strengthening exercises can be added. The graft leg is started on step-down exercises while continuing the previously described exercises. Our two-week goals for the reconstructed knee now include full hyperextension, 120° of flexion, and good quadriceps control. The patient should be able to perform an active heel lift by this visit. Patients do not receive formal continuous therapy sessions with a therapist (such as three visits per week). Instead, the patients are given a detailed home therapy program, and their progress is supervised and adjusted by the therapist (who is in close contact with the surgeon) on a regularly scheduled basis. The remainder of our rehabilitative program maintains the full hyperextension while progressing with strengthening and sport-specific exercises, and is beyond the scope of this chapter.[12, 21]

Treatment

The loss of full hyperextension is the key component for developing anterior knee pain after anterior cruciate ligament reconstruction. Type 1 arthrofibrosis (defined as less than 10° loss of knee extension) and type 2 (defined as greater than 10° loss of knee extension) are associated with anterior knee pain.[19] The treatment begins with a thorough history and physical examination. The length of time since surgery should be noted. Was the patient compliant with the postoperative protocol? Was there a reinjury to the knee? All these questions are important to ask, even if you were the operating surgeon on this patient. Proper radiographs should be done to evaluate the bone tunnels and graft placement. Possible impingement can be inferred from these studies. If the tunnels were appropriately placed and surgery was recent, regaining hyperextension can be easily obtainable. Regaining full hyperextension early will still allow the graft to conform to the intercondylar space as it continues to heal, allowing full range of motion and preventing further anterior knee pain. A lateral radiograph view of the knee can be used to evaluate for patella tendon contracture by measuring the distance between the tendinous attachment sites on the inferior patella and tibial tubercle. For patients who demonstrate a patella tendon contracture, decreased flexion will be observed and the patient will have an arthrofibrosis type 3 or 4. This loss of flexion is likely the result of the contracted patella tendon.

Nonoperative treatment should be instituted as soon as possible. The longer a flexion contracture exists, the more difficult it is to overcome. Early postoperative management includes formal therapist evaluation and implementation of a therapeutic exercise program designed to maximize the amount of knee hyperextension. Towel extension exercises, prone leg hangs, emphasis of both sitting and standing extension habits (described above), and the use of a hyperextension device should all be implemented. The hyperextension device (Figure 17.4) is a device that allows the patient to independently apply a long-duration stretch to the posterior knee several times throughout the day. This device consists of a pulley system that is connected to the knee that the patient can progressively tighten during the treatment. Since the patient is controlling the amount of stretch applied to the knee, he or she is able to better relax the musculature around the knee, making the stretch from the device more effective. The hyperextension stretch should be held for 10 to 12 minutes at a time. This routine of hyperextension device and therapeutic exercises should be performed 3 to 5 times throughout the day to fully maximize the patient's extension range of motion. If the deformity is chronic, correction will take a prolonged course and the patient should be properly educated about goals. The longer the flexion con-

traction has existed, the longer it will take to correct. It is important that the patient maintain a positive mental attitude during this long process. Often, patients have been to several medical providers that offer little or no help with their condition. This can easily lead to patients' frustration with the whole process. Consistent communication of goals and feedback on improvement will help focus the patients and help them strive to attain their goal of full range of motion. Often these patients complain not only of pain, but also of loss of strength. However, it is only after full motion is regained that the knee can be strengthened, and strengthening exercises should be avoided until full range of motion can be demonstrated. This simply is due to the biomechanical disadvantages that exist when the knee cannot fully extend.

Occasionally nonoperative means fail for types 1 and 2 arthrofibrosis, and surgical intervention must be offered. This is considered only after the patient has failed an appropriate therapy program as detailed above. Preoperative pain evaluation with forced extension should produce anterior pain only. If posterior pain is present, then posterior structures need to be addressed and this encompasses a different spectrum of pathology than is being discussed. Surgical intervention is most often performed with an arthroscopic procedure. Type 1 arthrofibrosis is treated by excising the cyclops lesion from the graft, which allows the graft to fit properly within the notch with the knee in full hyperextension. Type 2 arthrofibrosis requires resection of anterior scar tissue that forms in front of the graft and proximal tibia. If impingement persists with extension, a notchplasty is also performed. Patients are kept overnight in the hospital for a period of 2 nights to prevent postoperative hemarthrosis, allow for the continuous infusion of intravenous ketorolac, and to start postoperative rehabilitation immediately. Full weightbearing is allowed immediately, but only for bathroom privileges to reduce the chance of getting a hemarthrosis. No casting is performed at this time because this can lead to problems with hemarthrosis, decreased knee flexion, and most importantly decreased quadriceps control. Patients use the hyperextension device followed by towel stretches 3 to 5 times throughout the day to focus on maximizing extension. The focus is to regain full extension over the course of the 2- to 3-day stay in the hospital instead of regaining all hyperextension immediately. The patient remains on bedrest with bathroom privileges only with the leg in a CPM machine moving from 0° to 30°. This forces the patient to stay in a supine position with the leg elevated so that the knee is elevated above the level of the heart to avoid a hemarthrosis. Additionally, the Cryo/Cuff is worn consistently while in the hospital to provide cold and compression to the knee joint. Anti-embolism stockings are worn to prevent problems with postoperative blood clot and to provide knee joint compression. While the patient is in the hospital, daily visits are made by the physical therapist to ensure consistent improvement and to answer any questions the patient may have. When patients can demonstrate full hyperextension equal to the opposite knee and appropriate independence with their exercises, they are allowed to be discharged home. They are instructed to continue with the same exercise routine and should remain supine with their leg elevated in the CPM for another 3 days. Activity is restricted to bathroom privileges only even while at home. Consistent follow-up daily by phone is important to ensure continued maintenance of full hyperextension and is helpful in keeping the patient motivated during the postoperative process. Weekly follow-up is mandatory until hyperextension can be maintained actively.

Once full passive hyperextension is able to be maintained, the next goal is to maintain full extension actively with a quadriceps contraction. Leg control exercises are initiated when the patient demonstrated full hyperextension and include terminal knee extension with rubber tubing, step-ups onto a box, single-leg knee extensions, and step-downs. Continued focus though should be maintained on hyperextension exercises during this phase. When the patient can demonstrate a full, symmetric active heel lift equal to the opposite side, then exercises for flexion can be added only if full extension is maintained. If there is any loss of hyperextension, flexion exercises should be decreased until full hyperextension returns. Gentle strengthening exercises can be added once the patient has demonstrated full range of motion, both hyperextension and flexion. Strengthening exercises include leg press, step-downs, knee extensions, and low-impact conditioning exercise such as a stationary bicycle, Stairmaster, or elliptical cross trainer. Consistent follow-up is maintained until

the patient has return of full motion and strength equal to the opposite side. Of the patients that we have treated with type 1 or 2 arthrofibrosis using this protocol, all were able to achieve full hyperextension and anterior knee pain was eliminated.[19]

Summary

Anterior knee pain following reconstruction of the anterior cruciate ligament is a problem that has plagued many patients. After extensively studying patients with this problem and comparing them to those that do not suffer from this entity, we have concluded that this is most often due to a loss of full hyperextension. Prevention of this by proper preoperative, intraoperative, and postoperative management can be successfully performed. Prevention should be the number-one concern. If anterior knee pain after ACL reconstruction does occur, the symptoms can usually be alleviated through nonoperative means. Occasionally, surgical intervention may become necessary. Other causes for this pain syndrome are rare but with proper evaluation can easily be differentiated and treated.

References

1. Arnold, T, and KD Shelbourne. A Perioperative rehabilitation program for anterior cruciate ligament surgery. *Phys Sports Med* 2000; 28: 31–44.
2. Baszotta, H, and K Prunner. Refilling of removal defects: Impact on extensor mechanism complaints after use of a bone-tendon-bone graft for anterior cruciate ligament reconstruction. *Arthroscopy* 2000; 16: 160–164.
3. Fisher, SE, and KD Shelbourne. Arthroscopic treatment of symptomatic extension block complicating anterior cruciate ligament reconstruction. *Am J Sports Med* 1993; 21: 558–564.
4. Kartus, J, L Magnusson, S Stener et al. Complications following arthroscopic anterior cruciate ligament reconstruction: A 2- to 5-year follow-up of 604 patients with special emphasis on anterior knee pain. *Knee Surg Sports Traumatol, Arthrosc* 1999; 7: 2–8.
5. Kleipool, AE, T van Loon, and RK Marti. Pain after use of the central third of the patellar tendon for cruciate ligament reconstruction: 33 patients followed 2–3 years. *Acta Orthop Scand* 1994; 65: 62–66.
6. Laprade, J, E Culham, and B Brouwer. Comparison of five isometric exercises in the recruitment of the vastus medialis oblique in persons with and without patellofemoral pain syndrome. *J Orthop Sports Phys Ther* 1998; 27: 197–204.
7. Rosenberg, TD, JL Franklin, GN Baldwin et al. Extensor mechanism function after patellar tendon graft harvest for anterior cruciate ligament reconstruction. *Am J Sports Med* 1992; 20: 519–525.
8. Rubinstein, RA, Jr., and KD Shelbourne. Graft selection, placement, fixation, and tensioning for anterior cruciate ligament reconstruction. *Op Tech Sports Med* 1993; 1: 10–15.

9. Sachs, RA, DM Daniel, ML Stone et al. Patellofemoral problems after anterior cruciate ligament reconstruction. *Am J Sports Med* 1989; 17: 760–765.

10. Sanchis-Alfonso, V, E Rosello-Sastre, Martinez-Sanjuan. V. Pathogenesis of anterior knee pain syndrome and functional patellofemoral instability in the active young. *Am J Knee Surg* 1999; 12: 29–40.

11. Sheehy, P, RG Burdett, JJ Irrgang et al. An electromyographic study of vastus medialis oblique and vastus lateralis activity while ascending and descending steps. *J Orthop Sports Phys Ther* 1998; 27: 423–429.

12. Shelbourne, KD, and T Gray. Anterior cruciate ligament reconstruction with autogenous patellar tendon graft followed by accelerated rehabilitation: A two- to nine-year follow-up. *Am J Sports Med* 1997; 25: 786–795.

13. Shelbourne, KD, S Jari, and T Gray. Outcome of untreated traumatic articular cartilage defects of the knee: A natural history study. *J Bone Joint Surg (Supplement)* 2003; 85-A: 8-16.

14. Shelbourne, KD, and GE Johnson. Outpatient surgical management of arthrofibrosis after anterior cruciate ligament surgery. *Am J Sports Med* 1994; 22: 192–197.

15. Shelbourne, KD, TE Klootwyk, JH Wilckens et al. Ligament stability two to six years after anterior cruciate ligament reconstruction with autogenous patellar tendon graft and participation in accelerated rehabilitation. *Am J Sports Med* 1995; 23: 575-579.

16. Shelbourne, KD, and FJ Liotta. ACL reconstruction utilizing an abnormally thick autogenous patellar tendon graft. *Am J Knee Surg* 1999; 12: 79–81.

17. Shelbourne, KD, and P Nitz. Accelerated rehabilitation after anterior cruciate ligament reconstruction. *Am J Sports Med* 1990; 18: 292–299.

18. Shelbourne, KD, and DV Patel. Treatment of limited motion after anterior cruciate ligament reconstruction. *Knee Surg Sports Traumatol Arthrosc* 1999; 7: 85–92.

19. Shelbourne, KD, KV Patel, and DJ Martini. Classification and management of arthrofibrosis of the knee after anterior cruciate ligament reconstruction. *Am J Sports Med* 1996; 24: 857–862.

20. Shelbourne, KD, and RV Trumper. Preventing anterior knee pain after anterior cruciate ligament reconstruction. *Am J Sports Med* 1997; 25: 41–47.

21. Shelbourne, KD, and SE Urch. Primary anterior cruciate ligament reconstruction using the contralateral autogenous patellar tendon. *Am J Sports Med* 2000; 28: 651–658.

22. Siegel, MG, KA Siqueland, and FR Noyes. The use of computerized thermography in the evaluation of non-traumatic anterior knee pain. *Orthopedics* 1987; 10: 825–830.

23. Witonski, D. Anterior knee pain syndrome. *Int Orthop* 1999; 23: 341–344.

18

Lysis of Pretibial Patellar Tendon Adhesions (Anterior Interval Release) to Treat Anterior Knee Pain after ACL Reconstruction

Sumant G. Krishnan, J. Richard Steadman, Peter J. Millett, Kimberly Hydeman, and Matthew Close

Abstract

We report the clinical results of an anterior interval release for recalcitrant anterior knee pain associated with decreased patellar mobility after anterior cruciate ligament (ACL) reconstruction.

Thirty consecutive patients with recalcitrant anterior knee pain and decreased patellar mobility after ACL reconstruction underwent an arthroscopic lysis of adhesions and scar of the distal patella tendon from the proximal anterior tibia (anterior interval release). Anterior knee pain was initially treated nonoperatively. Failure of nonoperative treatment was defined by recalcitrant anterior knee pain and no improvement in functional outcome, assessed by Lysholm scores and patient questionnaires. Minimum clinical follow-up was 2 years. All anterior interval release procedures were also performed by the senior author using a high inferolateral viewing portal in order to arthroscopically evaluate the anterior interval between the patella tendon and tibia. Prior to anterior interval release, Lysholm score averaged 68 (range 18–90). Postoperative Lysholm score averaged 85 (range 68–100) (P < 0.0001). Postoperative range-of-motion did not change significantly. Postoperative instability examinations were all graded zero using the International Knee Documentation Committee (IKDC) system. Average patient satisfaction at follow-up was 8.0 (1 = very dissatisfied; 10 = very satisfied).

Early operative intervention with an anterior interval release has been shown in this series to result in significantly improved functional outcomes in the treatment of recalcitrant anterior knee pain after ACL reconstruction.

Introduction

Arthroscopic anterior cruciate ligament (ACL) reconstruction has become one of the most commonly performed procedures in orthopedic surgery and knee reconstruction.[13,14,21] Over the last decade, the results of arthroscopic ACL reconstruction have remained outstanding in most peer-reviewed series, regardless of surgical technique.[13,21] However, the published literature regarding postoperative complications after ACL reconstruction remains quite sparse.[5,6,10,38]

Anterior knee pain is a well-documented complication after arthroscopic ACL reconstruction and has been reported as the most common complaint after ACL surgery.[1,6,10,19,30,31,34,38] While the initial studies reported anterior knee pain after patellar tendon autograft reconstruction, recent work confirms a real incidence of anterior knee pain even after hamstring or allograft ACL reconstruction.[1,32] Consequently, the etiology of this anterior knee pain remains elusive and controversial.[6,12,24,27,32]

Paulos et al.[26,27] were the first to describe the "infrapatellar contracture syndrome (IPCS)," an "exaggerated pathologic fibrous hyperplasia" of soft tissue in the anterior knee after intra-articular surgery and specifically after ACL reconstruction. IPCS can create significant arthrofibrosis, loss of knee motion, decreased patellar mobility ("patellar entrapment"), and even patella infera. The diagnosis of IPCS according to these authors was based on a "decrease in patellar mobility as compared with the opposite knee," zero or negative passive patellar tilt, and less than 2 cm of superior/inferior patellar glide. Without appropriate identification and aggressive treatment, IPCS after ACL reconstruction results in significant functional morbidity.

Several others have also documented the incidence of adhesions of the patellar tendon to the anterior tibia after arthroscopic procedures.[2,4,8,15,16,20,22,26-29,33,36,37] Ahmad et al.[2] demonstrated the biomechanical effect of such patellar tendon adhesions to the anterior tibia. These authors documented an effective patella infera when the patellar tendon was adhesed to the anterior tibial cortex in this pretibial recess. The adhesions were shown to significantly alter both patellar and tibial kinematics and contact – potentially increasing patellofemoral and tibiofemoral contact forces that may eventually result in arthrosis.[2,8,15,35,41]

We have encountered a population of patients with recalcitrant anterior knee pain after ACL reconstruction that have failed conservative treatment and have subtle alterations in patellar mobility despite a full range of flexion and extension. To our knowledge, this clinical entity and its appropriate treatment have not yet been described. We report here the clinical results of an arthroscopic release of pathologic adhesions in the pretibial recess (anterior interval release) in these patients to treat the anterior knee pain.

Materials and Methods

Between 1992 and 1998, 30 consecutive patients with recalcitrant anterior knee pain after isolated ACL reconstruction underwent an arthroscopic anterior interval release by the senior author. All 30 patients had previously undergone arthroscopic ACL reconstruction by the senior author, using a 2-incision technique and an ipsilateral bone-patellar tendon-bone autograft with interference screw fixation. Mean age at the time of ACL reconstruction was 32 years (range 16–43 years). There were 14 men and 16 women patients. For all 30 patients, the ACL reconstruction was the first surgery performed on that knee. Mean duration between injury and ACL reconstruction was 6 weeks (range 2–16 weeks). No patient demonstrated abnormal posterior, posterolateral, varus, or valgus examinations. Criteria required before proceeding with ACL reconstruction included ability to perform a supine straight-leg raise, flexion greater than

90°, and no warmth of the knee relative to the contralateral side.[7,33] Intraoperatively, no patient demonstrated other ligament pathology in addition to the ACL injury. Seventeen patients underwent concurrent meniscus trephination, and no patients underwent a meniscus repair. Postoperative rehabilitation followed the same protocol: full passive and active range-of-motion exercises (with emphasis on terminal extension), crutches in the immediate postoperative period with progressive full weightbearing, and a hinged knee brace for the first 6 postoperative weeks. Strengthening exercises did not begin until full range-of-motion was achieved.

All 30 patients complained of disabling anterior knee pain within 6 weeks of the ACL reconstruction. All Lachman examinations were graded zero using the International Knee Documentation Committee system (IKDC). Physical examination demonstrated significantly restricted passive patellar and patellar tendon mobility relative to the contralateral side, both in medial/lateral and in superior/inferior excursion. All patients demonstrated less than 2 cm of superior/inferior passive patellar excursion, decreased medial/lateral passive patellar excursion relative to the contralateral side, and an inability to passively "tilt" the inferior pole of the patella away from the anterior tibial cortex (Figure 18.1).[20,28] Range-of-motion in all 30 patients averaged 0° of extension (range 5° of hyperextension to a 3° lack to full extension) and 140° of flexion (range 130°–155°). No patients demonstrated either a 10° or greater loss of knee extension or a 25° or greater loss of knee flexion.[20,28]

Initial treatment consisted of nonsteroidal anti-inflammatory (NSAID) medication, patellar mobilization exercises, and closed-chain quadriceps-strengthening exercises for a minimum of 12 weeks in all 30 patients. Failure of conservative treatment was identified by recalcitrant anterior knee pain and no further improvement in functional outcome as assessed by a standardized patient questionnaire and the scoring system of Lysholm and Gillquist.[39]

The anterior interval release was performed at a mean duration of 9 months after the ACL reconstruction (range 6–12 months). Postoperative rehabilitation consisted of immediate passive patellar mobilization exercises, immediate progressive weightbearing with crutches, and no brace.

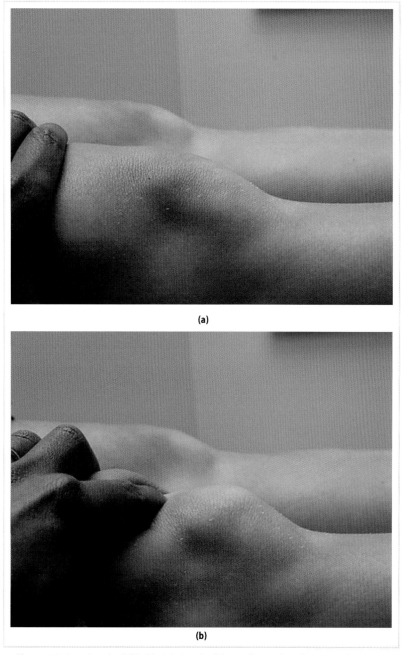

Figure 18.1. Normal passive "tilt" of the inferior pole of the patella away from the anterior tibial cortex.

Minimum clinical follow-up after the anterior interval release was 2 years. All patients were objectively examined by the senior author, functionally evaluated using the scoring system of Lysholm and Gillquist,[39] and subjectively evaluated using a standardized patient questionnaire. The questionnaire documents pain, stiffness, function during daily and sporting activities, and satisfaction based on a 10-point scale (1 point = very dissatisfied; 10 points = very satisfied). Statistical significance for data analysis was set at $P < 0.05$.

Surgical Technique for Arthroscopic Anterior Interval Release

Arthroscopy was performed with the arthroscope in an inferolateral portal relative to the patella and the working instruments in an inferomedial portal. In all cases, the inferolateral viewing portal was placed at the level of the patella with the knee in full extension (Figure 18.2). This high portal (originally described by Patel[23]) is approximately 1 cm proximal to the standard inferolateral arthroscopy portal and provides clear visualization of the anterior soft tissues in the retropatellar and pretibial regions.[23]

After standard arthroscopic evaluation of the knee and confirmation of an intact ACL graft, the infrapatellar and suprapatellar regions were evaluated. In all cases, the infrapatellar fat pad and patellar tendon were adhesed to the anterior tibial cortex below the inferior pole of the patella. These anterior interval adhesions prevented normal motion of the intermeniscal ligament over the tibial plateau during dynamic flexion and extension. An anterior interval release was performed by releasing this scar tissue (Figure 18.3) from medial to lateral just anterior to the peripheral rim of the anterior horn of each meniscus (Figure 18.4A). The release was performed either with electrocautery or with a thermal ablation device (Arthrocare, Arthrocare Corporation, Sunnyvale, California, USA). The release also proceeded from proximal (at the level of the meniscus) to approximately 1 cm distal along the anterior tibial cortex (Figure 18.4B). Great care was taken to avoid cauterizing or burning the bone of the anterior tibia or the patellar tendon. Meticulous hemostasis was obtained prior to completion of the procedure by cauterizing any bleeding vessels in the infrapatellar fat pad.

Results

Examination under anesthesia revealed all patients had less than 2 cm of superior/inferior passive patellar excursion, decreased medial/lateral passive patellar excursion relative to the contralateral side, and an inability to passively tilt the inferior pole of the patella away from the anterior tibial cortex. Intraoperative examination immediately after anterior interval release demonstrated that all patients had at least 2 cm of superior/inferior passive patellar excursion, equal medial/lateral patellar excursion relative to the contralateral side, and the ability to passively tilt the inferior pole of the patella away from the anterior tibial cortex.

Postoperative range-of-motion did not change significantly from the preoperative evaluation and averaged 0° of extension (range 5° of hyperextension to 2° lack to full extension) and 145° of flexion (range 140°–155°).

Postoperative stability examinations revealed IKDC grade zero Lachman, posterior drawer,

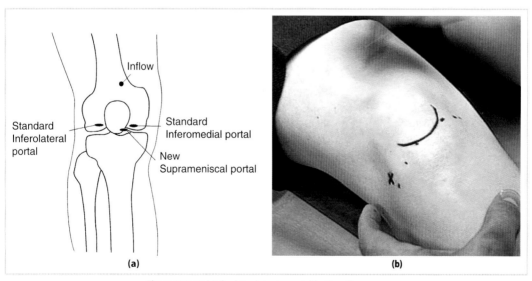

(a)   (b)

Figure 18.2. High inferolateral viewing portal for the arthroscope.

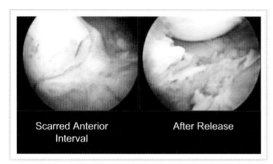

Figure 18.3. "Anterior interval release" from medial to lateral just anterior to the peripheral horn of each meniscus.

varus stress, and valgus stress tests. Postoperative posterolateral corner examination was normal in all patients.

After failure of nonoperative treatment, preoperative Lysholm score averaged 68 (range 18–90). After arthroscopic anterior interval release, postoperative Lysholm score significantly increased to an average of 85 (range 68–100) ($P < 0.0001$).

Based on the preoperative patient questionnaires, 74% of patients reported moderate to severe pain, 63% reported moderate to severe stiffness, and 58% reported that their knee functioned abnormally. Postoperatively, 21% reported moderate to severe pain, 5% reported moderate to severe stiffness, and 16% reported that their knee functioned abnormally.

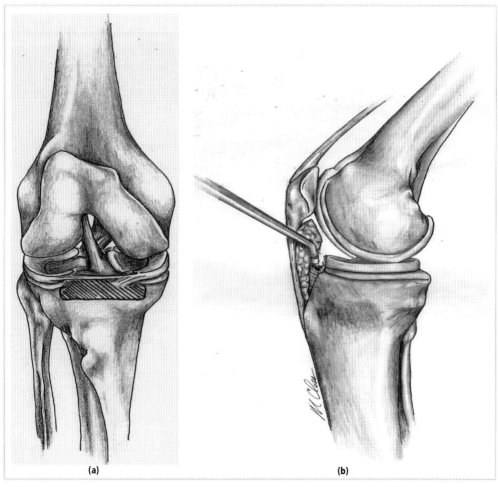

(a)   (b)

Figure 18.4. Drawing of anterior interval release, demonstrating area of medial-lateral release **(a)** and superior-inferior release from the level of the meniscus to approximately 1 cm distal along the anterior tibial cortex **(b)**.

Preoperatively, average patient satisfaction was 2.0 (range 1–5) while postoperatively, average patient satisfaction increased to 8.0 (range 5–10) (1.0 = very unsatisfied; 10 = highly satisfied).

Complications

Six of the 30 patients (20%) underwent reoperation within 1 year after the initial anterior interval release for recalcitrant anterior knee pain. Preoperative evaluation, as well as examination under anesthesia, revealed that patellar entrapment had recurred with less than 2 cm of passive superior/inferior excursion and an inability to passively tilt the inferior pole of the patella away from the anterior tibial cortex.[20,28] In all 6 cases, scar tissue had reformed in the anterior interval and was again released arthroscopically. Qualitatively, the scar tissue appeared to be less robust than the tissue identified in the initial anterior interval release procedure. Postoperative rehabilitation in these patients stressed patellar mobilization exercises. No other complications or reoperations occurred in this population of patients during the study period. No patients suffered from patellar tendonitis during the study period.

Discussion

Postoperative adhesions of the patellar tendon to the anterior tibia (anterior interval scarring) have been described by several authors.[2,4,8,15,16,20,22,26-29,33,36,37] The etiology of these adhesions remains unknown. Hughston[10] has proposed that iatrogenic injury to the infrapatellar fat pad and subsequent scarring is the responsible cause, and Rosenberg et al.[30] have documented this scarring via computed tomographic scan after patellar tendon graft harvest for ACL reconstruction. Still, the correlation between such anterior interval scarring and anterior knee pain after ACL reconstruction has remained controversial.

We hypothesized that the cause of recalcitrant knee pain after ACL reconstruction in this patient population was anterior interval scarring. Release of this scarring significantly improved functional outcome scores in the majority of patients. We postulate that the cause of this scarring after ACL reconstruction is the hematoma that necessarily forms in the soft tissues of the anterior knee after drilling of the tibial tunnel. Based on this same proposed mechanism, current investigation is underway evaluating the incidence of anterior interval scarring and recalcitrant anterior knee pain after either hamstring or allograft ACL reconstruction.

Noyes et al.[20] have proposed that patellar adhesions and associated subtle patella infera may lead to patellar pain due to increased stress on the patellofemoral cartilage. In a retrospective review, Rosenberg et al.[30] identified narrowing of the patellofemoral joint space in over 50% of their patients with ACL-reconstructed knees, relative to the contralateral uninjured side. Furthermore, Paulos et al.[26-28] have documented the clear association between patella infera and radiographic changes of patellofemoral arthrosis in patients with patellar entrapment and IPCS. These findings were confirmed by Millett et al.[16] who identified patella infera and patellofemoral arthrosis in cases of global arthrofibrosis. These reports suggest that abnormal stress on the patellofemoral articulation can be a leading cause of anterior knee pain after ACL reconstruction.

Ahmad et al.[2] have biomechanically demonstrated the alteration in contact position in the patellofemoral articulation due to anterior interval adhesions. Such altered contact appears to lead to altered stress in the cartilage and may lead to recalcitrant anterior knee pain.[8,15,35,41] Several authors have described the surgical management of these adhesions when associated with IPCS or arthrofibrosis of the knee.[3,4,7,11,16,17,22,29,36,37,40] Paulos et al.[26,28] recommend resecting all fibrous scar tissue between the inferior pole of the patella and the anterior tibial plateau and releasing the patellar tendon from the anterior tibial cortex (anterior interval release). Richmond et al.[29] describe arthroscopically resecting fibrotic areas of the infrapatellar fat pad and also releasing the adhesion of the fat pad to the anterior tibia (anterior interval release). In both of these published studies, anterior interval adhesions were associated with significant arthrofibrosis of the knee and significant preoperative limitations of motion in terminal extension and/or terminal flexion.

The group of patients in the present study represents a special population whose appropriate management, to our knowledge, has not yet been documented in the peer-reviewed literature. These patients all experienced recalcitrant anterior knee pain that was clearly refractory to conservative treatment, all demonstrated pathological restriction of patellar and patellar tendon mobility, but all patients maintained a preoperative range-of-motion that did not qualify for a diagnosis of IPCS based on the criteria published by Paulos et al.[28] In our opinion, this group of patients represents an earlier (perhaps less aggressive) stage of anterior interval scarring, which may eventually lead to full-blown IPCS. However, all patients experience significant functional morbidity due to this anterior interval scarring, despite a preserved arc-of-motion. It is the diagnosis and prompt treatment of these patients that is the focus of this study.

All 30 patients presented here suffered from recalcitrant anterior knee pain after ACL reconstruction. All failed at least 3 months of conservative treatment. One weakness of this retrospective study is the lack of a designated concurrent control group. However, those patients in our clinical experience with anterior knee pain after ACL reconstruction whose pain resolved and who regained patellar mobility after 3 months or less of conservative treatment became the inherent control group to aid in the decision to proceed to surgical management. Based on this clinical experience, we have arbitrarily identified a timeline of at least 3 months of failed conservative treatment and at least 6 months after the ACL reconstruction as the point at which surgical management should be considered.

All of the patients presented here demonstrated subtle finding of patellar entrapment: decreased superior/inferior passive patellar excursion (less than 2 cm), decreased medial/lateral passive patellar excursion, and inability to passively tilt the inferior pole of the patella and the patellar tendon away from the anterior tibial cortex.[20,28] Paulos et al.[26,28] describe limitation of flexion and/or extension along with the abnormality in patellar mobility. In our opinion, the study group presented here is too early in the natural course of anterior interval scarring to demonstrate restricted motion. The hallmark clinical signs described previously for abnormal patellar mobility remain important in our evaluation of all patients after ACL reconstruction, especially those with anterior knee pain. If the subtle signs of decreased passive patellar excursion and tilt are identified early, we remain confident that the majority of these patients can be managed with nonoperative methods for their anterior knee pain.

The findings of this study have led us to alter both our surgical technique during ACL reconstruction and our initial postoperative management of all patients undergoing ACL reconstruction. Intraoperatively during the reconstruction, we pay particular attention to avoiding injury to the infrapatellar fat pad and to obtaining meticulous hemostasis. Postoperatively, we now emphasize passive patellar mobility in the immediate and ensuing postoperative periods and also focus on obtaining terminal knee extension. Shelbourne et al.[32] have indicated that perhaps the incidence of anterior knee pain after ACL reconstruction may be reduced by obtaining full extension postoperatively. However, as demonstrated in the biomechanical model of Ahmad et al.,[2] anterior interval scarring and patellar tendon adhesions cause anterior tibial translation. In this clinical situation, emphasizing extension can be *detrimental* since full extension may excessively stress the ACL graft when anterior interval scarring is present, due to anterior tibial translation. These findings have led us to pay close attention to patella and patellar tendon mobility and excursion during the physical examination of any patient with an ACL reconstruction, to prevent these potential complications.

Six patients (20%) in this study developed recurrent intractable anterior knee pain after the initial anterior interval release procedure, requiring a second arthroscopic procedure. This is a significant portion of the patient population in this study group. Potential reasons for failure of the first anterior interval release procedure are either an error in appropriately diagnosing the etiology of the anterior knee pain or a technical failure to adequately perform the anterior interval scar tissue release. Both of these points highlight weaknesses in the present study design and patient population. However, all procedures were performed by the same experienced knee surgeon. Furthermore, we continue to encounter a subgroup of this patient population that requires a second anterior interval release procedure because the scarring and adhesions have reformed. In all of these cases, the scar tissue is clearly less abundant but still restricts patella mobility. Again, we cannot definitively conclude whether this scar tissue either was inadequately released in the first procedure or recurred secondary to the particular biology of each patient. Still, the fact that these 6 patients experienced initial pain relief after the first (and again after the second) anterior interval release is encouraging for the correctness of both diagnosis and surgical management.

During the surgical management of anterior interval scarring, we have identified certain key aspects of the anterior interval release. The most important technical point is the use of the infer-olateral arthroscopic viewing portal of Patel.[23] This portal (placed lateral to the patellar tendon at the level of the inferior pole of the patella with the knee in full extension) allows for a "bird's-eye" view of the anterior soft tissues of the knee. In our experience, if this high viewing portal is not used, the standard inferolateral portal (just above the level of the meniscus) prevents adequate evaluation of the anterior interval – possibly contributing to missed anterior interval pathological scarring.

Lastly, during the anterior interval release, it is important to clearly visualize the anterior horns of each meniscus during the division of scar tissue to prevent iatrogenic damage. In addition, the intermeniscal ligament should be clearly identified, both to demarcate the anterior interval and to prevent iatrogenic destabilization of the meniscal horns. The release should progress distally from the level of the meniscal horns by approximately 1 cm along the anterior tibial cortex. Care should be taken not to cauterize or burn the bone of the anterior tibia or the patellar tendon. In our experience, the release is complete when the intermeniscal ligament and the anterior horn of the medial meniscus moves more than 1 cm over the tibial plateau during full flexion and extension. Also, the infrapatellar fat pad can be seen to lift away from the anterior tibial cortex after adequate release.

Acknowledgments

The authors wish to thank Karen Briggs and the Clinical Research Department of the Steadman Hawkins Sports Medicine Foundation for their invaluable help with this study.

References

1. Aglietti, P, R Buzzi, S D'Andria et al. Patellofemoral problems after intraarticular anterior cruciate ligament reconstruction. *Clin Orthop* 1993; 288: 195–204.
2. Ahmad, CS, SD Kwak, GA Ateshian et al. Effects of patellar tendon adhesion to the anterior tibia on knee mechanics. *Am J Sports Med* 1998; 26: 715–724.
3. Christel, P, S Herman, S Benoit et al. A comparison of arthroscopic arthrolysis and manipulation of the knee under anesthesia and the treatment of postoperative stiffness of the knee. *French J Orthop Surg* 1988; 2: 348–355.
4. Del Pizzo, W, JM Fox, MJ Friedman et al. Operative arthroscopy for the treatment of arthrofibrosis of the knee. *Contemp Orthop* 10: 1985; 67–72.
5. DeLee, JC. Complications of arthroscopy and arthroscopic surgery: Results of a national survey. *Arthroscopy* 1985; 1: 214–220.
6. Graf, B, and F Uhr. Complications of intra-articular anterior cruciate reconstruction. *Clin Sports Med* 1988; 7: 835–848.
7. Harner, CD, JJ Irrgang, J Paul et al. Loss of motion after anterior cruciate ligament reconstruction. *Am J Sports Med* 1992; 20: 499–506.
8. Heegaard, J, PF Leyvraz, A Van Kampen et al. Influence of soft structures on patellar three-dimensional tracking. *Clin Orthop* 1994; 299: 235–243.
9. Huberti, HH, and WC Hayes. Patellofemoral contact pressures. The influence of q-angle and tendofemoral contact. *J Bone Joint Surg* 1984; 66A: 715–724.
10. Hughston, JC. Complications of anterior cruciate ligament surgery. *Orthop Clin North Am* 1985; 16: 237–240.
11. Jackson, DW, and RK Schaefer. Cyclops syndrome: Loss of extension following intra-articular anterior cruciate ligament reconstruction. *Arthroscopy* 1990; 6: 171–178.
12. Jacobsen, KE, and FC Flandry. Diagnosis of anterior knee pain. *Clin Sports Med* 1989; 8: 179–195.
13. Johnson, RJ, E Eriksson, T Haggmark et al. Five- to ten-year follow-up evaluation after reconstruction of the anterior cruciate ligament. *Clin Orthop* 1984; 183: 122–140.
14. Kaplan, N, TL Wickiewicz, and RF Warren. Primary surgical treatment of anterior cruciate ligament ruptures: A long-term follow-up study. *Am J Sports Med* 1990; 18: 354–358.
15. Meyer, SA, TD Brown, DR Pedersen et al. The effects of patella infera on patellofemoral contact stress. *Trans Orthop Res Soc* 1993; 18: 303.
16. Millett, PJ, RJ Williams, TL Wickiewicz. Open debridement and soft tissue release as a salvage procedure for the severely arthrofibrotic knee. *Am J Sports Med* 1999; 21: 552–561.
17. Mohtadi, NG, S Webster-Bogaert, PJ Fowler. Limitation of motion following anterior cruciate ligament reconstruction: A case-control study. *Am J Sports Med* 1991; 19: 620–624.
18. Noyes, FR, SD Barber, LA Mooar. A rationale for assessing sports activity levels and limitations in knee disorders. *Clin Orthop* 1989; 246: 238–249.
19. Noyes, FR, RE Mangine, and S Barber. Early knee motion after open and arthroscopic anterior cruciate ligament reconstruction. *Am J Sports Med* 1987; 15: 149–160.
20. Noyes, FR, EM Wojtys, and MT Marshall. The early diagnosis and treatment of developmental patella infera syndrome. *Clin Orthop* 265: 1991; 241–252.
21. O'Brien, SJ, RF Warren, H Pavlov et al. Reconstruction of the chronically insufficient anterior cruciate ligament with the central third of the patellar ligament. *J Bone Joint Surg* 1991; 73A: 278–286.
22. Parisien, JS. The role of arthroscopy in the treatment of postoperative fibroarthrosis of the knee joint. *Clin Orthop* 1988; 229: 185–192.
23. Patel, D. Proximal approaches to arthroscopic surgery of the knee. *Am J Sports Med* 1981; 9: 296–303.
24. Patel, D. Plica as a cause of anterior knee pain. *Orthop Clin North Am* 1986; 17: 273–277.
25. Paulos, L, FR Noyes, E Grood et al. Knee rehabilitation after anterior cruciate ligament reconstruction and repair. *Am J Sports Med* 1981; 9: 140–149.
26. Paulos, LE, TD Rosenberg, J Drawbert et al. Infrapatellar contracture syndrome: An unrecognized cause of knee stiffness with patella entrapment and patella infera. *Am J Sports Med* 1987; 15: 331–341.
27. Paulos, LE, DC Wnorowski, and CL Beck. Rehabilitation following knee surgery. Recommendations. *Sports Med* 1991; 11: 257–275.

28. Paulos, LE, DC Wnorowski, and AE Greenwald. Infrapatellar contracture syndrome: Diagnosis, treatment, and long-term follow-up. *Am J Sports Med* 1994; 22: 440–449.
29. Richmond, JC, and M al Assal. Arthroscopic management of arthrofibrosis of the knee, including infrapatellar contracture syndrome. *Arthroscopy* 1991; 7: 144–147.
30. Rosenberg, TD, JL Franklin, GN Baldwin et al. Extensor mechanism function after patellar tendon graft harvest for anterior cruciate ligament reconstruction. *Am J Sports Med* 1992; 20: 519–525.
31. Sachs, RA, DM Daniel, ML Stone et al. Patellofemoral problems after anterior cruciate ligament reconstruction. *Am J Sports Med* 1989; 17: 760–765.
32. Shelbourne, KD, and RV Trumper. Preventing anterior knee pain after anterior cruciate ligament reconstruction. *Am J Sports Med* 1997; 25: 41–47.
33. Shelbourne, KD, JH Wilckens, A Mollabashy et al. Arthrofibrosis in acute anterior cruciate ligament reconstruction: The effect of timing of reconstruction and rehabilitation. *Am J Sports Med* 1991; 19: 332–336.
34. Shino, K, S Nakagawa, M Inoue et al. Deterioration of patellofemoral articular surfaces after anterior cruciate ligament reconstruction. *Am J sports Med* 1993; 21: 206–211.

35. Singerman, R, DT Davy, and VM Goldberg. Effects of patella alta and patella infera on patellofemoral contact forces. *J Biomech* 1994; 27: 1059–1065.
36. Sprague, NF III, RL O'Connor, and JM Fox. Arthroscopic treatment of postoperative knee fibroarthrosis. *Clin Orthop* 1982; 166: 165–172.
37. Sprague, NF III. Motion-limiting arthrofibrosis of the knee: The role of arthroscopic management. *Clin Sports Med* 1987; 6: 537–549.
38. Strum, GM, MJ Friedman, JM Fox et al. Acute anterior cruciate ligament reconstruction: Analysis of complications. *Clin Orthop* 1990; 253: 184–189.
39. Tegner, Y, and J Lysholm. Rating systems in the evaluation of knee ligament injuries. *Clin Orthop* 1985; 198: 43–49.
40. Tria, AJ Jr, JA Alicea, and RP Cody. Patella baja in anterior cruciate ligament reconstruction of the knee. *Clin Orthop* 1994; 299: 229–234.
41. van Eijden, TM, E Kouwenhoven, and WA Weijs. Mechanics of the patellar articulation: Effects of patellar ligament length studied with a mathematical model. *Acta Orthop Scand* 1987; 58: 560–566.

19

Donor-Site Morbidity after Anterior Cruciate Ligament Reconstruction Using Autografts

Clinical, Radiographic, Histological, and Ultrastructural Aspects

Jüri Kartus, Tomas Movin, and Jon Karlsson

Abstract

Postoperative donor-site morbidity and anterior knee pain following ACL surgery may result in substantial impairment for the patient. The selection of graft, surgical technique and rehabilitation program can affect the occurrence of undesirable pain conditions.

The loss or disturbance of anterior sensitivity caused by intraoperative injury to the infrapatellar nerve(s) in conjunction with patellar tendon harvest is correlated with donor-site discomfort and an inability to kneel and knee walk.

The patellar tendon at the donor site displays significant clinical, radiographic, histological, and ultrastructural abnormalities several years after harvesting its central third. The donor-site discomfort correlates poorly with radiographic and histological findings after the use of patellar tendon autografts. The use of hamstring tendon autografts causes less postoperative donor-site morbidity and anterior knee problems than the use of patellar tendon autografts. There also appears to be a regrowth of the hamstring tendons within two years after the harvesting procedure. There is a lack of knowledge in terms of the course of the donor site after harvesting fascia lata autografts. Harvesting quadriceps tendon autografts appears to cause low donor-site morbidity.

Efforts should be made to spare the infrapatellar nerve(s) during ACL reconstruction using patellar tendon autografts as well as hamstring autografts. Reharvesting the patellar tendon cannot be recommended due to significant clinical, radiographic, histological, and ultrastructural abnormalities several years after harvesting its central third. It is important to regain full range of motion and strength after the use of any type of autograft to avoid future anterior knee pain problems.

Since randomized controlled trials have shown that the laxity measurements and clinical results following ACL reconstruction using hamstring tendon autografts are similar to those of patellar tendon autografts, we recommend the use of hamstring tendon autografts due to fewer donor-site problems.

Introduction

At the present time, arthroscopic ACL reconstruction is one of the most common surgical procedures in sports medicine. Every year, approximately 150,000 procedures are performed in the United States. After the introduction of the arthroscopic technique and the opportunity to perform reproducible anatomic replacements of the ruptured ACL, the results in terms of restored laxity and a return to sports activities have generally been found to be good.[1-3] However, persistent donor-site morbidity such as tenderness, anterior knee pain, disturbance in anterior knee sensitivity, and the inability to kneel and knee walk is still a problem and is present in approximately 40–60%, at least in patients who have undergone arthroscopic ACL reconstruction using patellar tendon autografts.[4-11] Despite efforts to utilize synthetic materials[12,13] and allografts,[14,15] the use of autografts probably remains the best option for the replacement of the torn ACL. Common autograft alternatives for reconstruction or augmentation of the ACL include the use of the iliotibial band,[16-20] the hamstring tendons,[21-26] the patellar tendon,[1,27-32] and the quadriceps tendon.[33-36]

Provided that the surgical technique was correctly used and no internal derangement of the knee has occurred, late problems related to the donor site after ACL reconstruction using autografts can be divided into three categories.

1. General pain and discomfort in the anterior knee region caused by a decrease in function such as range of motion (ROM) and muscular strength
2. Specific discomfort in terms of numbness, tenderness, and the inability to kneel or withstand pressure toward the donor-site area
3. Late tissue reactions in, or close to, the donor site

There are several ways of assessing the donor site and anterior knee region problems.

1. Clinically useful tools are measurements of strength using either functional tests such as the one-leg-hop test or dynamometers (e.g., Cybex®, Hoover Inc., Austin, Texas, USA), measurement of loss of motion, assessment of the kneeling or knee-walking ability, and measurement of the disturbance or loss of sensitivity in the donor-site area or in the area that is innervated by nerves passing the donor-site region.
2. Radiographic assessments using standard radiographs, computed tomography (CT), magnetic resonance imaging (MRI), and ultrasonography.
3. Histological, biochemical, and ultrastructural assessments of samples obtained from the donor-site area.

The amount of information about the donor site after the use of patellar tendon autografts is fairly extensive. Recently the amount of information about donor-site problems following the use of hamstring autografts has increased. Some information describing the problems that can occur after ACL reconstruction using quadriceps tendon autografts is available. However, there is very little information after using fascia lata autografts.

Postoperative Restriction in Range of Motion and Loss of Strength

There appears to be agreement in the literature that the restoration of full extension compared with the noninjured side after ACL reconstruc-

tion is essential in order to avoid postoperative discomfort in the anterior knee region. Irrgang and Harner,[37] Harner et al.,[38] Sachs et al.,[10] and Kartus et al.[39] have all stated that the loss of extension contributes to anterior knee pain. Shelbourne and Trumper[11] have stated that the restoration of full hyperextension is of major importance when it comes to avoiding anterior knee pain.

The influence of loss of flexion on anterior knee pain is controversial. Stapleton[40] and Kartus et al.[39] have stated that the loss of flexion causes significantly more anterior knee pain than the loss of extension and Aglietti et al.[41] reported that a loss of flexion exceeding 10° might be correlated with anterior knee pain. However, Irrgang and Harner[37] found that a loss of flexion rarely matters, unless the knee flexion is less than 110°.

Although these reports are all concerned with the use of patellar tendon autografts or allografts,[37] we can generalize and state that the return of full range of motion (ROM) including full hyperextension is essential to reduce anterior knee problems after ACL reconstruction using any type of graft.

In line with this information, we recommend that it is essential to regain normal strength in the lower extremity to avoid future pain in the anterior knee region. Risberg et al.[42] have reported that pain and strength are the most important variables, which affect the results after ACL reconstruction using patellar tendon autografts. Several reports on strength deficits after ACL reconstruction using autografts are found in the literature. Muneta et al.[43] reported that the patients' subjective evaluation of the results after ACL reconstruction using either hamstring or patellar tendon autografts was worse if the quadriceps or hamstring strength was decreased compared with the contralateral side. Hiemstra et al.[44] reported that at one year the patients had substantial strength deficits in extension both after reconstruction using patellar tendon and hamstring tendon grafts. Feller et al.[45] reported a quadriceps peak torque strength deficit up to one year after surgery after harvesting the patellar tendon compared with harvesting the hamstring tendons. Adachi et al.[46] reported that the harvest of both semitendinosus and gracilis tendons causes more loss of active flexion angle and peak torque than the harvest of semitendinosus alone. Correspondingly Tashiro et al.[47] recommended sparing the gracilis due to less loss of hamstring muscle strength at high knee flexion angles compared with harvesting both the semitendinosus and gracilis tendons.

After using the quadriceps tendon grafts Lee et al.[35] reported a loss of quadriceps strength of 13% compared with the contralateral side at one year after surgery.

After using iliotibial band augmentation for open primary ACL repair, Natri et al.[19] reported a peak torque loss of 14% in extension and 6% in flexion 2 to 5 years after surgery.

Dissection Studies in the Knee Region

Arthornthurasook and Gaew-Im,[48] Horner and Dellon,[49] Hunter et al.,[50] and Kartus et al.[51] (Figure 19.1) have shown in dissection studies that the infrapatellar nerve is in danger when incisions are made close to or above the tibial tubercle and the medial side of the knee joint. From anatomic descriptions of the prepatellar area it appears that the infrapatellar nerve can be damaged when incisions are made in the anterior knee region.[52-54] Correspondingly, medial knee incisions can jeopardize the saphenous nerve.[25] In a dissection study of 40 cadaver knees Boon et al.[55] have recommended using oblique incisions medial to the tibial tubercle

when harvesting hamstring tendons to avoid sensory nerve damage.

Knee Surgery and Sensory Nerve Complications

Johnson et al.,[56] Swanson,[57] and Tapper et al.[58] have described postoperative morbidity, such as numbness and problems with kneeling, after injury to the infrapatellar branch(es) of the saphenous nerve after open medial meniscectomies. Chambers[59] explored three patients because of pain and numbness after open medial meniscectomies and found scarring or neuroma of one infrapatellar branch of the saphenous nerve. Ganzoni and Wieland[60] have shown a difference in postoperative sensory loss, depending on whether the infrapatellar nerve(s) were protected during medial knee arthrotomies.

Mochida and Kikuchi[61] have described the possibility of injury to the infrapatellar nerve(s) during arthroscopic surgery and Poehling et al.[62] have described the development of reflex sympathetic dystrophy after sensory nerve injury in the knee region. The importance of the sensory nerves in the knee region was further stressed in the reports by Gordon[63] and

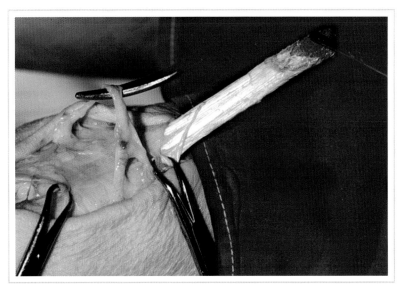

Figure 19.1. The infrapatellar nerve splits into two branches, right in the center of a central anterior 8 cm incision. The towel clamps indicate the paratenon. The patellar tendon autograft in this specimen was harvested using the two-incision technique with the aim of sparing the infrapatellar nerve(s) and the paratenon. In this specimen, the two incisions have been conjoined in order to examine the result of the harvesting procedure.[129] (Reproduced with permission from reference 51.)

Detenbeck[64] on prepatellar neuralgia after direct impacts to the anterior knee region, the report by House and Ahmed[65] on the entrapment of the infrapatellar nerve, and the report by Worth et al.[66] on the entrapment of the saphenous nerve in the knee region. Slocum et al.[67] have discussed the possibility of damage to the nerves in the anterior knee region during a pes anserinus transplantation, which requires an incision similar to the one used for harvesting hamstring tendon autografts.

There are only a few reports in the literature with regard to discomfort after injury to the infrapatellar nerve or its branches in conjunction with ACL surgery. Berg and Mjöberg[68] have reported that the difficulty in kneeling was cor-

related with the loss of sensitivity in the anterior knee region after open knee ligament surgery and they, therefore, recommend a lateral parapatellar skin incision. In two studies involving 90[69] and 604[39] patients respectively, Kartus et al. have reported that the inability to kneel and knee-walk (Figure 19.2) after arthroscopic ACL reconstruction using patellar tendon autografts harvested through a 7–8 cm vertical incision was correlated with the area of disturbed or lost anterior knee sensitivity (Figure 19.3). Mastrokalos et al.[70] reported lost or disturbed sensitivity in 85.4% of patients after harvesting ipsilateral patellar tendon autografts.

Mishra et al.[71] have reported that the use of two horizontal incisions while harvesting the central

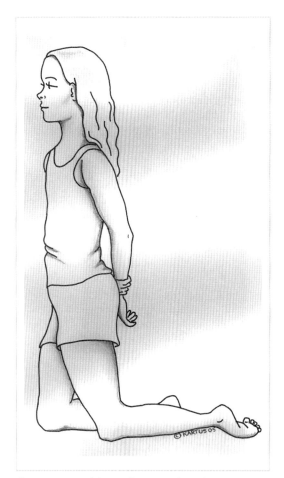

Figure 19.2. A simple knee-walking test can be used to determine the discomfort in the anterior knee region after ACL reconstruction.[73] (Copyright Catarina Kartus.)

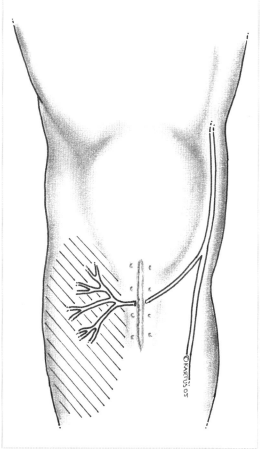

Figure 19.3. After the use of a central 7–8 cm incision to harvest a patellar tendon autograft, the discomfort during the knee-walking test correlated with the area of disturbed sensitivity in the anterior knee region.[39, 73] (Copyright Catarina Kartus.)

third of the patellar tendon may offer an opportunity to protect the infrapatellar nerve(s). No results in terms of nerve function have, however, been presented. Kartus et al.,[72] on the other hand, presented a method using two 25 mm vertical incisions to reduce the risk of injury to the infrapatellar nerve(s) when harvesting patellar tendon autografts (Figure 19.4). This technique was first tested in cadavers[51] and was subsequently proven in two clinical studies[73,74] to produce less loss of sensitivity and a tendency toward less knee-walking discomfort than the use of a vertical 7–8 cm incision. In a clinical study without a control group, Tsuda et al.[75] suggested patellar tendon harvest to be performed using two horizontal incisions in order to minimize postoperative anterior knee symptoms. In a dissection study, Tifford et al.[76] made similar findings and further recommended that incisions in the anterior knee region should be made with the knee in flexion in order to avoid injury to the infrapatellar nerve(s).

When hamstring tendon autografts are harvested, a branch of the infrapatellar branch of the saphenous nerve might also be jeopardized[25] and occasionally numbness in the skin area supplied by the saphenous nerve may also occur. Bertram et al.[77] in a case report described saphenous neuralgia after arthroscopically assisted ACL reconstruction using semitendinous and gracilis tendons. Eriksson[78] as well as Ejerhed et al.[79] have shown that the area of disturbed sensitivity after

harvesting either semitendinosus or patellar tendon autografts is comparable. However, both studies suggested that the area of disturbed sensitivity after harvesting semitendinosus autografts is of less clinical importance.

It appears that the same amount of disturbance in sensitivity in the knee region after harvesting hamstring tendon autografts causes fewer kneeling and knee-walking difficulties than after harvesting patellar tendon autografts. This can be due to the fact that, after patellar tendon harvest, the pressure when kneeling is applied directly on or close to the incision where the injured nerve is located as suggested by Ejerhed et al.[79] Spicer et al.[80] have reported that sensory changes in the whole anterior knee region after hamstring tendon harvest are possible and 50% of their patients reported such changes. However, this rarely limited the activity of their patients.

After harvesting fascia lata and quadriceps tendon autografts, the risk of nerve injuries appears to be low and no such reports are found in the literature to our knowledge.

Local Discomfort in the Donor Site Region

In a prospective, randomized study, Brandsson et al.[81] have shown that suturing the patellar tendon defect and bone grafting the defect in the

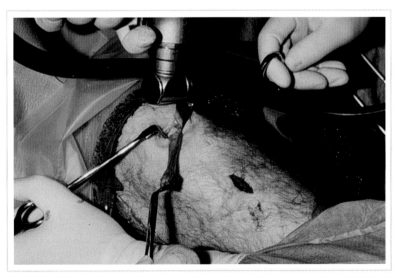

Figure 19.4. The use of the two-incision technique to harvest a patellar tendon autograft resulted in less discomfort during the knee-walking test than the use of the central one-incision technique. (Reproduced with permission from reference 51.)

patella did not reduce anterior knee problems or donor-site morbidity. Boszotta and Prünner[82] also found that bone grafting the patellar defect did not reduce kneeling complaints or patellofemoral problems. It therefore appears that suturing and bone grafting the defects after patellar tendon harvest is of minor importance when it comes to reducing donor-site problems. Tsuda et al.,[75] on the other hand, suggested bone grafting of the defects in order to decrease donor-site problems. However, in their study the grafts were harvested subcutaneously and no control group was available.

Kartus et al.[73] reported that 65% of the patients had difficulty or were unable to perform the knee-walking test two years after patellar tendon harvest using a central vertical 7–8 cm incision. The corresponding value after the use of a two-incision technique with the aim of sparing the infrapatellar nerve(s) was 47%.[73] Rubinstein et al.[83] found that the isolated donor-site morbidity was negligible after ACL surgery, when the contralateral patellar tendon was used as a graft. In contrast Mastrokalos et al.[70] found that more than 70% of the donor knees had knee-walking problems regardless whether the patellar tendon graft was harvested from the ipsi- or contralateral side.

Preoperatively, as well as two years after the use of hamstring autografts, approximately 20% of the patients reported that they had difficulty or were unable to perform the knee-walking test as shown by Ejerhed et al.[79] in their prospective randomized trial. Corry et al.[84] reported that only 6% of patients had kneeling pain two years after the use of hamstring tendon autografts, compared with 31% after the use of patellar tendon autografts. However, no preoperative data were presented. Yasuda et al.[85] reported that activity-related soreness had resolved by three months after harvesting the contralateral hamstring tendon graft. Eriksson et al.[78,86,87] have in prospective randomized studies shown that patients operated on using semitendinosus autografts have less anterior knee problems and donor-site morbidity than patients operated on using patellar tendon autografts, both in the short and long term. In a randomized study Feller and Webster[45] reported that 67% of patients operated on using patellar tendon autografts and only 26% of patients operated on using hamstring tendon grafts had kneeling pain at three years after surgery. These findings suggest that the use of hamstring autografts

causes only minor morbidity in the anterior knee region compared with the use patellar tendon autografts.

Bak et al.[18] reported that 8% of their patients complained of swelling and pain laterally on the thigh after harvesting a fascia lata autograft. Twenty percent of their patients also expressed slight cosmetic dissatisfaction with a lateral thigh herniation. Sensory loss and nerve injuries were, however, not discussed. Natri et al.[19] reported that 84% of their patients had no or only slight anterior knee pain after harvesting iliotibial grafts.

Chen et al.[33] reported that one in 12 patients reported mild harvest-site tenderness after an average of 18 months and Fulkerson and Langeland[34] reported no early quadriceps tendon morbidity in their series of 28 patients. Lee et al.[35] reported 12% moderate or severe anterior knee pain in their study involving 67 patients. Correspondingly, Noronha[36] and Theut et al.[88] in their studies as well as Santori et al.[89] in a review article regarded the quadriceps tendon as a low morbidity graft.

Radiographic Assessments

Reports by Coupens et al.,[90] Berg et al.,[91] Nixon et al.,[92] Liu et al.,[93] Meisterling et al.[94] and Kartus et al.[69,95,96] using MRI assessments of the patellar tendon at the donor site have all shown that the thickness of the patellar tendon increases, at least up to six years postoperatively, irrespective of whether or not the defect is sutured. Wiley et al.,[97] Kartus et al.,[98] and Hou et al.[99] have made corresponding findings using ultrasonography 1 to 2 years after the harvesting procedure.

Reports in the literature on the healing of the donor-site gap in the patellar tendon after harvesting its central third and leaving the defect open are contradictory. Using MRI assessments, Berg et al.[91] and Nixon et al.[92] claimed that the defect had healed, eight months and two years respectively after the index operation. Adriani et al.[100] have used ultrasonography to show that the healing of the patellar tendon defect with tendinous-like scar tissue can be expected approximately one year after harvesting its central third and Cerullo et al.[101] used CT to show that scarring of the open defect takes place within six months postoperatively. Rosenberg et al.[102] have demonstrated persistent defects using CT and MRI, approximately two years after the index operation. Kartus et al. have found persistent defects in several studies using MRI[69,74,95,98,103] and in one study using ultrasonography[98] after leaving the defect open (Figures 19.5 and 19.6). However, even if the defect was still present two years after the harvesting procedure it showed a significant decrease over time in the prospective studies by Kartus et al.[103] and Bernicker et al.[104] using MRI and by Wiley et al.[97] using ultrasonography. Liu et al.[93] using MRI have shown that there can be a persistent donor-site gap even 13 years after the harvesting procedure. After six years the defect had healed in the majority of patients; however, a thinning of the central part of the tendon was still present as shown by Svensson et al.[96] in a prospective long-term study of 17 patients (Figure 19.7). Koseoglu et al.[105] described that the defect had not healed up to 12 months after the harvesting procedure but appeared to heal in the long term. Kartus et al.[69,74] have shown that the kneeling and knee-walking problems did not correlate with any MRI findings in the patellar tendon at the donor site. The corresponding finding in terms of patellar tendon pain was made by Kiss et al.,[106] using ultrasonography.

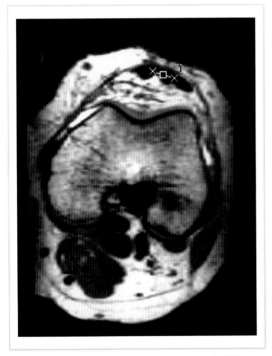

Figure 19.5. A persistent donor site gap is displayed on this MRI examination in the axial dimension obtained 26 months after harvesting a central third patellar tendon autograft. (Copyright Jüri Kartus.)

After harvesting hamstring tendon autografts, it appears that there is at least some regrowth in the semitendinosus and gracilis tendons. This has been reported in the literature by Cross et al.,[107] Simonian et al.,[108] and Eriksson et al.[78,109,110] using MRI. In their prospective ultrasonography study, Papandrea et al.[111] reported that the regrowth of the tendons appeared to be completed two years after the harvesting procedure. However, the insertion of the tendons was approximately 3–4 cm more proximal compared with the normal anatomical position.

No radiographic data on the donor site after harvesting, fascia lata and quadriceps tendon autografts are available to our knowledge.

Histological Examinations

Reports on donor-site histology in humans are few in number.[91,92,98,112] Histological descriptions of the donor-site area after ACL reconstruction using central patellar tendon autografts in a goat model have been given by Proctor et al.[113] They found ill-defined fascicles, woven collagen fibrils, poorly aligned with the longitudinal axis of the patellar ligament, in the central part of the tendon 21 months after the harvesting procedure. Correspondingly, in a study of lambs, Sanchis-Alfonso et al.[114] found that the regenerated tissue in the harvest-site defect did not have the histological appearance of normal patellar tendon. In a dog model, Burks et al.[115] found that the entire patellar tendon was involved in scar formation three and six months after harvesting its central third. In contrast, Nixon et al.[92] obtained biopsies from two patients two years after the harvesting procedure and found tissue that was indistinguishable from normal tendon using polarized light microscopy. In a human case report, Berg et al.[91] showed that the defect was filled with hypertrophic "tendon-like" tissue eight months after the harvesting procedure. Battlehner et al.[112] obtained open biopsies from eight humans, a minimum of 24 months after ACL reconstruction using patellar tendon autografts and found using light microscopy that the patellar tendon did not regain the appearance of normal tendon. However, in their study the donor-site gap was closed during the ACL reconstruction. In a biopsy study of 19 patients, 27 months after harvesting the central third of the patellar tendon and leaving the defect open, Kartus et al.[98] revealed tendon-like repair tissue in the donor site. However, histological abnormalities in

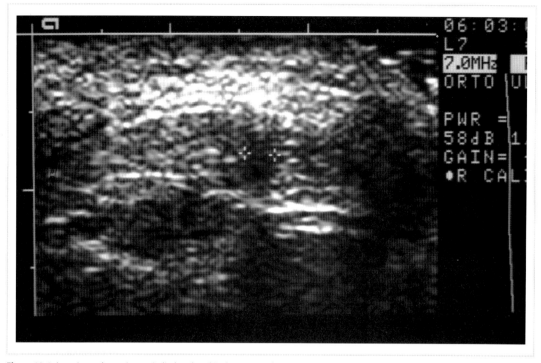

Figure 19.6. A persistent donor-site gap is displayed on this ultrasonography examination obtained 25 months after harvesting a central third patellar tendon autograft. (Copyright Jüri Kartus.)

terms of increased cellularity, vascularity, and nonparallel fibers were present in both the central and peripheral parts of the tendon. The same patients underwent biopsies once again at six years after the harvesting procedure and still the same pathology was found.[116] No correlation between the histological findings and the donor-site discomfort was found (Figures 19.8 and 19.9).[116]

The finding of histological abnormalities in the human patellar tendon up to six years after the primary harvest strongly suggests that reharvesting the central third of the patellar tendon cannot be recommended. This opinion is supported by the findings of LaPrade et al.,[117] who in a dog model reported inferior mechanical properties in the reharvested central third patellar tendon up to 12 months after the primary procedure, and by Scherer et al.,[118] who in a sheep model reported the corresponding finding in the remaining two-thirds of the patellar tendon. Moreover, in a clinical study by Kartus et al.,[95] patients who had undergone revision ACL reconstruction using reharvested patellar

tendon autograft displayed significantly worse results, especially in terms of anterior knee problems, than patients in whom the contralateral patellar tendon autograft was used.

Eriksson[78,109] obtained open biopsies from the regenerated tendon in five humans mean 20 months after the harvest of a semitendinosus autograft. Suprisingly, the biopsies revealed tissue resembling normal tendon.

No histological data from the donor site after harvesting fascia lata or quadriceps tendon autografts are available to our knowledge.

Ultrastructural Examinations

Proctor et al.[113] in a goat model reported abnormal tissue composition when biopsies were evaluated ultrastructurally in the transmission electron microscope (TEM) 21 months after the harvesting procedure. Correspondingly, Battlehner et al.[112] reported that the patellar tendon in humans does not restore *ad integrum* a minimum of two years after harvesting its central third. In a dog model using the electron microscope, LaPrade et al.[117] reported that the reharvested central third of the

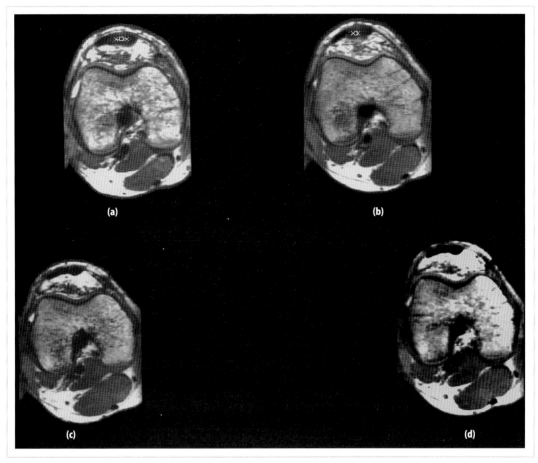

Figure 19.7a-d. The serial MRI examinations demonstrate that the donor-site gap was 7 mm at six weeks, 2 mm at six months, and completely healed at 27 and 71 months. Furthermore, the thickness of the patellar tendon decreased over time. This is a male patient who, at the time of the index operation, was 18 years old. (Copyright Jüri Kartus.)

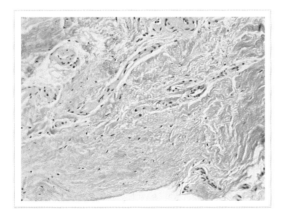

Figure 19.8. A high-power view of a biopsy obtained from the central part of the patellar tendon 72 months after the harvesting procedure showing increased cellularity, vascularity, and nonparallel fibers. (Hematoxylin and eosin staining; original magnification, X200.) (Reproduced from reference 116 with kind permission of Springer Science and Business Media.)

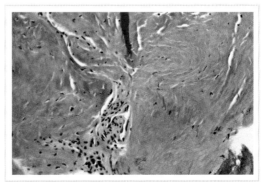

Figure 19.9. A high-power view of a biopsy obtained from the peripheral part of the patellar tendon 72 months after the harvesting procedure showing increased cellularity, vascularity, and nonparallel fibers. (Hematoxylin and eosin staining; original magnification, X200.) (Reproduced from reference 116 with kind permission of Springer Science and Business Media.)

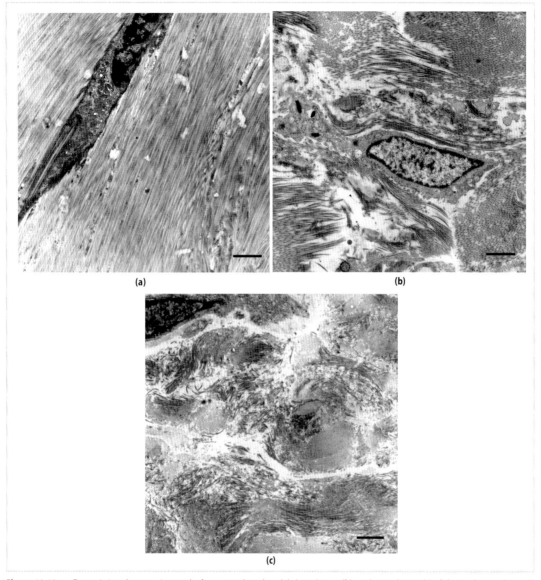

Figure 19.10a-c. Transmission electron micrographs from control tendons **(a)**, lateral parts **(b)**, and central parts **(c)** of the tendons in the study group. The fibrils were less regularly orientated in both the central and lateral part of the harvested tendon compared with normal tendon. (Bar = 2 μm.) (Copyright Jüri Kartus.)

patellar tendon displayed an increased fibril size and fibril packing at six months compared with control tendons. However, at 12 months, no significant differences were registered.

The patellar tendon did not regain a normal ultrastructure as seen on biopsies examined in TEM six years after the harvesting procedure. The fibrils were less regularly orientated and more small fibrils compared with normal control tendons were found (Figure 19.10) (Kartus et al. unpublished data).

Taken together, there is evidence in the literature to suggest that the patellar tendon does not regain normal ultrastructure after harvesting its central third in both animals and humans, at least not up to six years.

Biochemical Investigations

Sulphated glycosaminoglycans (GAGs) possess a very high water-retaining capacity and they appear in low concentrations in the normal patellar tendon.[119,120] Increasing concentrations of GAGs are seen in areas of tendons that are subjected to compression forces, as described by Vogel et al.,[121] in pathological scar tissue in the Achilles tendon, as described by Movin et al.,[122] and in the patellar tendon in "jumper's knee" (tendinosis) disease, as described by Khan et al.[123] and Green et al.[124] Furthermore, Kannus and Jozsa[125] have reported that increasing amounts of GAGs were found in ruptured tendons compared with healthy control tendons. Kartus et al.[98] showed that there were undetectable amounts of GAGs in the biopsies obtained from the patellar tendon 27 months as well as six years (Kartus et al. unpublished data) after the harvesting procedure. This suggests that factors other than retained water contributed to the increase in the cross-sectional area of the patellar tendon and, furthermore, that the repair tissue did not display similarities with the tendon pathology that has been found in achillodynia and jumper's knee.

The presence of collagen type III is associated with early collagen synthesis in a repair process in tendons, as described by Liu et al.[126] and Matsumoto et al.[127] in rat models. Collagen type III has the capacity rapidly to form cross-linked intermolecular disulphide bridges.[128,129] This capacity is supposed to be a great advantage in the development of repair tissue.[128] Collagen type III fibers are also known to be thin, with inferior mechanical properties, compared with collagen type I. Kartus et al.[98] failed to demonstrate increased amounts of collagen type III in the central and peripheral parts of the patellar tendon, which indicates that no early collagen synthesis was present 27 months after the harvesting procedure.

Eriksson has shown that the immunoreactivity for collagen types I and III in regenerated semitendinosus tendon was similar to that of normal tendon at mean 20 months after the harvesting procedure.[78,109]

Conclusions

- There is a lack of knowledge about the course of the donor site after harvesting, fascia lata and quadriceps tendon autografts. However, both graft types appear to have low harvest-site morbidity.

- Reduced strength and loss of ROM are correlated with anterior knee pain after ACL reconstruction using all kinds of autografts. Efforts should therefore be made during the surgical procedure and the rehabilitation process to regain full ROM and full strength after ACL reconstructions regardless of the type of graft used.

- Loss or disturbance of anterior knee sensitivity caused by intraoperative injury to the infrapatellar nerve(s) in conjunction with patellar tendon harvest are correlated with donor-site discomfort and inability to knee-walk. A similar nerve injury after harvesting hamstring tendon grafts does not appear to cause as many knee-walking problems.

- No correlations can be found between donor-site discomfort and radiographic or histological findings after the use of patellar tendon autografts.

- If the surgeon wishes to use patellar tendon autografts, efforts to spare the infrapatellar nerve(s) should be made during surgery.

- Due to radiographic, histological, and ultrastructural abnormalities in the patellar tendon after primary harvest, reharvesting cannot be recommended, at least not up to six years after the primary harvest.

- Since prospective randomized studies have shown that the use of hamstring tendon autografts for ACL reconstruction produces laxity restoration comparable to patellar tendon autografts, we recommend the use of hamstring tendon autografts due to fewer donor-site problems.

Acknowledgments

The authors thank Catarina Kartus for the illustrations.

References

1. Bach, BR, Jr., GT Jones, FA Sweet, and CA Hager. Arthroscopy-assisted anterior cruciate ligament reconstruction using patellar tendon substitution: Two- to four-year follow-up results. *Am J Sports Med* 1994; 22: 758–767.
2. Bach, BR, Jr., GT Jones, CA Hager, FA Sweet, and S Luergans. Arthrometric results of arthroscopically assisted anterior cruciate ligament reconstruction using autograft patellar tendon substitution. *Am J Sports Med* 1995; 23: 179–185.
3. Buss, DD, RF Warren, TL Wickiewicz, BJ Galinat, and R Panariello. Arthroscopically assisted reconstruction of the anterior cruciate ligament with use of autogenous patellar-ligament grafts: Results after twenty-four to forty-two months. *J Bone Joint Surg [Am]* 1993; 75: 1346–1355.

4. Breitfuss, H, R Fröhlich, P Povacz, H Resch, and A Wicker. The tendon defect after anterior cruciate ligament reconstruction using the midthird patellar tendon-a problem for the patellofemoral joint? *Knee Surg Sports Traumatol Arthrosc* 1996; 3: 194–198.

5. Graf, B, and F Uhr. Complications of intra-articular anterior cruciate reconstruction. *Clin Sports Med* 1988; 7: 835–848.

6. Kartus, J, S Stener, K Köhler, N Sernert, BI Eriksson, and J Karlsson. Is bracing after anterior cruciate ligament reconstruction necessary? A 2-year follow-up of 78 consecutive patients rehabilitated with or without a brace. *Knee Surg Sports Traumatol Arthrosc* 1997; 5: 157–161.

7. Kohn, D, and A Sander-Beuermann. Donor-site morbidity after harvest of a bone-tendon-bone patellar tendon autograft. *Knee Surg Sports Traumatol Arthrosc* 1994; 2: 219–223.

8. Mohtadi, NG, S Webster-Bogaert, and PJ Fowler. Limitation of motion following anterior cruciate ligament reconstruction: A case-control study. *Am J Sports Med* 1991; 19: 620–625.

9. Paulos, LE, TD Rosenberg, J Drawbert, J Manning, and P Abbott. Infrapatellar contracture syndrome: An unrecognized cause of knee stiffness with patella entrapment and patella infera. *Am J Sports Med* 1987; 15: 331–341.

10. Sachs, RA, DM Daniel, ML Stone, and RF Garfein. Patellofemoral problems after anterior cruciate ligament reconstruction. *Am J Sports Med* 1989; 17: 760–765.

11. Shelbourne, KD, and RV Trumper. Preventing anterior knee pain after anterior cruciate ligament reconstruction. *Am J Sports Med* 1997; 25: 41–47.

12. Dandy, DJ, JP Flanagan, and V Steenmeyer. Arthroscopy and the management of the ruptured anterior cruciate ligament. *Clin Orthop* 1982; 167: 43–49.

13. Engström, B, T Wredmark, and P Westblad. Patellar tendon or Leeds-Keio graft in the surgical treatment of anterior cruciate ligament ruptures: Intermediate results. *Clin Orthop* 1993; 295: 190–197.

14. Jackson, DW, ES Grood, JD Goldstein, MA Rosen, PR Kurzweil, JF Cummings, and TM Simon. A comparison of patellar tendon autograft and allograft used for anterior cruciate ligament reconstruction in the goat model. *Am J Sports Med* 1993; 21: 176–185.

15. Noyes, FR, and SD Barber-Westin. Reconstruction of the anterior cruciate ligament with human allograft: Comparison of early and later results. *J Bone Joint Surg [Am]* 1996; 78: 524–537.

16. Nicholas, JA, and J Minkoff. Iliotibial band transfer through the intercondylar notch for combined anterior instability (ITPT procedure). *Am J Sports Med* 1978; 6: 341–353.

17. Ekstrand, J. Reconstruction of the anterior cruciate ligament in athletes, using a fascia lata graft: A review with preliminary results of a new concept. *Int J Sports Med* 1989; 10: 225–232.

18. Bak, K, U Jörgensen, J Ekstrand, and M Scavenius. Results of reconstruction of acute ruptures of the anterior cruciate ligament with an iliotibial band autograft. *Knee Surg Sports Traumatol Arthrosc* 1999; 7: 111–117.

19. Natri, A, M Järvinen, and P Kannus. Primary repair plus intra-articular iliotibial band augmentation in the treatment of an acute anterior cruciate ligament rupture:
A follow-up study of 70 patients. *Arch Orthop Trauma Surg* 1996; 115: 22–27.

20. Laupattarakasem, W, and B Mahaisavariya. Iliotibial band for anterior cruciate ligament reconstruction: A new technique for graft augmentation, placement and fixation. *J Med Assoc Thai* 1994; 77: 343–350.

21. Aglietti, P, R Buzzi, PM Menchetti, and F Giron. Arthroscopically assisted semitendinosus and gracilis tendon graft in reconstruction for acute anterior cruciate ligament injuries in athletes. *Am J Sports Med* 1996; 24: 726–731.

22. Puddu, G. Method for reconstruction of the anterior cruciate ligament using the semitendinosus tendon. *Am J Sports Med* 1980; 8: 402–404.

23. Otero, AL, and L Hutcheson. A comparison of the doubled semitendinosus/gracilis and central third of the patellar tendon autografts in arthroscopic anterior cruciate ligament reconstruction. *Arthroscopy* 1993; 9: 143–148.

24. Siegel, MG, and SD Barber-Westin. Arthroscopic-assisted outpatient anterior cruciate ligament reconstruction using the semitendinosus and gracilis tendons. *Arthroscopy* 1998; 14: 268-277.

25. Brown, CH, Jr., ME Steiner, and EW Carson. The use of hamstring tendons for anterior cruciate ligament reconstruction: Technique and results. *Clin Sports Med* 1993; 12: 723–756.

26. Hamner, DL, CH Brown, Jr., ME Steiner, AT Hecker, and WC Hayes. Hamstring tendon grafts for reconstruction of the anterior cruciate ligament: Biomechanical evaluation of the use of multiple strands and tensioning techniques. *J Bone Joint Surg[Am]* 1999; 81: 549–557.

27. Alm, A, and J Gillquist. Reconstruction of the anterior cruciate ligament by using the medial third of the patellar ligament: Treatment and results. *Acta Chir Scand* 1974; 140: 289–296.

28. Clancy, WG, Jr., DA Nelson, B Reider, and RG Narechania. Anterior cruciate ligament reconstruction using one-third of the patellar ligament, augmented by extra-articular tendon transfers. *J Bone Joint Surg [Am]* 1982; 64: 352–359.

29. Eriksson, E. Reconstruction of the anterior cruciate ligament. *Orthop Clin North Am* 1976; 7: 167–179.

30. Jones, KG. Reconstruction of the anterior cruciate ligament. *J Bone Joint Surg [Am]* 1963; 45: 925–932.

31. Jones, KG. Reconstruction of the anterior cruciate ligament using the central one-third of the patellar ligament. *J Bone Joint Surg [Am]* 1970; 52: 838–839.

32. Marshall, JL, RF Warren, TL Wickiewicz, and B Reider. The anterior cruciate ligament: A technique of repair and reconstruction. *Clin Orthop* 1979; 143: 97–106.

33. Chen, CH, WJ Chen, and CH Shih. Arthroscopic anterior cruciate ligament reconstruction with quadriceps tendon-patellar bone autograft. *J Trauma* 1999; 46: 678–682.

34. Fulkerson, JP, and R Langeland. An alternative cruciate reconstruction graft: The central quadriceps tendon. *Arthroscopy* 1995; 11: 252–254.

35. Lee, S, SC Seong, H Jo, YK Park, and MC Lee. Outcome of anterior cruciate ligament reconstruction using quadriceps tendon autograft. *Arthroscopy* 2004; 20: 795–802.

36. Noronha, JC. Reconstruction of the anterior cruciate ligament with quadriceps tendon. *Arthroscopy* 2002; 18: E37.

37. Irrgang, JJ, and CD Harner. Loss of motion following knee ligament reconstruction. *Sports Med* 1995; 19: 150–159.

38. Harner, CD, JJ Irrgang, J Paul, S Dearwater, and FH Fu. Loss of motion after anterior cruciate ligament reconstruction. *Am J Sports Med* 1992; 20: 499–506.

39. Kartus, J, L Magnusson, S Stener, S Brandsson, BI Eriksson, and J Karlsson. Complications following arthroscopic anterior cruciate ligament reconstruction: A 2- to 5-year follow-up of 604 patients with special emphasis on anterior knee pain. *Knee Surg Sports Traumatol Arthrosc* 1999; 7: 2–8.

40. Stapleton, TR. Complications in anterior cruciate ligament reconstructions with patellar tendon grafts. *Sports Med Arthrosc Rev* 1997; 5: 156–162.

41. Aglietti, P, R Buzzi, S D'Andria, G Zaccherotti. Patellofemoral problems after intraarticular anterior cruciate ligament reconstruction. *Clin Orthop* 1993; 288: 195–204.

42. Risberg, MA, I Holm, H Steen, BD Beynnon. Sensitivity to changes over time for the IKDC form, the Lysholm score, and the Cincinnati knee score: A prospective study of 120 ACL reconstructed patients with a 2-year follow-up. *Knee Surg Sports Traumatol Arthrosc* 1999; 7: 152–159.

43. Muneta, T, I Sekiya, T Ogiuchi, K Yagishita, H Yamamoto, and K Shinomiya. Objective factors affecting overall subjective evaluation of recovery after anterior cruciate ligament reconstruction. *Scand J Med Sci Sports* 1998; 8: 283–289.

44. Hiemstra, LA, S Webber, PB MacDonald, and DJ Kriellaars. Knee strength deficits after hamstring tendon and patellar tendon anterior cruciate ligament reconstruction. *Med Sci Sports Exerc* 2000; 32: 1472–1479.

45. Feller, JA, and KE Webster. A randomized comparison of patellar tendon and hamstring tendon anterior cruciate ligament reconstruction. *Am J Sports Med* 2003; 31: 564–573.

46. Adachi, N, M Ochi, Y Uchio, Y Sakai, M Kuriwaka, and A Fujihara. Harvesting hamstring tendons for ACL reconstruction influences postoperative hamstring muscle performance. *Arch Orthop Trauma Surg* 2003; 123: 460–465.

47. Tashiro, T, H Kurosawa, A Kawakami, A Hikita, and N Fukui. Influence of medial hamstring tendon harvest on knee flexor strength after anterior cruciate ligament reconstruction: A detailed evaluation with comparison of single- and double-tendon harvest. *Am J Sports Med* 2003; 31: 522–529.

48. Arthornthurasook, A, and K Gaew-Im. Study of the infrapatellar nerve. *Am J Sports Med* 1988; 16: 57–59.

49. Horner, G, and AL Dellon. Innervation of the human knee joint and implications for surgery. *Clin Orthop* 1994; 301: 221–226.

50. Hunter, LY, DS Louis, JR Ricciardi, and GA O'Connor. The saphenous nerve: Its course and importance in medial arthrotomy. *Am J Sports Med* 1979; 7: 227–230.

51. Kartus, J, L Ejerhed, BI Eriksson, and J Karlsson. The localization of the infrapatellar nerves in the anterior knee region with special emphasis on central third patellar tendon harvest: A dissection study on cadaver and amputated specimens. *Arthroscopy* 1999; 15: 577–586.

52. Abbott, LC, and WF Carpenter. Surgical approaches to the knee joint. *J Bone Joint Surg [Am]* 1945; 27: 277–310.

53. Kennedy, JC, IJ Alexander, and KC Hayes. Nerve supply of the human knee and its functional importance. *Am J Sports Med* 1982; 10: 329–335.

54. von Lantz, T, and W Wachmuth. *Praktische Anatomie.* Berlin: Springer-Verlag, 1972.

55. Boon, JM, MJ Van Wyk, and D Jordaan. A safe area and angle for harvesting autogenous tendons for anterior cruciate ligament reconstruction. *Surg Radiol Anat* 2004; 26: 167–171.

56. Johnson, RJ, DB Kettelkamp, W Clark, and P Leaverton. Factors effecting late results after meniscectomy. *J Bone Joint Surg [Am]* 1974; 56: 719–729.

57. Swanson, AJ. The incidence of prepatellar neuropathy following medial meniscectomy. *Clin Orthop* 1983; 181: 151–153.

58. Tapper, EM, and NW Hoover. Late results after meniscectomy. *J Bone Joint Surg [Am]* 1969; 51: 517–526.

59. Chambers, GH. The prepatellar nerve: A cause of suboptimal results in knee arthrotomy. *Clin Orthop* 1972; 82: 157–159.

60. Ganzoni, N, and K Wieland. The ramus infrapatellaris of the saphenous nerve and its importance for medial parapatellar arthrotomies of the knee. *Reconstr Surg Traumatol* 1978; 16: 95–100.

61. Mochida, H, and S Kikuchi. Injury to infrapatellar branch of saphenous nerve in arthroscopic knee surgery. *Clin Orthop* 1995; 320: 88–94.

62. Poehling, GG, FE Pollock, Jr., and LA Koman. Reflex sympathetic dystrophy of the knee after sensory nerve injury. *Arthroscopy* 1988; 4: 31–35.

63. Gordon, GC. Traumatic prepatellar neuralgia. *J Bone Joint Surg [Br]* 1952; 34: 41–44.

64. Detenbeck, LC. Infrapatellar traumatic neuroma resulting from dashboard injury. *J Bone Joint Surg [Am]* 1972; 54: 170–172.

65. House, JH, and K Ahmed. Entrapment neuropathy of the infrapatellar branch of the saphenous nerve. *Am J Sports Med* 1977; 5: 217–224.

66. Worth, RM, DB Kettelkamp, RJ Defalque, and KU Duane. Saphenous nerve entrapment: A cause of medial knee pain. *Am J Sports Med* 1984; 12: 80–81.

67. Slocum, DB, and RL Larson. Pes anserinus transplantation: A surgical procedure for control of rotatory instability of the knee. *J Bone Joint Surg [Am]* 1968; 50: 226–242.

68. Berg, P, and B Mjöberg. A lateral skin incision reduces peripatellar dysaesthesia after knee surgery. *J Bone Joint Surg [Br]* 1991; 73: 374–376.

69. Kartus, J, S Stener, S Lindahl, B Engström, BI Eriksson, and J Karlsson. Factors affecting donor-site morbidity after anterior cruciate ligament reconstruction using bone-patellar tendon-bone autografts. *Knee Surg Sports Traumatol Arthrosc* 1997; 5: 222–228.

70. Mastrokalos, DS, J Springer, R Siebold, and HH Paessler. Donor site morbidity and return to the preinjury activity level after anterior cruciate ligament reconstruction using ipsilateral and contralateral patellar tendon autograft: A retrospective, nonrandomized study. *Am J Sports Med* 2005; 33: 85–93.

71. Mishra, AK, GS Fanton, MF Dillingham, and TJ Carver. Patellar tendon graft harvesting using horizontal incisions for anterior cruciate ligament reconstruction. *Arthroscopy* 1995; 11: 749–752.

72. Karlsson, J, J Kartus, S Brandsson, L Magnusson, O Lundin, and BI Eriksson. Comparison of arthroscopic one-incision and two-incision techniques for recon-

struction of the anterior cruciate ligament. *Scand J Med Sci Sports* 1999; 9: 233–238.

73. Kartus, J, L Ejerhed, N Sernert, S Brandsson, and J Karlsson. Comparison of traditional and subcutaneous patellar tendon harvest: A prospective study of donor site-related problems after anterior cruciate ligament reconstruction using different graft harvesting techniques. *Am J Sports Med* 2000; 28: 328–335.

74. Kartus, J, S Lindahl, S Stener, BI Eriksson, and J Karlsson. Magnetic resonance imaging of the patellar tendon after harvesting its central third: A comparison between traditional and subcutaneous harvesting techniques. *Arthroscopy* 1999; 15: 587–593.

75. Tsuda, E, Y Okamura, Y Ishibashi, H Otsuka, and S Toh. Techniques for reducing anterior knee symptoms after anterior cruciate ligament reconstruction using a bone-patellar tendon-bone autograft. *Am J Sports Med* 2001; 29: 450–456.

76. Tifford, CD, L Spero, T Luke, and KD Plancher. The relationship of the infrapatellar branches of the saphenous nerve to arthroscopy portals and incisions for anterior cruciate ligament surgery: An anatomic study. *Am J Sports Med* 2000; 28: 562–567.

77. Bertram, C, M Porsch, MH Hackenbroch, and D Terhaag. Saphenous neuralgia after arthroscopically assisted anterior cruciate ligament reconstruction with a semitendinosus and gracilis tendon graft. *Arthroscopy* 2000; 16: 763–766.

78. Eriksson, K. On the semitendinosus in anterior cruciate ligament reconstructive surgery. *Thesis* 2001; Karolinska Institutet.

79. Ejerhed, L, J Kartus, N Sernert, K Köhler, and J Karlsson. Patellar tendon or semitendinosus tendon autografts for anterior cruciate ligament reconstruction? A prospective randomized study with a two-year follow-up. *Am J Sports Med* 2003; 31: 19–25.

80. Spicer, DD, SE Blagg, AJ Unwin, and RL Allum. Anterior knee symptoms after four-strand hamstring tendon anterior cruciate ligament reconstruction. *Knee Surg Sports Traumatol Arthrosc* 2000; 8: 286–289.

81. Brandsson, S, E Faxén, BI Eriksson, P Kälebo, L Swärd, O Lundin, and J Karlsson. Closing patellar tendon defects after anterior cruciate ligament reconstruction: absence of any benefit. *Knee Surg Sports Traumatol Arthrosc* 1998; 6: 82–87.

82. Boszotta, H, and K Prunner. Refilling of removal defects: Impact on extensor mechanism complaints after use of a bone-tendon-bone graft for anterior cruciate ligament reconstruction. *Arthroscopy* 2000; 16: 160–164.

83. Rubinstein, RA, Jr., KD Shelbourne, CD VanMeter, JC McCarroll, and AC Rettig. Isolated autogenous bone-patellar tendon-bone graft site morbidity. *Am J Sports Med* 1994; 22: 324–327.

84. Corry, IS, JM Webb, AJ Clingeleffer, and LA Pinczewski. Arthroscopic reconstruction of the anterior cruciate ligament: A comparison of patellar tendon autograft and four-strand hamstring tendon autograft. *Am J Sports Med* 1999; 27: 444–454.

85. Yasuda, K, J Tsujino, Y Ohkoshi, Y Tanabe, and K Kaneda. Graft site morbidity with autogenous semitendinosus and gracilis tendons. *Am J Sports Med* 1995; 23: 706–714.

86. Eriksson, K, P Anderberg, P Hamberg, AC Löfgren, M Bredenberg, I Westman, and T Wredmark. A comparison of quadruple semitendinosus and patellar ten-

don grafts in reconstruction of the anterior cruciate ligament. *J Bone Joint Surg [Br]* 2001; 83: 348–354.

87. Eriksson, K, P Anderberg, P Hamberg, P Olerud, and T Wredmark. There are differences in early morbidity after ACL reconstruction when comparing patellar tendon and semitendinosus tendon graft: A prospective randomized study of 107 patients. *Scand J Med Sci Sports* 2001; 11: 170–177.

88. Theut, PC, JP Fulkerson, EF Armour, and M Joseph. Anterior cruciate ligament reconstruction utilizing central quadriceps free tendon. *Orthop Clin North Am* 2003; 34: 31–39.

89. Santori, N, E Adriani, and L Pederzini. ACL reconstruction using quadriceps tendon. *Orthopedics* 2004; 27: 31–35.

90. Coupens, SD, CK Yates, C Sheldon, and C Ward. Magnetic resonance imaging evaluation of the patellar tendon after use of its central one-third for anterior cruciate ligament reconstruction. *Am J Sports Med* 1992; 20: 332–335.

91. Berg, EE. Intrinsic healing of a patellar tendon donor site defect after anterior cruciate ligament reconstruction. *Clin Orthop* 1992; 278: 160–163.

92. Nixon, RG, GK SeGall, SL Sax, TE Cain, and HS Tullos. Reconstitution of the patellar tendon donor site after graft harvest. *Clin Orthop* 1995; 317: 162–171.

93. Liu, SH, DW Hang, A Gentili, and GA Finerman. MRI and morphology of the insertion of the patellar tendon after graft harvesting. *J Bone Joint Surg [Br]* 1996; 78: 823–826.

94. Meisterling, RC, T Wadsworth, R Ardill, H Griffiths, and CL Lane-Larsen. Morphologic changes in the human patellar tendon after bone-tendon-bone anterior cruciate ligament reconstruction. *Clin Orthop* 1993; 289: 208–212.

95. Kartus, J, S Stener, S Lindahl, BI Eriksson, and J Karlsson. Ipsi- or contralateral patellar tendon graft in anterior cruciate ligament revision surgery: A comparison of two methods. *Am J Sports Med* 1998; 26: 499–504.

96. Svensson, M, J Kartus, L Ejerhed, S Lindahl, and J Karlsson. Does the patellar tendon normalize after harvesting its central third? A prospective long-term MRI study. *Am J Sports Med* 2004; 32: 34–38.

97. Wiley, JP, RC Bray, DA Wiseman, PD Elliott, KO Ladly, and LA Vale. Serial ultrasonographic imaging evaluation of the patellar tendon after harvesting its central one third for anterior cruciate ligament reconstruction. *J Ultrasound Med* 1997; 16: 251–255.

98. Kartus, J, T Movin, N Papadogiannakis, LR Christensen, S Lindahl, and J Karlsson. A radiographic and histologic evaluation of the patellar tendon after harvesting its central third. *Am J Sports Med* 2000; 28: 218–226.

99. Hou, CH, CL Wang, and CC Lin. Ultrasound examination of patellar tendon after harvest for anterior cruciate ligament reconstruction. *J Formos Med Assoc* 2001; 100: 315–318.

100. Adriani, E, PP Mariani, G Maresca, and N Santori. Healing of the patellar tendon after harvesting of its mid-third for anterior cruciate ligament reconstruction and evolution of the unclosed donor site defect. *Knee Surg Sports Traumatol Arthrosc* 1995; 3: 138–143.

101. Cerullo, G, G Puddu, E Gianni, A Damiani, and F Pigozzi. Anterior cruciate ligament patellar tendon reconstruction: It is probably better to leave the tendon defect open! *Knee Surg Sports Traumatol Arthrosc* 1995; 3: 14–17.

102. Rosenberg, TD, JL Franklin, GN Baldwin, and KA Nelson. Extensor mechanism function after patellar tendon graft harvest for anterior cruciate ligament reconstruction. *Am J Sports Med* 1992; 20: 519–525.
103. Kartus, J, S Lindahl, K Köhler, N Sernert, BI Eriksson, and J Karlsson. Serial magnetic resonance imaging of the donor site after harvesting the central third of the patellar tendon: A prospective study of 37 patients after arthroscopic anterior cruciate ligament reconstruction. *Knee Surg Sports Traumatol Arthrosc* 1999; 7: 20–24.
104. Bernicker, JP, JL Haddad, DM Lintner, TC DiLiberti, and JR Bocell. Patellar tendon defect during the first year after anterior cruciate ligament reconstruction: Appearance on serial magnetic resonance imaging. *Arthroscopy* 1998; 14: 804–809.
105. Koseoglu, K, A Memis, M Argin, and R Arkun. MRI evaluation of patellar tendon defect after harvesting its central third. *Eur J Radiol* 2004; 50: 292–295.
106. Kiss, ZS, DP Kellaway, JL Cook, and KM Khan. Postoperative patellar tendon healing: An ultrasound study. VIS Tendon Study Group. *Australas Radiol* 1998; 42: 28–32.
107. Cross, MJ, G Roger, P Kujawa, and IF Anderson. Regeneration of the semitendinosus and gracilis tendons following their transection for repair of the anterior cruciate ligament. *Am J Sports Med* 1992; 20: 221–223.
108. Simonian, PT, SD Harrison, VJ Cooley, EM Escabedo, DA Deneka, and RV Larson. Assessment of morbidity of semitendinosus and gracilis tendon harvest for ACL reconstruction. *Am J Knee Surg* 1997; 10: 54–59.
109. Eriksson, K, LG Kindblom, P Hamberg, H Larsson, and T Wredmark. The semitendinosus tendon regenerates after resection: A morphologic and MRI analysis in 6 patients after resection for anterior cruciate ligament reconstruction. *Acta Orthop Scand* 2001; 72: 379–384.
110. Eriksson, K, H Larsson, T Wredmark, and P Hamberg. Semitendinosus tendon regeneration after harvesting for ACL reconstruction: A prospective MRI study. *Knee Surg Sports Traumatol Arthrosc* 1999; 7: 220–225.
111. Papandrea, P, MC Vulpiani, A Ferretti, and F Conteduca. Regeneration of the semitendinosus tendon harvested for anterior cruciate ligament reconstruction: Evaluation using ultrasonography. *Am J Sports Med* 2000; 28: 556–561.
112. Battlehner, CN, M Carneiro Filho, JM Ferreira, Jr., PH Saldiva, and GS Montes. Histochemical and ultrastructural study of the extracellular matrix fibers in patellar tendon donor site scars and normal controls. *J Submicrosc Cytol Pathol* 1996; 28: 175–186.
113. Proctor, CS, DW Jackson, and TM Simon. Characterization of the repair tissue after removal of the central one-third of the patellar ligament. An experimental study in a goat model. *J Bone Joint Surg [Am]* 1997; 79: 997–1006.
114. Sanchis-Alfonso, V, A Subias-Lopez, C Monteagudo-Castro, and E Rosello-Sastre. Healing of the patellar tendon donor defect created after central-third patellar tendon autograft harvest: A long-term histological evaluation in the lamb model. *Knee Surg Sports Traumatol Arthrosc* 1999; 7: 340–348.
115. Burks, RT, RC Haut, and RL Lancaster. Biomechanical and histological observations of the dog patellar tendon after removal of its central one-third. *Am J Sports Med* 1990; 18: 146–153.
116. Svensson, M, J Kartus, LR Christensen, T Movin, N Papadogiannakis, and J Karlsson. A long-term serial histological evaluation of the patellar tendon in humans after harvesting its central third. *Knee Surg Sports Traumatol Arthrosc* 2005; Feb 1 (Epub ahead of print).
117. LaPrade, RF, CD Hamilton, RD Montgomery, F Wentorf, and HD Hawkins. The reharvested central third of the patellar tendon: A histologic and biomechanical analysis. *Am J Sports Med* 1997; 25: 779–785.
118. Scherer, MA, HJ Fruh, R Ascherl, and W Siebels. Biomechanical studies of change in the patellar tendon after transplant removal. *Aktuelle Traumatol* 1993; 23: 129–132.
119. Amiel, D, JB Kleiner, and WH Akeson. The natural history of the anterior cruciate ligament autograft of patellar tendon origin. *Am J Sports Med* 1986; 14: 449–462.
120. Amiel, D, C Frank, F Harwood, J Fronek, and W Akeson. Tendons and ligaments: A morphological and biochemical comparison. *J Orthop Res* 1984; 1: 257–265.
121. Vogel, KG, A Ordog, G Pogany, and J Olah. Proteoglycans in the compressed region of human tibialis posterior tendon and in ligaments. *J Orthop Res* 1993; 11: 68–77.
122. Movin, T, A Gad, FP Reinholt, and C Rolf. Tendon pathology in long-standing achillodynia: Biopsy findings in 40 patients. *Acta Orthop Scand* 1997; 68: 170–175.
123. Khan, KM, F Bonar, PM Desmond, JL Cook, DA Young, PJ Visentini, MW Fehrmann, ZS Kiss, PA O'Brien, PR Harcourt, RJ Dowling, RM O'Sullivan, KJ Crichton, BM Tress, and JD Wark. Patellar tendinosis (jumper's knee): Findings at histopathologic examination, US, and MR imaging. Victorian Institute of Sport Tendon Study Group. *Radiology* 1996; 200: 821–827.
124. Green, JS, B Morgan, I Lauder, DB Finlay, and M Allen. Correlation of magnetic resonance imaging and histology in patellar tendinitis. *Sports Exercise and Injury* 1997; 3: 80–84.
125. Kannus, P, and L Jozsa. Histopathological changes preceding spontaneous rupture of a tendon: A controlled study of 891 patients. *J Bone Joint Surg [Am]* 1991; 73: 1507–1525.
126. Liu, SH, RS Yang, R al-Shaikh, and JM Lane. Collagen in tendon, ligament, and bone healing: A current review. *Clin Orthop* 1995; 318: 265–278.
127. Matsumoto, N, S Horibe, N Nakamura, T Senda, K Shino, and T Ochi. Effect of alignment of the transplanted graft extracellular matrix on cellular repopulation and newly synthesized collagen. *Arch Orthop Trauma Surg* 1998; 117: 215–221.
128. Burgeson, RE, and ME Nimni. Collagen types: Molecular structure and tissue distribution. *Clin Orthop* 1992; 282: 250–272.
129. Cheung, DT, P DiCesare, PD Benya, E Libaw, and ME Nimni. The presence of intermolecular disulfide crosslinks in type III collagen. *J Biol Chem* 1983; 258: 7774–7778.

II

Clinical Cases Commented

20

Complicated Case Studies

Roland M. Biedert

Introduction

Patellofemoral problems with anterior knee pain (AKP) represent a significant problem for the clinician with regard to diagnosis and conservative and operative treatment. Anterior knee pain can be caused by single trauma or may be cumulative. The patellofemoral joint (PFJ) can be painful during periods of rapid growth in adolescence, after increased repetitive activity of the knee during sports, or just in daily life, like long sitting in a car or walking down the stairs. This means, that each level of activity or all types of use of the knee during various occupations can cause AKP. Accordingly, the causes of complaints and the underlying pathologies are various. Therefore it seems logical that successful treatment can only be achieved with respect to the specific pathomorphology. This again presupposes the best possible diagnosis. A consolidated diagnosis is the key of long-term effective and successful therapy.

The two following complicated case studies represent a summation of my clinical experience including thoughts, critical opinions, and accomplishments of colleagues and experts in orthopedic surgery. Special attention has been given to the different possibilities of evaluating the patellofemoral relationship.

For an annual meeting presentation to the International Patellofemoral Study Group we evaluated the clinical histories and courses of 10 patients with the worst histories.[3] These 10 patients underwent altogether 124 operations to treat patellofemoral problems on one of their knees. We examined 8 females and 2 males with the mean age of 21 years (range 14–41 years) at the time of the first surgical intervention. The average number of operations was 12 (range 7–25). The initial diagnosis was in 5 cases a dislocation of the patella, 4 patients suffered from pain, and 1 patient had a direct contusion. The first surgical procedure was in 8 cases a transposition of the tibial tuberosity (medially, proximally, advancement or in combination), and all patients had one or several releases of the lateral retinaculum (n = 2–6). The evaluation showed that 5 patients had a proximal dysplastic trochlea but a distal correction. Seven patients suffered from an unequivocal medial subluxation of the patella following the lateral release. The last surgical procedure was in 4 cases a Re-Elmslie, 9 had a secondary reconstruction of the lateral retinaculum, 5 an elevation of a low lateral condyle, and 5 a resection of a hypertrophic synovial plica.

All patients with the initial diagnosis of patella dislocation had also a proximal dysplasic trochlea (low lateral condyle or short trochlea). Therefore the procedures on the tibial tuberosity were in 50% of cases probably not necessary. The necessity to perform a Re-Elmslie confirms this statement. The lateral retinaculum release (LRR) could not even help one patient as a single surgical procedure.

The medial subluxation with instability was a major problem in our chronic cases. Chondral damage was never the initial problem that started the series of operations. In conclusion, we found in this retrospective analysis no treatment strategies or clear concepts focusing on the underlying pathology. This explains the catastrophic long-term outcomes and the chronic complaints of the patients.

Two of these 10 patients are presented in the following as complicated case studies. The major problems and mistakes of diagnosis and treatment are summarized, and the missing or insufficient diagnostic investigations described and explained. Treatment concepts offer possibilities to escape the presented problems.

Case Study 1

History

A 19-year-old female patient suffered from unspecific bilateral AKP. The first operation was performed in the age of 19 years and consisted of an enlarged Roux procedure (medial transfer of the patellar tendon, release of lateral retinaculum, and plication of the medial retinaculum). At the age of 43 years she had a total of 24 operations on the same right knee. In addition to numerous arthroscopic revisions, a LRR was redone six times, different osteotomies (valgisation, flexion, varisation) performed, and different treatments on the tibial tuberosity (Roux, Bandi, Elmslie) added. The major problems included at the time of the first presentation in our clinic chronic pain, effusion and swelling, loss of strength, inability to perform almost all types of sport, and reduction in daily life.

Comments

Surgical treatment of unspecific AKP in the young female patient is a controversial problem. The excessively high number of contradictory operative interventions documents the inaccurate existing therapeutic concepts in resolving this pain problem surgically.

Course of Action

The physical examination of this patient showed tenderness and pain on palpation on the proximal lateral aspect of the patella, the medial facet of the patella and the medial femoral condyle, the tibial tuberosity, and the patellar tendon. A mild chronic effusion could be documented.

The range of motion was unlimited. The patella apprehension test was positive especially to the medial side but also laterally with pain and crepitation. The patella was locking during flexion and extension movements between 20° and 40° of flexion. The patella tendon was stuck to the head of the tibia. The Q-angle (measured in extension) was 8° on the right side (Figure 20.1A) and 15° on the left side (Figure 20.1B). One leg standing in flexion, like going downstairs, was painful and created continued limping.

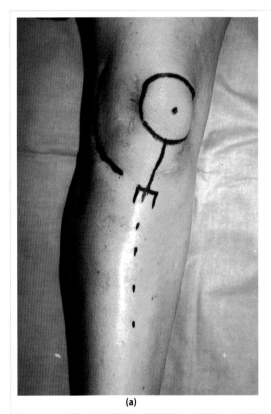
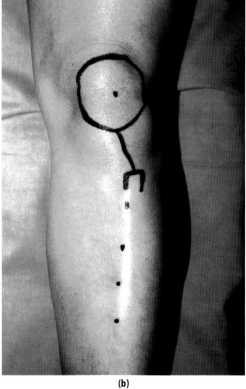

(a)   (b)

Figure 20.1. Excessive medialization of the patella following transposition of the tibial tubercle and repeated release of the lateral retinaculum (**a**). Situation on the nonoperated left knee (**b**).

Diagnostic Examinations

The most important diagnostic studies in these types of patellofemoral complaints are the physical examination and the axial computed tomography (CT) evaluation. The medial instability and the painful medial apprehension test document the significant medial subluxation of the patella. Performing axial CT-scans in extension with and without quadriceps contraction and in 30° of knee flexion is the best imaging procedure to evaluate the patellofemoral relationship near extension (Figures 20.2A, 20.2B);[4,5,7,9,17,28] 3D-CT-scans are also available and even improve the diagnostic value of this type of imaging (Figures 20.3A, 20.3B).[6]

Treatment Concepts

- What is the reason for the medial subluxation of the patella?
- Can this cause chronic pain, effusion, and locking?

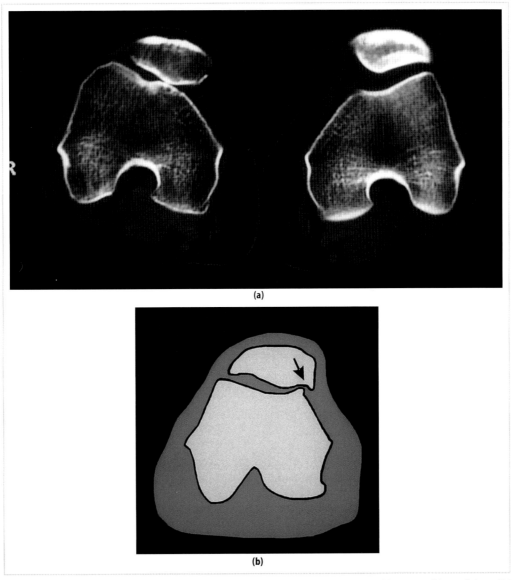

(a)

(b)

Figure 20.2. Axial CT-scans in extension **(a)**. Right knee: Overmedialization of the patella with subluxation and destruction of the patellofemoral joint. Left knee: Normal patella position in the trochlea despite high Q-angle value. Schematic diagram of the medial degenerative changes (→) due to malposition **(b)**.

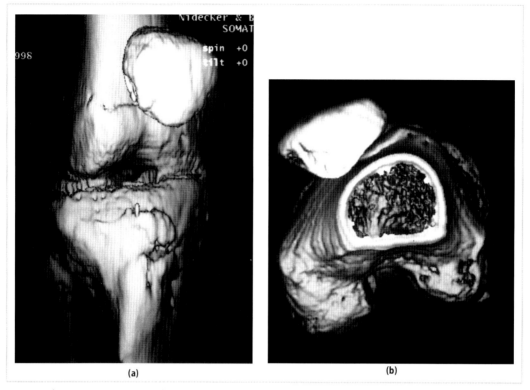

Figure 20.3. 3D-CT ap-view with medial patellar subluxation (right side) **(a)**. View from proximal to distal (right side) **(b)**.

- Which other structures are involved in the problem?
- What kind of procedure is necessary and how do we make the decision?

After 24 operations it is not possible to regain a good result. The goal must be to eliminate the medial subluxation and to improve the passive stability of the patella in the femoral groove. The clinical examination showed that the lateral retinaculum is no longer a functional passive structure. The increased mobility of the patella (more than 3 quadrants) to the medial side documents the secondary instability.[22] This is also visible on the axial CT-scans. The medial subluxation caused the overuse with degenerative changes on the medial patellofemoral joint. Strengthening of the vastus medialis obliquus muscle as a dynamic stabilizer of the patella cannot be successful as this increases the medial subluxation.

The first step of treatment must include the recentering of the patella in the trochlea in combination with increased ligament stabiliza-

tion. This can only be achieved by a Re-Elmslie procedure and a secondary reconstruction of the lateral retinaculum using either the local scar tissue or a tendon graft.[6,29] To decide how much we have to lateralize again the tibial tuberosity we can use the measurement and alignment of the nonoperated knee (if available). After the bony realignment has been performed, the lateral retinaculum is reconstructed with respect to a normal patella mobility of 1 to 2 quadrants.[3,22]

Discussion

Twenty-four operations on the right knee could not resolve the initial problem of unspecific pain. The local situation got worse and worse with each surgical procedure. Regarding the left knee, which was initially also painful but was never operated, one must conclude that probably no surgical intervention was ever necessary. Unspecific AKP without documented pathological patellofemoral relationship is primarily always a matter of conservative treatment. This consists of controlled adaptation of the individual load acceptance. Medications (analgesics, nonsteroidal anti-inflammatory drugs, intra-articular injections) can be helpful to relieve pain and inflammation. Physical therapy is needed for strengthening, stretching, and mobilization of the different structures. Clear pathological factors such as foot disorders, lateral muscle tightness, increased hip antetorsion, or lower back problems can be treated by adequate conservative therapy. Only a few pathological factors (like dysplastic femoral condyle, trochlear-bump, plicae syndrome, loose bodies) are indications for surgical treatment.[1,2]

The presented case study raises two questions:

1. Is an "abnormal" Q-angle an indication for a medialization of the tibial tuberosity?
2. When do we perform an LRR?

The indication for the transposition of the tibial tuberosity was in this case a Q-angle of 15°. Many authors use a so-called "pathological" Q-angle (measured in extension) as an indication for medialization.[27] But the diagnostic relevance of the Q-angle has never been established.[5,7] There exists not even a universally accepted method with detailed description of how to measure the Q-angle.[5,7] Messier and colleagues[24] measured the Q-angle using a goniometer and two anatomically defined lines: one line connecting the anterior-superior iliac spine (ASIS) and the mid-point of the patella, and a second line connecting the mid-point of the patella and the center of the tibial tuberosity in extension. He considered Q-angle values in excess of 16° to be significantly associated with patellofemoral pain.[24] Ford and Post[15] and Caylor and colleagues[9] defined the Q-angle in the same way. Q-angle values of 15° or less were considered to be normal and angles greater than 20° should be considered abnormal.[9] The question of how values between 16° and 19° should be regarded remained unanswered. Papagelopoulos and Sim[26] considered generally Q-angle values greater than 20° as abnormal and associated with patellofemoral pain. Caylor and colleagues[9] measured the Q-angle also in two different standing positions. Finally Guzzanti and colleagues[17] performed the examination of the Q-angle using CT-scans in 15° of knee flexion. They found average values of 19.4° in symptomatic patients and 20.2° in the healthy control group.[17]

In conclusion, there exists an immense controversy about how to measure the Q-angle and what are its normal values. Therefore it seems dangerous to draw the conclusion that an "abnormal" Q-angle is an etiological factor in AKP.[5,7]

The lateral patellar retinaculum is an important anatomical structure, which interplays with the intra-articular components and the dynamic structures to ensure patellofemoral stability.[14,16,21,25,31] This allows correct functioning of the joint. The position of the patella, the central pivotal point of the knee extensor mechanism, is thus controlled by the lateral patellar structures.[3,10,11,12,14,19,29,30] The resultant pulling force of the quadriceps muscle acts on the tibial tuberosity. Therefore, and due to a frequently present valgus axis about the knee, both a laterally directed force vector and the Q-angle are created.[21,25] The patella's tendency to dislocate laterally is counteracted by the horizontal portion of the vastus medialis obliquus muscle and the geometry of the trochlea, especially the shape of the lateral condyle. This underlines the importance of coronal, sagittal, and horizontal alignment in the lower extremity.[14,29]

The incision (release) of the lateral retinaculum results in biomechanical changes of the position of the patella and its gliding behavior in the trochlea.[8,13,22] Some authors explain the therapeutic effect as being due to reduction of the pressure in the patellofemoral joint. These authors attribute the positive results of the LRR to a temporary recovery of the cartilage resulting from a shift of the contact surface area of the patella with consecutive changes of local pressure points. Thus, it is assumed that there is no significant reduction in the pressure of the contact surfaces in the patellofemoral area but rather a change of the contact side area with highest-pressure forces.[18] The combination of LRR with medialization of the tibial tuberosity increases the risk of both medial subluxation of the patella and overloading of the medial patellofemoral joint, as described in our case study.[3,6] Kolowich and colleagues[22] found in 55% of their patients continued repetitive episodes of lateral dislocation following LRR for patellar dislocation. This problem will also be described in the second case study. Hughston and Deese[19] reported the increased possibility of medial subluxation in 50% of patients treated with LRR. Teitge[29,30] documented recurrent medial subluxations and dislocations of the patella after LRR using patellofemoral stress x-rays. We found in our series in 78% disabling medial subluxation of the patella with a severe imbalance of the patellofemoral gliding mechanism following LRR.[3] Additionally we documented the medial patellar instability following LRR performing quantitative gait analysis.[23] The gait analysis consisted of video recordings, three-dimensional motion analysis, dynamic electromyography, and sampling of the ground reaction forces.[23] Abnormal medial translation of the patella was observed during unloading of the leg while the knee was bending in preparation for the swing phase.[23] This is a phase during the gait cycle when the quadriceps muscle is silent and the patella position is guided by the passive structures. These findings weaken the argument of muscle imbalance as a cause for the patellar instability and stresses the importance of well-balanced passive structures. It explains why a muscular rehabilitation program is likely to fail as long as the passive structures allow the instability to occur.

Therefore lengthening of the lateral retinaculum is the therapy to choose. The lateral retinaculum consists of a superficial oblique and deep transverse part (Figure 20.4A). Lengthening is started incising longitudinally the superficial oblique retinaculum about 5 mm from its attachment to the lateral border of the patella, down to the ligamentum patellae. Then it is separated from the deep transverse retinaculum preparing with a knife in the dorsal direction (Figure 20.4B). As much dorsal as possible, then the deep transverse ligament is incised also longitudinally and the synovial layer opened (Figure 20.4C). This releases the increased tension of the lateral structures. The two parts of the lateral retinaculum are sutured together in 90° of knee flexion (Figure 20.4D). This makes it impossible that the retinaculum is too tight. The mobility of the patella should be 1 to 2 quadrants to the medial and the lateral side in full extension, guaranteeing a normal balance of the patella in the trochlea.

Summary

This case outlines the severe complications following the medial transposition of the tibial tuberosity in combination with LRR in a patient with unspecific AKP. Secondary instability of the patellar gliding mechanism and degenerative changes with overuse of the medial patellofemoral joint are the major problems creating chronic pain and disability.

Case Study 2
History

This female patient had undergone surgery performing an Elmslie procedure at the age of 15 years because of repetitive patellar dislocation. Nevertheless the dislocations continued and the medialization of the tibial tuberosity was at the end 28 mm. At the age of 42 years she had in total 15 operations including LRR, denervation, and shaving of the patellar cartilage. The major problems consisted of chronic pain on the medial femorotibial and patellofemoral joint, weakness and instability during loaded flexion, and disability in daily living.

Comments

The recurrent subluxation or dislocation in the young patient is a severe problem. Dislocations without primary traumatic etiology indicate an abnormal biomechanical situation. This includes, for example, dysplastic lateral femoral condyle, patella alta, tight lateral structures, or weakness of the vastus medialis obliquus muscle.[2,10,11,19,28]

Course of Action

The physical examination showed both medial and still lateral subluxation of the patella with painful apprehension tests in both directions. Severe crepitations were found in the medial patellofemoral joint with locking. The medial femorotibial joint line was painful with positive meniscus signs during rotation. The Q-angle was negative with minus 3°. The tibial tuberosity was palpated on the medial side of the tibial head. Varus instability and varus axis were increased in one leg standing.

Diagnostic Examinations

Full weight-bearing x-rays documented a severe medial subluxation of the patella and an excessive medialization of the tibial tuberosity (Figures 20.5A, 20.5B). Varus axis with advanced osteoarthritis of the medial femorotibial compartment was noted. Axial CT-scans documented overloading of the medial patellofemoral joint with degenerative changes in addition to a flat lateral condyle and a nonexisting trochlear groove (Figure 20.6).

Treatment Concepts

- How is it possible that the patella lies extremely on the medial side but still subluxates laterally?

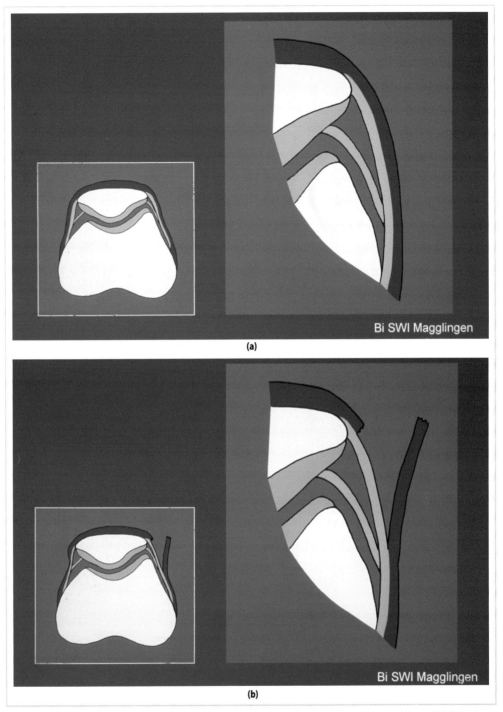

Figure 20.4. Schematic diagram showing the lengthening of the lateral retinaculum (technical note according to R.M. Biedert.)

(*continued*)

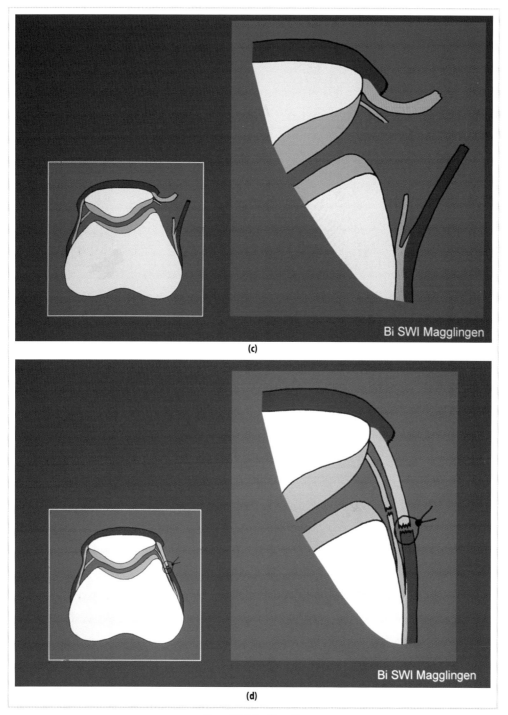

Figure 20.4. *(continued)*

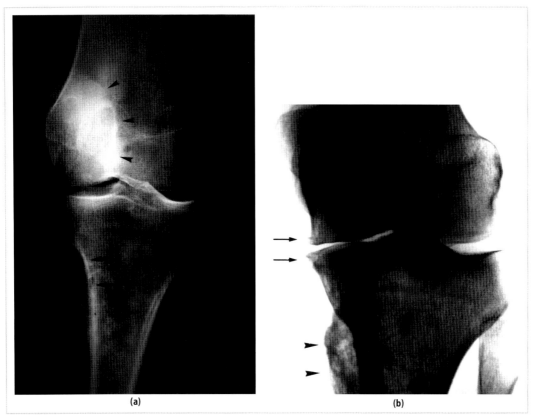

(a)
(b)

Figure 20.5. Long one-leg standing ap-x-ray with medial subluxation of the patella (◄), varus axis and medialization of the tibial tubercle (←) (left knee) **(a)**. Negative imaging x-ray showing the degenerative changes on the medial femorotibial joint (→) and the medialized tibial tubercle (►) (left knee) **(b)**.

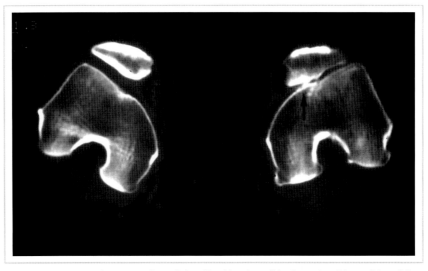

Figure 20.6. Axial CT-scans in extension documenting the medial patella subluxation and the destruction of the medial patellofemoral joint on the left side (↑).

- What is the reason for the medial pain?
- What kind of surgical treatment is necessary to eliminate the subluxation in both diametric directions?
- What do we do with the overmedialization of the tibial tuberosity?
- Has the varus axis a negative influence on the medial patellofemoral and femorotibial joint?

Our treatment of this patient consisted of four major steps:

1. Arthroscopy with partial medial meniscectomy and debridement of scar tissues.
2. Re-Elmslie with normal positioning of the tibial tuberosity according to the tibial shaft axis (Figures 20.7A, 20.7B).
3. High tibial valgisation osteotomy (new axis of 7° valgus) including high fibular osteotomy (Figure 20.8).
4. Elevation of the lateral femoral condyle using a self-locking bone wedge (taken from the

tibia) reconstructing a trochlear groove (Figures 20.9A, 20.9B). In Figure 20.10 you can see the steps to perform a trocheoplasty.

At 6 years follow-up, the result was subjectively and objectively positive with generally improved function of the knee joint (Figure 20.11). A new joint line was formed in comparison to the former situation (Figure 20.6).

Discussion

Twenty-eight millimeters medialization of the tibial tuberosity of twenty-eight millimeters could not eliminate the lateral subluxations of the patella near extension. But this excessive medialization created together with several LRR procedures severe medialization of the patella with degenerative changes of the patellofemoral joint and important weakness of the extensor and decellerator mechanism. The reason why the patella was still laterally subluxating was the low lateral femoral condyle. Therefore, the

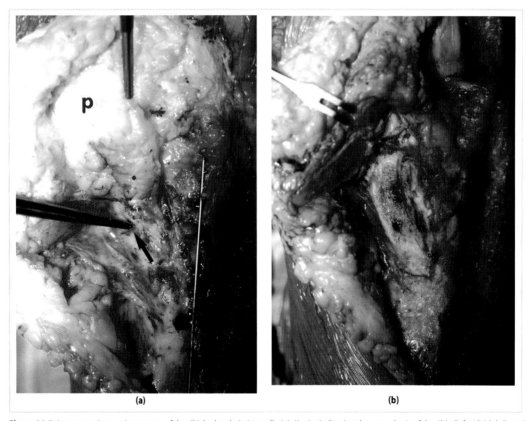

Figure 20.7. Intraoperative ap-view: center of the tibial tubercle (↑); patella (p); K-wire indicating the normal axis of the tibia (left side) **(a)**. Detached tibial tuberosity showing the amount of medialization before Re-Elmslie (left side) **(b)**.

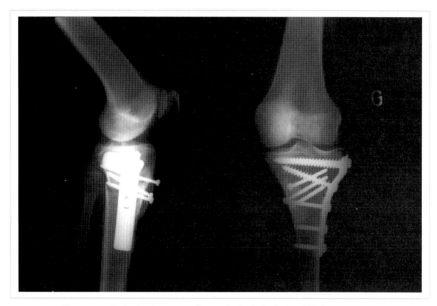

Figure 20.8. Sagittal and ap-x-rays after Re-Elmslie, high tibial, and fibular osteotomies.

osseous resistance of a normal lateral condyle was missing and the laterally directed force vector of the quadriceps muscle caused the lateral subluxation of the patella. The vastus medialis obliquus muscle, acting as an antagonist to this force, was not strong enough to pull the patella medially.[25] The medialization created at the same time a severe overloading of the medial femorotibial compartment, resulting in destruction of the medial meniscus, osteoarthritis of the joints, and varus deformity.[6]

This case study raises two questions:

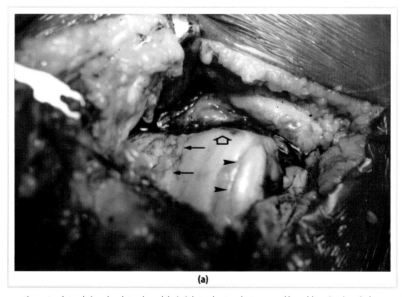

(a)

Figure 20.9. Intraoperative anterolateral view: low lateral condyle (↑), lateral osteophytes caused by subluxation (➤), degenerative changes of the medial patellofemoral joint (←) **(a)**.

(continued)

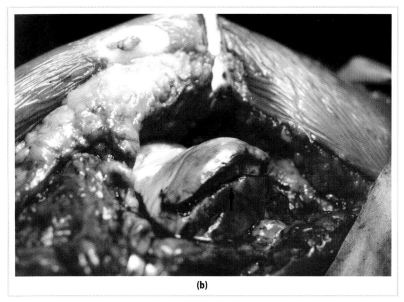

Figure 20.9. *(continued)* Intraoperative anterolateral view after elevation of the lateral condyle. Bone wedge (↑) **(b)**.

1. Which diagnostic imaging is necessary in young patients with recurrent patellar dislocation?
2. How can we treat recurrent patellar dislocation in adolescent or adult patients?

Correct lateral x-rays in 30° of knee flexion can be used to document form and depth of the trochlea.[10,11,12] The crossing sign is a simple and characteristic finding in dysplastic trochlea.[10,11] The dysplastic trochlea is in most cases an indication for surgical reconstruction. CT-scans are helpful in these cases for classification and determination of the type of surgery.[4,17,28] Sasaki and Yagi[28] and Biedert and Gruhl[6] demonstrated that the evaluation of the

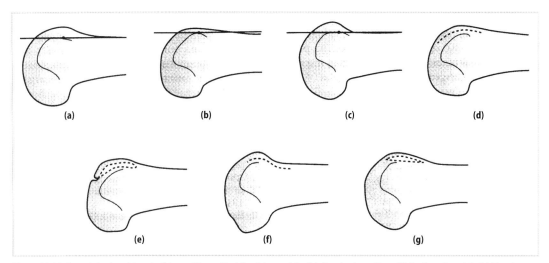

Figure 20.10. Normal depth and length of the trochlea and height of the condyles **(a)**. Dysplastic trochlea with flat lateral condyle **(b)**. Too short trochlea with normal height and depth **(c)**. Incomplete osteotomy of the lateral condyle (dotted line) about 5–7 mm from the cartilage down to the sulcus terminalis **(d)**. The lateral condyle (osteochondral flap) is raised with a chisel (carefully!) and the gap filled with cancellous bone (dotted area) taken from the lateral head of the tibia **(e)**. Dotted line showing the lateral incomplete osteotomy in a too short trochlea **(f)**. Situation after lengthening of a too short trochlea: Lengthening includes 10–15 mm of the lateral femoral shaft **(g)**.

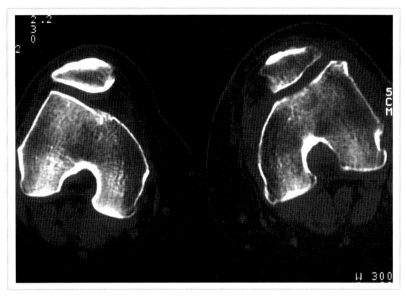

Figure 20.11. Axial CT-scans in extension 6 years postoperative with the reconstructed trochlear groove and the well-centered patella on the left side.

first 30° of knee flexion gives the most important diagnostic information about the patellofemoral congruence. This agrees with Goodfellow's biomechanical studies demonstrating that the most susceptible position for patella dysfunction is at the beginning of knee flexion.[16] At this position, the patella normally starts to center itself in the femoral trochlea.[25] The patella lies in extension more lateral and proximal in the femoral groove and the lateral condyle gives less osseous support to the patella. At this position, the patella must be guided by the normal shaped lateral condyle into the trochlear groove with increased flexion. This maneuver is missing in a short trochlea or a patella alta.

Patients presenting a low lateral condyle (crossing sign in x-ray) are therefore susceptible for recurrent patellar dislocation.[10,11] These patients need either elevation of the condyle or trochlear deepening plasty when they are out of adolescence.[1,2] Different treatment is necessary in young patients with open epiphyseal cartilage. Only soft tissue reconstruction (imbrication of the medial retinaculum and/or vastus medialis obliquus muscle or shortening/tightening of the medial patellofemoral ligament, lengthening of the lateral retinaculum) can be performed in young patients to avoid early epiphyseal fusion.

Summary

This case outlines unsuccessful treatment performing medialization of the tibial tuberosity in recurrent patellar dislocation in patients with dysplastic trochlea. A distal correction is not sufficient and adequate to treat a proximal pathological situation on the femur. In contrast, it can be dangerous creating secondary pathologies. The goal of the surgical reconstruction must be the elimination of the real pathology. The pathology in recurrent patellar dislocations is in most cases a dysplastic trochlea and only a few dislocations are really traumatic.[19] In addition to lateral normal x-rays, the axial CT-scans in 0° of knee flexion with and without quadriceps muscle contraction are the best imaging modality to demonstrate abnormal patellofemoral relationship.[4,17,28] Medialization of the tibial tuberosity always includes the risk of overloading the medial patellofemoral and femorotibial joint.

References

1. Albee, FH. The bone graft wedge in the treatment of habitual dislocation of the patella. *Med Rec* 1915; 88: 257–258.
2. Bereiter, H. Die Trochleaplastik bei Trochleadysplasie zur Therapie der rezidivierenden Patellaluxation. In Wirth, CJ, and M Rudert, eds., *Das patellofemorale Schmerzsyndrom.* Darmstadt: Steinkopff Verlag, 2000, pp. 162–177.
3. Biedert, RM. One hundred twenty-four operations to treat 10 patients suffering from patellofemoral pain:

What was wrong? *Proceedings International Patellofemoral Study Group,* Garmisch-Partenkirchen, Germany, 2000.

4. Biedert, RM. Korrelation zwischen Q-Winkel und Patellaposition: Eine klinische und computertomographische Evaluation. In Wirth, CJ, and M Rudert, eds., *Das patellofemorale Schmerzsyndrom.* Darmstadt: Steinkopff Verlag, 2000, pp. 78–86.

5. Biedert, RM, and NF Friederich. Failed lateral retinacular release: Clinical outcome. *J Sports Traumatol Rel Res* 1994; 16:162–173.

6. Biedert, RM, and C Gruhl. Axial computed tomography of the patellofemoral joint with and without quadriceps contraction. *Arch Orthop Trauma Surg* 1997; 116: 77–82.

7. Biedert, RM, and K Warnke. Correlation between the Q angle and the patella position: a clinical and axial CT evaluation. *Proceedings International Patellofemoral Study Group,* Lyon, France, 1998.

8. Busch, MT, and KE DeHaven. Pitfalls of the lateral retinacular release. *Clin Sports Med* 1989; 8: 279–290.

9. Caylor, D, R Fites, and TW Worrell. The relationship between quadriceps angle and anterior knee pain syndrome. *J Orthop Sports Phys Ther* 1993; 17: 11–15.

10. Dejour, H, G Walch, Ph Neyret et al. Dysplasia of the intercondylar groove. *French Journal Orthop Surg* 1990; 4: 113–122.

11. Dejour, H, G Walch, Ph Neyret et al. La dysplasie de la trochlée fémorale. *Rev Chir Orthop* 1990; 76: 45–54.

12. Dejour, H, G Walch, L Nové-Josserand et al. Factors of patellar instability: An anatomic radiographic study. *Knee Surg Sports Traumatol Arthroscopy* 1994; 2: 19–26.

13. Dzioba, RB. Diagnostic arthroscopy and longitudinal open lateral release. *Am J Sports Med* 1990; 18: 343.

14. Ficat, P. *Pathologie fémoro-patellaire.* Paris: Masson & Cie, 1970.

15. Ford, DH, and WR Post. Open or arthroscopic lateral release: Indications, techniques and rehabilitation. *Clin Sports Med* 1997; 16: 29–49.

16. Goodfellow, JW, DS Hungerford, and C Woods. Patellofemoral joint mechanics and pathology: 2. Chondromalacia patellae. *J Bone Joint Surg* 1976; 58-B: 291–299.

17. Guzzanti, V, A Gigante, A Di Lazzaro et al. Patellofemoral malalignment in adolescents: Computerized tomographic assessment with or without quadriceps contraction. *Am J Sports Med* 1994; 22: 55–60.

18. Hille, E, KP Schulitz, C Henrichs et al. Pressure and contact-surface measurements within the femoropatellar joint and their variations following lateral release. *Arch Orthop Trauma Surg* 1985; 104: 275–282.

19. Hughston, JC, and M Deese. Medial subluxation of the patella as a complication of lateral release. *Am J Sports Med* 1988; 16: 383–388.

20. Hughston, JC, WM Walsh, and G Puddu. Patellar subluxation and dislocation. *Saunders Monographs in Clin Orth,* Vol. V, 1984.

21. Kapandji, IA. Funktionelle Anatomie der Gelenke: Untere Extremität. Stuttgart: Enke-Verlag, 1985.

22. Kolowich, PA, LE Paulos, TD Rosenberg et al. Lateral release of the patella: Indications and contraindications. *Am J Sports Med* 1990; 18: 359–365.

23. Kramers de Quervain, IA, RM Biedert, and E Stüssi. Quantitative gait analysis in patients with medial patellar instability following lateral retinacular release. *Knee Surg Sports Traumatol, Arthrosc* 1997; 5: 95–101.

24. Messier, SP, SE Davis, WW Curl et al. Etiologic factors associated with patellofemoral pain in runners. *Med Sci Sports Exerc* 1991; 23: 1008–1015.

25. Müller, W. *Das Knie.* Heidelberg: Springer Verlag, 1982.

26. Papagelopoulos, PI, and FH Sim. Patellofemoral pain syndrome: Diagnosis and management. *Orthopaedics* 1997; 20: 148–157.

27. Rillmann, P, A Dutly, C Kieser et al. Modified Elmslie-Trillat procedure for instability of the patella. *Knee Surg Sports Traumatol Arthrosc* 1998; 6: 31–35.

28. Sasaki, T, and T Yagi. Subluxation of the patella: Investigation by computerized tomography. *Int Orthop* 1986; 10: 115–120.

29. Teitge, RA. Stress x-rays for patellofemoral instability. *Separatum,* 1988.

30. Teitge, RA, and WW Faerber. Stress radiographs of the patellofemoral joint. *J Bone Joint Surg* 1996; 78-A: 193–203.

31. Terry, GC. The anatomy of the extensor mechanism. *Clin Sports Med* 1989; 8: 163–177.

21

Failure of Patellofemoral Surgery: Analysis of Clinical Cases

Robert A. Teitge and Roger Torga-Spak

Introduction

Malfunction of the patellofemoral joint is the result of a failure of any one or a combination of three factors: alignment, stability, and articular cartilage.

An analysis of patellofemoral dysfunction best proceeds with an independent analysis of each of these elements. A more clear understanding of the clinical syndrome can be made if one first looks at each factor independently and then attempts to relate the factors sequentially and causally. As yet there exists no formula that can quantitatively determine the relative contributions of each of these components in such a way as to define the mechanics, the pathology, and the clinical picture. These three factors are not the same but are often related. It is important to think of the disease process as resulting from a combination of contributions of abnormality from each of these three components. There may be a failure of any one area individually, simultaneously, or sequentially. If the pathomechanics can be determined, then a revision surgery that first reverses the previous surgeries and then corrects the primary mechanical etiology has the best chances of success.

Alignment

The first factor to analyze in patellofemoral pain is the alignment. There are two common uses for the term alignment: (1) malposition of the patella on the femur, and (2) malposition of the axis of the knee joint on the limb with the subsequent effect of that malalignment on patellofemoral mechanics. Tracking is the change in position of the patella relative to the femur during knee flexion and extension.

Alignment refers to the overall anatomy, that is the lower extremity architecture, the geometrical relationship of all of its components, with the result effecting patellofemoral mechanics. It is a common mistake to consider alignment as referring only to the position of the patella on the femoral trochlea. Alignment refers to the changing relationship of all the bones of the lower extremity and might best be considered as the relationship of the patella to the body. Malalignment refers to a variation from the normal anatomy, considering normal that which is mechanically optimal; however, normal patterns have not been fully defined or quantified.

Bones have an optimal shape and juxtaposition that create optimal functional efficiency. A deviation from optimal geometry alters mechanical loading vectors that may result in symptomatic tissue overuse. It is important to look at the lower limb skeleton in each of three planes with respect to both: geometry of the single bone and of the relative positioning of adjacent bones.

Diagnosis

X-rays, including full-length limb alignment films as well as computed axial tomography (CAT) scan with determination of bone torsion, are necessary to evaluate the skeleton in three planes.

Stability

The second factor that can independently affect the patellofemoral joint is a failure of the normal stabilizing mechanism. It is clear that the stability is provided by a combination of bone and ligamentous restraints. Instability then must result from a failure of the patellofemoral ligaments contained within the retinaculum or the bony buttress. The contact area of bone surfaces, the total applied load, and the direction of the applied load create the friction necessary for stability. Thus, stability is the result of the restraining structures acting against the displacing forces (Table 21.1). Increasing the depth of the trochlea may convert an abnormal side-directed shearing force more perpendicular to the contact surface, thus reducing potential instability in a joint subjected to abnormal side force direction of load application; conversely in a patient with less intrinsic bony stability (trochlear dysplasia) greater responsibility for maintaining congruent surfaces falls on the ligaments. It is clear that insufficient ligamentous tissue either constitutionally or because of injury may render a susceptible joint unstable, while a joint with greater intrinsic stability through bony congruity may continue to function asymptomatically after a similar ligamentous injury.

Diagnosis

The diagnosis of instability needs to be made on the demonstration of pathologically increased sideward motion of the patella. X-rays with stress of the patellofemoral joint are needed to put in evidence ligament insufficiency. To obtain these stress x-rays the patient is positioned as for a routine Merchant x-ray view. If there is a knee flexion angle where medial or lateral subluxation stress applied to the patella produces greater apprehension or greater sideways excursion, then this position is selected for the axial x-ray with the line tangent to the joint determined by viewing the lateral x-ray. The examiner's hand supports the knee to keep it from rotating away

from the x-ray tube while stress is applied from the medial or the lateral side to the edge of the patella. A quantitative stress device had been used to standardize the displacement force (Medmetric Corp., San Diego, CA, USA). The usual stress applied is 15–18 lbs depending on the patient's ability to tolerate the pressure without contracting the muscles and an equal stress is applied to both patellae. A marked increase in displacement on one side is evidence of instability with subluxation.[1]

Cartilage

Cartilage damage may result from direct trauma (acute pressure increase such as dashboard injury or fall); chronic trauma (pressure increase) secondary to the imposed stress of malalignment without ligamentous failure and subluxation or dislocation which reduces contact pressure areas or from chronic overload on an anatomically sound knee (as weightlifting or obesity); or chronic overload from reduction in contact area and load sharing such as patella alta.[2,3] It is presumed that articular cartilage stays healthy when subjected to loads confined to a small range (3–5 mPa). A reduction of surface area or an increase in imposed load will elevate this to an unacceptable level, leading to chondromalacia and ultimately arthrosis. The presence of chondromalacia does not tell us what its etiology was.

Diagnosis

The condition of the cartilage may be seen well with double contrast arthrography and as this also reveals the thickness of the articular cartilage over the surface of the patella, contrast CT may be preferable to arthroscopy. Good magnetic resonance images can reveal the articular cartilage, but at times lower-quality studies do not, especially at the point of contact between the two surfaces.

Treatment

The treatment will be directed to correct the abnormality detected after the independent assessment of the three factors described above. Ideally the treatment should address the primary mechanical factor responsible for the condition (Table 21.2). However, in most cases the etiology is multifactorial and more than one factor or altered structure is observed during the examination. If that is the case we generally correct the factor that is more out of what is considered normal.

Table 21.1. Restraining structures acting against displacing forces

Displacing forces	Restraining structures
Trauma Body weight Limb malalignment	Medial patellofemoral ligament Lateral patellofemoral ligament Trochlear depth
• Increased femoral anteversion • Increased tibial external torsion • Valgus knee	
Patella alta Foot hyperpronation Tight Achilles	

Table 21.2. Procedures performed after independent analysis

Alignment		Stability		Cartilage	
Condition	Procedure	Condition	Procedure	Condition	Procedure
Genu valgum	Femoral varus osteotomy	Lateral instability	MPFL reconstruction	Focal lesion	Osteotomy or biological procedure
Genu varum	Tibial valgus osteotomy	Medial instability	LPFL reconstruction	Generalized lesion	Allograft or prosthetic replacement
Increased femoral anteversion	External rotation femoral ostetomy	Multidirectional instability (medial+lateral)	MPFL + LPFL reconstruction		
Increased tibial external torsion	Internal rotational tibial osteotomy	Trochlear dysplasia	Trochleoplasty or MPFL reconstruction		
Foot hyperpronation	Foot orthotics				
Patella alta	Distal tubercle displacement				
Lateral tibial tubercle (>20 mm)	Tibial tubercle medialization				
Medial tibial tubercle	Lateral tibial tubercle transfer				

Failed Surgery

The treatment of the complications depends on recognizing whether the complication was caused by incomplete or incorrect diagnosis or by selection of an inappropriate procedure. A common mistake that leads to failure is the local treatment of intra-articular lesions rather than the predisposing factors responsible for the pathology.

In the treatment of the patient with a failed patellofemoral surgery a two-step approach is necessary. First is to restore to the preoperative state the anatomy and the relations of the structures, which have been incorrectly modified by the procedure. Table 21.3 shows a list of common complications and the procedures we perform to restore the preoperative anatomy. Second is to detect and correct the predisposing factors that have led to the preoperative symptoms (Table 21.2).

Techniques in Revision Surgery

Lateral Patellofemoral Ligament Reconstruction

Medial dislocation or subluxation of the patella is a serious complication that can occur after an isolated arthroscopic lateral release, after an isolated open lateral release, or after lateral release in combination with tibial tubercle transfer or medial soft-tissue imbrications. The patient experiences pain and apprehension when the patella is stressed in a medial direction. Stress x-rays are very useful to quantify the medial displacement when compared to the contralateral side. In some extreme cases the patella can be dislocated outside the medial trochlea.

In our experience with lateral retinacular repair and imbrication, a noticeable increase in medial excursion usually would reappear after the first postoperative year. This led us to develop a technique for lateral patellofemoral ligament reconstruction,[4] following the principles of all ligament reconstruction: (1) selection of a sufficiently strong and stiff graft, (2) isometric graft placement, (3) adequate fixation, (4) correct tension, and (5) no condylar rubbing or impingement.

The quadriceps tendon provides a reliable graft but bone–patellar tendon–bone and Achilles

Table 21.3. Common complications and procedures to restore preoperative anatomy

Procedure	Complication	Treatment
Lateral retinacular release	Medial dislocation of the patella	Reconstruction of the lateral PF ligament
Medial retinacular repairs or reefings	Recurrent lateral instability	Medial PFL reconstruction
Lateral retinacular release	Multidirectional instability (combined medial and lateral instability)	Medial and lateral PFL reconstruction
Shaving chondroplasty	Patellofemoral arthrosis	Osteotomy +/− allograft
Medial tubercle transfer with normal TT–TG distance	Pathological external rotation of tibia and medial compartment overload	Lateralization of the distal tubercle

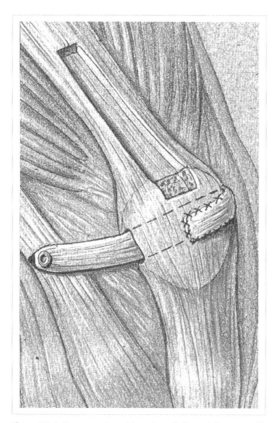

Figure 21.1. Reconstruction of lateral patellofemoral ligament with quadriceps tendon.

allograft can also be used (Figure 21.1). The graft must be located isometrically to avoid overstretching it to failure during joint motion or to avoid overconstraining patellar motion. A transverse hole is placed through the patella at about the mid-one-third height. We use a pneumatic isometer to determine the isometric point that is close to the lateral epicondyle. Once the isometric location is found, the graft must be fixed to the femur and to the patella. The bone block is countersunk into the femur and fixed with a 4.0 mm fully threaded lag screw. The tendon is pulled into the transverse tunnel drilled in the patella, out the medial side and turning it superficially onto the anterior surface of the patella, where it is sutured to the quadriceps expansion. We set the tension with the knee flexed 60° to 90° to avoid the risk of pulling too far lateral. The range of motion must be tested to ensure there is no restriction of patellar or knee motion. If impingement on the wall of the lateral femoral condyle is detected, the graft can be placed on the anterior surface of the

patella and pulled into the medial tunnel in a lateral direction.

Medial Patellofemoral Ligament Reconstruction

Reconstruction of the medial PF ligament is a very common procedure in our practice for the treatment of recurrent instability after failed patellar stabilization surgery. The medial patellofemoral ligament is the primary stabilizer against lateral dislocation or subluxation. Consequently if there is lateral patellar instability there is also an insufficient medial patellofemoral ligament. It is common to see persistent lateral instability of the patella after recovery from procedures that fail to address the insufficient ligament as the primary pathology. Procedures that intend to repair the failed medial structures may lead to an improvement in the symptoms during the first year postsurgery, but instability reappears after that period. We believe the reasons for the later failures are related to: (1) the material used to fix the medial ligament is inadequate, the failed retinacular tissue is extremely thin and friable leading to stretching over time, and (2) the medial structures are subject to greater than normal lateral displacement forces (skeletal malalignment, trochlear dysplasia, patella alta).

The fact that a direct repair of the medial structures gives a temporary improvement in symptoms can be used as a diagnostic tool when the diagnosis is in question. Certainly a reconstruction of the MPFL with a stronger structure will have greater chances to succeed.

The technique we postulate follows the same principles as the one described for reconstruction for the lateral PFL. In addition to the use of quadriceps tendon or bone-tendon or other allografts, the adductor magnus tendon or hamstring tendons have been used as grafts.[5] The adductor magnus with its insertion just proximal the medial epicondyle can be conveniently used to reconstruct the MPFL (Figure 21.2).

Tibial Tubercle Transfer

Distal tubercle transfer is indicated for patella alta, proximal displacement of the tubercle for patella baja, lateral tubercle transfer for inadequate Q-angle, and medial tubercle transfer for grossly excessive Q-angle.

Patella alta has been long recognized as associated with patellar instability. This is likely because the patella is not engaged in the trochlea

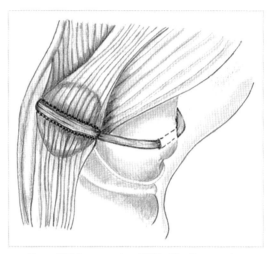

Figure 21.2. Reconstruction of MPFL with adductor tendon.

and thus receives neither the trochlear buttress support nor the necessary fulcrum for the medial patellofemoral ligament to operate efficiently during the twisting activity that usually causes patellar subluxation.

The transfer is planned on the lateral preoperative x-rays; the tubercle should be moved distally enough to create an Insall-Salvati ratio of 1. Great effort is taken not to alter a normal Q-angle. Through a lateral vertical incision, the tibial tubercle is exposed and the patellar tendon insertion is identified. An anteroposterior K-wire is placed just distal to the patellar tendon; then an anteroposterior hole (2.5 mm drill) is performed distally in line with the patellar tendon and parallel to the K-wire. The distance between the K-wire and the hole will determine the amount distalization and is calculated from the preoperative planning. A series of drill holes are placed from lateral to medial and connected with a chisel. The fragment should be at least 7 cm long and 15 mm thick at the proximal part in order to obtain a good contact surface and to reduce the risk of fracture at the time of fixation. The fragment is pulled distally so the proximal hole is aligned with the distal drill hole, and then a K-wire is used to maintain alignment while the fragment is fixed with 2 lag screws.

The same technique is used to lateralize the medial tubercle to restore the normal tibial tubercle–trochlear (TT-TG) groove distance in patients who have had an excessive medial transfer. It is not unusual to see in our practice patients who had medial transfers in knees with

previously normal TT-TG. Excessive medialization may contribute to medial subluxation or dislocation of the patella and to the development of medial patellofemoral osteoarthritis as well as medial compartment osteoarthritis due to overload of the medial compartment. Additionally, the tibia is externally rotated and the patients may walk with increased outward foot progression angle. This external rotation of the tibia on the femur stresses the tibiofemoral capsule and pain at the posteriomedial corner of the joint may be present. A symptomatic medially transferred tibial tubercle should be repositioned laterally so the TT-TG distance is between 10 and 20 mm.

Osteotomy of Long Bones

Skeletal alignment in all three planes has a great influence on patellar tracking and loading. The source of patellofemoral loading is extra-articular; this is the reason that operations limited to the knee joint frequently fail when skeletal malalignment is not recognized. The treatment of skeletal malalignment requires the correct bony operation. If there is genu valgum because of a short lateral femoral condyle, a femoral varus osteotomy is indicated. If the genu valgum is the result of a valgus bow to the tibia then a varus osteotomy of the tibia near the deformity is indicated. Genu varum with medial trochlear degeneration should be treated with tibial valgus osteotomy. Inward pointing knees with secondary lateral subluxation should be treated by with external rotation femoral osteotomy if it is caused by increased femoral anteversion, and internal rotation tibial osteotomy if it is caused by increased external tibial torsion. Combined deformities are not uncommon and the type of osteotomy and location depends on the deformity. A detailed description of the types and level of the osteotomies is presented in Chapter 11.

Osteochondral Allograft

If the articular cartilage has been lost and osteoarthritis develops, two alternatives are available: (1) restoration of the normal extra-articular anatomy and stability and (2) replacement of the articular cartilage. Options for articular cartilage replacement are biological or prosthetic. In the past 18 years, 11 patients have undergone 14 fresh patellar and trochlear allografts. The most frequently performed pre-replacement procedure in this series was shaving chondroplasty, leaving a painful patella with exposed subchondral patellar bone and progressive degenerative changes on the trochlear side. At an average 10 years follow-up we observed 3 failures and 11 good-to-excellent results. The results of our study suggest that, in young patients with isolated secondary patellofemoral arthrosis, fresh osteochondral allografts in conjunction with correction of predisposing factors may offer an alternative to patellectomy and delay prosthetic joint replacement.

Clinical Cases

Case 1

History. A 44-year-old woman was normal with no complaints in her knees until an automobile accident in which she was driving her car that was struck from the side by another car. She slid underneath the seat belt, striking both knees directly against the dashboard. Radiographs were negative. After physiotherapy she continued to have mild pain over the patella with no signs or symptoms of instability in the left knee. Six months after accident she underwent arthroscopy and an arthroscopic lateral release. Anterior knee pain was much more severe after surgery. Almost immediately she noted that a knee sleeve would push the patella out of place in the medial direction. She now had retropatellar crepitation, pain laterally, an effusion after walking for 20 minutes, limping, insecurity, difficulty going down stairs, a sense that the patella was out of place especially walking down hills, aching pain at night, collapsing of the knee, and inability to wear high-heel shoes.

Physical Exam. Knee motion 0°–150°, effusion, diffuse warmth, soft tissue swelling, crepitation with extension, a negative J-sign, marked increased medial and lateral mobility of the left patella compared with the nonoperated right, there was considerable apprehension with pressing the patella medially and a complete medial dislocation could be demonstrated with medial stress, the Q-angle was 15°, there was significant tenderness palpating the defect in the lateral retinaculum, the Ober test was negative, collateral and cruciate ligaments were normal, limb alignment in the frontal plane was clinically normal, prone examination revealed hip rotation 65° internal and 35° external, the foot thigh axis was normal, there was moderate pronation of the foot, the Achilles tendon was tight bilaterally.

Radiographs. AP, lateral, and axial radiographs were normal with normal height of the patella, normal tibiofemoral axis, and normal sulcus. Stress radiographs, however, revealed a complete medial dislocation of the patella, which moved medially 24 mm more than in the normal knee and laterally 5 mm more than in the normal knee, and tilted 14° more than in the normal knee. Figure 21.3 shows this abnormal displacement. Figure 21.4 shows (in another patient) clinically a medially dislocated patella.

Analysis. The complication is an iatrogenic medial patellar dislocation following an isolated arthroscopic lateral release. There is no evidence in this case to suggest that the lateral retinaculum was in any way contributing to the patient's symptoms. The normal lateral

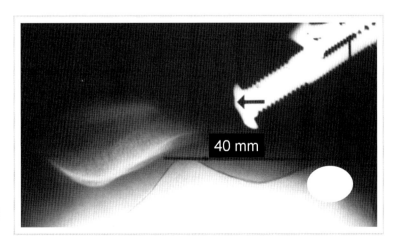

Figure 21.3. Medial dislocation of the patella after arthroscopic lateral patellar release.

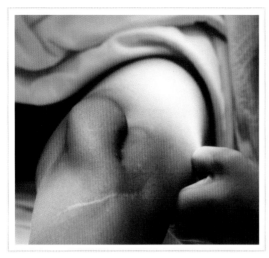

Figure 21.4. Example of medial dislocatable patella post realignment.

retinaculum contributes to stability in both the medial and in the lateral direction and prevents abnormal tilt.

Treatment. The correction was a reconstruction with quadriceps graft of the lateral patellofemoral ligament.

Case 2

History. A 26-year-old woman with disabling left knee pain and instability. At age 19 she was struck in the front of the knee by an opponent while playing baseball. She continued to play baseball but because of continued pain one year later she underwent diagnostic arthroscopy and subcutaneous lateral release. She was somewhat worse, so 3 months later underwent a repeat arthroscopy with chondroplasty of both the patella and femur to create bleeding bone for stimulation of cartilage growth. She was definitely worse and a consultant suggested repeating the lateral release. One year later she underwent an lnsall proximal realignment, repeat lateral release and drilling of the patella. She deteriorated further and began to experience medial dislocations of the patella. A second consultant recommended quadriceps exercises, which she performed 3 days a week for 3 years. A third consultant recommended 6 weeks of casting, which did not help. On at least 4 occasions a patellar dislocation medially required manipulative reduction, twice in the hospital. Seven years after the original injury a fourth

consultant recognized medial patellar dislocation. At this point she needed a railing to assist in going up and down stairs, with constant aching, pain at night, regular stiffness.

Physical Exam. Genu varum greater on the involved side, recurvatum, pronation of the feet and inward pointing or squinting of both patella, retropatellar crepitation with active knee extension bilaterally, a negative J-sign compared with a markedly positive J-sign on the asymptomatic side, increased medial-lateral patellar excursion, no apprehension moving the patella laterally but severe apprehension moving the patella medially, significant quadriceps atrophy, motion $-7°-145°$, pain at the medial joint line, pain at the lateral retinaculum, Q-angle = $20°$ bilaterally, negative Ober test, foot thigh axis $-10°$, tibia varum, no Achilles tightness, hip internal rotation $45°$, external rotation $50°$.

Radiographs. Narrowing of the patellofemoral joint, and a shallow sulcus, normal patellar height. CT arthrogram revealed complete loss of lateral articular cartilage with excellent preservation of medial patellar articular cartilage (Figure 21.5). Medial stress CT revealed a complete medial dislocation of the patella.

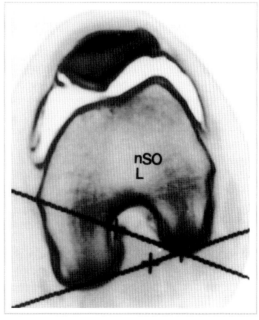

Figure 21.5. CT arthrogram. Loss lateral articular cartilage, shallow trochlea, post lateral release and arthroscopic chondroplasty.

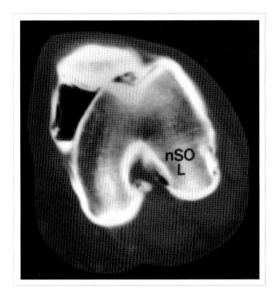

Figure 21.6. Medial dislocation patella post lateral release showing why medial dislocation causes lateral facet damage.

This film (Figure 21.6) clearly shows how the lateral cartilage could be injured with good preservation of the medial cartilage during medial dislocation.

Analysis. The complication is iatrogenic arthrosis through removal of articular cartilage and iatrogenic medial dislocation of the patella through repeated lateral releases plus medial imbrication.

Treatment. Lateral patellofemoral ligament reconstruction with a quadriceps tendon graft with the result being significant improvement as the instability was treated but ultimately not the cartilage loss.

Case 3

History. A 34-year-old woman with anterior knee pain unresponsive to arthroscopy 15 years ago. Four years prior to consultation had been injured by blunt trauma when a metal cart carrying 100 Kg struck the anterior knee near the patellar tendon. One year later underwent arthroscopy, which did not improve the knee, and after physiotherapy one year later underwent another arthroscopy. There was no change in the pain, swelling, and giving way, so she had a Maquet osteotomy with soft tissue breakdown requiring a gastrocnemius muscle flap for coverage (Figure 21.7).

Physical Exam. 183 cm tall, 121 Kg. Neutral alignment, pronated feet, squinting patellae,

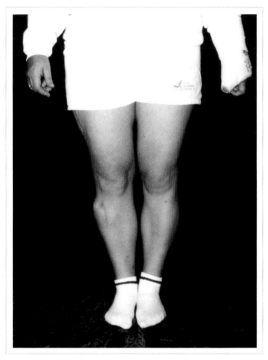

Figure 21.7. Thirty-four-year-old patient post right Maquet osteotomy with inpointing left patella. She is post-op right intertrochanteric 40° external rotation osteotomy.

circumduction gait. Squat only 30° because of pain, motion −5°–110° bilaterally, ligaments stable, meniscal signs negative, Q-angle 15° R and 20° L, no patellofemoral crepitation but weakness of the quadriceps, moderate thigh muscle atrophy, Ober tight at 4 cm without pain, prone hip internal rotation 70°, external rotation 50°.

Radiographs. AP, lateral, and axial radiographs were negative except for CT study for limb rotation showing femoral anteversion 54° (vs. normal 13°) (Figure 21.8).

Analysis. Complication was failure to recognize limitation of external hip rotation forcing the knee joint axis to be chronically facing inward.

Treatment. The treatment was external rotational femoral osteotomy (intertrochanteric). The result at four months was she noticed the operated knee moves straight forward while in the nonoperated limb the foot swings outward. The preoperative pain that had been present for over four years was gone and the operated limb now had less pain than the noninjured knee and she was anxious to have the same surgery on the noninjured limb.

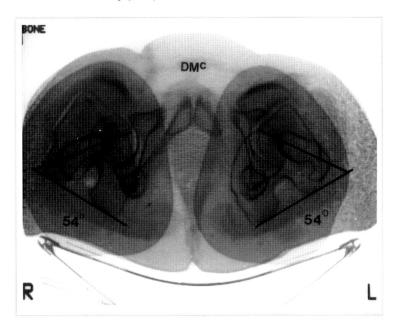

Figure 21.8. Pre-op CT rotational scan shows bilateral 54° femoral anteversion.

Case 4

History. A 37-year-old woman with 6 months of constant pain in both knees requiring narcotic medication. Anterior knee pain began 19 years earlier. Two years later, 17 years ago, she underwent a medial transfer of the left tibial tubercle. Fifteen years ago she underwent a medial transfer of the right tibial tubercle. A manipulation was required for limited motion post-op. Twelve years ago she underwent arthroscopy with lysis of adhesions followed shortly afterward with a manipulation. Ten years ago she had an arthroscopic synovectomy. Four years ago she underwent right arthroscopic medial meniscectomy, patellar chondroplasty by arthroscopic shaving, and lateral release. She was much worse after that procedure. There is constant pain that keeps her awake at night, pain walking, pain going up and down stairs, pain sitting, weakness, buckling, limping, insecurity, catching, and intermittent sharp pains.

Examination. Slight varus, inpointing of the patella (squinting), limited squatting, Motion R 0°–130°, L 0°–134°, L effusion, bilateral soft tissue swelling, retropatellar crepitation, increased lateral mobility bilaterally with apprehension on the right, not the left, increased medial mobility on the right, not the left, with apprehension on the right. Q-angle: 12° R and 14° L, cruciate and collateral ligaments intact, significant pain with palpation along the medial joint line on the right, prone internal hip rotation 50°, external rotation 25°. The tibial tubercles appeared to be located excessively medial and the feet were pointed outward.

Radiographs. The mechanical axis was neutral, flexion weight bearing showed equal joint space medial and lateral, both patellae were centered in the trochlea in the axial view, but there was narrowing with increased subchondral sclerosis of the medial patellofemoral joints. CT arthrography revealed loss of medial facet articular cartilage greater on the left (Figure 21.9) and CT studies for torsion showing increased anteversion bilaterally at 24° and 32° (Figure 21.10), with the tibial tubercle–trochlear groove distance 0 on the right and –5 mm on the left.

Analysis. The complication is medial patellofemoral arthrosis after medial tibial tubercle transfer. In addition the tibias are being rotated externally as a result of an external rotational pull from a medially transferred tibial tubercle, and it is felt that the medial compartments were being overloaded by the increased medial patellofemoral loading. There was no proof of

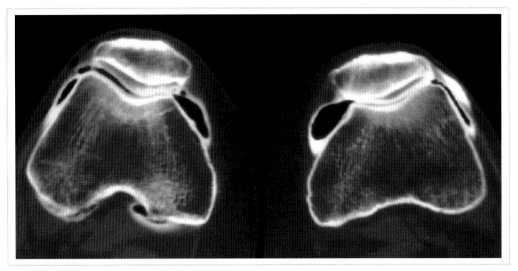

Figure 21.9. Doble contrast CT arthrogram showing loss medial patellofemoral cartilage bilaterally post-medial tibial tubercle transfer.

subluxation or dislocation in this patient. It was assumed that lateral patellar displacement was responsible for the anterior knee pain and it was assumed that a medial transfer of the tibial tubercle would reduce this subluxation and pain. It was assumed that lateral release, chondroplasty, and medial meniscectomy would improve the symptoms. It is likely that this made the situation worse.

Treatment. Lateral transfer of the tibial tubercles and external rotational osteotomy of the femurs. The patient remains improved at 6 years post-osteotomy, although she has intermittent pain along the left medial joint line that is felt to be due to an inadequate lateral transfer of the left tibial tubercle.

Case 5

History. A 33-year-old male hospital administrator was seen in consultation for bilateral anterior knee pain of increased severity of 3 months' duration after a painful bucking

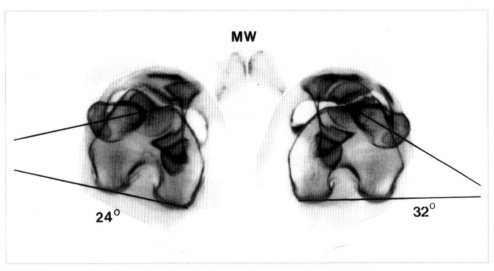

Figure 21.10. CT rotational study showing bilateral femoral anteversion. Treatment was lateral tibial tubercle transfer to unload medial facet and intertrochanteric external rotational osteotomy to treat rotational alignment.

episode while in church. He complained of limping, recurrent swelling, locking, buckling at least 6 times per day, pain going up and down stairs, pain with sitting, and a feeling of the patella slipping but not requiring manipulation for relocation. At age 20 (13 years earlier) he had realignment surgery (medial tubercle transfer, lnsall-type medial imbrication, and lateral release) bilaterally. Nine years earlier he had removal of loose bodies from the left knee.

Physical Exam. 193 cm tall, 119 Kg. Genu valgum, hyperpronation of feet, inability to squat because of pain and stiffness, motion 0°–130°, there is hypermobility of both patellae, there is hypersensitivity with this motion, pain with lateral subluxation bilaterally and pain with medial subluxation of the left patella, Q-angle 0°, medial facet tenderness bilaterally, increased articular grind with side motion of the patella, patella alta, 1+ laxity to varus stress bilaterally, thigh atrophy, Ober tight at 3 cm, prone hip internal rotation 60°, external rotation 20°, tight Achilles bilaterally.

Radiographs. Patella alta, normal congruence angle, narrowing of the medial patellofemoral joint, stress radiographs indicated no increased lateral excursion but almost a dislocation medially. CT arthrography revealed good quality articular cartilage superiorly on the patella with marked loss of distal and especially medial patellar articular cartilage; CT rotation study revealed femoral anteversion 36° (normal 13°).

Analysis. (1) Postsurgical arthrosis, (2) medial patellar instability, (3) trochlear dysplasia, (4) increased femoral anteversion, (5) mild increased external tibial torsion, (6) hyperpronation of feet, (7) mild genu valgum, (8) contracture of Achilles tendon, and (9) post-medial tibial tubercle transfer.

Treatment. (1) Distal and lateral transfer tibial tubercle, (2) external rotation varus osteotomy distal femur, and (3) imbrication of both the medial and lateral retinaculum. Postoperatively he described "a new sensation which is comfortable and confident," and at 1 ½ years postsurgery, "wonderful, the knee better than he could ever remember having it been." He requested the same procedure on the opposite knee and is now 5 years postsurgery on the right and 3 years postsurgery on the left. He continues to remain improved over the preoperative state. However, we have not addressed the loss of articular cartilage, tibial torsion,

trochlear dysplasia, Achilles contracture, or the patient's height and weight.

In each of these first 5 cases, limb alignment including varus-valgus, torsion of the femur and tibia, foot pronation, muscle contracture, trochlear dysplasia, patellar height, and patellofemoral ligament laxity need to be considered. A simple lateral release or tibial tubercle transfer fails to address the more important contributing variables.

Case 6

History. A 34-year-old female teacher was referred for consultation regarding recurrent dislocation of the patella starting at age 13. At age 30 because of pain and swelling she underwent arthroscopy followed by medial transfer of tibial tubercle (Elmslie-Trillat), lateral retinacular release, and chondroplasty. She now presents with pain, swelling, weakness, and slippage of the patella.

Physical Exam. Straight limb alignment, bilateral foot hyperpronation, motion 0°–150°. Unable to extend against gravity, with audible crepitation as she attempts this; Q-angle = 5° compared with 20° on the opposite side. Patella is hypermobile both to the medial and the lateral direction. Gross atrophy of the quadriceps, moderate effusion, collateral and cruciate ligaments are stable, McMurray negative, Ober test negative, prone hip internal rotation 40°, external rotation 30°.

Radiographs. Narrowing of articular cartilage space and osteoporosis. Slight patella alta with Insall ratio = 0.8. Stress radiographs show complete dislocation of the patella medially and hypermobility laterally.

Analysis. The complication is iatrogenic medial patellar dislocation due to combined lateral release and medial tubercle transfer, with arthrosis aggravated by chondroplasty.

Treatment. Lateral transfer of the tibial tubercle and lateral retinacular repair. She improved but at two years post-op redislocated the patella medially. The lateral retinaculum is frequently not of sufficient quality to create a permanent repair. At this stage she underwent lateral patellofemoral ligament reconstruction with a quadriceps tendon graft. This was effective in providing stability but further deterioration in the remaining articular cartilage occurred (Figures 21.11 and 21.12). Three

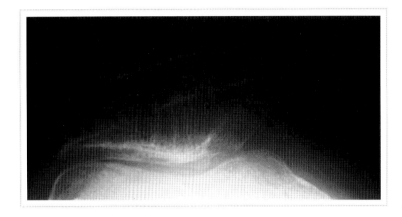

Figure 21.11. Post lateral PF ligament reconstruction development arthrosis PF joint.

years later she underwent patellar-trochlear fresh allograft replacement (Figures 21.13 to 21.18). She is now 9 years post-allograft and although the radiographs appear to show extensive abnormal bone changes the articular space still remains widened and her symptoms are still greatly improved over her earlier treatment (Figure 21.18).

Conclusion

In the treatment of patellofemoral complications, the surgical treatment should address the primary pathology as well as the changes induced by the failed procedure. Cutting normal ligaments, removing articular cartilage, or transferring tendons to an abnormal position usually create new problems and should be performed cautiously.

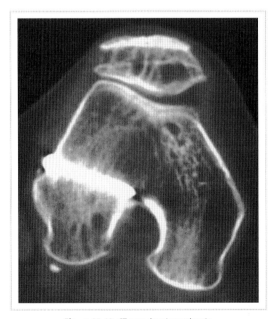

Figure 21.12. CT scan showing arthrosis.

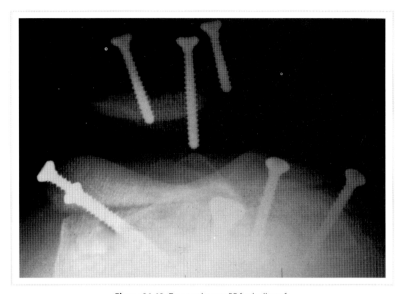

Figure 21.13. Two weeks post PF fresh allograft.

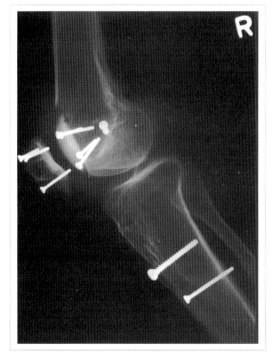

Figure 21.14. Two weeks post PF fresh allograft.

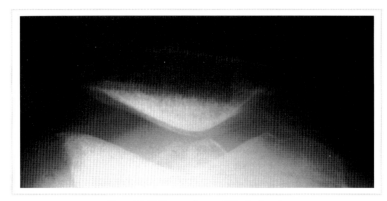

Figure 21.15. Ten months post PF fresh allograft.

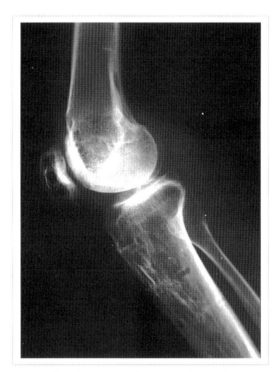

Figure 21.16. Ten months post PF fresh allograft.

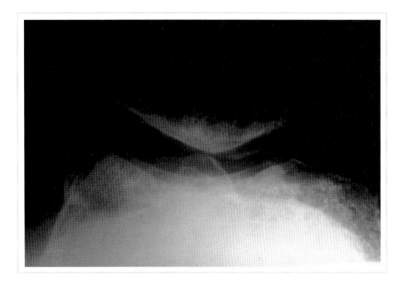

Figure 21.17. Five years post PF fresh allograft.

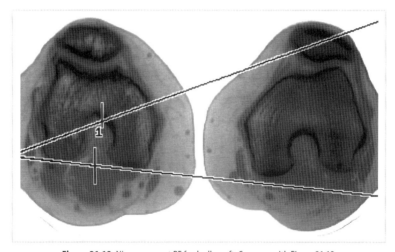

Figure 21.18. Nine years post PF fresh allograft. Compare with Figure 21.12.

References

1. Teitge, RA, WW Faerber, P Des Madryl, and TM Matelic. Stress radiographs of the patellofemoral joint. *J Bone Joint Surg Am* 1996; 78(2): 193–203.
2. Huberti, HH, and WC Hayes. Contact pressures in chondromalacia patellae and the effects of capsular reconstructive procedures. *J Orthop Res* 1988; 6(4): 499–508.
3. Huberti, HH, and WC Hayes. Patellofemoral contact pressures: The influence of Q-angle and tendofemoral contact. *J Bone Joint Surg Am* 1984; 66(5): 715–724.
4. Teitge, RA, and R Torga-Spak. Lateral patellofemoral ligament reconstruction. *Arthroscopy* 2004; 20(9): 998–1002.
5. Teitge, RA, and R Torga-Spak. Medial patellofemoral ligament reconstruction. *Orthopedics* 2004; Oct., 27(10):1037–1040.

22

Arthrofibrosis and Patella Infera

Christopher D. Harner, Tracy M. Vogrin, and Kenneth J. Westerheide

Case Report
History

A 37-year-old male farmer underwent an arthroscopic partial medial meniscectomy in his right knee at an outside center. Unfortunately following his surgery, the patient developed an acute staphylococcal infection, which was initially treated by arthroscopic irrigation and debridement, followed by an open irrigation and debridement two weeks later. He was placed on a six-week course of intravenous antibiotics and concurrently received physical therapy in an attempt to improve the range of motion of his stiff knee. Despite physical therapy, he continued to have swelling and decreased range of motion.

Approximately 18 months later, the patient was treated by another physician at an outside center with an arthroscopic lysis of adhesions, manipulation under anesthesia, and postoperative physical therapy for persistent stiffness. Subsequently, his range of motion reportedly improved to 5° to 120° of flexion. However, the patient reinjured his knee while performing exercises less than one year later. He again experienced a gradual loss of motion with intermittent swelling as well as medial-sided knee pain. The patient was then prescribed a course of Prednisone and Celebrex, which did not provide any significant relief.

The patient presented to our center with the primary complaint of right knee stiffness, particularly in flexion, which caused him difficulty working on his farm and stepping down stairs or inclines. He was also experiencing mild pain in the anterior and medial aspects of his knee, but the pain was tolerable. His past medical and social history were noncontributory.

Physical Examination

On examination, he was mildly overweight with a normal gait. His right knee was neutrally aligned and his left was in 2° of valgus. The squat was limited to 90° on the right side secondary to pain. His active and passive ranges of motion were equal, with a range of 3° to 90° for the right knee and 0° to 130° for the left. His right quadriceps muscle was 10% atrophied and he had no effusion. Patellar exam revealed a −10° tilt for his right patella compared with a 0° tilt for the left. For the right knee, patellar glide was 1+ laterally, and 0 medially, superiorly, and inferiorly. His left knee had a 2+ medial and lateral patellar glide. Ligamentous exam revealed a symmetric, stable knee. The patient had 2+ joint line tenderness of the right knee in the middle and posteromedial aspects and no lateral joint line tenderness. Flexion McMurray test was negative.

Imaging Studies

Knee flexion weightbearing, lateral, Merchant, and long-cassette radiographs and an MRI were obtained (Figures 22.1 and 22.2). The radiographs were significant for medial joint space narrowing and positive Fairbanks changes. Mild to moderate changes were noted in the patellofemoral compartment and the lateral compartment appeared normal. The lateral radiograph revealed 1 cm of patella infera on the right knee compared to the left. Abundant retropatellar scar tissue was observed on the MRI.

Diagnosis

1. Arthrofibrosis secondary to postoperative septic arthritis, including patellar entrapment and early patella infera.

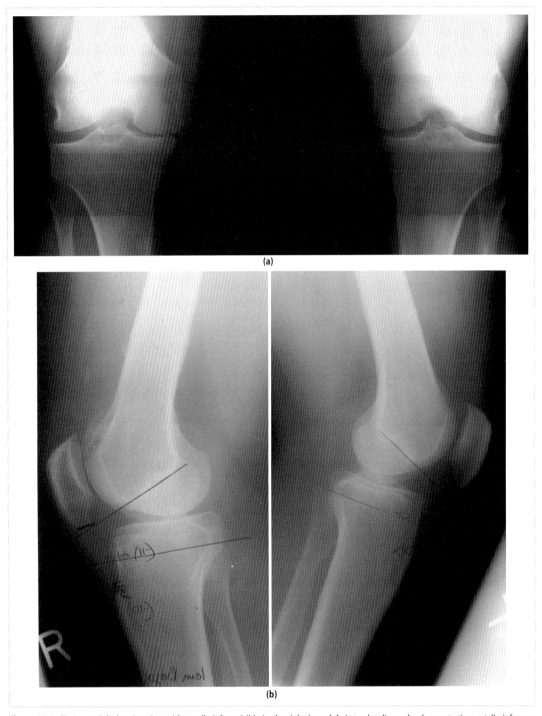

Figure 22.1. Flexion weight-bearing view with patella infera visible in the right knee **(a).** Lateral radiographs demonstrating patella infera on right knee **(b).**

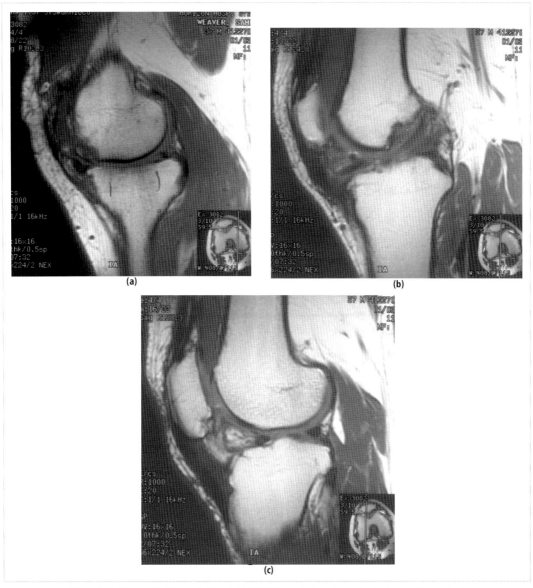

Figure 22.2. Three sagittal views of a T1-weighted MRI demonstrating retropatellar tendon scar tissue **(a,b,c).**

2. Moderate medial compartment degenerative joint disease and mild patellofemoral degenerative changes.

Initial Management

For treatment of the arthrofibrosis, alternatives discussed with the patient included splinting or bracing, physical therapy, CPM, and manipulation under anesthesia. It was recommended that arthroscopic or open excision of scar tissue be performed with the goal of increasing his flexion by 10 to 20 degrees. If this could not be achieved, the patellar tendon would be reconstructed using semitendinosus autograft. Following discussion of options, surgical techniques, and risks and benefits, the patient elected to undergo the surgery.

In addition, a medial unloader brace was recommended for treatment of the medial compartment degenerative changes. We believed that an osteotomy would be unlikely to provide significant benefits until his range of motion was improved.

Surgical Findings and Technique

Bilateral extremities were prepared and sterilely draped to enable intraoperative comparisons of range of motion and patellar height (Figure 22.3). The patient's previous midline incision was used and extended from 3 cm above the superior patellar pole down to the level of the tibial tubercle. Sharp dissection was continued down to the level of the fascia, preserving full thickness flaps (Figure 22.4). This enabled visualization of the entire width of the extensor mechanism, which revealed extremely poor patellar motion. Scar tissue was palpable throughout the extensor mechanism, as well as between the subcutaneous tissues and the tendon itself.

A medial arthrotomy was made, curving along the patella and paralleling the medial side of the patellar tendon. Abundant scar tissue was noted behind the patellar tendon and was resected, taking care to preserve the meniscus (Figure 22.5). Another arthrotomy was made along the lateral aspect of the patella in order to remove scar tissue from the retropatellar area and the lateral fat pad. The extensor mechanism

was found to be scarred down to the femur itself. Metzenbaum scissors were used to release this tissue and recreate the suprapatellar pouch as well as the medial and lateral gutters.

After releasing the scar tissue, knee flexion was improved but still not equal to the contralateral side. It was thought that central third of the patellar tendon was providing the majority of the restraint. Therefore, the decision was made to "pie-crust" the central third of the patellar tendon (Figure 22.6). Multiple relaxing incisions in a transverse orientation were first marked carefully using a pen and then made using a #11 blade. Upon flexion, the relaxing incisions lengthened, providing 120 degrees of flexion, which was slightly less than the contralateral side. A lateral release was performed to improve patellar mobility and tracking. After deflating the tourniquet and performing hemostasis, the arthrotomies were closed anatomically with the knee maximally flexed. A brace was applied and the knee was locked in full extension.

Post-Op Rehabilitation

Immediately postoperatively, the patient was locked in extension in order to protect the extensor mechanism, and allowed to weight-bear as tolerated. In order to maintain the flexion that

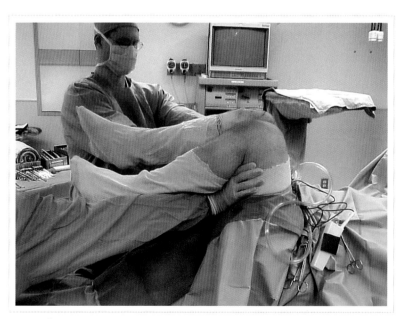

Figure 22.3. Intraoperative comparison demonstrating decreased flexion in the right knee.

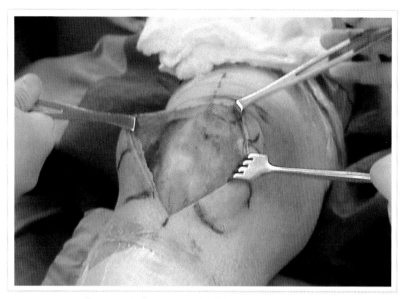

Figure 22.4. Midline incision with full thickness flaps for exposure.

was achieved, continuous passive motion was started immediately from 0 to 50 degrees of flexion for two sessions per day for two hours each. These sessions were increased by 5 degrees per session if tolerated, up to a maximum of 120 degrees. He was also directed to perform straight leg raises, quadriceps sets, and heel slides. Physical therapy was initiated in order to maintain his range of motion.

Case Discussion

Arthrofibrosis is a potentially severe complication of knee surgery or trauma, including arthroscopy, cruciate ligament reconstruction, prolonged immobilization, or septic arthritis as in this case example.[1-7] It is characterized by a wide spectrum of pathologies that result in a loss of motion due to inflammation and scarring. This may include intra-, peri- and extra-articular adhesions, with the resulting development of Cyclops lesions, patellar entrapment syndrome, patella infera, or infrapatellar contracture syndrome.[1-7]

Making the Correct Diagnosis

Prevention and early diagnosis are key for the successful treatment of an entrapped patella. Therefore, obtaining a complete history is critical, including the date of surgery, length and type of immobilization and rehabilitation, and onset of pain and stiffness. Typically, the patient will complain of knee stiffness and pain, with physical examination revealing alterations in gait, crepitation, and possibly quadriceps weakness. Patellar glides are often reduced due to entrapment. If patella infera is present, the knee may lose its rounded contour at 90 degrees of flexion; however, this may not be obvious if swelling is present.[3] If the patient is diagnosed and treated early (i.e., within three months), he or she can still be successfully treated.[7]

Pathoanatomy

Patella infera is a manifestation of severe arthrofibrosis, resulting in tightening of the extensor mechanism, increased articular pressures in the patellofemoral joint, and restricted knee flexion.[3] Inflammation in the joint results in fibrous proliferation behind the patellar tendon, which then adheres to the tibia. Subsequently, the patella may adhere to the fat pad, occupying the entire space between the notch and joint lines. The fatty tissue is replaced by a dense fibrotic tissue that is abundant anteriorly and in the medial and lateral gutters.[3] If the patella infera is present for more than six months, a pannus may form that impinges into the joint and may damage the cartilage. Tendon shortening may also occur, as in this case example, secondary to the fibrosis and quadriceps atrophy.[7]

Paulos and colleagues described the Infrapatellar Contracture Syndrome (IPCS), which is the combination of patellar entrapment due to arthrofibrosis and loss of both flexion and extension.[3] It may occur secondary to knee

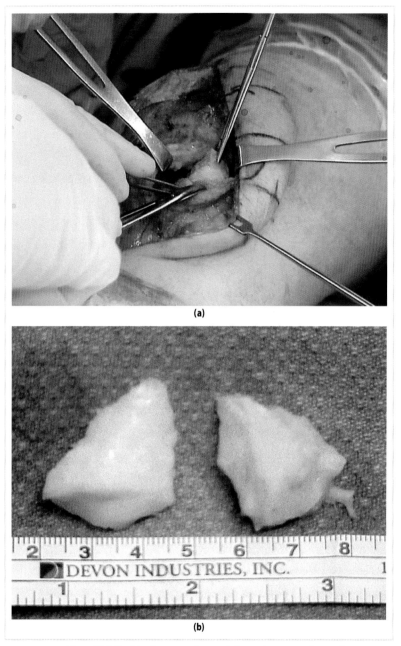

Figure 22.5. Medial arthrotomy and removal of extensive retropatellar scar tissue.

surgery, reflex sympathetic dystrophy, quadriceps insufficiency, neuromuscular disorder, or infection.[3,7] They described three stages that were indicative of prognosis: The early, or prodromal, stage (2–8 weeks) is characterized by induration of the synovium, fat pad, and retinaculum, and is manifested by painful range of motion, restricted patellar mobility, and quadriceps lag. Often a difficult, painful rehabilitation serves as a clue for diagnosis. In the active stage (6–20 weeks), the indurated tissues may form a shelf beneath the patella, further restricting patellar glides and tilts. The quadriceps lag disappears, but quadriceps atrophy and crepitus

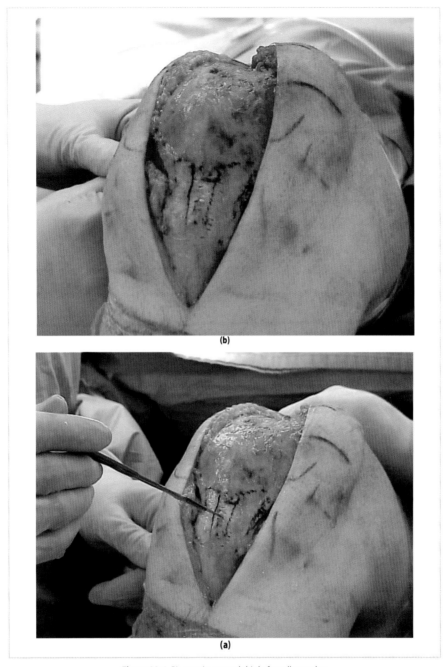

Figure 22.6. Pie-crusting central third of patellar tendon.

may be present and the patient cannot achieve full extension. After approximately 8 months, the third, or "burned out" stage is reached, in which the inflammation and induration have subsided and patella infera develops. There is a loss of both flexion and extension, quadriceps atrophy, severe crepitus, and diminished patellofemoral joint space. Although the patient in this case example did not have a severe loss of extension, it would appear based on his history and examination that the patient in this case example is in the early third stage.

Surgical Indications and Technical Pearls

For those diagnosed in the early stages of arthrofibrosis and patella infera, nonsurgical management can often be successful, such as daily physical therapy with early range of motion exercises, manual patellar mobilization, nonsteroidal anti-inflammatory drugs, corticosteroids, and electrical stimulation of the quadriceps.[3,7] Manipulation or a drop-out case can also assist in obtaining full extension.

If surgery is needed, it is usually important to wait for 4 to 12 weeks. In this time, the patient can improve quadriceps strength while pain, swelling, and inflammation diminish.[3] Manipulation and arthroscopic soft tissue release are usually the initial step taken, although repeated attempts to improve motion manually in the presence of fibrous adhesions may only cause further damage to the articular surface.[6] It is critical to assess the quadriceps function prior to surgery, as the extensor mechanism may be further inhibited and the patella infera will persist.[7]

When manipulation and soft tissue release fail, open debridement and release is required.[2,3,5] This enables adequate visualization so that all pathological structures can be debrided or excised.[2] Open debridement may include anterior, medial, and lateral extra-articular release and partial fat pad resection. The patella is freed intra-articularly in the medial, superior, and inferior directions; often a medial arthrotomy may be required to achieve this. The suprapatellar pouch and intracondylar notch are also debrided. Posterior surgical release to improve extension should not be performed unless the previous approach was also posterior and unless release of the tissue can account for the flexion contracture.[3]

It may be necessary to elevate and release the patellar tendon from the tibia or even reposition the tibial tubercle.[7] As the patellar tendon can also shorten secondary to the fibrosis and quadriceps atrophy, lengthening of the tendon may be required, as in this example. We prefer to "pie-crust" the tendon, making many small transverse incisions along its length. This results in fractional lengthening of the tendon without disrupting the extensor mechanism.

Expected Outcomes

If diagnosed and treated early – depending upon the severity – a successful outcome can be obtained. However, if the condition is not corrected, degenerative changes may occur in the patellofemoral articulating surface secondary to the abnormal joint loading. At this point in time, only a salvage procedure will be possible.[2,7] The prognosis does appear to depend on the etiology, as patients who develop arthrofibrosis secondary to ligament injuries have had better outcomes;[1] however, this is also likely a function of the population of younger, more athletic patients with ligamentous injuries.

In more severe cases, surgical treatment is required. Clinical outcome studies have indicated that debridement and soft tissue release can provide significant improvements in range of motion.[2,4,5] However, in one series of eight patients with arthrofibrosis, only one was able to return to his previous level of sports.[2] Additional risk factors identified included multiple ligament injuries, acute (within 1 month of injury) reconstruction, and septic arthritis.[2] In a series of 28 patients with IPCS, Paulos found that open debridement and soft tissue release provided an average extension increase of 12 degrees and a flexion increase of 35 degrees. However, even with these improvements in range of motion, 90% of the patients still had symptoms of patellofemoral arthrosis and 30% had crepitation. No athletes returned to their previous level of sports, nor were any manual laborers able to return to their previous level of employment.[4]

Avoiding Arthrofibrosis

The key to avoiding severe arthrofibrosis is prevention and early detection. Severe steps can be taken to prevent the development of arthrofibrosis following arthroscopic or ligament surgery. One critical factor is the timing of the surgery. By waiting several weeks, the effusion is reduced and the patient may receive physical therapy to improve range of motion, thereby decreasing the risk of arthrofibrosis. The postoperative period is critical as well, and prolonged immobilization should be avoided wherever possible. The peripatellar soft tissues should be mobilized as soon as possible following surgery and range of motion exercises should be started early for the tibiofemoral joint. It is also beneficial to start active quadriceps contractions within three days of surgery. Obtaining early lateral radiographs can also be helpful for the early detection of patella infera.[7]

Warning signs for the presence of arthrofibrosis and the development of early patella infera can include the inability to voluntarily contract the quadriceps 1 to 3 weeks following surgery, decreased medial-lateral and superior-inferior patellar mobility, a decrease in the palpable tension in the patellar tendon, failure of the patella to elevate with quadriceps contraction, and a distal malposition of the patella compared to the other side. Tenderness and warmth around the fat pad and peripatellar tissues can also suggest inflammation and early arthrofibrosis.

Conclusion

Arthrofibrosis includes a wide spectrum of pathologies that can result in loss of motion of varying degrees secondary to inflammation and scarring. Prevention and early detection of arthrofibrosis remains the key to successful clinical outcomes. In situations involving prolonged immobilization or severe inflammation, such as the case presented here, surgical intervention is required. Open debridement and release and tendon lengthening can be performed in order to restore range of motion.

References

1. Cosgarea, AJ, KE DeHaven, and JE Lovelock. The surgical treatment of arthrofibrosis of the Knee. *Am J Sports Med* 1994; 22: 184–191.
2. Millet, PJ, RJ Williams, and TL Wickiewicz. Open debridement and soft tissue release as a salvage procedure for the severely arthrofibrotic knee. *Am J Sports Med* 1999; 27: 552–561.
3. Paulos, LE, and JL Pinkowski. Patella infera: The Patellofemoral Joint. In Fox, JM, and W Del Pizzo, eds. New York: McGraw Hill, 1993.
4. Paulos, LE, TD Rosenberg, J Drawbert et al. Infrapatellar contracture syndrome: A recognized cause of knee stiffness with patella entrapment and patella infera. *Am J Sports Med* 1987; 15: 331–341.
5. Shelbourne, KD, DV Patel, and DJ Martini. Classification and management of arthrofibrosis of the knee after anterior cruciate ligament reconstruction. *Am J Sports Med* 1996; 24: 857–862.
6. Sprague, NF III, RL O'Connor, and JM Fox. Arthroscopic treatment of postoperative knee fibroarthrosis. *Clin Orthop* 1982; 166: 165–172.
7. Wojtys, EM, B Oakes, TN Lindenfeld, and BR Bach. Patella infera syndrome: An analysis of the patellar tendon pathology. *Instr Course Lect* 1997; 46: 241–250.

23

Neuromatous Knee Pain: Evaluation and Management

Maurice Nahabedian

Introduction

Chronic pain around the knee joint has been and continues to remain a challenging problem. This is primarily related to the fact that the neural pathways responsible for the pain have been poorly understood. However, recent anatomical studies detailing these neural pathways have facilitated our understanding of the sensory mechanisms responsible for pain around the knee joint.[1] This has greatly enhanced our ability to evaluate, diagnose, and manage patients with chronic and intractable knee pain. Unfortunately, there are only scattered reports in the literature describing these conditions and the appropriate treatments.

Denervation for chronic joint pain was initially described in 1958.[2,3] Early reports of total denervation for chronic pain about the elbow joint were not well accepted due to the untoward effects on extremity function. This is because both sensory and motor nerves were ablated. Thus, for many years, denervation was not considered a reasonable option. However, with the advent of selective denervation, the untoward sequellae have been eliminated because only the specific sensory nerves are excised.[4,5] Thus, in properly selected patients, a significant to complete reduction in pain is possible. It is important to realize, however, that selective denervation is primarily directed at patients with neuromatous pain. It is not recommended for chronic pain resulting from a nonneuromatous etiology.

Selective denervation for chronic neuromatous knee pain was initially described by Dellon et al. in 1995.[6] In his pilot study, 15 patients with persistent neuromatous pain following total knee arthroplasty were treated. All patients reported a reduction in pain. Mean follow-up was 12 months. In a subsequent study, 70 patients with chronic neuromatous knee pain following total knee arthroplasty, trauma, or osteotomy had selective denervation with a good to excellent outcome in 86% with a mean follow-up of 24 months.[7] These studies have provided the basis for further investigation.

Anatomic Basis for Selective Denervation

There are currently seven surgically identifiable sensory nerves around the knee joint (Figure 23.1).[8] The sensory innervation around the medial aspect of the knee includes the infrapatellar branch of the saphenous nerve, the medial retinacular nerve, and the medial and anterior cutaneous nerves of the thigh. The sensory innervation to the lateral aspect of the knee includes the tibiofibular branch of the peroneal nerve, the lateral retinacular nerve, and the lateral femoral cutaneous nerve. The medial and lateral retinacular nerves provide sensation to the knee joint whereas the other five nerves provide sensation to the cutaneous surface of the knee.

The anatomical location and paths of these nerves is generally constant; however, variations and anomalies can occur especially in the setting of prior operative procedures. The superficial nerves around the knee are located in the subcutaneous fat, whereas the deep nerves lie deep to the medial and lateral retinaculum. These nerves are located just distal to the

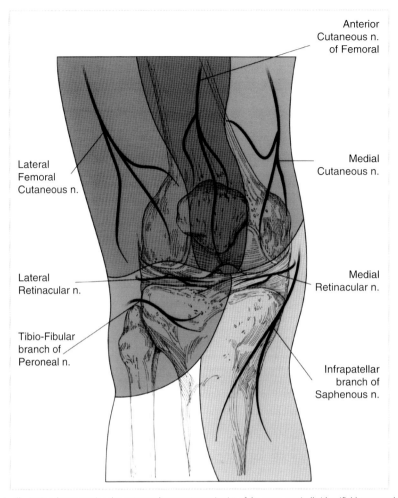

Figure 23.1. An illustration demonstrating the course and cutaneous territories of the seven surgically identifiable nerves about the knee.

medial and lateral vastus lateralis muscle respectively.

Technique of Selective Denervation

A critical component in the management of patients with chronic knee pain is to differentiate pain of neuromatous versus nonneuromatous origin. In general, neuromatous knee pain is characterized as sharp and localized whereas nonneuromatous knee pain is dull and diffuse. Determining whether the pain is of neuromatous origin is accomplished by obtaining a thorough history and physical examination, assessing the characteristics of the pain, and performing the appropriate diagnostic evaluation. This section

will review the initial consultation, diagnostic evaluation, and operative technique.

Initial Consultation

At the initial consultation, patients are thoroughly questioned regarding the mechanism responsible for the knee pain. This can be secondary to chronic disease states such as arthritis or chondromalacia as well as acute events such as trauma or prior operative procedures that may include total knee arthroplasty, arthroscopy, and extirpative procedures. Chronic disease states are rarely secondary to neuromata whereas pain of acute onset can be. The date of the onset is also important because many of these painful conditions are often self-limiting and resolve by 6 months. Pain of acute origin that is persistent beyond six months may be secondary to neuromata.

Other factors related to the pain that are important include the nature, intensity, location, duration, aggravating factors, relieving factors, and frequency. The nature of the pain is characterized as sharp or dull, constant or intermittent, and localized or diffuse. The location of the pain is documented on the surface of the knee as well as whether it is superficial or deep. Superficial pain is usually secondary to neuromata of the five cutaneous nerves that include the anterior, medial, and lateral femoral cutaneous nerves as well as the infrapatellar branch of the saphenous nerve and the tibiofibular branch of the peroneal nerve. Deep pain may be due to neuromata of the medial or lateral retinacular nerves that innervate the capsule of the knee joint. Some patients may also experience numbness or tingling on the lateral aspect of the leg due to compression of the common peroneal nerve. The severity of the pain is graded on a visual analog scale (VAS) ranging from 0 to 10.

Important aspects of the physical examination include location of scars, assessment of knee stability, range of motion, gait assessment, and the location of the pain. It is important to rule out any infectious or inflammatory etiology. The territories of pain corresponding to the surface of the knee are delineated (Figure 23.2). The most important finding for the diagnosis of a neuroma is the presence of a Tinels sign. This is identified by tapping on the surface of the knee and noting the response. The elicitation of a sharp pain that occasionally radiates is characteristic of neuromata (Figure 23.3). There may be an isolated or multiple Tinels signs around the knee. It is recommended that a photograph be obtained of these markings.

Diagnostic Evaluation

The diagnosis is based on ruling out nonneuromatous causes and ruling in a neuroma. Neuromata are ruled in by a successful response to a nerve block using 1% lidocaine. Several cc's of lidocaine is injected subcutaneously at the site of the potential neuroma formation. This can range from 1 to 7 sites based on the number of potential sites that a neuroma can form. After 5 to 10 minutes, pain intensity is again charted using a VAS. Ideally, when a true neuroma is present, the pain should completely resolve

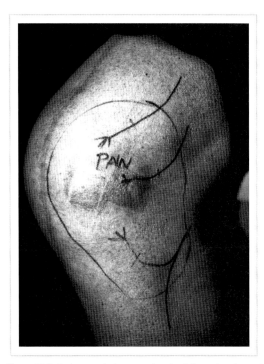

Figure 23.2. A photograph demonstrating the delineated territory of pain secondary to a neuroma of the infrapatellar branch of the saphenous nerve.

following the nerve block. At least a 5-point reduction in the VAS is recommended for a patient to be considered an appropriate candidate for selective denervation. It is important to assess gait before and after nerve blockade and document any changes. Usually the gait is improved following successful blockade of a neuroma. Pain that is not relieved by the lidocaine injection may be related to other causes such as arthritis, ligamentous instability, malalignment of the prosthesis, aseptic loosening, and polyethylene wear. Further orthopedic evaluation is recommended in these circumstances. A plain radiograph is necessary for all prospective patients (Figure 23.4). Electromyography and nerve conduction studies are not usually obtained for neuromatous knee pain.

For patients who are considered candidates for selective denervation, a discussion ensues regarding the risks and benefits of this operation. Candidates for this procedure understand that portions of the knee may be permanently anesthetic and rendered susceptible to other forms of trauma such as a burn. The success of the operation is variable with approximately

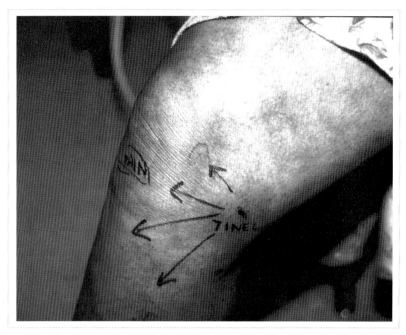

Figure 23.3. A photograph demonstrating the Tinels point and the paths of radiation.

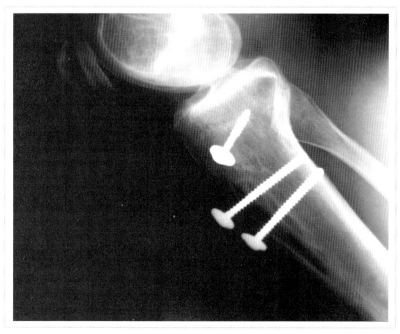

Figure 23.4. Radiograph demonstrating proximal tibial screws that resulted in a neuroma.

40% reporting an excellent improvement, 40% reporting a partial or good improvement, and 20% reporting no improvement. These results are based on personal experience in performing this operation. The response is quantified based on the reduction in the VAS. An excellent response is obtained when the VAS score is reduced to 0 to 1, a partial or good response is obtained when the VAS is reduced by 50%, and a poor response in obtained when there is no appreciable change in the VAS.

Operative Technique

Prior to the induction of regional or general anesthesia, the Tinels points are again marked and the bony and reticular landmarks are outlined. The incision sites and the usual course of the nerves are delineated. Following induction of anesthesia, a proximal thigh tourniquet is applied and inflated to 300 mm of mercury. It is recommended that the tourniquet not be inflated for greater than one hour. At least 3.5 power loupe magnification is recommended.

The techniques of excision of neuromata for the different nerves are different. The cutaneous nerves about the knee lie in the subcutaneous fat. Neuromata of the anterior, medial, and lat-eral cutaneous nerves as well as the infrapatellar branch of the saphenous nerve can be excised through a skin incision approximately 1 to 2 centimeters from the Tinels point along the usual course of the nerve. Dissection proceeds using fine scissors and bipolar cautery. Following identification of the nerve, traction is applied on the isolated segment to observe for skin retraction at the Tinels point. This maneuver confirms that the correct nerve has been isolated. The nerve is divided and the proximal stump of the nerve is buried in adjacent muscle to minimize the possibility of recurrence.

Neuromata of the tibiofibular branch of the common peroneal nerve are approached in a different manner (Figures 23.5, 23.6). The common peroneal nerve is exposed and released and the articular branches to the tibiofibular joint are isolated. It is helpful to use a nerve stimulator to ensure that motor branches to the peroneus longus muscle are not divided.

Neuromata of the deeper knee structures (i.e., medial and lateral retinacular nerves) require a different approach. Neuromata of the medial retinacular nerve are approached using a skin incision just distal to the vastus medialis muscle. The medial retinaculum is incised between the

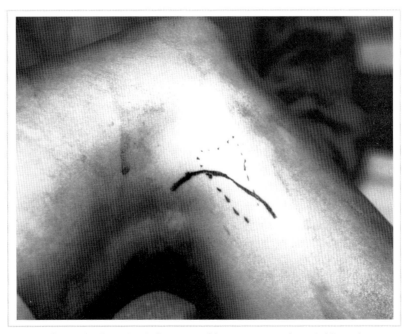

Figure 23.5. The incision site for exposure of the common peroneal nerve is delineated.

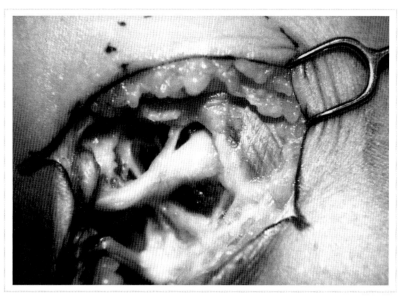

Figure 23.6. The common peroneal nerve is isolated and the tibiofibular branch is isolated as it traverses under the peroneus longus muscle.

patella and the medial epicondyle of the femur. The nerve is located under the retinaculum. Neuromata of the lateral retinacular nerve are approached using a skin incision distal to the vastus lateralis muscle. The lateral retinaculum is incised between the patella and iliotibial tract. The nerve is isolated and excised.

Case Examples
Case 1

A 44-year-old man presented with 2-year history of chronic right knee pain following total knee arthroplasty. The pain was localized to the infra-patellar regions of the medial and lateral knee (Figures 23.7, 23.8). The pain was described as sharp and constant and was confined to the cutaneous surface and did not involve the deeper structures of the knee. It was exacerbated by knee motion. Knee stability and gait was within normal limits. The patient also described numbness and tingling on the lateral surface of the knee. Physical therapy and analgesics were unsuccessful in ameliorating the pain. Pain severity was graded on a visual analog scale as 9. Radiographs revealed well-aligned knee pros-thesis.

On physical examination, a well-healed 20 centimeter midline knee incision was noted. There was no evidence of swelling or erythema.

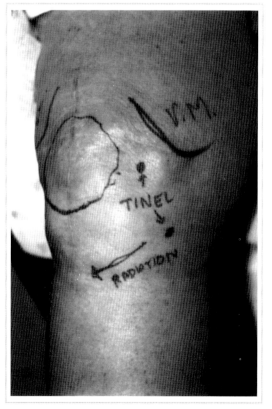

Figure 23.7. The medial aspect of the knee is depicted demonstrating the patella and vastus medialis muscle (VM). The Tinel points and path of radiation are outlined.

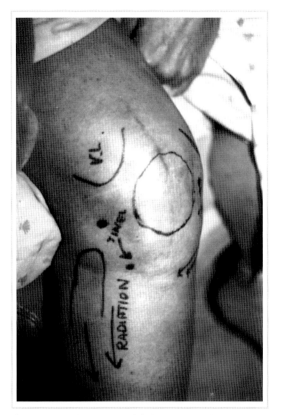

Figure 23.8. The lateral aspect of the knee is depicted demonstrating the fibular head and the vastus lateralis muscle (VL). The Tinel points are marked.

A Tinels sign was elicited on the infrapatellar aspect of the medial and lateral knee. In addition, there was diminished sensation along the lateral aspect of the leg extending from the fibular head to the lateral malleolus. Joint laxity or instability was not appreciated. The presumptive diagnosis was a neuroma of the infrapatellar branch of the saphenous nerve and the tibiofibular branch of the common peroneal nerve as well as compression of the common peroneal nerve. A nerve block using 1% lidocaine was performed at the point of the Tinels sign with complete resolution of pain within 5 minutes.

In the operating room, the infrapatellar branch of the saphenous nerve and the tibiofibular branch of the common peroneal nerve were identified and resected (Figure 23.9). The proximal nerve stump was buried in adjacent muscle. The common peroneal nerve was decompressed without incident.

Postoperatively, the pain was completely eliminated with a visual analog score of 0. The lateral leg dysesthesia resolved completely. The patient has classified this outcome as excellent with a two-year follow-up.

Case 2

A 28-year-old man presented with chronic knee pain of seven years' duration following a

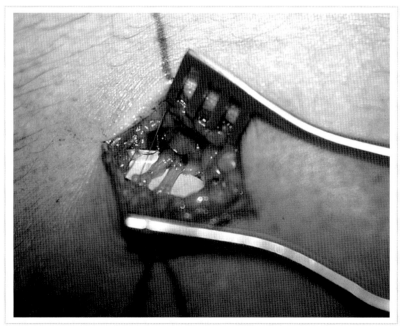

Figure 23.9. Two branches of the infrapatellar branch of the saphenous nerve are illustrated. These branches were excised and the proximal stumps buried in adjacent muscle.

traumatic injury. In total, seven prior operations had been performed that have contributed to the chronic pain. The pain was described as sharp, constant, and located in the superficial cutaneous territory of the superior knee. Pain severity was graded as an 8 on the visual analog scale. Physical therapy and analgesics did not ameliorate the pain. Radiographs demonstrated a well-aligned knee without arthritic changes.

On physical examination, all incisions were well-healed without signs of infection or inflammation. Ligamentous laxity was not demonstrated. A Tinels sign was elicited over the medial suprapatellar region. Nerve blockade successfully eliminated the pain reducing the pain severity score to 0. A neuroma of the medial cutaneous nerve of the knee was diagnosed (Figure 23.10). The neuroma was excised and the proximal nerve stump buried without incident.

Postoperatively, the patient reported complete resolution of pain in the medial suprapatellar territory; however, one week following the procedure, the patient reported new onset of anterior and lateral suprapatellar pain. This pain was described as sharp and intermittent with a visual analog score of 8 points. Nerve blockade successfully reduced the pain to 0. A second operation was performed four months

later and the anterior and lateral femoral cutaneous neuromata were excised. Postoperatively, the patient was pain free with 2-year follow-up.

Case 3

A 70-year-old man presented with left medial infrapatellar knee pain of 2-year duration following total knee arthroplasty. The pain was described as sharp, intermittent, localized, and superficial with a visual analog score of 7 points. The pain was exacerbated by prolonged periods of sitting and knee motion. There were no complaints of mechanical dysfunction and radiographs demonstrated a knee prosthesis that was well-aligned. Physical therapy and analgesics did not alleviate the pain.

On physical examination, the midline incision was well-healed and there was no evidence of swelling, inflammation, or infection. Knee stability was intact with normal range of motion and normal gait. A Tinels sign was localized to the medial infrapatellar region of the knee. Diagnostic nerve block reduced the pain to a 2 on the visual analog scale that was suggestive of a neuroma of the infrapatellar branch of the saphenous nerve. Although there was improvement in the pain, some discomfort remained.

In the operating room, the infrapatellar branch of the saphenous nerve was isolated, resected, and proximally buried in adjacent muscle.

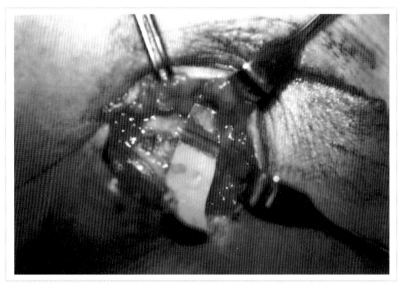

Figure 23.10. The medial cutaneous nerve of the knee is demonstrated.

Postoperatively, no substantial improvement in the pain was reported with a reduction in the visual analog score to 5 points. The patient graded this as a poor result at 2-year follow-up.

Discussion

Selective denervation for neuromatous knee pain is an excellent procedure in properly selected patients; however, its use remains controversial. This is primarily because denervation is considered an extreme maneuver and historically the clinical outcomes following denervation procedures have been mixed. However, selective denervation of the sensory nerves about the knee has been demonstrated in several studies to be safe and beneficial in the majority of properly selected patients. The three cases illustrated were selected because they represent situations and outcomes that the practicing surgeon is likely to encounter.

Case 1 represents a straightforward situation in which a single neuroma was responsible for the knee pain. The nerve block was effective at temporarily eliminating the pain and the excision of the single neuroma completely eliminated the pain. Case 2 appeared to be straightforward with identification of a single neuroma. However, following intraoperative identification and excision of the responsible nerve, adjacent pain ensued requiring a second selective denervation procedure. This case demonstrates that additional denervation procedures, although uncommon, may be necessary. Although unclear why the subsequent pain was not demonstrated at the initial consultation, it can be postulated that the adjacent neuromata elicited a less intense signal that was masked by the primary neuroma. Case 3 represents a situation in which there was an equivocal response to the nerve blockade. Although, the visual analog score was reduced from 7 to 2 following the nerve block, a mild amount of pain remained. Selective denervation did not effectively relieve the pain. This incomplete resolution of pain following nerve blockade may have occurred because of adjacent nerves that were not anesthetized. The persistence of pain following denervation may have been due to nonspecific reinnervation by adjacent nerves to the denervated territory.

In order to determine the true benefit of selective denervation, prospective studies are necessary. In our previous study, 43 patients with intractable knee pain were prospectively analyzed.[8] Only patients that met the criteria for selective denervation were included in the study. Inclusion required pain of at least 1 year's duration, failure of conservative management, pain localized at a Tinels point, and at least a 5-point reduction in the severity of pain based on a visual analog scale. Thirty patients met these criteria of which 25 had selective denervation. Thirteen patients did not meet the criteria. Of those that had selective denervation, the etiology of the pain was trauma in 15 patients and total knee arthroplasty in 10. The mean number of prior operations about the knee was 5.1 (range 0–20). A single neuroma was excised in 11 patients and multiple neuromata were excised in 14. A total of 62 nerves were excised in the 25 patients, which included the infrapatellar branch of the saphenous nerve (n = 24), the tibiofibular branch of the peroneal nerve (n = 5), the medial retinacular nerve (n = 12), the lateral retinacular nerve (n = 8), the medial cutaneous nerve (n = 6), the anterior cutaneous nerve (n = 3), and the lateral femoral cutaneous nerve (n = 4). Pain relief was complete in 11 patients (44%), partial in 10 patients (40%), and absent in 4 patients (16%). Follow-up ranged from 1 to 4 years. Patient satisfaction following the procedure was obtained in 21 of 25 patients (84%).

This study demonstrates that not all properly selected patients respond equally to selective denervation. Closer evaluation of the 11 patients who reported an excellent outcome reveals that the average preoperative score on the VAS was 8.5 points (range 5–10), the average post nerve block score was 0.4 points (range 0–1), and the average postoperative score was 0.5 points (range 0–2). Preoperative pain was localized to the medial aspect of the knee in 9 patients (82%) and to the medial and lateral aspect of the knee in 2 patients (18%). This outcome was obtained after a single operation in 9 patients (82%) and after a second operation in 2 patients (18%). The nerve most commonly excised was the infrapatellar branch of the saphenous nerve, which was excised in 10 patients (91%). More than one nerve was excised in 9 patients (82%).

A detailed evaluation of the 10 patients reporting a good outcome reveals that the average preoperative score on the VAS was 8.6 points (range 6–10), the average post nerve block score was 0.5 points (range 0–2), and the average postoperative score was 3.3 points (range 2–5). Preoperative pain was localized to the medial aspect of the knee in 5 patients (50%) and to the medial and lateral aspect of the knee in 5 patients (50%). This outcome was obtained after a single operation in 8 patients (80%) and after a second operation in 2 patients (20%). The nerve most commonly isolated was the infrapatellar branch of the saphenous nerve, which was excised in all 10 patients. More than one nerve was excised in 7 patients.

Detailed evaluation of the 4 patients reporting a poor outcome reveals that the average preoperative score on the VAS was 8.3 points (range 7–10), the average post nerve block score was 1.5 points (range 0–2), and the average postoperative score was 6.8 points (range 5–9). Preoperative pain was localized to the medial aspect of the knee in 2 patients and to the medial and lateral aspect in 2 patients. The nerve most commonly excised was the infrapatellar branch of the saphenous nerve, which was excised in 4 patients. More than one nerve was excised in 2 patients.

Outcomes that were considered less than excellent occurred in 14 of 25 patients (56%). In the group reporting a good outcome, patient complaints included new pain or migration of pain in 4 knees as well as persistent and deep pain in 6 knees. Predisposing factors to this outcome included a history of fracture or total knee arthroplasty in 7 patients, arthroscopy for ligamentous injury in 2 patients, and soft tissue trauma in 1 patient. Explanations included secondary neuroma formation, persistent pain from an unrecognized neuroma, overlapping nerve territories, and persistent pain from a nonneuromatous origin.

In the group reporting a poor outcome, predisposing factors included previous bone or joint surgery in 2 patients and knee joint arthroscopy in 2 knees. All four patients reported persistent and deep joint pain. Explanations include overlapping nerve territories and unrecognized or masked neuromata. The medial retinacular nerve was excised in 1 of these patients and the lateral retinacular nerve was excised in none of the patients. This decision was made based on the preoperative evaluation and the results of the lidocaine nerve block. Subsequent denervation procedures were not performed in this group of patients.

In conclusion, selective denervation for neuromatous pain about the knee joint can be a beneficial procedure. Proper patient selection is a critical component that impacts the success of the operation. The salient components include pain of at least 1-year duration unrelieved by conservative measures, the presence of a Tinels sign in the painful territory, and at least a 5-point reduction in the visual analog score following nerve blockade with 1% lidocaine. This procedure is not recommended for pain of nonneuromatous origin, pain that is less than 1-year duration, and for diffuse knee pain without a Tinels sign.

References

1. Horner, G, and AL Dellon. Innervation of the human knee joint and implications for surgery. *Clin Orthop Rel Res* 1994; 301: 221–226.
2. Wilhelm, A. Zur innervation der gelenke der oberen extremitat. *Z Anat Entwicklungs Geschechte* 1958; 120: 331–371.
3. Wilhelm, A. Die Gelenkdenervation und ihre anatomischen Grundlagen: Ein neues Behandlungsprinzip in der Habdchirurgie. *Hefte Unfallheilkd* 1966; 86: 1–109.
4. Dellon, AL. Partial dorsal wrist denervation: Resection of the distal posterior interosseous nerve. *J Hand Surg* 1985; 10A: 527–533.
5. Dellon, AL, SE MacKinnon, and A Daneshvar. Terminal branch of the anterior interosseous nerve as a source of wrist pain. *J Hand Surg* 1984; 9B: 316–322.
6. Dellon, AL, MA Mont, KA Krackow, and DS Hungerford. Partial denervation for persistent neuroma pain after total knee arthroplasty. *Clin Orthop Rel Res* 1995; 316: 145–150.
7. Dellon, AL, MA Mont, T Mullick, and DS Hungerford. Partial denervation for neuromatous knee pain around the knee. *Clin Orthop Rel Res* 1996; 329: 216–222.
8. Nahabedian, MY, and CA Johnson. Operative management of neuromatous knee pain: Patient selection and outcome. *Ann Plast Surg* 2001; 46: 15–22.

Epilogue

Scott F. Dye

As this work is published, at the beginning of the 21st Century, a new perspective of the classic orthopedic enigma of the patellofemoral pain problem is becoming increasingly accepted. It is clear that the decades-old paradigm of a pure structural and biomechanical explanation for the genesis of patellofemoral pain is inadequate, and that a new era has begun with biological factors now being given more consideration. A variable mosaic of pathophysiologic events (often due to simple overload) such as patellofemoral synovitis, retinacular neuromas, patellar tendonitis, and painful increased osseous remodeling of the patellofemoral joint - processes when taken together can be characterized by the term "loss of tissue homeostasis" - can be seen as providing new and alternative explanations for the conundrum of anterior knee pain. It clinically matters little what structural factors may be present in a given joint (such as chondromalacia, patellar tilt or a Q angle above a certain value) if the pain free condition of tissue homeostasis is achieved and maintained. Despite recent conceptual advances - represented by this newer biological perspective - much remains to be discovered regarding the patellofemoral joint before it can be said to be fully understood.

Better methods of determining dynamic patellofemoral joint reaction forces and kinematics need to be developed utilizing perhaps cine-CT or cine-MRI. Actual *in vivo* measurements are still required, particularly under real-time loading conditions to calibrate any non-invasive external assessment system that may be devised. Methods of geographically manifesting the homeostasis characteristics of all tissues, including soft tissues, need to be developed perhaps with techniques such as fMRI or CT-PET, which could help objectively evaluate the effectiveness of a variety of current and future non-operative and operative therapies. I envision a day when this information may be displayed in a dynamic three-dimensional hologram with the structural and tissue homeostasis characteristics of the patellofemoral joint being represented by different colors and intensities.

Before advanced imaging techniques can be properly interpreted, further work on the histopathology associated with the genesis of patellofemoral pain needs to be accomplished, such as that currently being carried out by Sanchis-Alfonso. Simple tools that may be helpful to the clinician in assessing a joint's degree of homeostasis, such as the accurate determination of surface temperature through inexpensive hand held devices, could be developed and calibrated. New methods of treatment aimed at addressing the pathophysiology of loss of tissue homeostasis, that may seem unorthodox from today's perspective, such as the use of the hormone calcitonin in patients with painful increased osseous metabolic activity manifested by an intensely positive bone scan may, in time prove useful -whereas the ill considered and indiscriminate use of the lateral retinacular release, may not.

Those of us with a specific interest in the research of the patellofemoral joint also face general problems common to all musculoskeletal systems including discovering the factors that result in the induction, persistence, and eventual resolution of muscle atrophy. Subtle but important neuromuscular mechanisms such as the proprioceptive , spinal, and cerebellar systems that determine to a great degree the adaptive temporal sequencing of motor unit contractions, could be better understood and ultimately controlled for therapeutic benefit.

Other mysteries of the patellofemoral joint remain to be answered including, determining why some patients may indefinitely remain asymptomatic despite obvious radiographically identifiable structural abnormalities such as advanced chondromalacia, substantial malalignment, and even established degenerative arthrosis. When the patellofemoral joint is eventually understood in greater depth, the insights discovered should be generally applicable to other sub-disciplines within the field of orthopaedic surgery and musculoskeletal medicine as well.

Index